EXS 100

Molecular, Clinical and Environmental Toxicology

Volume 2: Clinical Toxicology

Edited by Andreas Luch

Birkhäuser Verlag
Basel · Boston · Berlin

Editor

Andreas Luch
Federal Institute for Risk Assessment
Thielallee 88-92
14195 Berlin
Germany

Library of Congress Control Number: 2008938291

Bibliographic information published by Die Deutsche Bibliothek
Die Deutsche Bibliothek lists this publication in the Deutsche Nationalbibliografie;
detailed bibliographic data is available in the Internet at http://dnb.ddb.de

ISBN 978-3-7643-8337-4   Birkhäuser Verlag AG, Basel – Boston – Berlin

© 2010 Birkhäuser Verlag AG
Basel – Boston – Berlin
P.O. Box 133, CH-4010 Basel, Switzerland
Part of Springer Science+Business Media
Printed on acid-free paper produced from chlorine-free pulp. TCF ∞
Cover illustrations: by A. Luch, J. White, G.P. Rossini and P. Hess; with friendly permission

Printed in Germany
ISBN 978-3-7643-8337-4   e-ISBN 978-3-7643-8338-1

9 8 7 6 5 4 3 2 1   www. birkhauser.ch

Contents

List of contributors

Jennifer Acciani, Department of Emergency Medicine, Division of Medical Toxicology, Indiana University School of Medicine, 1050 Wishard Boulevard, Room 2200, Indianapolis, IN 46202, USA; e-mail: jacciani@iupui.edu

Anna Arroyo, Department of Emergency Medicine, Division of Medical Toxicology, Indiana University School of Medicine, 1050 Wishard Boulevard, Room 2200, Indianapolis, IN 46202, USA; e-mail: aarroyo@iupui.edu

Shahnaz Bakand, Department of Occupational Health, School of Public Health, Iran University of Medical Sciences, Tehran, Iran; Visiting Research Fellow, School of Risk and Safety Sciences, University of New South Wales, Sydney, NSW 2052, Australia; e-mail: s.bakand@unsw.edu.au

Michael R. Baldwin, Department of Molecular Microbiology and Immunology, University of Missouri, M616 Medical Sciences Building, Columbia, MO 65212, USA; e-mail: baldwinmr@health.missouri.edu

Joseph T. Barbieri, Medical College of Wisconsin, Department of Microbiology and Molecular Genetics, 8701 Watertown Plank Road, Milwaukee, WI 53151, USA; e-mail: jtb01@mcw.edu

Daniel Butzke, Center for Alternatives to Animal Experiments (ZEBET), Federal Institute for Risk Assessment, Thielallee 88-92, 14195 Berlin, Germany; e-mail: daniel.butzke@bfr.bund.de

John A. Curtis, Department of Emergency Medicine, Division of Medical Toxicology, Drexel University College of Medicine, Philadelphia, PA 19102, USA; e-mail: jac129@gmail.com

Olaf H. Drummer, Victorian Institute of Forensic Medicine, Department of Forensic Medicine, Monash University, 57-83 Kavanagh St, Southbank 3006, Australia; e-mail: olaf@vifm.org

Blake Froberg, Department of Pediatrics, Division of Medical Toxicology, Indiana University School of Medicine, 1050 Wishard Boulevard, Room 2200, Indianapolis, IN 46202, USA; e-mail: bfroberg@iupui.edu

Brent Furbee, Department of Emergency Medicine, Division of Medical Toxicology, Indiana University School of Medicine, 1050 Wishard Boulevard, Room 2200, Indianapolis, IN 46202, USA; e-mail: bfurbee@clarian.org

Michael I. Greenberg, Department of Emergency Medicine, Division of Medical Toxicology, Drexel University College of Medicine, Philadelphia, PA 19102, USA, mgreenbe@drexelmed.edu

Bryan A. Hanson, Department of Chemistry and Biochemistry, Julian Science and Mathematics Center, 602 S. College Ave., Room 363, DePauw University, Greencastle, IN 46135, USA; e-mail: hanson@depauw.edu

Amanda Hayes, Chemical Safety and Applied Toxicology (CSAT) Laboratories, School of Risk and Safety Sciences, The University of New South Wales, Sydney, NSW 2052, Australia; e-mail: a.hayes@unsw.edu.au

James S. Henkel, Medical College of Wisconsin, Department of Microbiology and Molecular Genetics, 8701 Watertown Plank Road, Milwaukee, WI 53151, USA; e-mail: jhenkel@mcw.edu

Philipp Hess, IFREMER, Department of Environment, Microbiology and Phycotoxins, 44311 Nantes Cedex 03, France; e-mail: philipp.hess@ifremer.fr

Louise Kao, Department of Emergency Medicine, Division of Medical Toxicology, Indiana University School of Medicine, 1050 Wishard Boulevard, Room 2200, Indianapolis, IN 46202, USA; e-mail: lkao@clarian.org

Kamil Kuča, Center of Advanced Studies and Department of Toxicology, Faculty of Military Health Sciences, University of Defence, Trebesska 1575, 50001 Hradec Kralove, Czech Republic; e-mail: kucakam@pmfhk.cz

Hugo Kupferschmidt, Swiss Toxicological Information Centre (STIC), Freiestrasse 16, 8032 Zürich, Switzerland; e-mail: hkupferschmidt@toxi.ch, hugo.kupferschmidt@usz.ch

Nelson Lima, Centre of Biological Engineering, IBB-Institute for Biotechnology and Bioengineering, Universidade do Minho, 4710-057 Braga, Portugal; e-mail: micoteca@deb.uminho.pt

Andreas Luch, Department of Product Safety, Center for Alternatives to Animal Experiments, Federal Institute for Risk Assessment, Thielallee 88-92, 14195 Berlin, Germany; e-mail: andreas.luch@bfr.bund.de

Hans H. Maurer, Department of Experimental and Clinical Toxicology, Institute of Experimental and Clinical Pharmacology and Toxicology, Saarland University Hospital, Building 46, 66421 Homburg (Saar), Germany; e-mail: hans.maurer@uks.eu

David J. McCann, Division of Pharmacotherapies and Medical Consequences of Drug Abuse, National Institute on Drug Abuse (NIDA), National Institutes of Health (NIH), 6001 Executive Boulevard, Bethesda, MD 20892, USA; e-mail: dmccann@nida.nih.gov

Ivan D. Montoya, Division of Pharmacotherapies and Medical Consequences of Drug Abuse, National Institute on Drug Abuse (NIDA), National Institutes of Health (NIH), 6001 Executive Boulevard, Bethesda, MD 20892, USA; e-mail: imontoya@mail.nih.gov

Robert R.M. Paterson, Centre of Biological Engineering, IBB-Institute for Biotechnology and Bioengineering, Universidade do Minho, 4710-057 Braga, Portugal; e-mail: russell.paterson@deb.uminho.pt

Miroslav Pohanka, Center of Advanced Studies and Department of Toxicology, Faculty of Military Health Sciences, University of Defence, Trebesska 1575, 50001 Hradec Kralove, Czech Republic; e-mail: rau@atlas.cz, pohanka@pmfhk.cz

Robert H. Poppenga, California Animal Health & Food Safety Laboratory System (CAHFS), School of Veterinary Medicine, University of California,

Davis, West Health Sciences Drive, Davis, CA 95616, USA, e-mail: rhpoppenga@ucdavis.edu

Christine Rauber-Lüthy, Swiss Toxicological Information Centre (STIC), Freiestrasse 16, 8032 Zürich, Switzerland; e-mail: christine.rauber@usz.ch

Gian Paolo Rossini, Università di Modena e Reggio Emilia, Dipartimento di Scienze Biomediche, Via Campi 287, 41100 Modena, Italy; e-mail: gianpaolo.rossini@unimo.it

Daniel E. Rusyniak, Department of Emergency Medicine, Division of Medical Toxicology, Indiana University School of Medicine, 1050 Wishard Boulevard, Room 2200, Indianapolis, IN 46202, USA; e-mail: drusynia@iupui.edu

Silas W. Smith, New York City Poison Control Center, New York University School of Medicine, NYU Department of Emergency Medicine, Bellevue Hospital Center, 462 First Avenue, Room A-345A, New York, NY 10016, USA; e-mail: silas.smith@nyumc.org

David Vearrier, Department of Emergency Medicine, Division of Medical Toxicology, Drexel University College of Medicine, Philadelphia, PA 19102, USA; e-mail: david.vearrier@drexelmed.edu

Julian White, Toxinology Department, Women's and Children's Hospital, 72 King William Road, North Adelaide, SA 5006, Australia; e-mail: julian.white@adelaide.edu.au

Preface

It is done! I am very pleased to deliver the second volume of the series on "Molecular, Clinical and Environmental Toxicology" to the public today. All authors, the editorial office of Birkhäuser and I have been working very hard during the past months to get the promise made at the end of last year into reality. After the first volume on molecular toxicology, this second part is dedicated to clinically relevant aspects of toxicology and thus focused on more immediate (acute) and fatal effects of compounds and preparations that people might be exposed to under certain circumstances. For this reason the aim of this volume is not only to discuss highly toxic synthetic chemicals, metals and pharmaceuticals but also to cover the field of naturally occurring (biogenic) toxins produced in particular organisms distributed across the entire biosphere; the scientific area dealing with the latter is usually referred to as toxinology.

As a medical discipline, toxicology has developed over time from the early observations and appreciation of the allegedly healing, but sometimes also toxic effects of extractions and preparations made from plants, mushrooms or animals. Since nature in general formed a much greater part of regular life of human beings in the pre-industrialized era, in those days natural sources embodying rich and complex chemistries and assumed to possess inherent ("God-given") advantageous properties were sought and collected in the organismic world right beyond the doorstep, ultimately with the goal of utilizing these to ease (or cease) tough and arduous living conditions and destiny. The belief in the positive, health and well-being promoting effects of everything that comes from "mother nature" has been conserved throughout the centuries up to the present time where people still place most trust, confidence and favor in "natural products", while synthetically produced chemicals or pharmaceuticals are usually perceived with suspicion, mistrust and sometimes irrational fear.

Given this view, however, an extremely compelling and contradictory awareness might come from the comparison of acute toxicities between certain biogenic toxins and those particular kinds of small molecules synthetically designed and created in the chemist's lab and supposed to effectively eradicate human life within minutes through an irreversible block of neuromuscular transmission, *i.e.*, chemical warfare agents such as VX or soman. Applying the mouse bioassay that has been established in the 1930s by Sommer and Meyer, and which determines the particular dose necessary to kill one out of two of those poor animals treated (lethal dose 50%, LD_{50}), the most deadliest compounds known today are actually proteins produced by bacteria belonging to the genus *Clostridium*. Compared to the VX agent (LD_{50} of ~15 µg/kg body weight), botulinum neurotoxin (LD_{50} ~ 0.001 µg/kg) or tetanus neurotoxin

(LD$_{50}$ ~0.002 µg/kg) are no less than 15 000- (!) and 7500-fold more potent in killing mice when injected intraperitoneally. This crude method also delivered some kind of idea on the ranking of the most toxic compounds on earth. Here it turns out that a wide range of biogenic compounds produced from bacteria, algae (*e.g.*, dinoflagellates), fungi (*e.g.*, *Aspergillus*, *Fusarium*), invertebrates such as cone snails or jellyfish, vertebrates such as snakes and poison dart frogs, and lectin-producing plants (*e.g.*, *Abrus*, *Ricinus*) are by far more toxic than the most potent synthetic toxins artificially created in the lab. Interestingly, among the "top 10" toxins, all of which are of biogenic origin, small molecules are scarce and actually only represented by two exceptionally sizeable compounds, *i.e.*, maitotoxin (LD$_{50}$ ~ 0.1 µg/kg) and palytoxin (LD$_{50}$ ~ 0.15 µg/kg), and by batrachotoxin (LD$_{50}$ ~ 2 µg/kg). By contrast, the remaining, usually well-known and more typical, small toxins (saxitoxin, tetrodotoxin, ciguatoxins, etc.) are in general less toxic and displaced by proteinaceous or polypeptic toxins such as those produced in bacteria, plants (abrin, ricin), cone snails (conotoxins), scorpions (α- and β-toxins), or snakes (*e.g.*, textilotoxin).

The second volume, in its final composition released today, encompasses a very exciting journey starting from the fields of naturally occurring toxic products produced by bacteria (bacterial toxins), fungi (mycotoxins), algae (phycotoxins), plants (phytotoxins), and animals (venoms, poisons). Later in the volume the clinical management of intoxication and (if available) the applicability of antidotes are discussed in the context of metals, pharmaceuticals, drugs, or such chemicals that can be typically found in the household. Since illicit drugs and psychedelic preparations represent an extremely important concern in clinical toxicology and a life-threatening issue all over the world, this topic is addressed further by two separate chapters in the course of this book. The editor felt strongly convinced that any comprehensive work on clinical toxicology should be enriched by special chapters on more general but central themes such as those covering the fields of analytical toxicology, inhalation toxicology, forensic toxicology, and – of course – the highly and publicly debated topics of chemical and biological warfare agents. While analytical and forensic toxicology are key in detecting and elucidating compound-induced tissue and organ damage or failure due to intoxication, poisoning and envenomation in living and dead patients alike, the chapter on inhalation toxicology is meant to put more emphasis on the role of the (fast) inhalation exposure route with respect to rapidly or immediately occurring fatalities based on chemical-triggered failure of vital functions such as respiration, systemic (cardiovascular) circulation and neuronal activity in the central nervous system.

At this point, there is nothing left than expressing again my sincere appreciation and gratitude to all authors who contributed to this volume with their great work and their extreme efforts to nicely and comprehensively cover a specific topic in the field of clinical toxicology (*resp.* toxinology). The main goal of this volume was to outline and to communicate the diversity in this field and the great and exciting story of highly potent biogenic and synthetic toxins, as well as the routine and advanced means applied in the clinics to battle against accidental or intended intoxication or poisoning. In this sense, I personally think that it would be not inappropriate to argue that the current volume is something very uncommon and special in terms of its composition and breadth. As with volume 1, which was released at pretty much the same time last year, I deeply hope that volume 2 will also be acknowledged and well circulated throughout the scientific community. I am confident that it is appropriately suited to serve as guide for students and professionals in medicine and natural sciences, interested in gaining more insight into how potent toxins work in the body and into the issue of adequate counteractions and remedies to be applied in the clinics to help patients survive the imminent danger executed by potentially deadly chemicals, peptides or proteins intruding into their body.

Last but not least, I want to express my special gratitude to the editorial office of Birkhäuser. I am indebted to Beatrice Menz and Kerstin Tüchert, who both provided the necessary constant guide and help to the editor, enabling him to get this volume appropriately compiled on time. Through their extremely hard work and dedication, two volumes of the series have now cleared all hurdles and have been successfully released onto the market. I am now very much looking forward to the third and final volume of the series focused on environmental toxicology to be published shortly.

Andreas Luch
Berlin, October 2009

Molecular, Clinical and Environmental Toxicology. Volume 2: Clinical Toxicology
Edited by A. Luch
© 2010 Birkhäuser Verlag/Switzerland

Toxins from bacteria

James S. Henkel[1], Michael R. Baldwin[2] and Joseph T. Barbieri[1]

[1] Medical College of Wisconsin, Department of Microbiology and Molecular Genetics, USA
[2] University of Missouri, Department of Molecular Microbiology and Immunology, USA

Abstract. Bacterial toxins damage the host at the site of bacterial infection or distant from the site. Bacterial toxins can be single proteins or oligomeric protein complexes that are organized with distinct AB structure-function properties. The A domain encodes a catalytic activity. ADP ribosylation of host proteins is the earliest post-translational modification determined to be performed by bacterial toxins; other modifications include glucosylation and proteolysis. Bacterial toxins also catalyze the non-covalent modification of host protein function or can modify host cell properties through direct protein-protein interactions. The B domain includes two functional domains: a receptor-binding domain, which defines the tropism of a toxin for a cell and a translocation domain that delivers the A domain across a lipid bilayer, either on the plasma membrane or the endosome. Bacterial toxins are often characterized based upon the secretion mechanism that delivers the toxin out of the bacterium, termed types I–VII. This review summarizes the major families of bacterial toxins and also describes the specific structure-function properties of the botulinum neurotoxins.

Introduction

Bacterial pathogens damage the host *via* invasive and toxic attributes. Invasion involves the ability of the bacterium to grow in the host, in either an extracellular or an intracellular environment. Invasive bacteria injure the host through the production of extracellular enzymes that damage host tissue, or through the modulation of the host response system such as the up-regulation of cytokine expression. In contrast, bacterial pathogens that damage the host through the action of toxins are often non-invasive and have limited capacity to disseminate in the host. Bacterial toxins often act at a distance from the site of infection. They are physically organized into distinct domains, termed A-B structure-function organization, that recognize receptors on the surface of sensitive cells and possess enzymatic capacity to modulate the action of an intracellular host target, often a protein (Fig. 1). The A domain, also described as an effector, is usually an enzyme or a factor that functions through protein-protein interactions within the cell. The B domain comprises the receptor-binding function, providing tropism to specific cell types through receptor binding capacity. The B domain also includes a domain that translocates the A domain across a lipid bilayer, either at the plasma membrane or within the endosomal compartment. Translocation of the A domain across the lipid bilayer is hypothesized in most cases to occur through a pore/channel formed by the B domain.

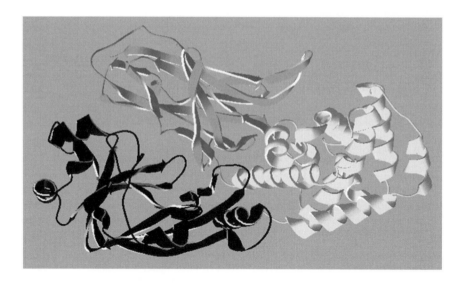

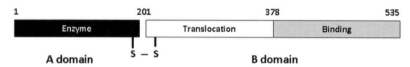

Figure 1. AB organization of bacterial toxins. Diphtheria toxin is an AB toxin where the N-terminal A domain (black) encodes an enzyme activity, an ADP-ribosyltransferase activity (NAD + EF-2 → ADP-r-EF-2 + nicotinamide + H^+). The C-terminal B domain encodes a receptor binding function (gray), which binds to a growth factor receptor and enters cells through receptor-mediated endocytosis, and a translocation function (white), which undergoes a pH-dependent conformational change where charged amino acids are protonated. This allows a pair of hydrophobic α helices to insert into the endosome membrane, which is responsible for the delivery of the A domain into the host cytosol. Structure is adapted from the Protein Databank (PDB): #1fol.

The B domain can be a single subunit (B) or an oligomeric (B5) form. The A and B domains may be linked by a disulfide bond or associated by non-covalent interactions. This review presents an overview of the properties of the major families of bacterial toxins and then describes in more detail the structure-function properties of the botulinum neurotoxins.

Heat-stable enterotoxins

Heat-stable enterotoxins (STs) are a family of conserved peptides expressed by pathogenic strains of *Escherichia coli*. STs elicits fluid accumulation in the intestine [1, 2], which is often responsible for diarrhea in travelers, young children, and domesticated animals in developing countries. STs includes two subfamilies, STa and STb.

The STa subfamily that intoxicates humans (STah) and porcine (STap) [3, 4] comprises ~18-amino acid peptides, including an N-terminal α-helix, a type I β-turn in the central region, and a type II β-turn at the C terminus of the peptide [5]. STa binds the guanylate cyclase C (GC-C) receptor on the surface of epithelial cells of the small intestine and colon. STa binding to the GC-C receptor mimics guanylin, a protein ligand of GC-C, where residues between Cys^5 and Cys^{17} (termed the central region) of STa are essential for binding. These residues are conserved within the STa subfamily, and comprise three disulfide bonds within the central region that are necessary for functional binding [6]. The central β-turn (Asn^{11}–Cys^{14}) interacts with three residues (Thr^{389}, Phe^{390}, Trp^{392}) of the extracellular domain of the GC-C receptor [7–9]. Peptides comprising residues 5–17 and 6–18 possess equivalent biological and immunological activities as native STa, showing that the central region is necessary and sufficient to elicit toxicity [10, 11]. STa-bound GC-C activates protein kinase G (PKG) and protein kinase C (PKC), increasing IP_3-mediated calcium to elevate intracellular cyclic GMP (cGMP) [12]. Increased cGMP activates phosphorylation of the Cl^- ion channel, the cystic fibrosis transmembrane regulator, increasing the concentration of Cl^- ions in the extracellular space and causing fluid accumulation within the lumen of the intestine [3, 13].

STb is a 48-amino acid peptide that causes diarrhea in porcine and humans [14, 15]. Despite the similarity of nomenclature, STb does not have primary amino acid homology with STa. STb is composed of two anti-parallel α-helices connected by a glycine-rich loop. It is stabilized by two disulfide bonds that are necessary for cellular intoxication [16–18]. STb binds to sulfatide, a glycosphingolipid on epithelial cells [19], and internalization is required for intoxication. While the molecular mechanism remains to be determined, STb does not cause cGMP elevation as observed with STa [20]. STb stimulates fluid accumulation through a pertussis toxin-sensitive GTP-binding regulatory protein, which has been proposed to stimulate the elevation of intracellular calcium through an unidentified ligand-gated Ca^{2+} channel [21]. Recent studies observed that STb forms multimeric complexes and enhances membrane permeability, implicating a pore-forming toxin-like activity [14, 17].

While details of the structure-function properties of the STs were resolved shortly after the identification of this family of toxins, recent studies address how ST peptides contribute to the pathology of the enterotoxigenic *E. coli* (ETEC). For example, Moxley and co-workers [22] utilized isogenic strains of ETEC to address the role of STb and other virulence factors in gnotobiotic piglets, while Lucas et al. [23] recently addressed the role of STa in the elicitation of distanced effects on fluid absorption in the intestine of rats.

Pore forming toxins

Bacterial pore-forming toxins (PFTs) are a large group of protein toxins that form pores in the membranes of bacteria, plants, and mammals, causing membrane permeability and ion imbalance. Bacteria release PFTs as soluble sub-units that form stable multimeric complexes on the membranes of various tar-get membranes, and translocate across lipid membranes through several mech-anisms. PFTs are classified into two groups based on the multimeric structure involved in membrane insertion. α-PFTs describe those PFTs that insert into membranes as an α-helix, while β-PFTs insert into the membrane as β-sheets [24, 25].

Examples of α-PFTs are colicins, which are produced in *E. coli* and share structural organization with diphtheria toxin. Colicins are cytotoxic for *E. coli* and other closely related species. Colicins encode α-helices that are utilized for translocation of the catalytic domains across a bacterial outer membrane. The mechanism of membrane insertion and translocation of the colicin cata-lytic domain has been proposed from early biochemical studies, the crystal structure of colicin E (ColE) bound to the BtuR receptor [26], and the crystal structure of OmpR, the putative pore utilized for translocation of the catalytic domain across the outer membrane [27]. ColE3 has 551 amino acids with an internal receptor binding domain, an N-terminal translocation domain, and an ~96-amino acid C-terminal sequence that functions as an endoribonuclease. Entry of ColE into the bacterial cell involves the binding of the internal recep-tor binding domain to the ButR protein, which concentrates into the outer membrane to coordinate the subsequent binding of the translocation domain into the translocator, OmpF. Translocation involves the association of residues within an α-helix of the translocation domain with internal regions of OmpF [27], and the subsequent movement of the nicked catalytic domain across the bacterial inner membrane *via* a TonB-dependent mechanism.

While not considered a PFT, the delivery mechanism that diphtheria toxin utilizes to translocate the catalytic subunit across the endosome membrane and into the host cytosol has properties that are analogous to those of the α-PFTs. Diphtheria toxin is a single chain protein that elicits a lethal pheno-type in humans through the ADP-ribosylation of elongation factor-2. Diphtheria toxin is a 535-amino acid AB toxin; the N terminus encodes the ADP-ribosyltransferase activity and the C terminus comprises a translocation domain and a C-terminal receptor binding domain. Diphtheria toxin binds to a growth factor receptor to traffic into early endosomes *via* receptor-mediated endocytosis where hydrophobic α-helixes of the translocation domain insert into the endosomal membrane by a pH-dependent mechanism [28]. Insertion of these helices into the bilayers opens a channel, analogous to the channel formed by the α-PFTs, that facilitates the translocation of an extended form of the N-terminal catalytic domain across the membrane. The catalytic domain refolds within the cytosol, and ADP-ribosylation of elongation fac-tor-2 occurs, which inhibits protein synthesis. Recent studies have implicated a role for host chaperones in the A domain translocation event [29]. The crys-tal structure of native diphtheria toxin, along with biophysical studies, pro-vides a model describing the molecular basis for the translocation of the cata-lytic domain of diphtheria toxin across the endosome membrane, where hydrophilic loops, containing several charged amino acids with pH-sensitive ionizable R-groups, stabilize hydrophobic α-helices within the B domain of diphtheria toxin (Fig. 1).

β-PFTs are produced as soluble proteins that oligomerize into multimeric complexes on the mammalian plasma membrane; there, one or two amphipathic β-hairpins on a monomeric subunit contribute to the organization of the pore [30]. These β-hairpins contain a hydrophobic outer surface, which favors insertion into the membrane [31, 32]. The pores are organized in a variety of subunit numbers (7–50) and sizes (2–50 nm) [33–35]. The largest group of β-PFTs are the cholesterol-dependent cytolysins (CDCs), which are primarily produced by Gram-positive, pathogenic bacteria such as *Listeria* sp., *Streptococcus pneumoniae,* and *Bacillus anthracis*, but are also found in the mammalian immune system [36–38]. CDC pore complex formation occurs before protein insertion into the membrane and is pH independent [39]. The mechanism of pore insertion includes steps that involve soluble monomer association with the plasma membrane, lateral diffusion of monomers with the membrane, pre-pore monomer oligomerization, pore formation, and insertion of the oligomer into the membrane [39]. CDC monomers are organized into four distinct domains (termed D1–D4), which control monomer-receptor binding, monomer to oligomer association, and membrane interactions. For most CDCs, the D4 domain is responsible for interactions with cholesterol through a tryptophan-rich area called the undecapeptide, which inserts a short distance into the membrane. Cholesterol-bound monomers concentrate and then associate through lateral diffusion on the membrane surface. A conformational change in D3, triggered by D4 domain-membrane interaction, exposes β-strand 4 of D3 domain, and hydrogen bonding between β-strand 4 of D3 domain with the β-strand 1 of D3 domain in the adjacent monomer initiates pre-pore formation [40–43]. The D3 domain also undergoes a second conformational change that causes rearrangement of three α-helices into two β-hairpins for each monomer, which represents the transmembrane component of the pore. These β-hairpins stabilize interactions with neighboring β-hairpins through π-bond stacking with tyrosine and phenylalanine residues. Once the pre-pore complex has assembled on the membrane, a conformational change occurs in which the complex inserts into the membrane due to β-barrel pore formation.

Superantigens

Superantigens (SAgs) are a group of secreted protein toxins produced by an increasing number of bacteria, including *Staphylococcus aureus*, *Streptococcus* sp., *Mycoplasma arthritidis*, and *Yersinia pseudotuberculosis* [44, 45]. SAgs bind to major histocompatibility complex II (MHC II) and stimulate peptide-independent MHC II/T cell receptor (TCR) interaction and immune activation. SAgs are responsible for the toxic shock syndrome (TSS) and food poisoning [46]. A second group of SAgs are the SAg-like toxins (SSLs), which possess much of the conserved domain structure of the SAgs, but do not bind MHC II or activate T cells, but do target the innate immune system [47]. SAgs and SSLs contain two conserved structures at the N-terminal and C-terminal domains. The N-terminal domain contains a conserved oligonucleotide-OB fold, whereas the C-terminal domain contains a β-grasp fold. The OB-fold and the β-grasp fold are closely packed, which contributes to protein stability upon heating, a property of SAgs. Within the family of SAgs, the N terminus includes a groove formed between the OB-fold and the β-grasp fold that comprise the TCR binding domain [47]. Members of the SAg family possess a variety of structures that bind MHC II. *Yersinia* SAgs (YPM-A, YPM-B, and YPM-C) are unique and contain a single domain that comprises a jelly-roll motif consisting of two β-strands [48]. The SAg of *M. arthritidis* (MAM) creates an 'L' structure through the assembly of ten α-helices. While the SSL toxins show an overall conserved structure relative to the SAgs, the surfaces for MHC II and TCR binding are altered [49–51]. In contrast to SAgs, SSLs do not bind to the MHC II complex or TCR. Binding sites and function vary among SSLs, demonstrated by SSL 11 binding sialyllactosamine and SSL 7 binding C5 and IgA [51, 52]. Crystallized SSL 11 has an elongated β-strand within the β-grasp fold that allows dimerization to occur, to presumably increase affinity for cellular glycoproteins [51].

SAgs can bind MHC II by several mechanisms and are classified by how each binds MHC II. TSST-1 binds the MHC II α-chain and a region of the β-chain by extending over the presented peptide (class I) [53]. *Staphylococcus* and *Streptococcus* SAgs bind the MHC II α-chain through the OB domain and do not contact the peptide (class II) [53]. Classes IV and V SAgs bind through the C-terminal domain to the β-chain of MHC II, utilizing a coordinated zinc site as well as the presented peptide [54, 55]. MAM binds in a different fashion by binding the MHC II α1-helix and β1-helix, causing the dimerization of the two MHC II molecules [56].

Binding to MHC II and TCR by SAgs appears to be sequential, based on kinetic binding data [47]. SAgs affinity to MHC II is between 10- and 100-fold higher than to TCR proteins [57]. This determined *in vitro* affinity is most likely a low estimation, since antigen-presenting cells bind SAgs in a stable conformation for over 30 hours [58]. SAg binding to TCR molecules for non-peptide-specific activation occurs through the β-chain, *via* diverse mechanisms that include binding to the CDR2 loop of TCR Vβ [59]. This interaction is sufficient to activate up to 20% of T cells [60]. Most SAgs, however, have an increased specificity to TCR that is defined by specific interactions with the TCR hypervariable areas surrounding the CDR2 loop (Fig. 2) [59]. Another action of SAgs is to directly block TCR interaction with the presented peptide, keeping the TCR and MHC II dimers physically separated; SAgs wedge between the two receptors (class II), allowing only minimal contact (TCR α-chain and MHC II β-chain), and physically block peptide interaction (class I), or bind to cause a sharp angle in between TCR and MHC II/peptide inter-

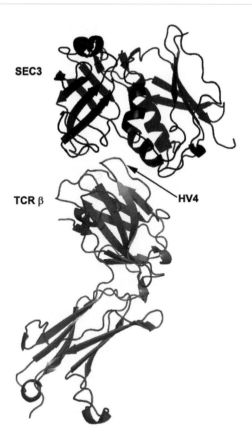

Figure 2. Binding of superantigen SEC3 to TCR β. *Staphylococcus aureus* superantigen SEC3 binds to the β chain of TCR through the hypervariable domain 4 (HV4), acting as a wedge to encourage TCR and MHC II interaction and activation lacking foreign peptide. Arrow indicates HV4 loop on TCR β. Structure: PDB: #1jck.

face (class V) [57]. Current studies on SAgs involve development of structural mimics to neutralize pathology in animal models [61] and to determine the specificity of immune stimulation by SAgs of clinical bacterial isolates [62].

Secretion of toxins from the bacterium

Bacterial toxins are transported across the bacterial membranes through co-translational and post-translational mechanisms to reach their targets. Toxin transport occurs by multiple mechanisms, which have been characterized in Gram-negative and Gram-positive bacteria. Most secretion systems utilize active transport, needing at least one energy-requiring step. For example, Types II, III, and IV secretion systems contain an oligomeric ring of ATPases on the cytoplasmic side of the secretion system's inner membrane complexes. While signal sequences often coordinate the secretion process, signal sequences are not universal. The following section describes the general properties of the Type I–VII secretion systems as related to the secretion of bacterial toxins.

Type I secreted toxins

Type I secretion is observed in Gram-negative and Gram-positive bacteria and transports a variety of proteins across the bacterial inner membrane into the periplasmic space in an active, single-step process. Proteins secreted *via* the Type I pathway contain glycine-rich repeats, usually at the C terminus, which bind calcium [63–65]. The organization of the Type I secretion complex is similar to the ABC family of membrane transporters, composed of a tripartite protein complex that includes an inner membrane transporter, a membrane fusion protein within the periplasm, and an outer membrane pore protein [65]. Central to Type I secretion is the inner membrane transporter that is a transmembrane protein and encodes an ATP-binding domain for recognition of the secretion signal. The membrane fusion protein exists within the periplasmic space and also contains a region that spans the inner membrane. This is exposed to the cytoplasm [66, 67] and links inner and outer membrane-spanning proteins. The outer membrane pore protein is a trimer that forms a channel for direct access of the extracellular space. This trimer assembles into the secretion complex when the ATP-binding domain recognizes a signal sequence contained by the secreted protein [67]. Current studies on Type I secretion address the physical link between energy utilization (ATP) and protein transport [62].

The adenylcyclase-hemolysin (CyaA) of *Bordetella pertussis* is a Type I secreted toxin [68]. Entry into the host cell, *via* the $\alpha(M)\beta(2)$ integrin (CD11b/CD18) cell receptor [69], involves a two-step process with insertion into the membrane and calcium-dependent unfolding of the N terminus of CyaA [70–72]. Upon entry into the cytosol of a host cell, CyaA is activated by the cofactor, calmodulin, and catalyzes the conversion of ATP to cAMP. Elevated intracellular cAMP disrupts signaling events within the cell and inhibits the ability of phagocytes to respond to *B. pertussis* infections [70]. Specifically, de-regulation of cell signaling by CyaA affects protein kinase A, which modulates neutrophil migration, cytokine synthesis, oxidative bursts and organization of the actin cytoskeleton [73, 74]. CyaA is an ~200 kDa protein with two functional domains, a 400-amino acid N-terminal domain that expresses adenylate cyclase activity, and a C-terminal domain that contains the hemolytic activity [75]. Current studies on CyaA involve characterization of structural organization [76] and functional properties [77] of the protein's multiple activities.

Type II secreted toxins

Type II secretion is facilitated by the Sec system and comprises protein complexes that span the bacterial inner and outer membranes. Sec secretion includes three groups of proteins, a protein complex that spans the inner membrane, a periplasm-spanning protein complex, and outer membrane-associated proteins. Type II secretion involves recognition of an N-terminal signal peptide on the nascent protein within the sequence recognition particle, which is analogous to eukaryotic protein secretion in the endoplasmic reticulum [78]. Upon recognition and docking, the growing polypeptide undergoes co-translational secretion and folding to a mature state in the periplasm where the protein is then translocated through the outer membrane [79]. The signal sequence consists of positively charged N-terminal amino acids, internal hydrophobic amino acids, and a C-terminal domain with prolines and glycine [80, 81]. Type II secretion is an active process, requiring a hexameric ATPase associated with the cytoplasmic portion of the inner membrane protein complex and periplasmic proteins that link the inner membrane complex with the outer membrane-associated proteins. One group of periplasmic proteins is homologous to pilin-like structures (known as pseudopilins) and regulatory proteins of the Type IV secretion system, suggesting that these proteins interact to make a tube spanning the periplasmic space [82] and may be involved in the transfer of the secreted protein to the outer membrane complex.

Cholera toxin (CT) of *Vibrio cholerae* is a Type II secreted toxin. CT is an AB_5 toxin, where the A domain (~27.4 kDa) consists of two components, CT-A_1 and CT-A_2, and the B domain (~58 kDa) is a homo-pentameric protein complex [83]. CT-A_1 ADP-ribosylates the G_α-subunit of the heterotrimeric protein G_s. CT-A_1 associates with the CT-A_2 *via* a disulfide bond where CT-A_2 inserts into the channel within the center of the B_5. The B_5 domain binds specifically to the ganglioside GM_{1a} on the surface of intestinal epithelial cells [84]. Once bound, CT enters the cell through both clathrin-dependent and non-clathrin-dependent vesicle mechanisms involving lipid rafts [85]. After internalization, CT traffics to the endoplasmic reticulum (ER) *via* a KDEL-like sequence on the C terminus of A_2 (note the KDEL sequence is not absolutely required for the intracellular trafficking of CT). The A_1 subunit utilizes a retro-translocation mechanism to cross the ER membrane through a degradation pathway that recycles misfolded host proteins called ERAD [86]. Cytosolic CT-A_1 binds the ADP-ribosylation factor (ARF), and the activated CT-A_1 mono-ADP-ribosylates Arg^{201} of $G_{s\alpha}$, which blocks intrinsic GTPase activity and constitutively activates $G_{s\alpha}$ [87, 88]. $G_{s\alpha}$ is a positive regulator of adenylate cyclase. Increased intracellular cAMP activates protein kinase A (PKA), which phosphorylates the cystic fibrosis transmembrane conductance regulator (CFTR), increasing active secretion of chloride ions [89]. Inhibition of the $Na^+/K^+/2Cl^-$ co-transporter at the same time increases the unidirectional flow of chloride into the gut lumen, causing osmotic water flow into the gut lumen, the pathological outcome of cholera [90]. Current studies on CT involve the utilization of the toxin as an adjuvant in vaccine development [91] and as a tool to study intracellular protein trafficking [85].

Type III secreted toxins

The Type III secretion system (TTSS) is a bacterial virulence factor that injects cytotoxins (also termed effectors) in an unfolded or semi-folded state into a host cell. Like Type II secretion, TTSS comprises inner and outer membrane protein complexes, but includes a hollow, pilin-like structure that extends beyond the outer membrane ring complex. The genetic material encoding the TTSS is a gene duplication of the inner and outer membrane ring complexes of the bacterial flagella protein complex [92]. The inner membrane complex is comprised of two interacting ring structures, each composed of a different oligomeric protein [93]. Like Type II secretion, the cytoplasmic domain of the inner membrane complex associates with an ATPase, which assembles in a hexameric ring to provide the energy for the unfolding and secretion of cytotoxins. The outer membrane structure is also similar to the Type II secretion system outer membrane ring and the Type IV pilus. Extracellular components of the TTSS include a needle, needle extension, and translocation pore, which deliver cytotoxins into the cytoplasm of host cells. The needle is a single protein oligomer that forms a hollow tube. This has direct interactions between the head and tail of the protein subunits and has been implicated in the secretion process upon conformational changes [94]. The needle tip proteins appear to be adaptors that link the translocator proteins within the host membrane to the needle body for efficient transfer of cytotoxins. Translocator proteins form a host membrane-spanning pore for the TTSS effectors [95]. The translocon protein complex prevents cytotoxin secretion before contact with the host cell by physically blocking the hollow channel of the needle complex [96].

ExoS is a Type III secreted cytotoxin. ExoS is a 453-amino acid protein produced by *Pseudomonas aeruginosa* and is a dual function toxin, containing a Rho GTPase activating protein (Rho GAP) activity in the N terminus (96–219) and an ADP-ribosylation domain in the C terminus (234–453) (Fig. 3). The ExoS Rho GAP domain increases γ-phosphate hydrolysis of GTP bound to

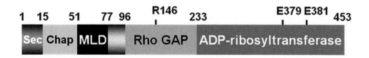

Figure 3. Functional organization of the type III cytotoxin of *Pseudomonas aeruginosa*. ExoS is a bifunctional toxin and is organized into discrete functional domains (amino acids): secretion domain (1–15), chaperone binding domain (16–51), membrane localization domain (51–77), Rho GAP domain, active site residue R146 (96–219), and ADP-ribosyltransferase domain; active site residues E379, E381 (234–453).

Rho GTPases, and inactivates RhoA, Rac1, and Cdc42 [97, 98]. Structural studies showed that the ExoS Rho GAP domain is a molecular mimic of the host Rho GAP, implicating a convergent mechanism of protein evolution for ExoS and their mammalian counterparts [99]. The C-terminal ADP-ribosylation domain of ExoS has the capacity to ADP-ribosylate multiple substrates including Ras at Arg^{41}, which blocks association with the guanine nucleotide exchange factor leading to an inactivation of Ras signaling [100]. Recently, ExoS has also been shown to ADP-ribosylate Rab proteins, such as Rab5, where the ADP-ribosylation of Rab5 uncoupled clathrin-mediated endocytosis [101] and ADP-ribosylation of ezrin/radixin/moesin caused cytoskeletal defects [102]. ExoS binds a cellular cofactor to express ADP-ribosyltransferase activity. The factor was termed 'factor activating exoenzyme S' (FAS) and later identified as a 14-3-3 protein [103]. Activation of a cytotoxin upon binding to a host protein is becoming a common feature of toxin action. Current studies on ExoS involve characterization of how ExoS traffics within host cells to efficiently target intracellular substrates [104], the determination of the role of ExoS and other Type III cytotoxins in *P. aeruginosa* pathogenesis [105], and the development of diagnostics for clinical therapy based upon the seroconversion of cystic fibrosis patients to components of the TTSS upon initial infection by *P. aeruginosa* [106].

Type IV secreted toxins

The Type IV secretion system is a multi-functional protein complex, which transfers DNA between bacteria through conjugation (Type IVA), and transports effector proteins into host cells to regulate host responses to bacterial infection (Type IVB). Type IV transport of effectors across the inner and outer bacterial membranes can follow a single- or two-step process [107]. DNA is transferred as a complex bound to transfer proteins, which bind by a C-terminal signal to DNA [108]. The VirT IVA secretion system in *Agrobacterium tumefaciens* is the best characterized Type IV secretion system; this transfers DNA and proteins into plants to cause disease. VirB contributes to the transfer of effectors into the host cell through the Type IV secretion apparatus [109]. DNA transfer requires a protein relaxase, which binds covalently to the 5' end of ssDNA and causes secretion specifically in a 5' to 3' direction. VirB11 is an ATPase that provides energy for the secretion process analogous to other secretion systems [110, 111]. Pilin homologs form an outer connecting transfer tube between the bacteria and the target cell or other bacteria [108]. Recent structural studies suggest that the inner membrane protein complex spans the majority of the periplasmic space [112]. In addition, Type IV secretion contributes to the pathogenesis of several intracellular bacterial pathogens, including *Legionella, Brucella* and *Coxiella* [113, 114].

SidC is a Type IV effector of *Legionella pneumophila,* the causative agent of Legionnaire's disease [115]. SidC localizes to legionella-containing vesicles *via* phosphatidylinositol-4 phosphate; deletion of SidC interferes with the recruitment of ER-derived vesicles to the legionella-containing vesicles. This is required for the maturation of the legionella-containing vesicles with lysosomal marker proteins.

Type V secreted toxins

The Type V secretion system, also termed the autotransporter secretion group, includes three transport secretion mechanisms: termed Va, Vb, and Vc. Va group autotransporters are translated as a single protein composed of an N-terminal signal peptide sequence for transport by the Sec system, the effector domain, and a C-terminal outer membrane translocation domain [116]. The N-terminal secretion signal utilizes Sec for transport into the periplasm, where the inner membrane secretion signal is cleaved by a periplasmic peptidase. While early models predicted that transported protein folded in mature configuration, recent studies suggest that an unfolded conformation is necessary for transport of the effector across the outer membrane [117]. The C-terminal translocation domain forms a β-barrel [118, 119] that utilizes a co-secreted chaperone protein to protect against proteases and premature folding and to fold effectors upon secretion [120]. A role for ATP has not been determined. A detailed investigation of effector transport through the Type V secretion system is underway [121–123]. The Vb two-partner secretion subgroup follows a mechanism similar to that for Va, involving a Sec-dependent pathway of two distinct proteins [124, 125] in which the translocation protein is predicted to contain β-strands and to interact with effector proteins for efficient translocation across the outer membrane [126–128].

IgA1 protease is a Type V secreted protein that is produced by several genera of bacteria that cleave mammalian IgA [129]. The IgA1 protease group contains a general structure containing a protease and a β-barrel-forming domain. This protease group cleaves proline-threonine and proline-serine bonds in the hinge region of human IgA1 [130].

Type VI and Type VII secretion systems

A Type VI secretion system has been proposed in *V. cholerae* [131] and *P. aeruginosa* [132]. Type VI effectors do not possess N-terminal signal peptides and are Sec secretion independent, implicating a unique mechanism for effector transport relative to the Type I–V secretion systems. Recently, a secretion system was identified in mycobacteria, which was classified as the Type VII secretion for Gram-positive bacteria [133]. Current studies are addressing the identification of mechanisms for effector protein secretion by these new secretion systems.

Botulinum neurotoxin

The botulinum neurotoxins (BoNTs) are the most toxic proteins for humans and have been characterized as Category A agents by the Center for Disease Control and Prevention (CDC). BoNTs block neurotransmitter signal transduction in peripheral α-motor neurons, causing flaccid paralysis, termed botulism [134]. Botulism poisoning in humans is typified by slurred speech, dry mouth, blurred or double vision, peripheral muscle weakness and paralysis. There are seven serotypes of the BoNTs, termed A–G.

Three types of human botulism include wound, ingestion, and infant. Wound botulism occurs upon the delivery of clostridial spores into a deep, anaerobic wound where the spores germinate into vegetative cells that produce BoNT. BoNT circulates in the bloodstream to target α-motor neurons. Food botulism results from the ingestion of preformed toxin in improperly cooked or stored food that allows growth of clostridial and subsequent production of BoNT. Ingested BoNT transcytoses across endothelial cells of the small intestine and migrates to the α-motor neurons. Infant botulism is caused by ingestion of clostridial spores by a child with an underdeveloped intestinal microbiota system. This provides a metabolic niche for the spores to germinate to vegetative cells that produce BoNT, which transcytoses epithelial barrier to cause paralysis. One potential source of clostridial spores for infant botulism appears to be raw or pasteurized honey in children <2 years of age [135]. A medically important characteristic of botulism intoxication is the extended duration of the toxin within neuron cells. The recommended treatment for botulism poisoning is a trivalent (ABE) equine antitoxin serum, obtainable through the CDC.

BoNT as a clinical therapeutic agent

BoNT/A holotoxin is also a clinically useful reagent, commercially available as BoTox®. The medical importance of BoTox transcends superficial cosmetic treatments and is used for a large range of muscle-induced impairments, as well as pain management [136]. Myobloc® is the commercial version of BoNT/B, which can be utilized as an alternative to BoTox treatment [137]. Despite the low immunoreactivity, there are reports of α-BoNT/A and α-BoNT/B antibodies developing in patients after long-term use of the toxin [138, 139]. Determining the antigenic epitopes in medically relevant BoNT and how these epitopes affect toxin action is an important area of research for development of non-reactive clinical BoNT therapies in the future.

BoNT-producing clostridial species

BoNT is produced by a heterogeneous group of clostridial species. While antigenic nomenclature separates the BoNTs by antibody cross-neutralization, clostridia that produce BoNT are differentiated into four groups based on physiology, Groups I–IV [140]. *Clostridium botulinum, C. butyricum, C. baratii,* and *C. argentinense* all produce BoNTs. BoNT genes are found on a variety of genetic elements with BoNT/A, B, E, and F encoded on the chromosome, plasmids, and bacteriophages in various clostridia. BoNT/C and D are found primarily in bacteriophage elements [141].

BoNT operon organization and secretion

BoNT is transcribed and translated as a single ~150 kDa protein with little proteolytic activity. BotR is a positive regulator of BoNT and an associated gene cluster, which is often transcribed as a set of three polycistronic transcripts [142]. BoNT forms complexes with non-toxinogenic proteins transcribed and translated together with the BoNT gene. These proteins include hemagglutinin-active components, which associate with BoNT as a noncovalent, pH-stable complex, but are not necessary for full toxicity [143–145]. The most basic BoNT protein complex is the M complex (~300 kDa), consisting of BoNT and a non-hemagglutinin protein, which is found in BoNT-producing strains except BoNT/G [146]. Other BoNT-containing protein complexes include the L complex (~500 kDa), which encodes a number of proteins associated with BoNT, and hemagglutinin activity. The genes encoding the hemagglutinin-active proteins are located upstream of the non-hemagglutinin protein, and are found in clostridia producing BoNT serotypes A, B, C, D and G [146]. The gene encoding the non-hemagglutinin protein is located upstream of the BoNT gene [147]. The hemagglutinin-active proteins were once hypothesized to protect the BoNT against acid damage during passage through the stomach, but ingested holotoxin without accessory proteins has demonstrated equal toxicity [148]. Currently, these proteins are hypothesized to increase access to the bloodstream (discussed below).

BoNTs are single-chain proteins, which are cleaved to di-chain proteins that are linked by a disulfide bond with AB structure-function properties [149] (Fig. 4). The N-terminal A domain (light chain, LC) is an ~50 kDa zinc metalloprotease with the characteristic thermolysin-family zinc coordination motif (HEXXH) [134]. The ~100 kDa C-terminal B domain (heavy chain, HC) is composed of two functional domains that are involved in receptor recognition (HCR) and translocation of the LC across the endosomal membrane (HCT) [149]. Antibody cross-neutralization differentiates BoNTs into seven serotypes, A–G.

BoNT accessing the bloodstream

There is debate on whether or not the hemagglutinin components of the BoNT protein complexes disrupt the intestinal barrier to contribute to BoNT transport

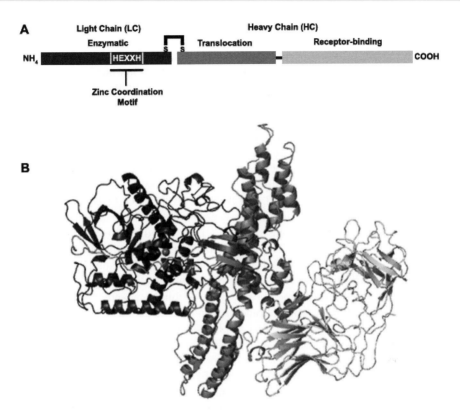

Figure 4. Schematic and structure of BoNT/A. A. Schematic of BoNT/A as an A/B toxin, linked by a disulfide bond between the light (LC) and heavy (HC) chain. B. Crystal structure of BoNT/A. LC (black) is the catalytically active domain and contains a HEXXH motif for coordination of the Zn^{2+} ion. The HC contains the N-terminal translocation (gray) domain and the C-terminal receptor-binding domain (light gray). Gray sphere represents zinc atom within LC active site. Colors between schematic and structure are coordinated with each domain. Structure: PDB: #3bta.

[150, 151]. Trans-epithelial cell transport progresses through a temperature-dependent transport system that can be utilized by BoNT holotoxin alone, suggesting that hemagglutinin and non-hemagglutinin components may increase the permeability of the epithelial barrier, but are not necessary for active BoNT transport to the bloodstream [152, 153]. Clathrin- and dynamin-dependent internalization and transport mechanisms have been implicated in BoNT entry into epithelial cells to an EEA-1-positive, non-acidified vesicle [154, 155]. The saturable nature of HC/A binding suggests that specific receptors are necessary for BoNT binding and trans-epithelial transport. Gangliosides and host synaptic vesicle proteins have been implicated in binding and internalization in the peripheral α-motor neurons, but it is unclear how these components contribute to trans-epithelial transport.

BoNT neuronal specificity

BoNT/HC is composed of two domains, the N-terminal translocation domain and the C-terminal receptor-binding domain (HCR). While there is considerable variability in the primary amino acid sequence of the BoNT/HCR among serotypes A–G, the BoNT/HCR have two conserved jelly-roll and β-trefoil folding motifs. The HCR domain binds neurons *via* several mechanisms that are serotype specific, but include a general dual receptor model for binding and entry into peripheral α-motor neurons. In this model, BoNT/HCR binds to gangliosides on the surface of a neuron, and this complex binds to protein receptors as a high-affinity complex. Gangliosides consist of a polysaccharide group linked to a ceramide lipid, and BoNT/A, B, C, E, G, and tetanus neurotoxin (TeNT) require the binding to ganglioside to associate with neurons [156]. Active synaptic vesicle recycling is required for internalization of BoNTs, except for BoNT/C. This activity-dependent internalization supports a model where receptor(s) for BoNT are located within the luminal domain of the synaptic vesicle and exposed to the extracellular milieu after synaptic vesicle fusion with the plasma membrane. BoNT/A binds synaptic vesicle protein SV2 on loop 4 of the transmembrane protein and the ganglioside GT1b [157]. A role for glycosylation has been implicated in recent studies on BoNT/E binding to SV2 [158]. BoNT/B and BoNT/G utilize synaptotagmin (I or II) as the protein component for neuron receptors [159, 160]. BoNT/C HCR binds GT1b and GD1b, but the protein receptor has not been resolved [161]. TeNT binds two molecules of gangliosides, but a role for a protein receptor component remains to be determined [162]. HCR/A binding to ganglioside demonstrates an increase in affinity over time, suggesting a conformational change in the ganglioside binding site to a higher affinity interaction [163], but how this conformational change modulates affinity to the protein receptor is not clear. BoNT/D HCR associates with phosphatidylethanolamine and shows a ganglioside-independent toxicity of cerebellar granule cells, suggesting a difference in binding specificity compared to the other BoNT serotypes [161]. Recent research suggests that a third binding site, with specificity to lipids, may exist within the N-terminal domain of the HCR [164]. BoNT/A HCR was shown to bind phosphatidylinositol phosphates; however, the binding site was not defined through mutational binding experiments and the structural model needed to be adjusted to accommodate the suggested receptor binding model; therefore how this domain is utilized during BoNT binding and internalization is unclear [164].

BoNT-neuronal cell interactions

BoNT entry into neurons is activity dependent, except for BoNT/C, demonstrating the necessity of vesicle recycling for BoNT uptake into neurons [157, 160]. SV2 and synaptotagmin (I and II) on the synaptic vesicle are integral components of synaptic vesicle fusion with the plasma membrane [165, 166]. Recent studies implicate the binding of the BoNT/HCRs to a protein complex in synaptic vesicles that includes the proton ATPase, synaptophysin, SV2 and synaptotagmin [167]. After fusion with the plasma membrane, the BoNT-receptor complex is endocytosed in a clathrin- and dynamin-dependent pathway [165]. The N terminus of the HC is involved in translocation of the LC from the endosome into the cytosol. The translocation event is pH dependent, which suggests that pore formation or LC translocation requires a conformational change to BoNT structure [168]. Indirect evidence through chimeras of BoNT/A and BoNT/E suggests that translocation speed can vary depending on the HC involved [169]. Recent research suggests that the isolated translocation domain of BoNT inserts into the membrane independent of pH, but acidification may be required to unfold and transport the LC through the HC pore [170, 171].

Mechanism of BoNT action in neurons

BoNTs share ~65% primary amino acid similarity and ~35% amino acid identity with TeNT [172]. BoNT/A, E, and C cleave SNAP25; BoNT/C also cleaves syntaxin 1a; and BoNT/B, D, F, G, and TeNT cleave VAMP-2 [173–175] (Tab. 1). Cleavage sites within each SNARE (soluble N-ethylmaleimide-sensitive factor attachment receptor) substrate differ among the BoNTs, suggesting specific residues on the LC are necessary for recognition of substrate. Recent studies have identified amino acids necessary for substrate recognition by LC/A, LC/B, LC/D, LC/E, LC/F, and TeNT [176–185], mechanistically supporting a crystal structure of a non-catalytic LC/A bound to SNAP25 through exosite and active site interactions [179, 180, 185]. Initial interactions of LC/A with SNAP25 were predicted with the LC/A-SNAP25 co-crystal, and functionally showed that LC/A interacts with a long stretch of amino acids

Table 1. Botulinum neurotoxins (BoNTs) and tetanus neurotoxin (TeNT) SNARE (soluble $\underline{N}$-ethyl-maleimide-sensitive factor $\underline{a}$ttachment $\underline{r}$eceptor) substrates and cleavage sites

Toxin	Substrate	Cleavage site	References
BoNT/A	SNAP25	Q^{197}/R^{198}	[173]
BoNT/B	VAMP-2	Q^{76}/F^{77}	[194]
BoNT/C	SNAP25/syntaxin1a,b	R^{198}/A^{199}: K^{253}/A^{254}	[195, 196]
BoNT/D	VAMP-2	K^{59}/L^{60}	[197]
BoNT/E	SNAP25	R^{180}/I^{181}	[173]
BoNT/F	VAMP-2	Q^{58}/K^{59}	[198]
BoNT/G	VAMP-2	A^{81}/A^{82}	[199]
TeNT	VAMP-2	Q^{76}/F^{77}	[194]

N-terminal to the cleavage site (Q197/R198) of SNAP25. Structural and bio-chemical studies suggest that SNAP25 wraps around the LC *via* a mechanism that mimics the binding of the HC loop to LC [186]. The LC-HC interaction is proposed to inactivate cleavage activity until the LC is released into the cytoplasm of the host cell. Kinetic data utilizing mutagenized SNAP25 iden-tified specific amino acids N-terminal to the active site that contribute to SNAP25 binding, as well as amino acids immediately surrounding the active site that orient SNAP25 within the active site and contribute to cleavage activ-ity. Corresponding studies involving mutations in LC/A demonstrated specif-ic amino acid interactions with SNAP25 along with the minimum length of substrate, defining the specificity of cleavage [180]. LC/E showed a similar mechanism of recognition for SNAP25, in which amino acids N-terminal to the LC/E active site on SNAP25 were identified as well as amino acids imme-diately surrounding the cleavage site that, when mutated, affected catalysis [179]. LC/B, which cleaves VAMP, demonstrated a slightly different mecha-nism of recognition and catalysis with amino acids N-terminal to the cleavage site (Q76/F77) affecting binding and catalysis when mutated. TeNT, which cleaves VAMP-2 at the same residue as BoNT/B and has ~40% primary amino acid homology with BoNT/B, showed similar substrate recognition, but included an extension of the binding domain upstream of the cleavage site [177]. These combinations of amino acid interactions involved in binding and catalysis as a mechanism for substrate recognition seems to explain the speci-ficity of neurotoxin substrate recognition and cleavage site specificity among BoNT serotypes and TeNT, despite a highly identical tertiary structure.

BoNT subtypes

Each BoNT serotype comprises subtypes that can vary between 3 and 32% at the primary amino acid level [187] (Fig. 5). Currently, BoNT/A includes five subtypes, termed A1–A5. BoNT/A1 and BoNT/A2 showed similar cleavage of SNAP25 and possessed ~95% primary amino acid homology [188]. DNA

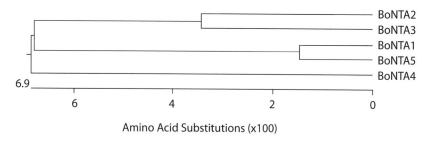

Figure 5. Phylogenetic dendrogram of BoNT/A1–A5 amino acid identity. Dendrogram constructed using DNAStar® MegAlign.

Table 2. Protein similarity of BoNT/A1–A4. Similarity of BoNT/A2–A4 compared to BoNT/A1

BoNTA1 versus	Holotoxin	LC 1-425	HC 438–1295	H_N subdomain 438–872	H_{CN} subdomain 873–1093	H_{CC} subdomain 1094–1295
A2	89	95	87	87	83	90
A3	84	76	86	85	82	90
A4	89	84	89	87	85	97

Adapted with permission from Arndt et al. [188].

sequencing analyses revealed two additional subtypes of BoNT/A: BoNT/A3 and BoNT/A4 [188, 189]. Clostridia producing BoNT/A3 were isolated from a botulism outbreak in Scotland in 1922, while clostridia producing BoNT/A4 were isolated from a case of infant botulism in 1988 [190, 191]. LC/A3 shows 76% identity to LC/A1, while LC/A4 shows 84% identity to LC/A1 [188] (Tab. 2). Phylogenetic analysis of the four subtypes suggested that residue changes in LC/A3 and LC/A4 could potentially affect binding (K_m) and catalysis (k_{cat}) of these two subtypes relative to LC/A1 [189]. Previous modeling studies suggested that LC/A3 and LC/A4 may possess different catalytic activities for SNAP25 relative to LC/A1 [188]. Biochemical studies showed that LC/A3 had similar kinetic properties to LC/A1, and amino acids that differed with LC/A1 within the binding site did not change the binding or catalytic activity of LC/A3 for SNAP25, while LC/A4 showed a ~80-fold decrease in catalytic activity compared to LC/A1, suggesting a defect in SNAP25 cleavage. This change in catalytic activity is believed to be due to a single residue substitution indirectly causing a loss of coordination with the catalytic zinc in the active site, as a point mutation to LC/A4 restores catalytic activity to the level of LC/A1 [192]. Another phenotype of LC/A1, autocatalysis, is observed with LC/A2, but not LC/A3 and LC/A4, demonstrating a difference in self-substrate recognition. Finally, a synthetic diagnostic peptide replicating the substrate cleavage site, SNAPtide™, demonstrates differences in cleavage activity between the subtypes, potentially suggesting differences in substrate recognition [192]. Thus, while LC/A subtypes retained the capacity to cleave SNAP25, efficiency and mechanisms for the cleavage reactions appear different, which will influence the ability to generate serotype-specific inhibitors of catalysis, challenging that ability to establish common steps in catalysis that can be targeted for inactivation. The HCs of BoNT/A subtypes are ~87% identical and polyclonal antisera to HCR/A1 neutralizes BoNT/A1 and BoNT/A2 [187, 193], but there are sufficient amino acid differences so that neutralizing monoclonal antibodies against BoNT/A1 are not effective in neutralizing BoNT/A2 [187]. Current vaccine strategies involve recombinant hepta-HC serotype vaccination, producing a polyclonal antibody response against the seven BoNT serotypes [193].

These data indicate that, while many of the properties of the subtypes of BoNT/A are similar, there are unique properties. Continued characterization of the BoNT serotypes may provide useful information on the development of strategies to generate vaccines and therapies against botulism and to develop novel BoNT derivatives that can extend the therapeutic utility.

Prospects

Since the first discovery in the 19th century of protein toxins as virulence factors of bacterial pathogens, scientific investigation has defined the biochemical and cellular aspects of toxin action, which was facilitated by the resolution of the structural properties of protein toxins. The determination that protein toxins were often organized into discrete domains, which comprise a catalytic, receptor binding, and translocation domain, allowed rapid development of vaccines to control disease. The next chapter in the study of protein toxin action is to utilize our understanding of toxin structure function to develop toxins for immunological and therapeutic intervention of human disease.

Acknowledgments
This work was supported by a grant from the Great Lakes Regional Center of Excellence to J.T.B. (NIH-NIAID U54 AI057153) and a grant to M.R.B. (NIH-NINDS K99 NS061763)

References

1 Field M, Graf LH Jr, Laird WJ, Smith PL (1978) Heat-stable enterotoxin of *Escherichia coli*: *In vitro* effects on guanylate cyclase activity, cyclic GMP concentration, and ion transport in small intestine. *Proc Natl Acad Sci USA* 75: 2800–2804

2 Giannella RA (1981) Pathogenesis of acute bacterial diarrheal disorders. *Annu Rev Med* 32: 341–357

3 Crane JK, Wehner MS, Bolen EJ, Sando JJ, Linden J, Guerrant RL, Sears CL (1992) Regulation of intestinal guanylate cyclase by the heat-stable enterotoxin of *Escherichia coli* (STa) and protein kinase C. *Infect Immun* 60: 5004–5012

4 Takao T, Hitouji T, Aimoto S, Shimonishi Y, Hara S, Takeda T, Takeda Y, Miwatani T (1983) Amino acid sequence of a heat-stable enterotoxin isolated from enterotoxigentic *Escherichia coli* strain 18D. *FEBS Lett* 152: 1–5

5 Ozaki H, Sato T, Kubota H, Hata Y, Katsube Y, Shimonishi Y (1991) Molecular structure of the toxic domain of heat-stable enterotoxin produced by enterotoxigenic *Escherichia coli*. *J Biol Chem* 266: 5934–5941

6 Hidaka Y, Kubota H, Yoshimura S, Ito H, Takeda Y, Shimonishi Y (1988) Disulfide linkages in heat-stable enterotoxin (STp) produced by a porcine strain of enterotoxigenic *Escherichia coli*. *Bull Chem Soc Jpn* 61: 1265–1271

7 Waldman SA, O'Hanley P (1989) Influence of a glycine or proline substitution on the functional properties of a 14-amino acid analog of *Escherichia coli* heat-stable enterotoxin. *Infect Immun* 57: 2420–2424

8 Yamasaki S, Sato T, Hidaka Y, Ozaki H, Ito H, Hirayama T, Takeda Y, Sugimura T, Tai A, Shimonishi Y (1990) Structure-activity relationship of *Escherichia coli* heat-stable enterotoxin: Role of Ala residue at position 14 in toxin-receptor interaction. *Bull Chem Soc Jpn* 63: 2063–2070

9 Hasegawa M, Shimonishi Y (2005) Recognition and signal transduction mechanism of *Escherichia coli* heat-stable enterotoxin and its receptor, guanylate cyclase C. *J Peptide Res* 65:

261–271

10 Yoshimura S, Ikemura H, Watanabe H, Aimoto S, Shimonishi Y, Hara S, Takeda T, Miwatani T, Takeda Y (1985) Essential structure for full enterotoxigenic activity of heat-stable enterotoxin produced by enterotoxigenic *Escherichia coli*. *FEBS Lett* 181: 138–142

11 Ikemura H, Takagi H, Inouye M (1987) Requirement of pro-sequence for the production of active subtilisin E in *Escherichia coli*. *J Biol Chem* 262: 7859–7864

12 Gupta DD, Saha S, Chakrabarti MK (2005) Involvement of protein kinase C in the mechanism of action of *Escherichia coli* heat-stable enterotoxin (STa) in a human colonic carcinoma cell line, COLO-205. *Toxicol Appl Pharmol* 206: 9–16

13 Goldstein JL, Sahi J, Bhuva M, Layden TJ, Rao MC (1994) *Escherichia coli* heat-stable enterotoxin-mediated colonic Cl-secretion is absent in cystic fibrosis. *Gastroenterology* 107: 950–956

14 Goncalves C, Vachon V, Schwartz JL, Dubreuil JD (2007) The *Escherichia coli* enterotoxin STb permeabilizes piglet jejunal brush border membrane vesicles. *Infect Immun* 75: 2208–2213

15 Handl CE, Flock JI (1992) STb producing *Escherichia coli* are rarely associated with infantile diarrhea. *J Diarrhoeal Dis Res* 10: 37–38

16 Arriaga YL, Harville BA, Dreyfus LA (1995) Contribution of individual disulfide bonds to biological action of *Escherichia coli* heat-stable enterotoxin B. *Infect Immun* 63: 4715–4720

17 Labrie V, Harel J, Dubreuil JD (2001) Oligomerization of *Escherichia coli* enterotoxin b through its C-terminal hydrophobic α-helix. *Biochim Biophys Acta* 1535: 128–133

18 Okamoto K, Baba T, Yamanaka H, Akashi N, Fujii Y (1995) Disulfide bond formation and secretion of *Escherichia coli* heat-stable enterotoxin II. *J Bacteriol* 177: 4579–4586

19 Rousset E, Harel J, Dubreuil JD (1998) Sulfatide from the pig jejunum brush border epithelial cell surface is involved in binding of *Escherichia coli* enterotoxin b. *Infect Immun* 66: 5650–5658

20 Kennedy DJ, Greenberg RN, Dunn JA, Abernathy R, Ryerse JS, Guerrant RL (1984) Effects of *Escherichia coli* heat-stable enterotoxin STb on intestines of mice, rats, rabbits, and piglets. *Infect Immun* 46: 639–643

21 Dreyfus LA, Harville B, Howard DE, Shaban R, Beatty DM, Morris SJ (1993) Calcium influx mediated by the *Escherichia coli* heat-stable enterotoxin B (STb). *Proc Natl Acad Sci USA* 90: 3202–3206

22 Erume J, Berberov EM, Kachman SD, Scott MA, Zhou Y, Francis DH, Moxley RA (2008) Comparison of the contributions of heat-labile enterotoxin and heat-stable enterotoxin b to the virulence of enterotoxigenic *Escherichia coli* in F4ac receptor-positive young pigs. *Infect Immun* 76: 3141–3149

23 Lucas ML, Duncan NW, O'Reilly NF, McIlvenny TJ, Nelson YB (2008) Lack of evidence *in vivo* for a remote effect of *Escherichia coli* heat stable enterotoxin on jejunal fluid absorption. *Neurogastroenterol Motil* 20: 532–538

24 Gouaux E (1997) Channel-forming toxins: Tales of transformation. *Curr Opin Struct Biol* 7: 566–573

25 Lesieur C, Vecsey-Semjen B, Abrami L, Fivaz M, van der Goot FG (1997) Membrane insertion: The strategy of toxins. *Mol Membr Biol* 14: 45–64

26 Kurisu G, Zakharov SD, Zhalnina MV, Bano S, Eroukova VY, Rokitskaya TI, Antonenko YN, Wiener MC, Cramer WA (2003) The structure of BtuB with bound colicin E3 R-domain implies a translocon. *Nat Struct Biol* 10: 948–954

27 Yamashita E, Zhalnina MV, Zakharov SD, Sharma O, Cramer WA (2008) Crystal structures of the OmpF porin: Function in a colicin translocon. *EMBO J* 27: 2171–2180

28 Choe S, Bennett MJ, Fujii G, Curmi PM, Kantardjieff KA, Collier RJ, Eisenberg D (1992) The crystal structure of diphtheria toxin. *Nature* 357: 216–222

29 Ratts R, Zeng H, Berg EA, Blue C, McComb ME, Costello CE, van der Spek JC, Murphy JR (2003) The cytosolic entry of diphtheria toxin catalytic domain requires a host cell cytosolic translocation factor complex. *J Cell Biol* 160: 1139–1150

30 Tilley SJ, Saibil HR (2006) The mechanism of pore formation by bacterial toxins. *Curr Opin Struct Biol* 16: 230–236

31 Iacovache I, Paumard P, Scheib H, Lesieur C, Sakai N, Matile S, Parker MW, van der Goot FG (2006) A rivet model for channel formation by aerolysin-like pore-forming toxins. *EMBO J* 25: 457–466

32 Nassi S, Collier RJ, Finkelstein A (2002) PA63 channel of anthrax toxin: An extended β-barrel. *Biochemistry* 41: 1445–1450

33 Moniatte M, van der Goot FG, Buckley JT, Pattus F, van Dorsselaer A (1996) Characterisation of

the heptameric pore-forming complex of the *Aeromonas* toxin aerolysin using MALDI-TOF mass spectrometry. *FEBS Lett* 384: 269–272

34 Parker MW, Feil SC (2005) Pore-forming protein toxins: From structure to function. *Prog Biophys Mol Biol* 88: 91–142

35 Sekiya K, Satoh R, Danbara H, Futaesaku Y (1993) A ring-shaped structure with a crown formed by streptolysin O on the erythrocyte membrane. *J Bacteriol* 175: 5953–5961

36 Park JM, Ng VH, Maeda S, Rest RF, Karin M (2004) Anthrolysin O and other gram-positive cytolysins are toll-like receptor 4 agonists. *J Exp Med* 200: 1647–1655

37 Rosado CJ, Kondos S, Bull TE, Kuiper MJ, Law RH, Buckle AM, Voskoboinik I, Bird PI, Trapani JA, Whisstock JC, Dunstone MA (2008) The MACPF/CDC family of pore-forming toxins. *Cell Microbiol* 10: 1765–1774

38 Rossjohn J, Polekhina G, Feil SC, Morton CJ, Tweten RK, Parker MW (2007) Structures of perfringolysin O suggest a pathway for activation of cholesterol-dependent cytolysins. *J Mol Biol* 367: 1227–1236

39 Tweten RK (2005) Cholesterol-dependent cytolysins, a family of versatile pore-forming toxins. *Infect Immun* 73: 6199–6209

40 Tweten RK (2005) Cholesterol-dependent cytolysins, a family of versatile pore-forming toxins. *Infect Immun* 73: 6199–6209

41 Ramachandran R, Tweten RK, Johnson AE (2005) The domains of a cholesterol-dependent cytolysin undergo a major FRET-detected rearrangement during pore formation. *Proc Natl Acad Sci USA* 102: 7139–7144

42 Rosado CJ, Kondos S, Bull TE, Kuiper MJ, Law RH, Buckle AM, Voskobolnlk I, Bird PI, Trapani JA, Whisstock JC, Dunstone MA (2008) The MACPF/CDC family of pore-forming toxins. *Cell Microbiol* 10: 1765–1774

43 Tilley SJ, Orlova EV, Gilbert RJ, Andrew PW, Saibil HR (2005) Structural basis of pore formation by the bacterial toxin pneumolysin. *Cell* 121: 247–256

44 Yoshino K, Abe J, Murata H, Takao T, Kohsaka T, Shimonishi Y, Takeda T (1994) Purification and characterization of a novel superantigen produced by a clinical isolate of *Yersinia pseudotuberculosis*. *FEBS Lett* 356: 141–144

45 McCormick JK, Yarwood JM, Schlievert PM (2001) Toxic shock syndrome and bacterial superantigens: An update. *Annu Rev Microbiol* 55: 77–104

46 Bergdoll MS (1983) Enterotoxins. In: CSF Easmon, C Adlam (eds): *Staphylococci and Staphylococcal Infections*. Academic Press, London, 559–598

47 Fraser JD, Proft T (2008) The bacterial superantigen and superantigen-like proteins. *Immunol Rev* 225: 226–243

48 Donadini R, Liew CW, Kwan AH, Mackay JP, Fields BA (2004) Crystal and solution structures of a superantigen from *Yersinia pseudotuberculosis* reveal a jelly-roll fold. *Structure* 12: 145–156

49 Al-Shangiti AM, Naylor CE, Nair SP, Briggs DC, Henderson B, Chain BM (2004) Structural relationships and cellular tropism of staphylococcal superantigen-like proteins. *Infect Immun* 72: 4261–4270

50 Arcus VL, Langley R, Proft T, Fraser JD, Baker EN (2002) The three-dimensional structure of a superantigen-like protein, SET3, from a pathogenicity island of the *Staphylococcus aureus* genome. *J Biol Chem* 277: 32274–32281

51 Chung MC, Wines BD, Baker H, Langley RJ., Baker EN, Fraser JD (2007) The crystal structure of staphylococcal superantigen-like protein 11 in complex with sialyl Lewis X reveals the mechanism for cell binding and immune inhibition. *Mol Microbiol* 66: 1342–1355

52 Langley R, Wines B, Willoughby N, Basu I, Proft T, Fraser JD (2005) The staphylococcal superantigen-like protein 7 binds IgA and complement C5 and inhibits IgA-Fc α RI binding and serum killing of bacteria. *J Immunol* 174: 2926–2933

53 Kim J, Urban RG, Strominger JL, Wiley DC (1994) Toxic shock syndrome toxin-1 complexed with a class II major histocompatibility molecule. *Science* 266: 1870–1874

54 Gunther S, Varma AK, Moza B, Kasper KJ, Wyatt AW, Zhu P, Rahman AK, Li Y, Mariuzza RA, McCormick JK, Sundberg EJ (2007) A novel loop domain in superantigens extends their T cell receptor recognition site. *J Mol Biol* 371: 210–221

55 Li Y, Li H, Dimasi N, McCormick JK, Martin R, Schuck P, Schlievert PM, Mariuzza RA (2001) Crystal structure of a superantigen bound to the high-affinity, zinc-dependent site on MHC class II. *Immunity* 14: 93–104

56 Zhao Y, Li Z, Drozd SJ, Guo Y, Mourad W, Li H (2004) Crystal structure of *Mycoplasma arthri-*

tidis mitogen complexed with HLA-DR1 reveals a novel superantigen fold and a dimerized super-antigen-MHC complex. *Structure* 12: 277–288

57 Sundberg EJ, Deng L, Mariuzza RA (2007) TCR recognition of peptide/MHC class II complexes and superantigens. *Semin Immunol* 19: 262–271

58 Pless DD, Ruthel G, Reinke EK, Ulrich RG, Bavari S (2005) Persistence of zinc-binding bacterial superantigens at the surface of antigen-presenting cells contributes to the extreme potency of these superantigens as T-cell activators. *Infect Immun* 73: 5358–5366

59 Sundberg EJ, Li H, Llera AS, McCormick JK, Tormo J, Schlievert PM, Karjalainen K, Mariuzza RA (2002) Structures of two streptococcal superantigens bound to TCR β chains reveal diversity in the architecture of T cell signaling complexes. *Structure* 10: 687–699

60 Sundberg EJ, Deng L, Mariuzza RA (2007) TCR recognition of peptide/MHC class II complexes and superantigens. *Semin Immunol* 19: 262–271

61 Yang X, Buonpane RA, Moza B, Rahman AK, Wang N, Schlievert PM, McCormick JK, Sundberg EJ, Kranz DM (2008) Neutralization of multiple staphylococcal superantigens by a single-chain protein consisting of affinity-matured, variable domain repeats. *J Infect Dis* 198: 344–348

62 Thomas D, Dauwalder O, Brun V, Badiou C, Ferry T, Etienne J, Vandenesch F, Lina G (2009) *Staphylococcus aureus* superantigens elicit redundant and extensive human Vβ patterns. *Infect Immun* 77: 2043–2050

63 Ostolaza H, Soloaga A, Goni FM (1995) The binding of divalent cations to *Escherichia coli* α-haemolysin. *Eur J Biochem* 228: 39–44

64 Wolff N, Ghigo JM, Delepelaire P, Wandersman C, Delepierre M (1994) C-terminal secretion signal of an *Erwinia chrysanthemi* protease secreted by a signal peptide-independent pathway: Proton NMR and CD conformational studies in membrane-mimetic environments. *Biochemistry* 33: 6792–6801

65 Allenby NE, O'Connor N, Pragai Z, Carter NM, Miethke M, Engelmann S, Hecker M, Wipat A, Ward AC, Harwood CR (2004) Post-transcriptional regulation of the *Bacillus subtilis* pst operon encoding a phosphate-specific ABC transporter. *Microbiology* 150: 2619–2628

66 Delepelaire P (2004) Type I secretion in gram-negative bacteria. *Biochim Biophys Acta* 1694: 149–161

67 Letoffe S, Delepelaire P, Wandersman C (1996) Protein secretion in gram-negative bacteria: Assembly of the three components of ABC protein-mediated exporters is ordered and promoted by substrate binding. *EMBO J* 15: 5804–5811

68 Glaser P, Danchin A, Ladant D, Barzu O, Ullmann A (1988) *Bordetella pertussis* adenylate cyclase: The gene and the protein. *Tokai J Exp Clin Med* 13 Suppl: 239–252

69 Guermonprez P, Khelef N, Blouin E, Rieu P, Ricciardi-Castagnoli P, Guiso N, Ladant D, Leclerc C (2001) The adenylate cyclase toxin of *Bordetella pertussis* binds to target cells *via* the α(M)β(2) integrin (CD11b/CD18). *J Exp Med* 193: 1035–1044

70 Weingart CL, Mobberley-Schuman, PS, Hewlett, EL, Gray, MC, Weiss AA (2000) Neutralizing antibodies to andenylate cyclase toxin promote phagocytosis of *Bordetella pertussis* by human neutrophils. *Infect Immun* 68: 7152–7155

71 Rogel A, Hanski E (1992) Distinct steps in the penetration of adenylate cyclase toxin of *Bordetella pertussis* into sheep erythrocytes. Translocation of the toxin across the membrane. *J Biol Chem* 267: 22599–22605

72 Cheung GY, Kelly SM, Jess TJ, Prior S, Price NC, Parton R, Coote JG (2009) Functional and structural studies on different forms of the adenylate cyclase toxin of *Bordetella pertussis*. *Microb Pathog* 46: 36–42

73 Arnoff DM, Canetti C, Serezani CH, Luo M, Peters-Golden M (2005) Cutting edge: Macrophage inhibition by cyclic AMP (cAMP): Differential roles of protein kinase A and exchange protein directly activated by cAMP-1. *J Immunol* 174: 595–599

74 Galgani M, De Rosa V, De Simone S, Leonardi A, D'Oro U, Napolitani G, Masci AM, Zappacosta S, Racioppi L (2004) Cyclic AMP modulates the functional plasticity of immature dendritic cells by inhibiting Src-like kinases through protein kinase A-mediated signaling. *J Biol Chem* 279: 32507–32514

75 Ehrmann IE, Gray MC, Gordon VM, Gray LS, Hewlett EL (1991) Hemolytic activity of adenylate cyclase toxin from *Bordetella pertussis*. *FEBS Lett* 278: 79–83

76 Chenal A, Guijarro JI, Raynal B, Delepierre M, Ladant D (2009) RTX calcium binding motifs are intrinsically disordered in the absence of calcium: Implication for protein secretion. *J Biol Chem* 284: 1781–1789

77 Kamanova J, Kofronova O, Masin J, Genth H, Vojtova J, Linhartova I, Benada O, Just I, Sebo P (2008) Adenylate cyclase toxin subverts phagocyte function by RhoA inhibition and unproductive ruffling. *J Immunol* 181: 5587–5597

78 Watanabe M, Blobel G (1989) SecB functions as a cytosolic signal recognition factor for protein export in *E. coli*. *Cell* 58: 695–705

79 Johnson TL, Abendroth J, Hol WG, Sandkvist M (2006) Type II secretion: From structure to function. *FEMS Microbiol Lett* 255: 175–186

80 Henderson IR, Navarro-Garcia F, Desvaux M, Fernandez RC, Ala'Aldeen D (2004) Type V protein secretion pathway: The autotransporter story. *Microbiol Mol Biol Rev* 68: 692–744

81 Martoglio B, Dobberstein B (1998) Signal sequences: More than just greasy peptides. *Trends Cell Biol* 8: 410–415

82 Yanez ME, Korotkov KV, Abendroth J, Hol WG (2008) Structure of the minor pseudopilin EpsH from the Type 2 secretion system of *Vibrio cholerae*. *J Mol Biol* 377: 91–103

83 Bachert C, Zhang N, Patou J, van Zele T, Gevaert P (2008) Role of staphylococcal superantigens in upper airway disease. *Curr Opin Allergy Clin Immunol* 8: 34–38

84 Van Heyningen S (1974) Cholera toxin: Interaction of subunits with ganglioside G_{M1}. *Science* 183: 656–657

85 Chinnapen DJ, Chinnapen H, Saslowsky D, Lencer WI (2007) Rafting with cholera toxin: Endocytosis and trafficking from plasma membrane to ER. *FEMS Microbiol Lett* 266: 129–137

86 Rodighiero C, Tsai B, Rapoport TA, Lencer WI (2002) Role of ubiquitination in retro-translocation of cholera toxin and escape of cytosolic degradation. *EMBO Rep* 3: 1222–1227

87 Moss J, Manganiello VC, Vaughan M (1976) Hydrolysis of nicotinamide adenine dinucleotide by choleragen and its A protomer: Possible role in the activation of adenylate cyclase. *Proc Natl Acad Sci USA* 73: 4424–4427

88 Gill DM (1975) Involvement of nicotinamide adenine dinucleotide in the action of cholera toxin *in vitro*. *Proc Natl Acad Sci USA* 72: 2064–2068

89 Cheng SH, Rich DP, Marshall J, Gregory RJ, Welsh MJ, Smith AE (1991) Phosphorylation of the R domain by cAMP-dependent protein kinase regulates the CFTR chloride channel. *Cell* 66: 1027–1036

90 Halm DR, Rechkemmer GR, Schoumacher RA, Frizzell RA (1988) Apical membrane chloride channels in a colonic cell line activated by secretory agonists. *Am J Physiol* 254: C505–511

91 Nystrom-Asklin J, Adamsson J, Harandi AM (2008) The adjuvant effect of CpG oligodeoxynucleotide linked to the non-toxic B subunit of cholera toxin for induction of immunity against *H. pylori* in mice. *Scand J Immunol* 67: 431–440

92 Plano GV, Day JB, Ferracci F (2001) Type III export: New uses for an old pathway. *Mol Microbiol* 40: 284–293

93 Marlovits TC, Kubori T, Sukhan A, Thomas DR, Galan JE, Unger VM (2004) Structural insights into the assembly of the type III secretion needle complex. *Science* 306: 1040–1042

94 Kenjale R, Wilson J, Zenk SF, Saurya S, Picking WL, Picking WD, Blocker A (2005) The needle component of the type III secreton of *Shigella* regulates the activity of the secretion apparatus. *J Biol Chem* 280: 42929–42937

95 Veenendaal AK, Hodgkinson JL, Schwarzer L, Stabat D, Zenk SF, Blocker AJ (2007) The type III secretion system needle tip complex mediates host cell sensing and translocon insertion. *Mol Microbiol* 63: 1719–1730

96 Picking WL, Nishioka H, Hearn PD, Baxter MA, Harrington AT, Blocker A, Picking WD (2005) IpaD of *Shigella flexneri* is independently required for regulation of Ipa protein secretion and efficient insertion of IpaB and IpaC into host membranes. *Infect Immun* 73: 1432–1440

97 Goehring UM, Schmidt G, Pederson KJ, Aktories K, Barbieri JT (1999) The N-terminal domain of *Pseudomonas aeruginosa* exoenzyme S is a GTPase-activating protein for Rho GTPases. *J Biol Chem* 274: 36369–36372

98 Krall R, Sun J, Pederson KJ, Barbieri JT (2002) *In vivo* rho GTPase-activating protein activity of *Pseudomonas aeruginosa* cytotoxin ExoS. *Infect Immun* 70: 360–367

99 Wurtele M, Wolf E, Pederson KJ, Buchwald G, Ahmadian MR, Barbieri JT, Wittinghofer A (2001) How the *Pseudomonas aeruginosa* ExoS toxin downregulates Rac. *Nat Struct Biol* 8: 23–26

100 Ganesan AK, Vincent TS, Olson JC, Barbieri JT (1999) *Pseudomonas aeruginosa* exoenzyme S disrupts Ras-mediated signal transduction by inhibiting guanine nucleotide exchange factor-catalyzed nucleotide exchange. *J Biol Chem* 274: 21823–21829

101 Deng Q, Barbieri JT (2008) Modulation of host cell endocytosis by the type III cytotoxin, *Pseudomonas* ExoS. *Traffic* 9: 1948–1957

102 Maresso AW, Deng Q, Pereckas MS, Wakim BT, Barbieri JT (2007) *Pseudomonas aeruginosa* ExoS ADP-ribosyltransferase inhibits ERM phosphorylation. *Cell Microbiol* 9: 97–105

103 Fu H, Coburn J, Collier RJ (1993) The eukaryotic host factor that activates exoenzyme S of *Pseudomonas aeruginosa* is a member of the 14-3-3 protein family. *Proc Natl Acad Sci USA* 90: 2320–2324

104 Zhang Y, Barbieri JT (2005) A leucine-rich motif targets *Pseudomonas aeruginosa* ExoS within mammalian cells. *Infect Immun* 73: 7938–7945

105 Roy-Burman A, Savel RH, Racine S, Swanson BL, Revadigar NS, Fujimoto J, Sawa T, Frank DW, Wiener-Kronish JP (2001) Type III protein secretion is associated with death in lower respiratory and systemic *Pseudomonas aeruginosa* infections. *J Infect Dis* 183: 1767–1774

106 Corech R, Rao A, Laxova A, Moss J, Rock MJ, Li Z, Kosorok MR, Splaingard ML, Farrell PM, Barbieri JT (2005) Early immune response to the components of the type III system of *Pseudomonas aeruginosa* in children with cystic fibrosis. *J Clin Microbiol* 43: 3956–3962

107 Burns DL (2003) Type IV transporters of pathogenic bacteria. *Curr Opin Microbiol* 6: 29–34

108 Christie PJ, Atmakuri K, Krishnamoorthy V, Jakubowski S, Cascales E (2005) Biogenesis, architecture, and function of bacterial type IV secretion systems. *Annu Rev Microbiol* 59: 451–485

109 Saier MH (2006) Protein secretion and membrane insertion systems in Gram-negative bacteria. *J Membr Biol* 214: 75–90

110 Planet PJ, Kachlany SC, DeSalle R, Figurski DH (2001) Phylogeny of genese for secretion NTPases: Identification of the widespread tadA subfamily and development of a diagnostic key for gene classification. *Proc Natl Acad Sci USA* 98: 2503–2508

111 Savvides SN, Yeo HJ, Beck MR, Blaesing F, Lurz R, Lanka E, Buhrdorf R, Fischer W, Haas R, Waksman G (2003) VirB11 ATPases are dynamic hexameric assemblies: New insights into bacterial type IV secretion. *EMBO J* 22: 1969–1980

112 Fronzes R, Schafer E, Wang L, Saibil HR, Orlova EV, Waksman G (2009) Structure of a type IV secretion system core complex. *Science* 323: 266–268

113 Backert S, Meyer TF (2006) Type IV secretion systems and their effectors in bacterial pathogenesis. *Curr Opin Microbiol* 9: 207–217

114 De Felipe KS, Glover RT, Charpentier X, Anderson OR, Reyes M, Pericone CD, Shuman HA (2008) *Legionella* eukaryotic-like type IV substrates interfere with organelle trafficking. *PLoS Pathog* 4: e1000117

115 Ragaz C, Pietsch H, Urwyler S, Tiaden A, Weber SS, Hilbi H (2008) The *Legionella pneumophila* phosphatidylinositol-4 phosphate-binding type IV substrate SidC recruits endoplasmic reticulum vesicles to a replication-permissive vacuole. *Cell Microbiol* 10: 2416–2433

116 Henderson IR, Navarro-Garcia F, Desvaux M, Fernandez RC, Ala'Aldeen D (2004) Type V protein secretion pathway: The autotransporter story. *Microbiol Mol Biol Rev* 68: 692–744

117 Henderson IR, Navarro-Garcia F, Nataro JP (1998) The great escape: Structure and function of the autotransporter proteins. *Trends Microbiol* 6: 370–378

118 Loveless BJ, Saier MH (1997) A novel family of channel-forming, autotransporting, bacterial virulence factors. *Mol Membr Biol* 14: 801–807

119 Yen MR, Peabody CR, Partovi SM, Zhai Y, Tseng YH, Saier MH (2002) Protein-translocating outer membrane porins of Gram-negative bacteria. *Biochim Biophys Acta* 1562: 6–31

120 Oliver DC, Huang G, Nodel E, Pleasance S, Fernandez RC (2003) A conserved region within the *Bordetella pertussis* autotransporter BrkA is necessary for folding of its passenger domain. *Mol Microbiol* 47: 1367–1383

121 Brunder W, Schmidt H, Karch H (1997) EspP, a novel extracellular serine protease of enterohaemorrhagic *Escherichia coli* O157:H7 cleaves human coagulation factor V. *Mol Microbiol* 24: 767–778

122 Leininger E, Roberts M, Kenimer JG, Charles IG, Fairweather N, Novotny P, Brennan MJ (1991) Pertactin, an Arg-Gly-Asp-containing *Bordetella pertussis* surface protein that promotes adherence of mammalian cells. *Proc Natl Acad Sci USA* 88: 345–349

123 St Geme JW, Cutter D (2000) The *Haemophilus influenzae* Hia adhesin is an autotransporter protein that remains uncleaved at the C terminus and fully cell associated. *J. Bacteriol* 182: 6005–6013

124 Henderson IR, Cappello R, Nataro JP (2000) Autotransporter proteins, evolution and redefining protein secretion. *Trends Microbiol* 8: 529–532

125 Jacob-Dubuisson F, Locht C, Antoine R (2001) Two-partner secretion in Gram-negative bacteria: A thrifty, specific pathway for large virulence proteins. *Mol Microbiol* 40: 306–313

126 Grass S, St Geme JW (2000) Maturation and secretion of the non-typable *Haemophilus influenzae*HMW1 adhesin: Roles of the N-terminal and C-terminal domains. *Mol Microbiol* 36: 55–67

127 Guedin S, Willery E, Tommassen J, Fort E, Drobecq H, Locht C, Jacob-Dubuisson F (2000) Novel topological features of FhaC, the outer membrane transporter involved in the secretion of the *Bordetella pertussis* filamentous hemagglutinin. *J Biol Chem* 275: 30202–30210

128 Jacob-Dubuisson F, Buisine C, Willery E, Renauld-Mongenie G, Locht C (1997) Lack of functional complementation between *Bordetella pertussis* filamentous hemagglutinin and *Proteus mirabilis* HpmA hemolysin secretion machineries. *J Bacteriol* 179: 775–783

129 Klauser T, Pohlner J, Meyer TF (1993) The secretion pathway of IgA protease-type proteins in gram-negative bacteria. *Bioessays* 15: 799–805

130 Frangione B, Franklin EC (1972) Chemical typing of the immunoglobulins IgM, IgA1 and IgA2. *FEBS Lett* 20: 321–323

131 Pukatzki S, Ma AT, Sturtevant D, Krastins B, Sarracino D, Nelson WC, Heidelberg JF, Mekalanos JJ (2006) Identification of a conserved bacterial protein secretion system in *Vibrio cholerae* using the *Dictyostelium* host model system. *Proc Natl Acad Sci USA* 103: 1528–1533

132 Mougous JD, Cuff ME, Raunser S, Shen A, Zhou M, Gifford CA, Goodman AL, Joachimiak G, Ordonez CL, Lory S, Walz T, Joachimiak A, Mekalanos JJ (2006) A virulence locus of *Pseudomonas aeruginosa* encodes a protein secretion apparatus. *Science* 312: 1526–1530

133 Abdallah AM, Gey van Pittius NC, Champion PA, Cox J, Luirink J, Vandenbroucke-Grauls CM, Appelmelk BJ, Bitter W (2007) Type VII secretion–Mycobacteria show the way. *Nat Rev Microbiol* 5: 883–891

134 Schiavo G, Rossetto O, Santucci A, DasGupta BR, Montecucco C (1992) Botulinum neurotoxins are zink proteins. *J Biol Chem* 267: 23479–23483

135 Tanzi MG, Gabay MP (2002) Association between honey consumption and infant botulism. *Pharmacotherapy* 22: 1479–1483

136 Dastoor SF, Misch CE, Wang HL (2007) Botulinum toxin (Botox) to enhance facial macroesthetics: A literature review. *J Oral Implantol* 33: 164–171

137 Callaway JE (2004) Botulinum toxin type B (Myobloc): Pharmacology and biochemistry. *Clin Dermatol* 22: 23–28

138 Dressler D, Munchau A, Bhatia KP, Quinn NP, Bigalke H (2002) Antibody-induced botulinum toxin therapy failure: Can it be overcome by increased botulinum toxin doses? *Eur Neurol* 47: 118–121

139 Dressler D, Bigalke H (2002) Botulinum toxin antibody type A titres after cessation of botulinum toxin therapy. *Mov Disord* 17: 170–173

140 Suen JC, Hatheway CL, Steigerwalt AG, Brenner DJ (1988) Genetic confirmation of identities of neurotoxigenic *Clostridium baratii* and *Clostridium butyricum* implicated as agents of infant botulism. *J Clin Microbiol* 26: 2191–2192

141 Popoff MR, Marvaud JC (1999) Structural and genomic features of clostridial neurotoxins. In: JE Alouf, JH Freer (eds): *The Comprehensive Sourcebook of Bacterial Protein Toxins*. Academic Press, London, 174–201

142 Dineen SS, Bradshaw M, Karasek CE, Johnson EA (2004) Nucleotide sequence and transcriptional analysis of the type A2 neurotoxin gene cluster in *Clostridium botulinum*. *FEMS Microbiol Lett* 235: 9–16

143 Oguma K, Inoue K, Fujinaga Y, Yokota K, Watanabe T, Ohyama T, Takeshi K, Inoue K (1999) Structure and function of *Clostridium botulinum* progenitor toxin. *J Toxicol Toxin Rev* 18: 17–34

144 Quinn CP, Minton NP (2001) Clostridial neurotoxins. In: H Bahl, P Dürre (eds): *Clostridia. Biotechnology and Medical Applications*. Wiley-VCH, Weinheim, 211–250

145 Sharma SK, Ramzan MA, Singh BR (2003) Separation of the components of type A botulinum neurotoxin complex by electrophoresis. *Toxicon* 41: 321–331

146 Rodriguez Jovita M, Collins MD, East AK (1998) Gene organization and sequence determination of the two botulinum neurotoxin gene clusters in *Clostridium botulinum* type A(B) strain NCTC 2916. *Curr Microbiol* 36: 226–231

147 East AK, Richardson PT, Allaway D, Collins MD, Roberts TA, Thompson DE (1992) Sequence of the gene encoding type F neurotoxin of *Clostridium botulinum*. *FEMS Microbiol Lett* 75: 225–230

148 Sugii S, Ohishi I, Sakaguchi G (1977) Correlation between oral toxicity and *in vitro* stability of *Clostridium botulinum* type A and B toxins of different molecular sizes. *Infect Immun* 16: 910–914

149 Bandyopadhyay S, Clark AW, DasGupta BR, Sathyamoorthy V (1987) Role of the heavy and light chains of botulinum neurotoxin in neuromuscular paralysis. *J Biol Chem* 262: 2660–2663

150 Couesnon A, Pereira Y, Popoff MR (2007) Receptor-mediated transcytosis of botulinum neurotoxin A through intestinal cell monolayers. *Cell Microbiol* 10: 375–387

151 Jin Y, Takegahara Y, Sugawara Y, Matsumura T, Fujinaga Y (2009) Disruption of the epithelial barrier by botulinum haemagglutinin (HA) proteins–Differences in cell tropism and the mechanism of action between HA proteins of types A or B, and HA proteins of type C. *Microbiology* 155: 35–45

152 Maksymowych AB, Simpson LL (1998) Binding and transcytosis of botulinum neurotoxin by polarized human colon carcinoma cells. *J Biol Chem* 273: 21950–21957

153 Park JB, Simpson LL (2003) Inhalational poisoning by botulinum toxin and inhalation vaccination with its heavy-chain component. *Infect Immun* 71: 1147–1154

154 Couesnon A, Pereira Y, Popoff MR (2008) Receptor-mediated transcytosis of botulinum neurotoxin A through intestinal cell monolayers. *Cell Microbiol* 10: 375–387

155 Couesnon A, Shimizu T, Popoff MR (2009) Differential entry of botulinum neurotoxin A into neuronal and intestinal cells. *Cell Microbiol* 11: 289–308

156 Kitamura M, Takamiya K, Aizawa S, Furukawa K (1999) Gangliosides are the binding substances in neural cells for tetanus and botulinum toxins in mice. *Biochim Biophys Acta* 1441: 1–3

157 Dong M, Yeh F, Tepp WH, Dean C, Johnson EA, Janz R, Chapman ER (2006) SV2 is the protein receptor for botulinum neurotoxin A. *Science* 312: 592–596

158 Dong M, Liu H, Tepp WH, Johnson EA, Janz R, Chapman ER (2008) Glycosylated SV2A and SV2B mediate the entry of botulinum neurotoxin E into neurons. *Mol Biol Cell* 19: 5226–5237

159 Rummel A, Karnath T, Henke T, Bigalke H, Binz T (2004) Synaptotagmins I and II act as nerve cell receptors for botulinum neurotoxin G. *J Biol Chem* 279: 30865–30870

160 Dong M, Richards DA, Goodnough MC, Tepp WH, Johnson EA, Chapman ER (2003) Synaptotagmins I and II mediate entry of botulinum neurotoxin B into cells. *J Cell Biol* 162: 1293–1303

161 Tsukamoto K, Kohda T, Mukamoto M, Takeuchi K, Ihara H, Saito M, Kozaki S (2005) Binding of *Clostridium botulinum* type C and D neurotoxins to ganglioside and phospholipid. Novel insights into the receptor for clostridial neurotoxins. *J Biol Chem* 280: 35164–35171

162 Rummel A, Bade S, Alves J, Bigalke H, Binz T (2003) Two carbohydrate binding sites in the H(CC)-domain of tetanus neurotoxin are required for toxicity. *J Mol Biol* 326: 835–847

163 Yowler BC, Schengrund CL (2004) Botulinum neurotoxin A changes conformation upon binding to ganglioside GT1b. *Biochemistry* 43: 9725–9731

164 Muraro L, Tosatto S, Motterlini L, Rossetto O, Montecucco C (2009) The N-terminal half of the receptor domain of botulinum neurotoxin A binds to microdomains of the plasma membrane. *Biochem Biophys Res Commun* 380: 76–80

165 Jung N, Haucke V (2007) Clathrin-mediated endocytosis at synapses. *Traffic* 8: 1129–1136

166 Morgans CW, Kensel-Hammes P, Hurley JB, Burton K, Idzerda R, McKnight GS, Bajjalieh SM (2009) Loss of the synaptic vesicle protein SV2B results in reduced neurotransmission and altered synaptic vesicle protein expression in the retina. *PLoS ONE* 4: e5230

167 Baldwin MR, Barbieri JT (2009) Association of botulinum neurotoxins with synaptic vesicle protein complexes. *Toxicon* 54: 570–574

168 Fischer A, Mushrush DJ, Lacy DB, Montal M (2008) Botulinum neurotoxin devoid of receptor binding domain translocates active protease. *PLoS Pathog* 4

169 Wang J, Meng J, Lawrence GW, Zurawski TH, Sasse A, Bodeker MO, Gilmore MA, Fernandez-Salas E, Francis J, Steward LE, Aoki KR, Dolly JO (2008) Novel chimeras of botulinum neurotoxins A and E unveil contributions from the binding, translocation, and protease domains to their functional characteristics. *J Biol Chem* 283: 16993–17002

170 Fischer A, Montal M (2007) Single molecule detection of intermediates during botulinum neurotoxin translocation across membranes. *Proc Natl Acad Sci USA* 104: 10447–10452

171 Montal M (2008) Translocation of botulinum neurotoxin light chain protease by the heavy chain protein-conducting channel. *Toxicon* 54: 565–569

172 Lacy DB, Stevens RC (1999) Sequence homology and structural analysis of the clostridial neurotoxins. *J Mol Biol* 291: 1091–1104

173 Binz T, Blasi J, Yamasaki S, Baumeister A, Link E, Südhof TC, Jahn R, Niemann H (1994)

Proteolysis of SNAP-25 by types E and A botulinal neurotoxins. *J Biol Chem* 269: 1617–1620

174 Foran P, Lawrence GW, Shone CC, Foster KA, Dolly JO (1996) Botulinum neurotoxin C1 cleaves both syntaxin and SNAP-25 in intact and permeabilized chromaffin cells: Correlation with its blockade of catecholamine release. *Biochemistry* 35: 2630–2636

175 Schiavo G, Shone CC, Bennett MK, Scheller RH, Montecucco C (1995) Botulinum neurotoxin type C cleaves a single Lys-Ala bond within the carboxyl-terminal region of syntaxins. *J Biol Chem* 270: 10566–10570

176 Arndt JW, Yu W, Bi F, Stevens RC (2005) Crystal structure of botulinum neurotoxin type G light chain: Serotype divergence in substrate recognition. *Biochemistry* 44: 9574–9580

177 Chen S, Hall C, Barbieri JT (2008) Substrate recognition of VAMP-2 by botulinum neurotoxin B and tetanus neurotoxin. *J Biol Chem* 283: 21153–21159

178 Ahmed SA OM, Ludivico ML, Gilsdorf J, Smith LA (2008) Identification of residues surrounding the active site of type A botulinum neurotoxin important for substrate recognition and catalytic activity. *Protein J* 27: 151–162

179 Chen S, Barbieri JT (2006) Unique substrate recognition by botulinum neurotoxins serotypes A and E. *J Biol Chem* 281: 10906–10911

180 Chen S, Kim JP, Barbieri JT (2007) Mechanism of substrate recognition by botulinum neurotoxin serotype A. *J Biol Chem* 282: 9621–9627

181 Rigoni M, Caccin P, Johnson EA, Montecucco C, Rossetto O (2001) Site-directed mutagenesis identifies active-site residues of the light chain of botulinum neurotoxin type A. *Biochem Biophys Res Commun* 288: 1231–1237

182 Schmidt JJ, Stafford RG (2005) Botulinum neurotoxin serotype F: Identification of substrate recognition requirements and development of inhibitors with low nanomolar affinity. *Biochemistry* 44: 4067–4073

183 Sikorra S, Henke T, Swaminathan S, Galli T, Binz T (2006) Identification of the amino acid residues rendering TI-VAMP insensitive toward botulinum neurotoxin B. *J Mol Biol* 357: 574–582

184 Arndt JW, Chai Q, Christian T, Stevens R (2006) Structure of botulinum neurotoxin type D light chain at 1.65 A resolution: Repercussions for VAMP-2 substrate specificity. *Biochemistry* 45: 3255–3262

185 Breidenbach MA, Brunger AT (2004) Substrate recognition strategy for botulinum neurotoxin serotype A. *Nature* 432: 925–929

186 Chen S, Kim JJ, Barbieri JT (2007) Mechanism of substrate recognition by botulinum neurotoxin serotype A. *J Biol Chem* 282: 9621–9627

187 Smith TJ, Lou J, Geren IN, Forsyth CM, Tsai R, LaPorte SL, Tepp WH, Bradshaw M, Johnson EA, Smith LA, Marks JD (2005) Sequence variation within botulinum neurotoxin serotypes impacts antibody binding and neutralization. *Infect Immun* 73: 5450–5457

188 Arndt JW, Jacobson MJ, Abola EE, Forsyth CM, Tepp WH, Marks JD, Johnson EA, Stevens RC (2006) A structural perspective of the sequence variability within botulinum neurotoxin subtypes A1–A4. *J Mol Biol* 362: 733–742

189 Hill KK, Smith TJ, Helma CH, Ticknor LO, Foley BT, Svensson RT, Brown JL, Johnson EA, Smith LA, Okinaka RT, Jackson PJ, Marks JD (2007) Genetic diversity among botulinum neurotoxin-producing clostridial strains. *J Bacteriol* 189: 818–832

190 Edmond BJ, Guerra FA, Blake J, Hempler S (1977) Case of infant botulism in Texas. *Tex Med* 73: 85–88

191 Leighton GR (1923) Report to the Scottish Board of Health. H.M. Stationery Office, London

192 Henkel JS, Jacobson M, Tepp W, Pier C, Johnson EA, Barbieri JT (2009) Catalytic properties of botulinum neurotoxin subtypes A3 and A4 (dagger). *Biochemistry* 48: 2522–2528

193 Baldwin MR, Tepp WH, Przedpelski A, Pier CL, Bradshaw M, Johnson EA, Barbieri JT (2008) Subunit vaccine against the seven serotypes of botulism. *Infect Immun* 76: 1314–1318

194 Schiavo G, Benfenati F, Poulain B, Rossetto O, Polverino de Laureto P, DasGupta BR, Montecucco C (1992) Tetanus and botulinum-B neurotoxins block neurotransmitter release by proteolytic cleavage of synaptobrevin. *Nature* 359: 832–835

195 Schiavo G, Shone CC, Bennett MK, Scheller RH, Montecucco C (1995) Botulinum neurotoxin type C cleaves a single Lys-Ala bond within the carboxyl-terminal region of syntaxins. *J Biol Chem* 270: 10566–10570

196 Williamson LC, Halpern JL, Montecucco C, Brown JE, Neale EA (1996) Clostridial neurotoxins and substrate proteolysis in intact neurons: Botulinum neurotoxin C acts on synaptosomal-asso-

ciated protein of 25 kDa. *J Biol Chem* 271: 7694–7699

197 Schiavo G, Rossetto O, Catsicas S, Polverino de Laureto P, DasGupta BR, Benfenati F, Montecucco C (1993) Identification of the nerve terminal targets of botulinum neurotoxin serotypes A, D, and E. *J Biol Chem* 268: 23784–23787

198 Schiavo G, Shone CC, Rossetto O, Alexander FC, Montecucco C (1993) Botulinum neurotoxin serotype F is a zinc endopeptidase specific for VAMP/synaptobrevin. *J Biol Chem* 268: 11516–11519

199 Schiavo G, Malizio C, Trimble WS, Polverino de Laureto P, Milan G, Sugiyama H, Johnson EA, Montecucco C (1994) Botulinum G neurotoxin cleaves VAMP/synaptobrevin at a single Ala-Ala peptide bond. *J Biol Chem* 269: 20213–20216.

Molecular, Clinical and Environmental Toxicology. Volume 2: Clinical Toxicology
Edited by A. Luch
© 2010 Birkhäuser Verlag/Switzerland

Toxicology of mycotoxins

Robert R. M. Paterson and Nelson Lima

IBB-Institute for Biotechnology and Bioengineering, Universidade do Minho, Portugal

Abstract. Humans are exposed to mycotoxins *via* ingestion, contact and inhalation. This must have occurred throughout human history and led to severe outbreaks. Potential diseases range from akakabio-byo to stachybotryotoxicosis and cancer. The known molecular bases of toxicology run the gamut of 23 compounds, from aflatoxins (AFs) to zearalenone, ochratoxin A and deoxynivalenol. Ergotism is one of the oldest recognized mycotoxicosis, although mycotoxin science only commenced in the 1960s with the discovery of AFs in turkey feed. AFs are carcinogenic. Some others are suspected carcinogens. The effects of mycotoxins are acute or chronic in nature. Mycotoxins are well known in the scientific community, although they have a low profile in the general population. An incongruous situation occurs in United States where mycotoxins from "moldy homes" are considered to be a significant problem, although there is a general debate about seriousness. This contrasts with the thousands of deaths from mycotoxins that occur, even now, in the technologically less developed countries (e.g., Indonesia, China, and Africa). Mycotoxins are more toxic than pesticides. Studies are moving from whole animal work to investigating the biochemical mechanisms in isolated cells, and the mechanisms of toxicity at the molecular level are being elucidated. The stereochemical nature of AFs has been shown to be important. In addition, the effect of multiple mycotoxins is being increasingly investigated, which will more accurately represent the situation in nature. It is anticipated that more fungal metabolites will be recognized as dangerous toxins and permitted statutory levels will decrease in the future.

Introduction

Mycotoxins are fungal metabolites that cause sickness or death in people and other animals when ingested, inhaled and/or absorbed. A crucial point is that they are active at low concentrations, which is of course "all" in toxicology. They occur naturally and are the most prevalent source of food-related health risk in field crops. Consumption of high levels can be fatal: Long-term exposure can, among other things, increase cancer risk and suppress the immune system.

Filamentous fungi are ubiquitous in nature and unavoidable, although they can be controlled: Those that produce mycotoxins are common. A recurring theme of many studies on fungal metabolites is the immature state of the systematics of fungi. It is worth recalling that Hawksworth's figure of 1.5 million fungal species of which only a small number (ca. 5%) have been identified [1], can be multiplied by "various whole numbers" to indicate the number of fungal natural products remaining to be discovered. However, it is difficult to obtain definitive information as to which fungi produce which metabolites.

The most convincing evidence of historical reports of mycotoxicosis is a
disease that affected many parts of Europe in the tenth century referred to as
St Anthony's or Holy fire, and is considered to have been caused by the consumption of rye contaminated with ergot alkaloids from *Claviceps purpurea*
[2]. Further accounts suggest that other contaminated grains have been responsible for major outbreaks of disease (e.g., the *Ten Plagues of Egypt* [3]).
Mycotoxins attract worldwide scientific, political and economic attention
because of the significant economic losses associated with negative impacts on
human health, animal productivity and international trade. They are also considered as weapons because of the ease of production of the toxic compounds
that could enter the food chain by this route [4].

A scientific approach to food contamination with mycotoxins has only been
undertaken since the 1960s, when aflatoxins (AFs) caused diseases of animals
in England. The toxic compound from *Aspergillus flavus* was discovered in the
feeds and many diseases are now considered to be caused by this and other
mycotoxins (Tab. 1). Mycotoxins can cause vomiting, abdominal pains, pul-

Table 1. Some human diseases in which analytic and/or epidemiologic data suggest or implicate
mycotoxin involvement

Disease	Species	Substrate	Etiologic agent
Akakabio-byo	Human	Wheat, barley, oats, rice	*Fusarium* spp.
Alimentary toxic aleukia (ATA or septic angina)	Human	Cereal grains (toxic bread)	*Fusarium* spp.
Balkan nephropathy	Human	Cereal grains	*Penicillium*
Cardiac beriberi	Human	Rice	*Aspergillus* spp., *Penicillium* spp.
Celery harvester's disease	Human	Celery (Pink rot)	*Sclerotinia*
Dendrodochiotoxicosis	Horse, human	Fodder (skin contact, inhaled fodder particles)	*Dendrodochium toxicum*
Ergotism	Human	Rye, cereal grains	*Claviceps purpurea*
Esophageal tumors	Human	Corn	*Fusarium moniliforme*
Hepatocarcinoma (acute aflatoxicosis)	Human	Cereal grains, peanuts	*Aspergillus flavus, A. parasiticus*
Kashin Beck disease, "Urov disease"	Human	Cereal grains	*Fusarium*
Kwashiorkor	Human	Cereal grains	*Aspergillus flavus, A. parasiticus*
Onyalai	Human	Millet	*Phoma sorghina*
Reye's syndrome	Human	Cereal grains	*Aspergillus*
Stachybotryotoxicosis	Human, horse, other livestock	Hay, cereal grains, fodder (skin contact, inhaled haydust)	*Stachybotrys atra*

monary edema, convulsions, coma, and death. Notable outbreaks were the death of 3 people in Taiwan in 1967 and 100 people in India in 1974 from AFs in rice and corn, respectively. Deaths were recorded in Kenya in a surprising contemporary outbreak [5] given the accumulated knowledge that we now have. Also, long-term effects are extremely important (*e.g.*, cancer and immune deficiency). Finally, mycotoxins cause high economic losses ($1.4 billion per annum in the USA [2]).

Filamentous fungi produce thousands of toxic compounds (see [6] for some), although only perhaps hundreds could conceivably be found in diets. Of these, a small number are taken seriously as mycotoxins and an estimate of ten would be reasonable. The more important mycotoxins belong to species of *Aspergillus*, *Fusarium*, *Penicillium* and *Claviceps*. The mycotoxins of prime importance are AFs, ochratoxin A (OTA), deoxynivalenol (DON), fumonisin (FUM), nivalenol (NIV), ergot alkaloids, T-2 toxin, patulin and zearalenone [2], approximately in that order of seriousness. The chemical structures of selected compounds are demonstrated in Figure 1, and Table 2 indicates which fungi produce the important mycotoxins.

There are limitations to the original "systems" approach for classification of mycotoxins. Research has advanced from large-dose, complete-animal, to small-dose, subcellular/molecular responses. This makes the systems approach for mycotoxin classification increasingly difficult as the variation or multiplicity in systems affected has become evident. For example, trichothecenes (e.g., DON, NIV, T-2 toxin) affect productivity, liver, kidney, hematopoietic system, CNS, and the immune system. FUMs "impact" brain, kidney, liver, and lung. The study of animal mycotoxicoses has become complex because of the interaction of the systems affected, the basic metabolic pathways affected,

Table 2. Some mycotoxins most commonly associated with particular fungi

Fungus	Mycotoxin
Aspergillus carbonarius, A. ochraceus	Ochratoxin A (OTA)
A. flavus	Aflatoxin B_1 (AFB$_1$), AFB$_2$
A. parasiticus	AFB$_1$, AFB$_2$, AFG$_1$, AFG$_2$
A. niger	OTA, fumonisins (FUMs)
A. terreus, A. clavatus	Patulin
Byssochlamys fulva, B. nivea	Patulin
Fusarium cerealis, F. poae	Nivalenol (NIV)
F. culmorum, F. graminearum	NIV, deoxynivalenol (DON)
F. equiseti	Zearalenone
F. sporotrichioides	T-2 toxin
F. verticillioides (= F. moniliforme)	Fumonisin B_1 (FUMB$_1$)
Penicillium expansum, P. roqueforti	Patulin
P. verrucosum	OTA

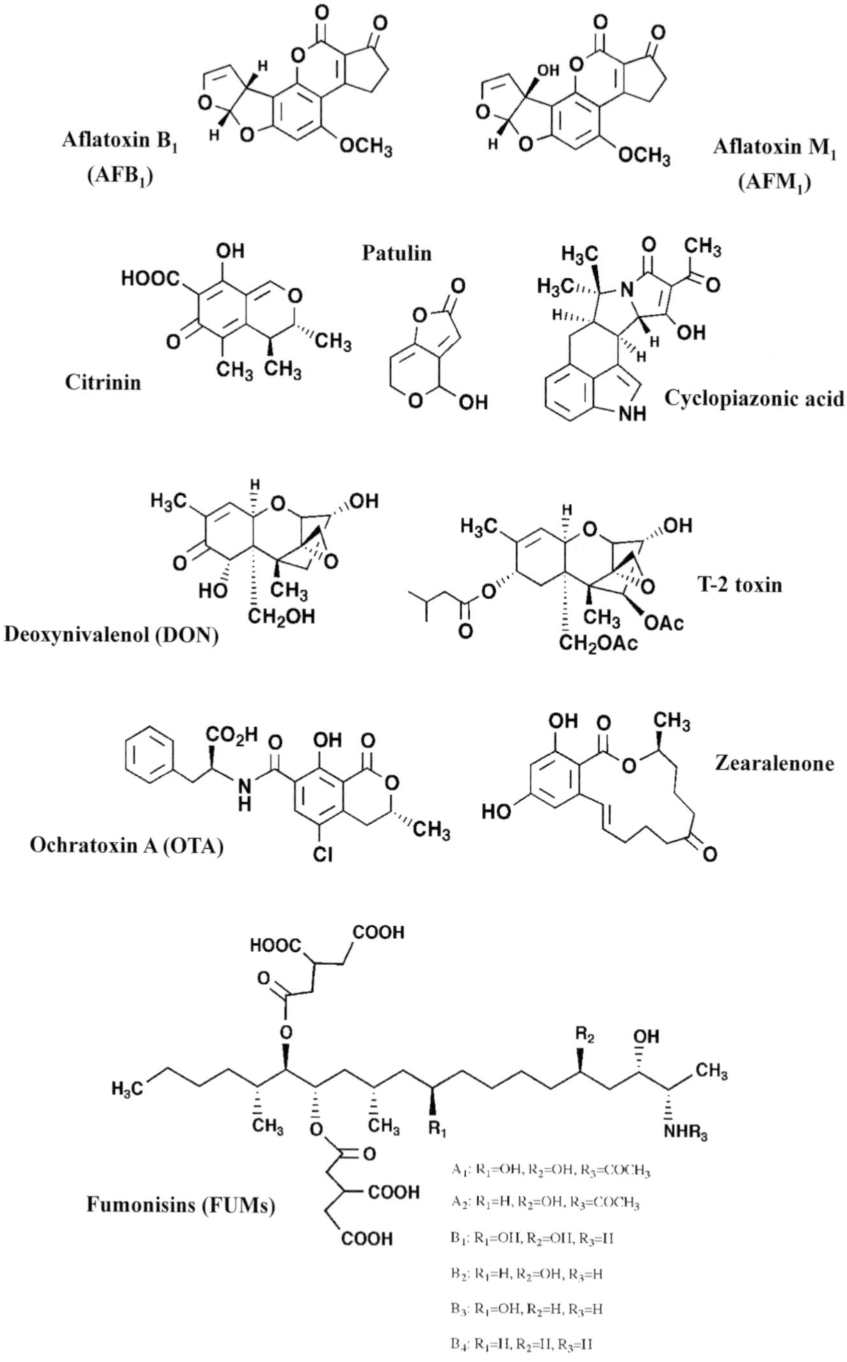

Figure 1. Chemical structures of selected mycotoxins.

and the physiopathological nature of intoxications. Furthermore, it is essential that the synergistic effects of mycotoxins are appreciated. Combinations of AFs and FUMB$_1$, and vomitoxin and zearalenone commonly occur together in the same grain. When mycotoxins are fed in combination, interactive effects can be classified as additive, less than additive, synergistic, potentiative, or even antagonistic [7]. Hence, in effect, many of the studies described below provide only a partial view.

Effect on humans

Mycotoxins are classified by the International Agency for Research on Cancer (IARC) according to their toxicity, with AFs being the only ones proven to be carcinogenic to humans [8]. Accumulated evidence for the others enables their classification in various lesser categories (Tabs 1–3). There is growing concern within medicine about mycotoxin involvement in human diseases. The diseases may be manifested as acute to chronic, and range from rapid death to tumor formation. More occult disease may occur when the mycotoxin interferes with immune processes, rendering the patient more susceptible to infectious diseases. This may explain why few data are available on mycotoxins being implicated in immunosuppressive illnesses. The following section discusses mycotoxicoses for which there is considerable evidence for involvement of a specific mycotoxin(s) (Tab. 3).

Aflatoxicosis

Acute aflatoxicosis
AF ingestion has been manifested in humans as acute hepatitis [9] associated with highly contaminated foodstuffs (*e.g.*, corn). Furthermore, the compounds have been detected in tissues. Histopathological evidence is adequate for diagnosing aflatoxicosis, and includes jaundice, low-grade fever, depression, anorexia, diarrhea and fatty degenerative changes in the liver. In outbreaks in India, mortality reached 25% and livers were shown to contain AFB$_1$. Furthermore, in Kenya, acute AF-caused hepatitis was observed, in which ascites (peritoneal fluid excess) sometimes developed [10]. Surprisingly, fatal outbreaks have also occurred recently in Kenya [5].

A disease known as kwashiorkor has been linked to consumption of AF-contaminated foods. Animals fed AFs possessed fatty liver, hypoalbuminemia, and immunosuppression similar to symptoms seen in kwashiorkor. Also, AFs were detected in liver specimens taken at autopsy from 36 children with kwashiorkor [11], adding additional weight to the hypothesis. The involvement of AFs in Reye's syndrome had not been proven, although AFB$_1$ produced a similar disease in monkeys.

Table 3. Probable primary biochemical lesions and the early cellular events in the flow of cellular events leading to toxic cell injury or cellular deregulation in mycotoxicosis [2]

Mycotoxin	Initial lesion–event cascade
Aflatoxins	Metabolic activation $\rightarrow$ DNA modification $\rightarrow$ cell deregulation $\rightarrow$ cell death transformation (metabolic activation $\rightarrow$ disruption of macromolecular synthesis $\rightarrow$ cell deregulation $\rightarrow$ apoptotic cell death)
Adenophostins	ER IP$_3$ receptor $\rightarrow$ Ca^{2+} release $\rightarrow$ cell deregulation $\rightarrow$ unknown consequences
Anthraquinones	Mitochondrial uncoupler $\rightarrow$ loss of respiratory control $\rightarrow$ cell death (possibly apoptotic)
Beauvericin	K$^+$ ionophore $\rightarrow$ K$^+$ loss $\rightarrow$ cell deregulation $\rightarrow$ cell death/apoptosis (inhibition of cholesterol acyltransferase $\rightarrow$ disruption of cholesterol metabolism $\rightarrow$ unknown consequences)
Citrinin	Loss of selective membrane permeability $\rightarrow$ cell deregulation $\rightarrow$ cell death (possibly apoptotic) (disruption of macromolecular synthesis $\rightarrow$ unknown consequences)
Cyclopiazonic acid	ER and SR Ca^{2+}-ATPase $\rightarrow$ disruption of Ca^{2+} homeostasis $\rightarrow$ cell deregulation $\rightarrow$ cell death
Cytochalasins	Cytoskeleton $\rightarrow$ disruption of endocytosis $\rightarrow$ cell deregulation $\rightarrow$ cell death
Deoxynivalenol	Inhibition of protein synthesis $\rightarrow$ disruption of cytokine regulation $\rightarrow$ altered cell proliferation $\rightarrow$ cell death (possibly apoptotic)
Fumonisins	Sphinganine N-acyltransferase $\rightarrow$ disrupted lipid metabolism $\rightarrow$ cell deregulation $\rightarrow$ cell death/apoptosis (disrupted delta-6-desaturase activity $\rightarrow$ disrupted fatty acid and arachidonic acid metabolism $\rightarrow$ cell death)
Gliotoxin	Calcium homeostasis $\rightarrow$ zinc homeostasis $\rightarrow$ endonuclease activation $\rightarrow$ apoptosis (radical mediated damage $\rightarrow$ oxidative stress $\rightarrow$ cell death) (inhibition of protein synthesis $\rightarrow$ possibly apoptotic)
Griseofulvin	Cytoskeleton $\rightarrow$ deregulation of cytoskeletal control $\rightarrow$ cell death
Luteoskyrin	Radical mediated damage $\rightarrow$ oxidative stress $\rightarrow$ lipid peroxidation $\rightarrow$ cell death (possibly apoptotic)
Moniliformin	Pyruvate and α-ketoglutarate decarboxylation $\rightarrow$ loss of respiratory control $\rightarrow$ cell death
Ochratoxin	Disruption of phenylalanine metabolism $\rightarrow$ reduced PEPCK $\rightarrow$ reduced gluconeogenesis $\rightarrow$ cell death (metabolic activation $\rightarrow$ inhibition of protein/DNA synthesis $\rightarrow$ apoptosis?) (altered membrane permeability $\rightarrow$ disrupt calcium homeostasis $\rightarrow$ cell deregulation $\rightarrow$ cell death)
Patulin	Nonprotein sulfhydryl depletion $\rightarrow$ altered ion permeability and/or altered intercellular communication $\rightarrow$ oxidative stress $\rightarrow$ cell death (inhibition of macromolecular biosynthesis $\rightarrow$ cell death)
Sphingofungin and ISP1	Serine palmitoyltransferase $\rightarrow$ decrease sphingolipids $\rightarrow$ cell deregulation $\rightarrow$ cell death/apoptosis
Sporidesmin	Radical mediated damage $\rightarrow$ oxidative stress $\rightarrow$ thiol depletion $\rightarrow$ cell death (disrupt calcium homeostasis $\rightarrow$ zinc homeostasis $\rightarrow$ endonuclease activation $\rightarrow$ apoptosis)
Swainsonine	Mannosidase II $\rightarrow$ disrupted glycoprotein processing $\rightarrow$ cell deregulation $\rightarrow$ cell death

(continued on next page)

Table 3. (continued)

Mycotoxin	Initial lesion–event cascade
Tremorgens (indole alkaloids)	GABA receptors → altered Cl⁻ permeability → disrupted neuromuscular control → ?
T-2 toxin	Inhibition of protein synthesis → ? → cell death (apoptotic?); transient Ca^{2+} elevation → endonuclease activation → apoptosis (altered membrane); structure → disruption of membrane function → cell deregulation → cell death
Wortmannin	Inhibition of phosphatidylinositol 3-kinase → responsiveness to insulin/growth factors/and apoptosis (inhibition of myosin light chain kinase → inhibition of IP_3 signaling pathway → ?) (Inhibition of phospholipase A_2 → ?)
Zearalenone	Cytosolic estrogen receptor → estrogenic response → disruption of hormonal control → ?

? = some uncertainty; ER, endoplasmic reticulum; SR, sarcoplasmic reticulum; PEPCK, phosphoenolpyruvate carboxy kinase.

Chronic aflatoxicosis

AFs were initially suspected of contributing to human hepatocellular carcinoma (HCC) (see Fig. 2 for actual involvement). However, the studies could not account for additional factors such as hepatitis B virus (HBV). Epidemiological studies in localities with high incidence of liver cancer compared the relevance of dietary AF [12]. Autrup et al. [13] found AFB_1-guanine in urine from individuals from high liver cancer risk areas who were presumably exposed to AFs. Some studies were criticized for not considering exposure of the populations to HBV: most found an AF effect independently of the prevalence of HBV surface antigen [14]. Campbell et al. [15] did not correlate AF exposure to liver cancer in China.

The development of AF detection has been crucial in determining the involvement of AFs in disease. There was a significant increase in detectable AF-albumin adducts and high levels of AF metabolites in urine in HBV-

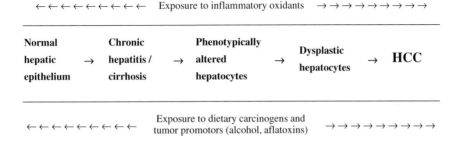

Figure 2. Human hepatocellular carcinoma (HCC). From healthy to HCC over a 5–30-year period.

infected males in Taiwan. A second study observed a dose-response relationship between urinary AFM_1 levels and HCC in chronic HBV carriers. The HCC risk associated with AFB_1 exposure was more striking among the HBV carriers with detectable AFB-N7-guanine adducts in urine. Studies of the prevalence of codon 249 mutations in HCC cases from patients in areas of high or low exposure to AFs suggested that a $G{\rightarrow}T$ transition at the third base is associated with AF exposure. The majority of codon 249 mutations are found in patients with an HBV infection, implicating an association. The mutation only occurred in areas of high AFB_1 exposure in comparison to codon 249 mutations in regions of high HBV infection but varying levels of AFB_1 exposure.

Reproductive effects of aflatoxins
AFs are implicated in affecting human males with (a) delayed testicular development, (b) testicular degeneration, (c) decreased reproductive potential, (d) morphological regressive changes in the testis, (e) reduction in size and weight of testis with mild testicular degeneration to complete disappearance of cellular components, (f) decrease in meiotic index, (g) marked decrease in the percentage of live sperm and greater sperm abnormalities, (h) degeneration and desquamation of seminiferous epithelium and decrease in its thickness, (i) decrease in plasma testosterone concentration, and (j) impairment of Leydig cell function [2] – so rather widespread.

Ochratoxicosis

A study compared the morphological effects of OTA on lymphocytes and neutrophils from the circulation of healthy subjects and patients with esophageal and breast carcinomas [16]. Leukocyte death was evident in the decrease in cell survival when exposed. In general, mycotoxins (a) impair immune functions of immunocytes (leukocytes) and the immune messengers (cytokines), and (b) increase susceptibility to chronic disease and carcinogenesis. The study supports the theory that homeostasis of the immune system is compromised in cancer patients exposed to fungal toxins, including those with breast cancer [16].

Fusarium toxins

In general, DON can disrupt cell signaling, differentiation, macromolecular synthesis and growth. This contributes to its impact on gastrointestinal homeostasis, neuroendocrine function, and immunity. There are marked species differences that relate to differences in metabolism, toxicokinetics, and feeding habits. The metabolite does not accumulate in tissues or appear at high con-

centrations as residues in animal foods. The emetic response is most sensitive
to low levels and swine are susceptible to extremely low doses of DON. It is
reasonable to speculate that humans are as sensitive to DON as pigs.

The sesquiterpenoid trichothecenes are the largest family of mycotoxins
and are associated with alimentary toxic aleukia (ATA). *Fusarium* is associated most with trichothecenes, although other genera are important producers,
e.g., *Trichothecium, Trichoderma, Myrothecium,* and *Stachybotrys*. ATA was
reported in Siberia in 1913 and subsequent outbreaks have occurred elsewhere. DON was detected abundantly and frequently in wheat samples from
China following a human red mold intoxication episode in studies related to
gastroenteritis. NIV and 15-acetyl-DON were also found in 20 samples.
Zearalenone co-occurred in a similar number (see below). ATA occurred in
Russia during the first half of the 20th century. Patients experienced abdominal pain, vomiting, diarrhea, and burning in the gastrointestinal tract soon after
consuming food contaminated with *Fusarium*. Most signs of ATA have been
documented in animals given T-2 toxin, the major toxic component of two
fungi isolated from the overwintered grain [17]. Furthermore, *Stachybotrys* is
associated with indoor health problems particularly in the United States.
Trichothecenes from cereal grains with red mold disease (akakabi-byo) and
black-spot disease (kokuten-byo) gave rise to headache, vomiting, and diarrhea symptoms [18, 19].

Zearalenone
Little conclusive information is available regarding the effects of zearalenone
on humans. However, despite this, there is currently considerable concern
about estrogenic effects in water systems [20]. Premature puberty may have
occurred in 7- and 8-year old children from consumption [21]. Hsieh [22] suggested that zearalenone was involved in human cervical cancer and premature
thelarche. Zearalenone mimics the effects of estrogen and induces feminiza-
tion at dietary concentrations of less than 1 mg/kg, while higher concentrations
interfere with conception, ovulation, implantation, fetal development, and the
viability of newborn animals. Szuets et al. [23] measured zearalenone in 5 of
36 children exhibiting early thelarche and found high concentrations of zearalenol in the cereal foods of the patients. They discovered that zearalenone and
zearalenol bind to estrogen receptors of human myometrial tissue.

Fusarin C
An association between consumption of moldy corn and the high human
esophageal cancer rates found in southern Africa and China has been known
for some time and is associated with FUMs (see below). *Fusarium* produces a
number of mycotoxins including the highly mutagenic compound fusarin C
[24], which has received attention as a possible carcinogen and may in fact be
a contributing factor [25].

Fumonisins

High human esophageal cancer rates associated with FUMs have been found
in China [26], Southern Africa [27], and Italy [28] especially after consumption of home-grown contaminated corn. These mycotoxins were discovered by
Gelderblom et al. [29] from fusaria. The occurrence of $FUMB_2$ from *Aspergillus niger* [30] is of considerable concern. $FUMB_1$ has been studied thoroughly as the most common homologue of those from *Fusarium*.

$FUMB_1$ inhibited growth and induced morphological features consistent
with apoptosis of human cells *in vitro* [31]; hence, FUMs may cause esophageal epithelial apoptosis. FUMs are involved in human diseases other than
esophageal cancer, but its role is not yet resolved. FUM derivatives may also
be toxic and exert effects by indirect mechanisms. The IARC concluded that
there is "inadequate evidence" for carcinogenicity in humans from oral exposure to $FUMB_1$ [8] and a role for FUMs in other human disease is unproven.

As mentioned above for OTA, a study was designed to determine and compare the morphological effects of $FUMB_1$ on lymphocytes and neutrophils
from patients with esophageal and breast carcinomas [16].

Stachybotryotoxicosis

Stachybotryotoxicosis occurs in humans and other animals and is caused by
toxins of *Stachybotrys chartarum*. For example, the disease occurred in horses and cattle that consumed *Stachybotrys*-contaminated hay [32]. The horse
(and cattle) disease is neurological in character with tremors, "incoordination",
impairment or loss of vision, dermonecrosis, leukopenia, and gastrointestinal
ulceration and hemorrhage. Somewhat tenuously, extrapolation has implicated
the macrocyclic trichothecenes from this genus in illnesses of humans in contaminated buildings [33].

Citreoviridin toxicosis

Acute cardiac beriberi or "shoshin kakke", a disease that occurred for centuries
in Japan and other Asian countries, was characterized by palpitations, nausea,
vomiting, rapid and difficult breathing, rapid pulse, abnormal heart sounds,
low blood pressure, restlessness, and violent mania leading to respiratory failure and death [34]. Citreoviridin was implicated, and has been detected from
various aspergilli and penicillia.

Ergotism

Convulsive and gangrenous ergotisms are separate symptoms from ingestion
of ergots [35]. The gangrenous form may result from the vasoconstrictive

action of certain alkaloids from *Claviceps* belonging primarily to the ergota-mine group and is associated with wheat and rye. The ergot of pearl millet involved in an outbreak of the convulsive form in India in 1975 contained alka-loids of the clavinet group. In Africa, 93 cases of gangrenous ergotism were reported involving grain infected with *C. purpurea* [36], and 78 cases of gas-trointestinal ergotism involving millet infected with *C. fusiformis* occurred in India [37].

Gliotoxin toxicosis

Gliotoxin may be involved in the mycosis referred to as aspergillosis. Gliotoxin is produced in (a) mice experimentally infected with *A. fumigatus*, (b) natural bovine udder infection, and (c) experimentally and naturally infect-ed turkeys. The compound was found in vaginal secretions of women with *Candida vaginitis*. Gliotoxin could be an important factor because of its immunosuppressive nature, which may exacerbate infection and be a virulence factor [38].

Effect on animals

The effects of mycotoxins are usually more obvious in domesticated animals and extrapolations to humans are often based on these observations. They are supported by laboratory-based animal studies. Chronic effects such as (a) decreased productivity, (b) subtle but chronic damage to vital organs and tis-sues, (c) increased disease incidence because of immune suppression, and (d) interference with reproductive capacity are much more prevalent than acute livestock death. At least one mycotoxin affects each system in the animal body *via* direct or indirect mechanisms of toxicity. Several important mycotoxins can affect the same system, e.g., the immune system, and a given mycotoxin may affect several systems. The true nature of such intoxications requires a more holistic comprehension of the complexities of the chemical, biochemi-cal, metabolic, molecular and environmental bases for mycotoxicoses. Finally, nursing animals may be affected by exposure to AF metabolites secreted in the milk.

Ochratoxicosis

In animals, OTA (a) damages kidneys, (b) causes intestinal necrosis and hemo-rrhage, (c) suppresses immunity, and (d) is carcinogenic. Changes in the renal function of pigs exposed to OTA include impairment of proximal tubular func-tion, altered urine excretion, and increased excretion of urine glucose [39]. Carcinogenicity was evident in rats/mice.

Fusarium toxins

The trichothecene mycotoxins (a) cause necrosis and hemorrhage throughout the digestive tract, (b) depress blood regenerative processes in the bone marrow and spleen, and (c) cause changes in reproductive organs. Affected animals show signs of anorexia, weight loss, poor feed utilization, vomiting, bloody diarrhea, and abortion; some die. Significant features of trichothecene intoxications include dysregulated immune and neuroendocrine function. Histological lesions consist of hemorrhage and necrosis in proliferating tissues of the intestinal mucosa, bone marrow, spleen, testis, and ovary.

All animal species tested were susceptible to DON [40]. However, only acute exposure to extremely high DON concentrations produced marked tissue injury or mortality. Acute exposure to low doses can induce emesis in swine, the most sensitive species. Monogastric animals are extremely sensitive to growth and weight-gain suppression due to subchronic/chronic toxicity (cf. below). DON is capable of inducing reproductive/teratogenic effects in mice and rabbits. Similar doses to those that produced adverse reproductive effects produced maternal toxicity (feed refusal or reduced weight gain).

Fumonisins

FUMs affect sphingolipid metabolism and cause diseases in a species-specific fashion. Ingestion of FUM-contaminated feed causes (a) neurotoxic effects in horses, (b) pulmonary edema in swine, and (c) liver and kidney damage including tumors and cancer in some species. $FUMB_1$ attributed to *F. verticillioides* causes diseases including leukoencephalomalacia in horses (cf. below). $FUMB_1$ and other FUMs with a primary amino group are liver cancer promoters in rats. $FUMB_1$ was a kidney carcinogen when fed to Fischer 344/N/Netr rats, causing renal tubule adenomas and carcinomas in males. Only at higher doses, or after longer exposures also other features of FUM toxicity become evident, e.g., overt necrosis, mitogenesis and regeneration, fibrosis.

Cyclopiazonic acid

Clinical signs of intoxication include weight loss, anorexia, diarrhea, dehydration, pyrexia, ataxia, immobility, and extensor spasm at death in dogs, rats, pigs, laying hens, sheep and chickens [41]. The possible role of cyclopiazonic acid in diagnosed aflatoxicoses should be explored due to co-occurrence in feed.

Immunology

AFs in the low ppm range are immunomodulatory. They are capable of lowering the resistance of animal species to fungal, bacterial, and parasitic infections [42]. Cell-mediated responses are particularly sensitive, as reflected by decreased thymus weight and lower peripheral T lymphocyte numbers in chickens fed AFB_1. AFB_1 depressed macrophage function in chicks, and oral administration in rats depressed macrophage number and function. Indications were that AFB_1 decreased phagocytic activity of the reticuloendothelial system in chicks [43]. The data also indicated suppression of phagocytic activity in chickens and rats.

Trichothecenes approximate AFs in the extent of causing immunosuppression, apparently by protein synthesis inhibition. Depression of host resistance by trichothecenes may involve suppression of several cellular functions and they can suppress or stimulate immunoglobulin production. Exposure to trichothecenes impairs murine antibody responses to challenge with sheep red blood cells [44]. Immunostimulatory effects at low doses are problematic, but may conceivably be a hormesis effect.

OTA may have an effect on immunoglobulins and phagocytic cells [45]. $FUMB_1$-treated chicken peritoneal macrophages show morphological alterations, and decreases in cell viability and phagocytic potential. Zearalenone can inhibit mitogen-stimulated lymphocyte proliferation and induce thymic atrophy and macrophage activation. Patulin inhibits multiple aspects of macrophage function *in vitro*. Interestingly, oral administration of patulin decreased the mortality of mice experimentally infected with *Candida albicans* [46]. The mycotoxin increased circulating neutrophils, which could have contributed to increased resistance. Neutrophilia in rats administered patulin orally was attributed to gastrointestinal inflammation by McKinley et al. [47]. Gliotoxin has both antimicrobial and immunosuppressive capabilities. The compound is produced in infected animal tissue strengthening its actual involvement in pathogenesis. Fescue and ergot alkaloids affected cattle grazing in tall fescue pastures infected with the endophyte and had a suppressed antibody response when immunized with tetanus toxoid [48].

Hematopoietic effects

Hemorrhagic anemia syndrome in poultry was linked to the presence of AFs in feed; this may also affect hemostasis in embryos. Chicks had significantly decreased cell counts, hematocrits, and hemoglobin concentrations [49]. Macrophages, lymphocytes, and erythrocytes may be decreased with prolonged exposure to trichothecenes. Erythrocyte numbers also can be decreased by trichothecene-induced hemolysis [50]. T-2 toxin caused a complete hemolysis of rat erythrocytes following a lag period dependent on the concentration of T-2 toxin.

Hepatotoxicity

AFs cause hemorrhage, jaundice, and diarrhea, along with decreased performance, which may be evident in affected animals with acute disease. OTA can cause liver damage particularly at higher doses. FUMs are hepatotoxic [29]. Sporidesmin is a hepatotoxic mycotoxin produced by *Pithomyces chartarum* on certain grasses. This can cause a photosensitization disease, facial eczema [51], which results from destruction of bile duct epithelial cells, with blocking of the bile ducts causing phylloerythin to accumulate in the circulating blood. Rubratoxin has been suspected as the cause of hepatotoxic, hemorrhagic disease of cattle and pigs. Phomopsins cause a lupinosis, which is a hepatotoxic condition characterized by severe liver damage and icterus [52].

Nephrotoxicity

OTA can cause kidney damage in dogs, rats, and swine. The impaired renal function results in glucosuria and proteinuria, with casts evident in the urine. Absorption of this mycotoxin occurs in the proximal and distal tubules of the kidney. DON and NIV are associated indirectly with a nephropathy in mice. Animals fed $FUMB_1$ exhibit altered renal histopathology, kidney weight, urine volume, proteinuria, enzymuria, and ion transport [53] *via* altered sphingolipid biosynthesis.

Reproductive effects

AFs are implicated in effects on animal males similar to those assumed in humans (see above 'Effects on humans'). The major effects of zearalenone are estrogenic and primarily involve the urogenital system [54]. Abortion may occur with ergot ingestion and ergot also inhibits prolactin secretion in pregnant swine. Other mycotoxins also have reproductive effects, e.g., T-2 toxin and diacetoxyscirpenol. OTA, rubratoxin B, secalonic acid D, and sterigmatocystin are all reported to affect embryonic survival.

Teratogenic effects

AFB_1, OTA, rubratoxin B, T-2 toxin, sterigmatocystin, and zearalenone are teratogenic in experiments with at least one mammalian species.

Vomiting and neurotoxicity

Gastric relaxation and/or delayed gastric emptying are important components of both emesis and food intake [55]. At lower doses DON induces feed refusal, and at high acute doses vomiting. It has anorexic and emetic potencies. However, T-2 toxin is at least ten times more lethal. Equine leukoencephalomalacia was shown to be caused by FUMs [56]. The mechanisms may be related to their ability to inhibit sphingolipid synthesis.

Tremorgens

Many fungal secondary metabolites (e.g., indole alkaloids) elicit a tremorgenic response in animals [51] and penitrem A (tremortin) is a well-known example. Convulsions may also occur from ergot ingestion [57].

Carcinogenesis

AFB_1 and AFM_1 (present in cow milk), aflatoxicol, and AFG_1 induce hepatic, renal, and colonic neoplasms in numerous animals [58]. In mice, pulmonary neoplasms were produced by AFB_1. Sterigmatocystin, a precursor of AFs, has lower toxicity but its carcinogenic potential is significant. Sterigmatocystin covalently binds to DNA at approximately 20–30% of the level observed with AFB_1. Although mutagenicity of OTA has not been established, tumorigenesis/carcinogenesis was reported in laboratory animals [19]. FUMs with a free primary amino group have been shown to be liver cancer promoters in rats [59], and they have been confirmed to be carcinogenic in rats.

Dermal toxicity

Several trichothecene mycotoxins are skin irritants [18]. T-2 toxin, the most potent compound tested, caused erythema on the shaved backs of guinea pigs.

Mechanisms of toxicity

Mycotoxins interacting with biomolecules or preventing biosynthesis are well known (Tab. 3) [2]. Investigating the mechanism of action is important to (1) reveal the initial biochemical lesion leading to diseases, (2) differentiate between biological effects that occur at high, from those at environmentally relevant dosages, (3) predict downstream biochemical effects developing from the initial biochemical lesion, and (4) predict potential chronic toxicity and interaction with other mycotoxins or bioactive agents, e.g., toxins and drugs.

Understanding the mechanism of action in animal cells may help to provide methods to decrease the toxicity of mycotoxins that are virulence factors, because biochemical targets can be similar in all eukaryotic cells. This information could be used to engineer biochemical target molecules that do not interact with the toxin, or bioactive derivatives that are metabolized or eliminated rapidly. These studies also provide insight to develop testable hypotheses concerning the role of mycotoxins in pathogenesis.

Mycotoxins as a group cannot be classified according to their mechanism of action, which is not surprising when the diversity of chemical structures is considered (Fig. 1). The potential for extremely complex toxin interactions is also great given the large number of mycotoxins and the diversity of the action mechanisms. Mycotoxins with similar modes of action would be expected to have at least additive effects. Conversely, some interactions could have subtractive effects. For example, cyclopiazonic acid prevents the lipid peroxidation induced by patulin [60].

Understanding the mechanism of action in *in vitro* systems can provide a rational basis for predicting toxin, drug, and/or nutritional interactions. Discovery of those interactions that pose a health risk from consumption of contaminated foods or feeds will be made more likely by coupling this approach with the known co-occurrence of mycotoxins. For example, those with dissimilar actions are (a) hepatotoxic FUMs and AFs, which co-occur on corn, and (b) nephrotoxic DON, FUMs, and OTA, which commonly contaminate foods (Tabs 1 and 2). The actual combined health risk from mycotoxin exposure is unknown because many mycotoxins are undiscovered (presumably). Furthermore, functional "food toxicology" would screen suspected feeds and foods for mechanisms known to be underlying causes of chronic disease. The number of possible biochemical targets is great and unraveling the source of the biological activity would be possible. Screening fungal isolates would pinpoint those biological activities of fungal origin.

Mutagenicity

A section on the mutagenic effects of myctoxins is merited due the importance of the field. These can be direct (e.g., changing bases) and/or indirect (e.g., inhibiting enzymes [61]) involved in stabilizing nucleic acids [62]. Mycotoxins with carcinogenic effects include AFs, sterigmatocystin, OTA, FUMs, zearalenone, citrinin, luteoskyrin, patulin, and penicillic acid produced by a wide range of fungi. All are DNA-damaging agents except for FUMs, which may act *via* disturbing signal transduction pathways.

It appears axiomatic that chemical carcinogens induce tumorigenesis by interactions with subcellular components that are involved intimately in mediating the basic heritable loss of growth control, assuming that cancer derives from clonal expansion of a single cell. These interactions may be (i) noncovalent and reversible, or (ii) covalent and reversible only in the case where repair mechanisms restore the original structure. To react with cellular macromolecules most carcinogens require enzymatic activation. The parent compounds are considered as precarcinogens/indirect carcinogens with the potential of being activated into carcinogenic forms. However, some compounds do not bind to DNA and remain capable of inducing tumors *via* nongenotoxic pathways. Some change expression levels of numerous proteins involved in cell and tissue homeostasis, i.e., cellular growth, proliferation, differentiation, and apoptosis. Luch [63] provides an excellent review of the complexities of the molecular action of organic carcinogens.

Aflatoxins
AFs (i) induce DNA damage, (ii) negatively affect the amelioration of damage, and (iii) alter DNA base compositions of genes. The mutagenicity of AFB_1 has been demonstrated in many systems. AFB_1 induces chromosomal aberrations, micronuclei, sister chromatid exchange, unscheduled DNA synthesis, and chromosomal strand breaks, and forms adducts in rodent/human cells. AFs contain an unsaturated terminal furan ring that can bind covalently to DNA, hence forming an epoxide. One dose of AFB_1 to rats can cause a measurable increase in AFB_1-DNA adducts. Furthermore, covalent binding of AFB_1 to adenosine and cytosine in DNA *in vitro* has been reported. AFB_1–DNA adducts can (i) form further repair-resistant adducts, (ii) undergo depurination, and/or (iii) lead to error-prone DNA repair yielding single-strand breaks, base pair substitution, and/or frame shift mutations. Mispairing of the adduct could induce transversion and transition mutations. AFB_1 induced GC→TA and GC→AT mutations when activated to its epoxide by microsomes, or as the 8,9-dichloride. Hot spots for AFB_1 mutagenesis were found predominantly in relatively GC-rich regions of DNA. AFB_1–8,9-epoxide (the active metabolite of AFB_1) caused base substitution mutations at G:C pairs with only approximately 50% GC→TA transversions. An oligonucleotide containing a single AFB_1–N7-guanine adduct yielded a mutation frequency of 4%. The predominant mutation was G→T, identical to the principal mutation in human liver tumors induced by AFs [2].

The major metabolite resulting from cytochrome P450-dependent epoxidation of AFB_1 or AFG_1, in relation to hepatotoxicity, is the 8,9-epoxide. This product forms an adduct with DNA involved in the carcinogenic activity of AFs. Binding of the epoxide intermediate with proteins could be important in the acute hepatic toxicity of AFs. The impact of stereochemistry is of crucial importance [63]. The cytochrome P450-dependent monooxygenase (CYP)-mediated toxification of AFB_1 occurs at its 8,9-position. Formation of an 8,9-epoxide intermediate was observed based on the isolation of the main DNA adduct (at N7 in guanine bases). The most important enzyme involved in AFB_1 activation in human liver, CYP3A4, exclusively forms the *exo* isomer, and CYP1A2 may add low concentrations of the diastereomeric *endo* epoxide. The *exo*-8,9-oxide is 1000-fold more genotoxic than the *endo* diastereomer due to the spatial configuration of the epoxide moiety within the AFB_1 *exo*-8,9-oxide-DNA complex. Hence, intercalation of the furanocoumarine residue between DNA bases directs the *exo* epoxide rings in a favorable position for S_N2 attacks by the N7 atoms of the guanines. Follow-up products of the main N7-DNA adducts of AFB_1 then result from depurination or ring opening of the purine bases. The "slow" pathological consequences are generally due to the adduction with lysine of proteins, whereas carcinogenesis and mutagenesis are due to adduction of AFB_1 8,9-epoxide with guanine of DNA.

A critical metabolic pathway of AFB_1 in relation to carcinogenesis entails formation of AFB_1 dialdehyde from the 8,9-epoxide. The protein adduct forming capabilities of AFB_1 dialdehyde has the mechanism of binding attributed to Schiff base formation with basic amino acid residues in proteins (e.g., lysine). The nuclear histone proteins are also targets. The *in vivo* biological consequences of protein adduction by AFB_1 dialdehyde are unknown. Protein adducts may contribute to risk by altering (a) the functions of adducted proteins, and (b) critical signal transduction pathways under protein control given the small attributable risk of DNA adducts in AFB_1-induced carcinogenesis. AFB_1 aldehyde reductase is important in controlling the level of the AF dialdehyde. This enzyme reduces AFB_1 dialdehyde by NADPH to alcohol products that are biologically inert and incapable of protein adduction; hence, it is AF detoxifying.

Support for the involvement of AFs in HCC etiology derives from (a) mutation studies in the p53 tumor suppressor gene, (b) the evidence from epidemiological studies, and (c) the use of biomarkers of biologically effective doses. The p53 gene is characterized by G→T transversion at the third base of codon 249 observed in HCC patients from high AF exposure regions, and *in vitro* data support this hypothesis. A majority of codon 249 mutations were found in patients with an HBV infection. The mutation only occurs in areas of high AFB_1 exposure and in regions of high HBV infection but varying levels of AFB_1 exposure. Hence, HBV may cause preferential selection of cells harboring the mutation. No codon 249 mutations were detected in countries with low AF exposure (e.g., Europe, Japan, and the United States [64]). Detection of the AF-nucleic acid adduct (AFB_1–N7-guanine) in urine was associated with an elevation in the risk of developing HCC. Finally, the use of the codon 249 mutation as a marker of exposure to AFs requires evidence from studies measuring AFB_1 adducts and mutations in the same individual [65].

Although unrelated to mutagenesis per se, the involvement of AFs in reproduction has produced some other interesting data. AFB_1 produced abundant symplastic spermatids in the seminiferous epithelium of mice, and these were traced to opening of cytoplasmic bridges, which then collapsed resulting in spherical symplasts. The study provided the first direct evidence for opening of cytoplasmic bridges as the mechanism underlying the origin of spermatid symplasts. Cytoskeletal proteins actin and tubulin have been demonstrated in the walls of the cytoplasmic bridges, and these could be targets of agents that disrupt cytoplasmic bridges between spermatids. Hence, the target for AFB_1 in the seminiferous epithelium could be actin microfilaments. Alternatively, AFB_1 treatment would bring about oxidative damage to the cells and the disruption of the cytoskeletal element in the cytoplasmic bridge as a consequence of this damage [66]. AFs caused a decrease of cell-mediated immunity in which production of cytokines are important. They have an important effect on levels of nonspecific humoral factors such as complement, interferon, and bactericidal serum components.

Sterigmatocystin

The toxigenic precursor to AFs, sterigmatocystin covalently binds to DNA forming DNA adducts.

Ochratoxin A

OTA is one of the most potent carcinogens in rats and is classified as a possible human carcinogen by the IARC. OTA adducts were found in kidney, liver, and spleen of mice treated with OTA and the DNA adduct level was dose dependent and time related. There was insufficient understanding of whether OTA acts as a direct genotoxic carcinogen or whether its carcinogenicity is related to indirect mechanisms (e.g., inhibition of stability enzymes). However, direct DNA binding of OTA has been reported. Evidence of OTA-mediated DNA damage is the induction of DNA single-strand breaks and form-amidopyrimidine-DNA glycosylase-sensitive sites. In agreement is the unscheduled DNA synthesis in primary human urothelial cultures, primary hepatocytes, and rat and mouse cell lines. Importantly, mutagenic activity by OTA has also been reported (e.g., in murine cells). OTA increases the process involved in spontaneous mutagenesis. Finally, the metabolite induces an increase of mutation frequency at two gene loci *via* a mechanism that is independent of biotransformation [67].

OTA biotransformations are cytochrome P450 dependent in animals and humans, resulting in the formation of metabolic intermediates that contribute to carcinogenesis. Both the phenylalanine and dihydroisocoumarin moieties are structural components of OTA probably involved in the complex toxic activities. The phenylalanine residue likely contributes to inhibition of enzyme reactions related to nephrotoxicity.

Administration of OTA to male rats resulted in a dose- and time-dependent increase in the expression of kidney injury molecule-1 (Kim-1), metalloproteinase-1 (Timp-1), lipocalin-2, osteopontin (OPN), clusterin, and vimentin. Gene expression changes were correlated with progressive histopathological alterations and preceded effects on clinical parameters indicative of impaired kidney function. Induction of Kim-1 mRNA expression was the earliest and most prominent response observed [68]. OTA was shown to bind to an $\alpha 2u$-globulin. It should be pointed out that some experimental nephrotoxicological data may not be appropriate for human risk assessment as potential internalized delivery of OTA to proximal tubule epithelia by the carrier was specific only to adult male rats. Re-examination of female rat renal tumor histopathology of the high-dose OTA study showed all carcinomas were clinically insignificant at the end stage [69].

A role for basal cell lymphoma-extra large (Bcl-xL) (an anti-apoptotic protein) in OTA-induced apoptosis in human lymphocytes has been demonstrated. Human peripheral blood lymphocytes and cells of the lymphoid T cell line

Kit 225 underwent apoptosis in a time- and dose-dependent manner. The indication was that caspases were responsible for the induction of apoptosis. OTA triggered mitochondrial transmembrane potential loss and caspase-9 and caspase-3 activation. Interestingly, Bcl-xL protein expression was decreased by OTA treatment, whereas Bcl-2 protein level was unaffected. Down-regulation of Bcl-xL mRNA was not observed in cells treated with OTA. Overexpression of Bcl-xL in Kit 225 cells protected them against mitochondrial perturbation and retarded the appearance of apoptotic cells. Mitochondria are a crucial component in OTA-induced apoptosis and the loss of Bcl-xL may participate in OTA-induced cell death [70].

Patulin

Patulin induces DNA–DNA cross-links. Mutations of cells by patulin might be from an indirect mutagenic mechanism (e.g., inhibition of enzymes [62]). Finally, also direct reactivity to DNA has been demonstrated [71].

Nivalenol and fusarenon X

NIV damaged nuclear DNA, demonstrating that it is a direct mutagen [72]. DNA damage appeared in the kidney and bone marrow of mice after oral dosing. NIV showed organ-specific genotoxicity in mice as a direct mutagen in a time and intensity related manner. NIV and fusarenon X caused DNA damage after 24- and 72-h exposure and damage was observed dose dependently. Furthermore, fusarenon X increased DNA strand breaks [73].

Zearalenone

Zearalenone showed a DNA damaging effect in recombination tests with *Bacillus subtilis*. The compound also induced (i) polyploidy in CHO cells, (ii) sister chromatid exchange, and (iii) chromosomal aberration *in vitro*. Treatment of mice led to the formation of several DNA adducts in the liver and kidney [74].

Fusarin C

Fusarin C is mutagenic and is produced from *Fusarium moniliforme* [75].

Toxicity mechanism of trichothecenes

A considerable weight of data has been produced on the mechanisms of toxicity of trichothecene mycotoxins apart from mutagenicity. Neuroendocrine effects may be mediated by the serotoninergic system based on increased levels of serotonin or its metabolites in DON-treated animals [76]. This is further supported by the capacity of serotonin receptor antagonists to prevent DON-induced emesis [77]. In particular this applies to anorectic and emetic responses. DON modulates serotonin activity [78], which suggests a link between DON-induced emesis and the serotoninergic mechanism. DON also inhibits small-intestinal motility in rodents, mediated through 5-HT$_3$ receptors. Prelusky and Trenholm [77] suggest that at least part of the mechanism of action of DON is mediated through action on the peripheral 5-HT$_3$ receptors found in the gastrointestinal tract.

Trichothecenes such as DON may also modulate immune function [79]. At low concentrations they potentiate or attenuate expression of cytokines, which can disrupt normal regulation of immune functions positively or negatively. At high concentrations they induce leukocyte apoptosis and produce pronounced immunosuppression. DON enhances differentiation of immunoglobulin A (IgA)-secreting cells at the Peyer's patch level and this affects the systemic immune compartment. The potential for enhanced IgA production exists in lymphocytes after a single oral exposure, perhaps related to the increased capacity to secrete the helper cytokines interleukin (IL)-2, IL-5, and IL-6 [80]. T cells expressing surface protein CB4 (CD4$^+$) and macrophages appear to be involved in this process [81]. Thus, increased cytokine expression may be responsible for up-regulation of IgA secretion in mice.

Superinduction of cytokine gene expression by DON is mediated *via* transcriptional and/or post-transcriptional mechanisms [80]. For example, DON increases DNA binding of the transcription factors NF-κB and AP-1 in T cell and macrophage cultures. In part, increased cytokine mRNA expression by DON was also found to be due markedly to enhanced mRNA stabilities in the T cell and IL-6/tumor necrosis factor (TNF) in the macrophage. DON significantly induced the mRNAs for (a) T helper 2 (T$_H$2) cytokines (IL-4 and IL-10), (b) T$_H$1 cytokines [interferon (IFN)-γ and IL-2] and (c) proinflammatory cytokines (IL-1β, IL-6, and TNF-α). IL-12 p40 was also induced, but not IL-12 p35 mRNA. DON increased the relative abundance of IL-1β, IL-6, TNF-α, IL-12 p35, IL-12 p40, IL-2, and IL-10 mRNAs with dose dependency, whereas IFN-γ and IL-4 mRNAs were unchanged, suggesting that the ability of DON to dysregulate cytokine expression was cumulative.

High doses of trichothecenes promoted rapid leukocyte apoptosis to yield immunosuppression. DON inhibited or enhanced apoptosis in a concentration-dependent manner in T, B, and IgA$^+$ cells isolated from spleen, Peyer's patches, and thymus [82]. Bacterial lipopolysaccharide (LPS) potentiation of DON-induced lymphocyte apoptosis in thymus, Peyer's patches, spleen, and bone marrow has been linked to elevated corticosterone [83], which is driven by superinduction of IL-1β [84].

Toxicity of trichothecenes is explained partially by binding to eukaryotic ribosomes and inhibition of protein synthesis [85]. Other toxic mechanisms include deregulation of calcium homeostasis, impaired membrane function and altered intercellular communication. Trichothecenes inhibit DNA (see [62]), also explaining toxicity. Dietary DON causes marked elevation of serum IgA, with concurrent decreases in IgM and IgG in the mouse; serum IgA elevation indicates immunopathological effects. The lowering of immune function can be explained by a potent capacity to inhibit protein synthesis. In addition, superinduction of cytokines has been demonstrated using trichothecenes (see above). Mechanisms may include interference with synthesis of high turnover proteins that limit transcription or the half-life of IL mRNA. Analogous mechanisms can also be proposed at the level of translation. Dysregulation of IgA production is induced apparently by macrophage- and T cell-mediated polyclonal differentiation of B cells to IgA secretion at the level of the Peyer's patch [81]. Trichothecenes induce mitogen-activated protein kinases (MAPKs) and other critical cellular kinases involved in signal transduction related to proliferation, differentiation, and apoptosis [86].

Early alterations in cell signaling may be critical to trichothecene toxicity particularly at the level of MAPKs [87]. A "ribotoxic stress response" has been demonstrated for translation inhibitors such as T-2 toxin. Alteration of 28S rRNA by this inhibitor was postulated to be a signal for activation of SAPK/JNK (an MAPK). This activity drives activation of transcription factors promoting cytokine production, cyclooxygenase 2 expression and induces apoptosis [88]. Upstream kinases were involved in the ribotoxic stress response using DON and the RAW 264.7 macrophage as models. DON induced phosphorylation of c-Jun N-terminal protein kinase (JNK), extracellular signal-regulated kinase (ERK), and p38 MAPKs. MAPK phosphorylation occurred early. Protein phosphatase-1 (PP1) suppressed DON-induced phosphorylation of the MAPK substrates c-jun, ATF-2, and p90Rsk. PP1 also reduced DON-induced increases in nuclear levels and binding activities of several transcription factors (NF-κB, AP-1, and C/EBP), which corresponded to decreases in TNF-α production, caspase-3 activation, and apoptosis. Tyrosine phosphorylation of hematopoietic cell kinase (Hck, an Src-family tyrosine kinase), was detectable after DON addition, and this was suppressed by PP1. Knockdown of Hck expression with siRNAs confirmed involvement of this Src in DON-induced TNF-α production and caspase activation. Activation of Hck is likely to be a critical signal that precedes MAPK activation and induction of resultant downstream events by DON [89] and other Src family tyrosine kinases may be involved. Double-stranded RNA-activated protein kinase (PKR) is a possible upstream signal transducer for MAPK activation by DON [90].

Inhibition of Hck blocks MAPK activation, transcription factor activation, and cytokine expression [91]. The potential also exists for a receptor to transduce these signals upon binding of DON. A third intermediate signal between trichothecene mycotoxins and MAPK activation might be the generation of reactive oxygen species (ROS). In support of this contention, trichothecene mycotoxins produce lipid peroxidation, and their adverse effects can be inhibited by antioxidants such as vitamin E and N-acetylcysteine [92]. However, the possibility of "cross-talk" between ROS and ribotoxic stress signals cannot be excluded in any explanation of the mechanism of trichothecene-induced MAPK activation [86].

The immunomodulating effects of DON were investigated in human peripheral blood mononuclear (PBM) cells. DON inhibited concanavalin A (Con A)-, phytohemagglutinin (PHA)-induced lymphocyte blast transformation (T lymphocyte proliferation), and the antibody-dependent cell-mediated cytotoxicity of monocyte-free PBM cells. DON also inhibited natural killer cell activity and increased apoptosis in human peripheral blood lymphocytes [93]. In conclusion, exposure of various human cells to DON resulted in stimulation (cytokines) or an impairment (apoptosis) of immune function.

DON-induced expression of the CXC chemokine IL-8, a neutrophil chemoattractant, was observed in human cell cultures. Human monocytes were the effector population. Comprehending the mechanisms by which DON up-regulates this chemokine is of potential toxicological significance since IL-8 is implicated in diseases from rheumatoid arthritis to inflammatory bowel disease. IL-8 up-regulation has been linked to elevated transcription, and/or increased mRNA stability. Work is required to test whether DON-induced IL-8 in monocytes is mediated transcriptionally through activation of multiple transcription factors or post-transcriptionally by increasing IL-8 mRNA stability. Human U937 cells originating from an individual with diffuse histiocytic lymphoma were employed to test this hypothesis. These cells markedly express IL-8 in response to DON and, thus, mimic primary monocytes. Indications were that DON-induced IL-8 expression in monocytes was driven, in part, by NF-κB-mediated transcription but did not involve mRNA stabilization. How DON mediated NF-κB activation in the monocyte is unknown [94].

The capacities of DON and T-2 toxin to promote 28S rRNA cleavage have been compared [95]. DON and T-2 did not depurinate yeast 28S rRNA and hence had no N-glycosidase activity in a cell-free model. Incubation of RAW 264.7 macrophages with DON or T-2 generated 28S rRNA-specific products consistent with cleavage sites near the 3' terminal end of murine 28S rRNA. DON and T-2 did promote cleavage at A3560 and A4045, although they did not damage the α-sarcin/ricin (S/R)-loop (A4256). Also, incubation of the cells with DON or T-2 induced RNase activity, RNase L mRNA and protein expression. These data suggest that DON and T-2 promoted intracellular 28S rRNA cleavage by facilitating the action of endogenous RNases and/or by up-regulating RNase expression.

Growth

Growth is another parameter that is particularly sensitive to DON. Reduction in weight appears to result from reduced feed intake (anorexia) and is reversible once DON is removed. The anorectic response could derive from disturbances in the serotonergic system, and up-regulation of proinflammatory cytokines such as TNF-α that are known to produce cachexia. DON affects reproduction, which appears to result from maternal toxicity associated with feed refusal and weight loss. However, the primary human safety concern for DON should be induction of acute gastroenteritis and concurrent vomiting. The mechanisms for this effect may be related to dysregulation of immune and/or neuroendocrine function. In addition, there is potential for chronic effects on growth (and immune function and reproduction) based on animal studies [86].

Fertility and reproduction

DON has been reported to reduce fertility. It inhibited oocyte maturation and caused 34% of the oocytes to form aberrant spindles. Maturation in the presence of DON was not compatible with development. Malekinejad et al. [96] concluded that DON can lead to less fertile oocytes and embryos with abnormal ploidy. The effects of zearalenone (see below) and DON were not synergistic. The mutagenic potential of DON does not represent a considerable risk, although it may be genotoxic [97]. DON treatment produced increased chromosomal aberrations using rat cells [86].

Toxicity mechanisms of zearalenone and derivatives

Reproductive effects of zearalenone (and derivatives) involve displacement of estradiol from its uterine binding protein, eliciting an estrogenic response. Szuets et al. [23] discovered that zearalenone and zearalenol bind to estrogen receptors of human myometrial tissue. Zearalenone has been reported to reduce fertility. The presence of zearalenone during maturation reduced the percentages of oocytes that cleaved and formed blastocysts by 50% [96].

Toxicity mechanisms of fumonisins

FUMs have pronounced effects on cellular sphingolipid metabolism because they inhibit the enzyme ceramide synthase, which may alter sphingolipid-mediated regulatory processes related to cell survival and replication. $FUMB_1$ inhibits *N*-acyltransferase, a key enzyme in sphingolipid metabolism in relation to hepatotoxicity. This enzyme is involved in the conversion of sphingosine and sphinganine to ceramide, which is subsequently converted to sphingolipid. Disruption of this pathway can produce several outcomes because the basic process is involved, amongst others, in cellular regulation [98].

Toxicity mechanisms of patulin

Protein synthesis was inhibited in rat alveolar macrophages exposed to patulin and cell membrane function was compromised [99]. Patulin suppressed the oxidative burst in rat and rabbit peritoneal macrophages [61], and decreased O_2 production, phagosome-lysosome fusion, and lysosomal enzyme activity in mouse peritoneal macrophages [100].

Tremorgens

The mode of action of fungal tremorgens is by release of neurotransmitters from synaptosomes in the CNS and in peripheral nerves at the neuromuscular junction. Although many tremorgens affect the high-conductance Ca^{2+}-activated K^+ channels in the release of neurotransmitters, this alone may not be the mechanism for the tremorgenic activity as some non-tremorgenic mycotoxins have similar activity [101].

Cyclopiazonic acid

Cyclopiazonic acid has the ability to chelate metal cations due to the structure of the tetramic acid moiety [102]. The chelation of cations such as calcium, magnesium, and iron may play an important role in cyclopiazonic acid toxicity.

Animal nutrition

AFs affect rumen function *in vitro* and *in vivo* by decreasing cellulose digestion, volatile fatty acid formation, and proteolysis [103]. In chickens, clinical responses include hypoproteinemia, decreased hemoglobin, and decreased serum triglycerides, phospholipids, and cholesterol [104]. AFs can decrease activities of several enzymes important to digestion of starches, proteins, lipids, and nucleic acids in broiler chickens [105]. The decreased activities of pancreatic amylase, trypsin, lipase, RNase, and DNase could contribute to the malabsorption of nutrients associated with aflatoxicoses.

Enzyme inhibition

Many mycotoxins function as enzyme inhibitors [62]. Enzymes inhibited include acetylcholinesterase, NF-κB, protein kinase, tyrosine kinase, aromatase and sulfatase, matrix metalloproteinases, cyclooxygenase, DNA polymerase/topoisomerases and glycosidases. Mycelianamide is a case in point. This compound is a mycotoxin and a treatment for reducing cholesterol by inhibiting butyrylcholinesterase (for patients with high cholesterol). β-Nitropropionic acid inhibits succinate dehydrogenase and hence provides a useful model for neurodegeneration comprehension; this is a common compound from the penicillia and aspergilli. Dehydroaltenusin from *Penicillium verruculosum* is an anti-cancer drug that acts *via* DNA polymerase inhibition. Furthermore, gliotoxin from *Gliocladium fimbriatum*, *Aspergillus*, *Penicillium* (and *Candida*) is another example. Low concentrations of gliotoxin specifically inhibited the activation of NF-κB. The compound appeared to prevent degradation of IκB α, which is the inhibitory subunit of NF-κB. Inhibitors of

MAPK protein kinase signaling pathways act on the tyrosine kinase activity. Three major MAPK cascades have been identified in mammalian cells. 1-Methoxy-agroclavine from a *Penicillium* and 7-triprenyl phenol type sesqui-terpenoid derivatives from *Stachybotrys chortarum* are inhibitors of tyrosine kinases. Phosphoinositide 3-kinase (PI3K) is inhibited by wortmannin produced from *P. wortmanni* [62].

Indoor fungal exposure

The controversial issue (in the United States at least) of the mycotoxic effects of indoor fungi are considered here. A debate was generated by Bush et al. [106], although the authors concede they may have been "overly conservative" [107]. Lieberman et al. [108] wondered, "Whose ox is being gored?". What the position paper does not mention is that mycotoxins have in fact been documented in small fragments released by mold growth indoors [109], where numerous other salient points are raised. For example, "mold" has been found to reside in the upper and lower airways of many persons with chronic respiratory disease. Hardin et al. [110], who are firmly in the no-evidence-of-a-problem camp, cite the other evidence-based statements and a (US) Institute of Medicine report. However, what is unfortunate is that two such different views can arise from the same available information. The impartial reader can only suggest that the truth lies between the extremes.

Combined effects

Hundreds of mycotoxins are known and detected frequently in plant-derived products. In all the above considerations on individual mycotoxins, it needs to be appreciated that various mycotoxins may occur simultaneously, depending amongst other things, on the environmental and substrate conditions. It is very likely that humans and animals are exposed to mixtures rather than to individual compounds. For example, future risk assessments should consider mixture toxicity data. OTA and citrinin are common mycotoxins that occur jointly in a wide range of food commodities. Bouslimi et al. [111] assessed the combined effects on cell proliferation and DNA fragmentation in cultured Vero cells and *in vivo* by monitoring the induction of chromosome aberrations. Results demonstrated that cultured renal cells respond to combined OTA and citrinin with increased inhibition of cell viability. Similar results were found for DNA fragmentation and chromosome aberrations (i.e., genotoxicity). OTA and citrinin combination effects are clearly synergistic. The synergistic induction of DNA damage observed with OTA and citrinin could help explain the molecular basis of the renal diseases and "tumorigenesis" induced by mycotoxins. Orsi et al. [112] discovered that combined administration of AFB_1 and $FUMB_1$ resulted in synergistic toxic effects both in the liver and in the kidney, but hepatic injuries were more marked in rabbits. Tammer et al. [113] examined predicted, specified and evaluated combined effects of patulin, gliotoxin, citrinin and OTA on the functional activity of human competent immune cells using stimulated human PBM cells. The mixture suppressed cytokine production in a concentration-dependent manner when compared to the individual mycotoxins. They conclude that low and weak-effect concentrations of mycotoxins may cause strong inhibitory effects on immune functions when occurring together.

Similarly, the combined effects of $FUMB_1$, beauvericin and OTA on cell viability, lipid peroxidation and intracellular glutathione (GSH) were studied on porcine kidney epithelial cells (PK15) [114]. Combined treatment resulted mostly in additive effects especially after a 24-h exposure, although synergistic as well as antagonistic interactions could not be excluded depending on toxin concentrations and time of exposure. This was the first report on beauvericin-induced effects on lipid peroxidation and GSH in animal cells, and may have relevance to the application of biological control agents. *Beauvaria bassiana* produces this compound, which may contaminate food originating from crops for which pest control may have been attempted [4]. OTA, ochratoxin B, citrinin and patulin were used as examples by Heussner et al. to study the interactive effects *in vitro* [115], using porcine renal cell line LLC-PK1 and the MTT reduction test as a cytotoxicity endpoint. The results obtained in this study confirm a potential for interactive (synergistic) effects of citrinin and OTA and possibly other mycotoxins in cells of renal origin. The possible combined effect of various mycotoxins is presented in Figure 3.

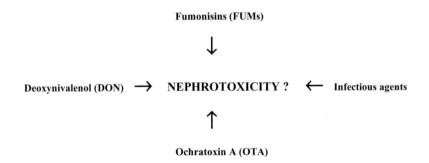

Figure 3. Theoretical example of mycotoxins and infectious agents acting to initiate or exacerbate renal dysfunction. Sphingolipid metabolism is disrupted and cytokine signaling pathways changed by fumonisins acting as a nephrotoxin. A fumonisin-sensitive sphingolipid receptor may then internalize a Shiga toxin from *Escherichia coli*, which initiates renal dysfunction *via* a cytokine pathway. An increased cytokine response could be elicited by DON acting as a nephrotoxin. Finally, OTA acts as a nephrotoxin.

Conclusions

In many ways mycotoxins remain a silent threat. It is surprising just how compelling the evidence of the toxicology of mycotoxins is, considering that the occurrence of high levels in food only occasionally makes headline news. This may relate to the fact that they are often considered to be under control in the technologically developed world but much less so elsewhere. The issue of fungi in indoor environments really needs to be carefully assessed particularly in the United States. Greater use of cell-free systems to test mycotoxins is required and the hidden effects of mycotoxins (e.g., impaired immune system) require more work. Testing individual mycotoxins can only provide limited information when it is realized that multiple mycotoxins will be present in the relevant commodities. It is essential that the influence of climate change on mycotoxins is being considered [116]. The awareness of the effects of mycotoxins will increase due to consumer demands for healthier foods and life styles in developed countries, at the same time leading to improvements in quality in developing nations that export many of the susceptible products.

Acknowledgments
R.R.M.P. is grateful for grant SFRH/BPD/34879/2007 from Fundaçao para a Ciência e a Tecnologia, Portugal, and the research position in the FCT framework, Commitment to Science ref. C2008-UMIN-HO-CEB-2.

References

1 Hawksworth DL (2001) The magnitude of fungal diversity: The 1.5 million species estimate revisited. *Mycol Res* 105: 1422–1432

2 CAST (2003) *Mycotoxins: Risks in Plant, Animal, and Human Systems*. Council for Agricultural Science and Technology, Ames, IA

3 Marr JS, Malloy CD (1996) An epidemiologic analysis of the ten plagues of Egypt. *Caduceus* 12: 7–24

4 Paterson RRM (2006) Fungi and fungal toxins as weapons. *Mycol Res* 110: 1003–1010

5 Lewis L, Onsongo M, Njapau H, Schurz-Rogers H, Luber G, Kieszak S, Nyamongo J, Backer L, Dahiye A, Misore A, DeCock K, Rubin C (2005) Aflatoxin contamination of commercial maize products during an outbreak of acute aflatoxicosis in Eastern and Central Kenya. *Environ Health Perspect* 113: 1763–1767

6 Cole RJ, Jarvis BB, Schweikert MA (2003) *Handbook of Secondary Fungal Metabolites, 3 Vols*, Academic Press, The Netherlands

7 Klaassen CD, Eaton DL (1991) Principles of Toxicology. In: MO Amdur, J Doull, CD Klaassen (eds): *Casarett and Doull's Toxicology. The Basic Science of Poisons*. Pergamon Press, New York, 12–49

8 IARC (1993) *Monographs on the Evaluation of Carcinogenic Risks to Humans, Some Naturally Occurring Substances: Food Items and Constituents, Heterocyclic Aromatic Amines, and Mycotoxins*. International Agency for Research on Cancer, Lyon, 56, 489–521

9 Krishnamachari KAVR, Bhat RV, Nagarajan V, Tilak TBG (1975) Hepatitis due to aflatoxicosis. An outbreak in Western India. *Lancet* 1: 1061–1063

10 Ngindu A, Johnson BK, Kenya PR, Ngira JA, Ocheng DM, Nandwa H, Omondi TN, Jansen AJ, Ngare W, Kaviti JN, Gatei D, Siongok TA (1982) Outbreak of acute hepatitis caused by aflatoxin poisoning in Kenya. *Lancet* 1: 1346–1348

11 Hendrickse RG (1984) The influence of aflatoxins on child health in the tropics with particular reference to kwashiorkor. *Trans R Soc Trop Med Hyg* 78: 427–435

12 Henry SH, Bosch FX, Troxell TC, Bolger PM (1999) Reducing liver cancer – Global control of aflatoxin. *Science* 286: 2453–2454.

13 Autrup H, Bradley KA, Shamsuddin AKM, Wakhisi J, Wasunna A (1983) Detection of putative

adduct with fluorescence characteristics identical to 2,3-dihydro-2-(7'-guanyl)-3-hydroxyaflatoxin B$_1$ in human urine collected in Murang'a district, Kenya. *Carcinogenesis* 4: 1193–1195

14 Yeh FS, Yu MC, Mo CC, Luo S, Tong MJ, Henderson BE (1989) Hepatitis B virus, aflatoxins, and hepatocellular carcinoma in southern Guangxi, China. *Cancer Res* 49: 2506–2509

15 Campbell TC, Chen J, Liu C, Li J, Parpia B (1990) Nonassociation of aflatoxin with primary liver cancer in a cross-sectional ecological survey in the People's Republic of China. *Cancer Res* 50: 6882–6893

16 Odhav B, Adam JK, Bhoola KD (2008) Modulating effects of fumonisin B$_1$ and ochratoxin A on leukocytes and messenger cytokines of the human immune system. *Int Immunopharmacol* 8: 799–809

17 Joffe ZA, Yagen B (1977) Comparative study of the yield of T-2 toxic produced by *Fusarium poae*, *F. sporotrichioides* and *F. sporotrichioides* var. *tricinctum* strains from different sources. *Mycopathologia* 60: 93–97

18 Ueno Y (1984) Toxicological features of T-2 toxin and related trichothecenes. *Fund Appl Toxicol* 4: S124–132

19 Ueno Y (1985) The toxicology of mycotoxins. *Crit Rev Toxicol* 14: 99–132

20 Bucheli TD, Wettstein FE, Hartmann N, Erbs M, Vogelgsang S, Forrer HR, Schwarzenbach RP (2008) *Fusarium* mycotoxins: Overlooked aquatic micropollutants? *J Agric Food Chem* 56: 1029–1034

21 Painter K (1997) Puberty signs evident in 7- and 8-year old girls. *USA Today*, April 8, A-1

22 Hsieh DPH (1989) Potential human health hazards of mycotoxins. In: S Natori, K Hashimoto, Y Ueno (eds): *Mycotoxins and Phycotoxins 1988*. Elsevier, The Netherlands, 69–80

23 Szuets P, Mesterhazy A, Falkay G, Bartok T (1997) Early thelarche symptoms in children and their relations to zearalenone contamination in foodstuffs. *Cereal Res Commun* 25: 429–436

24 Gelderblom WCA, Thiel PG, van Der Merwe KJ (1988) The role of rat liver microsomal enzymes in the metabolism of the fungal metabolite, fusarin C. Food and Chemical Toxicology. *Food Chem Toxicol* 26: 31–36

25 Zhu B, Jeffrey AM (1992) Stability of fusarin C: Effects of the normal cooking procedure used in China and pH. *Nutr Cancer* 18: 53–58

26 Li M, Lu S, Jin C, Wang Y, Wang M, Cheng S, Tian G (1980) Experimental studies on the carcinogenicity of fungus contaminated food from Linxian County. In: HV Gelboin (ed.): *Genetic and Environmental Factors in Experimental Human Cancer*. Japan Science Society Press, Tokyo, 139–148

27 Marasas WFO (1996) Fumonisins: History, world-wide occurrence and impact. In: LS Jackson, JW DeVries, LB Bullerman (eds): *Fumonisins in Food*. Plenum Press, New York, 1–17

28 Franceschi S, Bidoli E, Baron AE, La Vecchia C (1990) Maize and risk of cancers of the oral cavity, pharynx, and esophagus in northeastern Italy. *J Natl Cancer Inst* 82: 1407–1411

29 Gelderblom WCA, Jaskiewicz K, Marasas WFO, Thiel PG, Horak RM, Vleggaar R, Kriek, NPJ (1988) Fumonisins – Novel mycotoxins with cancer-promoting activity produced by *Fusarium moniliforme*. *Appl Environ Microbiol* 54: 1806–1811

30 Frisvad JC, Smedsgaard J, Samson RA, Larsen TO, Thrane U (2007) Fumonisin B$_2$ production by *Aspergillus niger*. *J Agric Food Chem* 55: 9727–9732

31 Tolleson WH, Melchior WB Jr, Morris SM, McGarrity LJ, Domon OE, Muskhelishvili L, Sjill J, Howard PC (1996) Apoptotic and anti-proliferative effects of fumonisin B$_1$ in human keratinocytes, fibroblasts, esophageal epithelial cells and hepatoma cells. *Carcinogenesis* 17: 239–249

32 Forgacs J (1972) Stachybotryotoxicosis. In: S Kadis, A Ceigler, S Ajl (eds): *Microbial Toxins. Volume VIII*. Academic Press, New York, 95–128

33 Dearborn DG, Yike I, Sorenson WG, Miller MJ, Etzel RA (1999) Overview of investigations into pulmonary hemorrhage among infants in Cleveland, Ohio. *Environ Health Perspect* 107: 495–499

34 Ueno Y (1974) Citreoviridin from *Penicillium citreoviride* Biourge. In: IFH Purchase (ed.): *Mycotoxins*. Elsevier, New York, 283–302

35 Beardall JM, Miller JD (1994) Diseases in humans with mycotoxins as possible causes. In: JD Miller, HL Trenholm (eds): *Mycotoxins in Grains: Compounds Other than Aflatoxins*. Eagan Press, MN, 487–539

36 Demeke T, Kidane Y, Wuhib E (1979) Ergotism – A report on an epidemic, 1977–78. *Ethiop Med J* 17: 107–113

37 Krishnamachari KAVR, Bhat RV (1976) Poisoning by ergoty bajra (pearl millet) in man. *Indian J Med Res* 64: 1624–1628

38 Richard JL (1991) Mycotoxins as immunomodulators in animal systems. In: GA Bray, DH Ryan (eds): *Mycotoxins, Cancer, and Health*. Pennington Center Nutrition Series, Louisiana State University Press, LA, 197–220

39 Krogh P (1976) Epidemiology of mycotoxic porcine nephropathy. *Nord Vet Med* 28: 452–458

40 Prelusky DB, Hamilton RMG, Trenholm HL, Miller JD (1986) Tissue distribution and excretion of radioactivity following administration of ^{14}C-labeled deoxynivalenol to white leghorn hens. *Fundam Appl Toxicol* 7: 635–645

41 Bryden WL (1991) Occurrence and biological effects of cyclopiazonic acid. In: K Mixe, JL Richard (eds): *Emerging Problem Resulting from Microbial Contamination*. National Institute of Hygienic Science, Tokyo, 127–147

42 Pier AC (1986) Immunomodulation in aflatoxicosis. In: JL Richard, JR Thurston (eds): *Diagnosis of Mycotoxicoses*. Martinus Nijhoff Publishers, The Netherlands, 143–148

43 Kadian SK, Monga DP, Goel MC (1988) Effect of aflatoxin B_1 on the delayed type hypersensitivity and phagocytic activity of reticuloendothelial system in chickens. *Mycopathologia* 104: 33–36

44 Robbana-Barnat S, Lafarge-Frayssinet C, Cohen H, Neish GA, Frayssinet C (1988) Immunosuppressive properties of deoxynivalenol. *Toxicology* 48: 155–166

45 Burns RB, Dwivedi P (1986) The natural occurrence of ochratoxin A and its effects in poultry. A review. Part II. Pathology and immunology. *World's Poultry Sci J* 42: 48–55

46 Escoula L, Thomsen M, Bourdiol D, Pipy B, Peuriere S, Roubinet F (1988) Patulin immunotoxicology: Effect on phagocyte activation and the cellular and humoral immune system of mice and rabbits. *Int J Immunopharmacol* 10: 983–989

47 McKinley ER, Carlton WW, Boon GD (1982) Patulin mycotoxicosis in the rat: Toxicology, pathology and clinical pathology. *Food Chem Toxicol* 20: 289–300

48 Dawe DL, Stuedemann JA, Hill NS, Thompson FN (1997) Immunosuppression in cattle with fescue toxicosis. In: CW Bacon, NS Hill (eds): *Neotyphodium/Grass Interactions*. Plenum Press, New York, 411–412

49 Dietert RR, Bloom SE, Qureshi MA, Nanna UC (1983) Hematological toxicology following embryonic exposure to aflatoxin B_1. *Proc Soc Exp Biol Med* 173: 481–485

50 Segal R, Milo Goldzweig I, Joffe AZ, Yagen B (1983) Trichothecene-induced hemolysis. 1. The hemolytic activity of T-2 toxin. *Toxicol Appl Pharmacol* 70: 343–349

51 Richard JL (1998) Mycotoxins, toxicity and metabolism in animals – A systems approach overview. In: M Miraglia, H van Egmond, C Brera, J Gilbert (eds): *Mycotoxins and Phycotoxins – Developments in Chemistry, Toxicology and Food Safety*. Alaken Inc, CO, 363–397

52 Edgar JA, Culvenor CCJ (1985) Aspects of the structure of phomopsin A, the mycotoxin causing lupinosis. In: AA Seawright, MP Hegarty, LF James, RF Keeler (eds): *Plant Toxicology*. Queensland Poisonous Plants Committee, Yeerongpilly, Australia, 589–594

53 Voss KA, Chamberlain WJ, Bacon CW, Herbert RA, Walters DB, Norred WP (1995) Subchronic feeding study of the mycotoxin fumonisin B_1 in B6C3F1 mice and Fischer 344 rats. *Fund Appl Toxicol* 24: 102–110

54 Hagler WM Jr, Towers NR, Mirocha CJ, Eppley RM, Bryden WL (2001) Zearalenone: Mycotoxin or mycoestrogen? In: BA Summerell, JF Leslie, D Backhouse, WL Bryden, LW Burgess (eds): *Fusarium: Paul E. Nelson Memorial Symposium*. APS Press, MN, 321–331

55 Hunt JN (1980) A possible relation between the regulation of gastric emptying and food intake. *J Physiol* 239: 61–64

56 Norred WP, Voss KA (1994) Toxicity and role of fumonisins in animal diseases and human esophageal cancer. *J Food Protect* 57: 522–527

57 Marasas, WFO, Nelson PE (1987) *Mycotoxicology*. Pennsylvania State University Press, PA

58 Eaton DL, Groopman JD (1994) *The Toxicology of Aflatoxins: Human Health, Veterinary and Agricultural Significance*. Academic Press, New York

59 Gelderblom WCA, Cawood ME, Snyman D, Vleggaar R, Marasas WFO (1993) Structure-activity relationships of fumonisins in short-term carcinogenesis and cytotoxicity studies. *Food Chem Toxicol* 31: 407–414

60 Riley RT, Showker JL (1991) The mechanism of patulin's cytotoxicity and the antioxidant activity of indole tetramic acids. *Toxicol Appl Pharmacol* 109: 108–126

61 Paterson RRM (2008) Fungal enzyme inhibitors as pharmaceuticals, toxins, and scourge of PCR. *Curr Enzyme Inhib* 4: 46–59

62 Paterson RRM, Lima N (2009) Mutagens manufactured in fungal culture may affect DNA/RNA

of producing fungi. *J Appl Microbiol* 106: 1070–1080

63 Luch A (2008) The mode of action of organic carcinogens on cellular structures. In: LP Bignold (ed.): *Cancer: Cell Structures, Carcinogens and Genomic Instability.* Birkhäuser, Switzerland 65–95

64 Groopman JD, Kensler TW (2005) Role of metabolism and viruses in aflatoxin-induced liver cancer. *Toxicol Appl Pharmacol* 206: 131–137

65 Groopman JD, Johnson D, Kensler TW (2005) Aflatoxin and hepatitis B virus biomarkers: A paradigm for complex environmental exposures and cancer risk. *Cancer Biomark* 1: 5–14

66 Faridha A, Faisal K, Akbarsha MA (2007) Aflatoxin treatment brings about generation of multinucleate giant spermatids (symplasts) through opening of cytoplasmic bridges: Light and transmission electron microscopic study in Swiss mouse. *Reprod Toxicol* 24: 403–408

67 Palma N, Cinelli S, Sapora O, Wilson SH, Dogliotti E (2007) Ochratoxin A-induced mutagenesis in mammalian cells is consistent with the production of oxidative stress. *Chem Res Toxicol* 20: 1031–1037

68 Rached E, Hoffmann D, Blumbach K, Weber K, Dekant W, Mally A (2008) Evaluation of putative biomarkers of nephrotoxicity after exposure to ochratoxin A *in vivo* and *in vitro*. *Toxicol Sci* 103: 371–381

69 Mantle PG, Nagy JM (2008) Binding of ochratoxin A to a urinary globulin: A new concept to account for gender difference in rat nephrocarcinogenic responses. *Int J Mol Sci* 9: 719–735

70 Assaf H, Azouri H, Pallardy M (2004) Ochratoxin A induces apoptosis in human lymphocytes through down regulation of Bcl-xL. *Toxicol Sci* 79: 335–344

71 Schumacher DM, Müller C, Metzler M, Lehmann L (2006) DNA-DNA cross-links contribute to the mutagenic potential of the mycotoxin patulin. *Toxicol Lett* 166: 268–275

72 Tsuda S, Kosaka Y, Murakami M, Matsuo H, Matsusaka N, Taniguchi K, Sasaki YF (1998) Detection of nivalenol genotoxicity in cultured cells and multiple mouse organs by the alkaline single-cell gel electrophoresis assay. *Mutat Res* 415: 191–200

73 Bony S, Olivier-Loiseau L, Carcelen M, Devaux A (2007) Genotoxic potential associated with low levels of the *Fusarium* mycotoxins nivalenol and fusarenon X in a human intestinal cell line. *Toxicol In Vitro* 21: 457–465

74 Wang JS, Groopman JD (1999) DNA damage by mycotoxins. *Mutat Res* 424: 167–181

75 Gelderblom WCA, Thiel PG, van der Merwe KJ (1984) Metabolic activation and deactivation of fusarin C, a mutagen produced by *Fusarium moniliforme*. *Biochem Pharmacol* 33: 1601–1603

76 Prelusky DB (1996) A study on the effect of deoxynivalenol on serotonin receptor binding in pig brain membranes. *J Environ Sci Health B* 31: 1103–1117

77 Prelusky DB, Trenholm HL (1993) The efficacy of various classes of anti-emetics in preventing deoxynivalenol-induced vomiting in swine. *Nat Toxins* 1: 296–302

78 Prelusky DB (1993) The effect of low-level deoxynivalenol on neurotransmitter levels measured in pig cerebral spinal fluid. *J Environ Sci Health* B 28: 731–761

79 Bondy GS, Pestka JJ (2000) Immunomodulation by fungal toxins. *J Toxicol Environ Health B* 3: 109–143

80 Wong SS, Zhou HR, Marin-Martinez ML, Brooks K, Pestka JJ (1998) Modulation of IL-1β, IL-6 and TNF-α secretion and mRNA expression by the trichothecene vomitoxin in the RAW 264.7 murine macrophage cell line. *Food Chem Toxicol* 36: 409–419

81 Yan D, Zhou HR, Brooks KH, Pestka JJ (1998) Role of macrophages in elevated IgA and IL-6 production by Peyer's patch cultures following acute oral vomitoxin exposure. *Toxicol Appl Pharmacol* 148: 261–273

82 Pestka JJ, Yon D, King LE (1994) Flow cytometric analysis of the effects of *in vitro* exposure to vomitoxin (deoxynivalenol) on apoptosis in murine T, B and IgA⁺ cells. *Food Chem Toxicol* 32: 1125–1136

83 Islam Z, King LE, Fraker PJ, Pestka JJ (2003) Differential induction of glucocorticoid-dependent apoptosis in murine lymphoid subpopulations *in vivo* following coexposure to lipopolysaccharide and vomitoxin (deoxynivalenol). *Toxicol Appl Pharmacol* 187: 69–79

84 Islam Z, Pestka JJ (2003) Role of IL-1β in endotoxin potentiation of deoxynivalenol-induced corticosterone response and leukocyte apoptosis in mice. *Toxicol Sci* 74: 93–102

85 Ueno Y (1983) Trichothecenes: Chemical, biological, and toxicological aspects. In: Y Ueno (ed.): *Trichothecenes*. Elsevier Press, Amsterdam, 135–146

86 Pestka JJ, Smolinski AT (2005) Deoxynivalenol: Toxicology and potential effects on humans. *J Toxicol Environ Health B Crit Rev* 8: 39–69

87 Yang GH, Jarvis BB, Chung YJ, Pestka JJ (2000) Apoptosis induction by the satratoxins and other trichothecene mycotoxins: Relationship to ERK, p38 MAPK, and SAPK/JNK activation. *Toxicol Appl Pharmacol* 164: 149–160

88 Zhou HR, Islam Z, Pestka JJ (2003) Rapid, sequential activation of mitogen-activated protein kinases and transcription factors precedes proinflammatory cytokine mRNA expression in spleens of mice exposed to the trichothecene vomitoxin. *Toxicol Sci* 72: 130–142

89 Zhou HR, Jia Q, Pestka JJ (2005) Ribotoxic stress response to the trichothecene deoxynivalenol in the macrophage involves the Src family kinase Hck. *Toxicol Sci* 85: 916–926

90 Zhou HR, Lau AS, Pestka JJ (2003) Role of double-stranded RNA-activated protein kinase R (PKR) in deoxynivalenol-induced ribotoxic stress response. *Toxicol Sci* 74: 335–344

91 Pestka JJ, Zhou HR (2003) Hck- and PKR-dependent mitogen-activated protein kinase phosphorylation and AP-1, C/EBP and NF-κB activation precedes deoxynivalenol-induced TNF-α and MIP-2 expression. *Toxicologist* 72: 121

92 Rizzo AF, Atroshi F, Ahotupa M, Sankari S, Elovaara E (1994) Protective effect of antioxidants against free radical-mediated lipid peroxidation induced by DON or T-2 toxin. *Zentralbl Veterinärmed A* 41: 81–90

93 Sun XM, Zhang XH, Wang HY, Cao WJ, Yan X, Zuo LF, Wang JL, Wang FR (2002) Effects of sterigmatocystin, deoxynivalenol and aflatoxin G_1 on apoptosis of human peripheral blood lymphocytes *in vitro*. *Biomed Environ Sci* 15: 145–152

94 Gray JS, Pestka JJ (2007) Transcriptional regulation of deoxynivalenol-induced IL-8 expression in human monocytes. *Toxicol Sci* 99: 502–511

95 Li M, Pestka JJ (2008) Comparative induction of 28S ribosomal RNA cleavage by ricin and the trichothecenes deoxynivalenol and T-2 toxin in the macrophage. *Toxicol Sci* 105: 67–78

96 Malekinejad H, Schoevers EJ, Daemen IJJM, Zijlstra C, Colenbrander B, Fink-Gremmels J, Ro BAJ (2007) Exposure of oocytes to the *Fusarium* toxins zearalenone and deoxynivalenol causes aneuploidy and abnormal embryo development in pigs. *Biol Reprod* 77: 840–847

97 Knasmuller S, Bresgen N, Kassie F, Mersch-Sundermann V, Gelderblom W, Zohrer E, Eckl PM (1997) Genotoxic effects of three *Fusarium* mycotoxins, fumonisin B1, moniliformin and vomitoxin in bacteria and in primary cultures of rat hepatocytes. *Mutat Res* 391: 39–48

98 Wang E, Norred WP, Bacon CW, Riley RT, Merrill AH Jr (1991) Inhibition of sphingolipid biosynthesis by fumonisins: Implications for diseases associated with *Fusarium moniliforme*. *J Biol Chem* 266: 14486–14490

99 Sorenson WG, Simpson J, Castranova V (1985) Toxicity of the mycotoxin patulin for rat peritoneal macrophages. *Environ Res* 38: 407–416

100 Bourdiol D, Escoula L, Salvayre R (1990) Effect of patulin on microbicidal activity of mouse peritoneal macrophages. *Food Chem Toxicol* 28: 29–33

101 Knaus HG, McManus OB, Lee SH, Schmalhofer WA, Garcia-Calvo M, Helms LMH, Sanchez M, Giangiacomo K, Reuben JP, Smith AB, Kaczorowski GJ, Garcia ML (1994) Tremorgenic indole alkaloids potently inhibit smooth muscle high-conductance calcium-activated potassium channels. *Biochemistry* 33: 5819–5828

102 Gallagher RT, Richard JL, Stahr HM, Cole RJ (1978) Cyclopiazonic acid production by aflatoxigenic and nonaflatoxigenic strains of *Aspergillus flavus*. *Mycopathologia* 66: 31–36

103 Dvorak R, Jagos J, Bouda J, Piskac A, Zapletal O (1977) Changes in the clinico-biochemical indices in the rumen liquor and urine in cases of experimental aflatoxicosis in dairy cows. *Vet Med (Prague)* 22: 161–169

104 Tung HT, Donaldson WE, Hamilton PB (1972) Altered lipid transport during aflatoxicosis. *Toxicol Appl Pharmacol* 22: 97–104

105 Osborne DJ, Hamilton PB (1981) Decreased pancreatic digestive enzymes during aflatoxicosis. *Poultry Sci* 60: 1818–1821

106 Bush RK, Portnoy JM, Saxon A, Terr AI, Wood RA (2006) The medical effects of mold exposure. *J Allergy Clin Immunol* 117: 326–333

107 Wood RA, Bush RK (2006) Reply. *J Allergy Clin Immunol* 118: 767

108 Lieberman A, Rea W, Curtis L (2006) Adverse health effects of indoor mold exposure. *J Allergy Clin Immunol* 118: 763

109 Strickland MHV (2006) How solid is the Academy position paper on mold exposure? *J Allergy Clin Immunol* 118: 763–764

110 Hardin BD, Kelman BJ, Saxon A (2007) Reply. *J Allergy Clin Immunol* 119: 256–257

111 Bouslimi A, Bouaziz C, Ayed-Boussema I, Hassen W, Bacha H (2008) Individual and combined

effects of ochratoxin A and citrinin on viability and DNA fragmentation in cultured Vero cells and on chromosome aberrations in mice bone marrow cells. *Toxicology* 251: 1–7

112 Orsi RB, Oliveira CAF, Dilkin P, Xavier JG, Direito GM, Corrêa B (2007) Effects of oral administration of aflatoxin B_1 and fumonisin B_1 in rabbits (*Oryctolagus cuniculus*). *Chem Biol Interact* 170: 201–208

113 Tammer B, Lehmann I, Nieber K, Altenburger R (2007) Combined effects of mycotoxin mixtures on human T cell function. *Toxicol Lett* 170: 124–133

114 Klarić MŠ, Pepeljnjak S, Domijan AM, Petrik J (2007) Lipid peroxidation and glutathione levels in porcine kidney PK15 cells after individual and combined treatment with fumonisin B_1, beauvericin and ochratoxin A. *Basic Clin Pharmacol Toxicol* 100: 157–164

115 Heussner AH, Dietrich DR, O'Brien E (2006) *In vitro* investigation of individual and combined cytotoxic effects of ochratoxin A and other selected mycotoxins on renal cells. *Toxicol In Vitro* 20: 332–341

116 Paterson RRM, Lima N (2009) How will climate change affect mycotoxins in food. *Food Res Int*, *in press*

Molecular, Clinical and Environmental Toxicology. Volume 2: Clinical Toxicology
Edited by A. Luch

Phycotoxins: chemistry, mechanisms of action and shellfish poisoning

Gian Paolo Rossini[1] and Philipp Hess[2]

[1] *Università di Modena e Reggio Emilia, Dipartimento di Scienze Biomediche, Italy*
[2] *IFREMER – Institut Français de Recherche pour l'Exploration de la Mer, Centre de Nantes, Département Environnement, Microbiologie et Phycotoxines, France*

Abstract. Phycotoxins are natural metabolites produced by micro-algae. Through accumulation in the food chain, these toxins may concentrate in different marine organisms, including filter-feeding bivalves, burrowing and grazing organisms, herbivorous and predatory fish. Human poisoning due to ingestion of seafood contaminated by phycotoxins has occurred in the past, and harmful algal blooms (HABs) are naturally occurring events. Still, we are witnessing a global increase in HABs and seafood contaminations, whose causative factors are only partially understood. Phycotoxins are small to medium-sized natural products and belong to many different groups of chemical compounds. The molecular mass ranges from ~300 to over 3000 Da, and the compound classes represented include amino acids, alkaloids and polyketides. Each compound group typically has several main compounds based on the same or similar structure. However, most groups also have several analogues, which are either produced by the algae or through metabolism in fish or shellfish or other marine organisms. The different phycotoxins have distinct molecular mechanisms of action. Saxitoxins, ciguatoxins, brevetoxins, gambierol, palytoxins, domoic acid, and, perhaps, cyclic imines, alter different ion channels and/or pumps at the level of the cell membrane. The normal functioning of neuronal and other excitable tissues is primarily perturbed by these mechanisms, leading to adverse effects in humans. Okadaic acid and related compounds inhibit serine/threonine phosphoprotein phosphatases, and disrupt major mechanisms controlling cellular functions. Pectenotoxins bind to actin filaments, and alter cellular cytoskeleton. The precise mechanisms of action of yessotoxins and azaspiracids, in turn, are still undetermined. The route of human exposure to phycotoxins is usually oral, although living systems may become exposed to phycotoxins through other routes. Based on recorded symptoms, the major poisonings recognized so far include paralytic, neurotoxic, amnesic, diarrheic shellfish poisonings, ciguatera, as well as palytoxin and azaspiracid poisonings.

Marine biotoxins in a changing environment

The term phycotoxin indicates natural metabolites produced by unicellular micro-algae (protists). Most phycotoxins are produced by dinoflagellates, although cyanobacteria have also been reported to produce saxitoxin; domoic acid is produced by diatoms. Some of the toxins were initially identified in associated organisms, e.g., okadaic acid in the sponge *Halichondria okadaii* [1], domoic acid in the red macroalga *Chondria armata* [2–5], or palytoxin in the soft coral *Palythoa toxica* [6].

Through accumulation in the food chain, these toxins may concentrate in a variety of marine organisms including filter-feeding bivalves, burrowing and grazing organisms (tunicates and gastropods) as well as herbivorous and predatory fish. All marine biotoxins described in this chapter have been selected because they are found in seafood and have been identified as bioactive compounds potentially causing seafood poisoning.

Human poisoning due to ingestion of seafood contaminated by phycotoxins has occurred in the past, and historical records as well as the habits of some populations in coastal and tropical areas show that harmful algal blooms (HABs) are naturally occurring events [7]. In the last 30 years HABs have attracted increasing attention from the scientific community and the society. The occurrence of episodes of human poisoning due to ingestion of toxic seafood involving tens or hundreds of people in several areas of the world [7] has certainly called for more attention to HABs and their consequences on human health. The increased awareness has supported more research efforts in the area, which are contributing to a better understanding of HABs and contamination of seafood by algal toxins, as well as the chemistry, mechanisms of action and toxicity of phycotoxins. The accumulation of information in this field has led to the conclusion that we are witnessing a global increase in HABs and seafood contamination, and more effective and complex measures to prevent human intoxications are being developed and implemented worldwide.

The increased recording of occurrence of toxic algae and HABs in coastal waters in several areas in the world is certainly a result of a deeper attention paid to the phenomenon. Other factors, however, are being recognized as contributing to the increasing frequency of HAB outbreaks, their appearance in areas of the world where they had not been recorded in the past, as well as the intensity and duration of HABs, with their possible consequences on seafood contamination and human intoxications/poisoning [7].

The ongoing changes can be exemplified by the trend of recording of *Ostreopsis* species in the Mediterranean Sea, which has been essentially anecdotic in the past century, in keeping with the mainly tropical distribution of these algal species. Over the last 5 years, blooms of *Ostreopsis* in several parts of Mediterranean Sea have been recorded (**Fig.** 1), and in some cases these have been accompanied by human intoxications involving up to two hundred people, e.g., in Italy in 2005 [8, 9].

The factors proposed to be involved in the global increase in HABs include the eutrophication of coastal waters as a consequence of increased aquaculture and fertilizer runoff from agriculture, as well as other economic activities linked to urbanization, the changes in climatic conditions, the transportation of toxic algae and their cysts from one coastal area to another as a consequence of their presence in the ballast water of ships or through the movement of shellfish stocks [7]. Furthermore, a recent meta-analysis of published data and historical records provided indications that the regional loss of species diversity and ecosystem services in coastal oceans increases the occurrence of algal blooms [10]. HABs and the contaminations of seafood, undoubtedly represent relevant social issues, because of the problems they pose to human

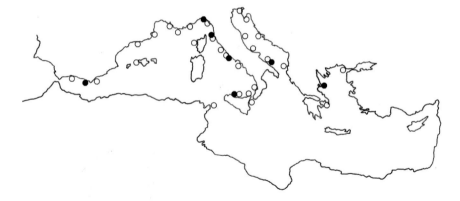

Figure 1. Records of *Ostreopsis* blooms in coastal areas of the Mediterranean Sea in the years 2000–2008. The map has been compiled on the basis of data reported in literature and of information kindly communicated by the Italian National Reference Laboratory for Marine Biotoxins (Cesenatico, Italy). The detection of *Ostreopsis* species is indicated by open symbols, whereas the record of health problems and intoxications that are suspected to be caused by the *Ostreopsis* blooms are indicated by the black symbols.

health, economic activities, recreation and tourism. The many facets of the phenomenon and their complexity represent a powerful drive for a better understanding of the chemistry and biology of phycotoxins, as a basis for a more effective protection of human health and the support of several human activities.

In this chapter we summarize available information on the chemistry, mechanisms of action of phycotoxins and the human poisoning they may cause. The complexity of the subject approached here, and the vast literature devoted to it, constrain our account to major issues. We apologize to the many scientists whose contributions have not been directly quoted in this chapter, and point the interested reader to excellent reviews devoted to specific topics, whenever appropriate.

Chemistry of marine biotoxins

Firstly, we should note that marine biotoxins are naturally produced compounds and, therefore, many enzymatic systems in nature are capable of metabolizing them. This characteristic puts them in contrast to man-made compounds such as polychlorinated biphenyls (PCBs) and pesticides many of which are extremely stable compounds for which nature has no metabolic processes foreseen. Similar to PCBs, dioxins or polycyclic hydrocarbons, most groups of marine toxins have also many analogues. Thus, between naturally produced analogues and metabolites of these, marine biotoxins constitute a vast array of bioactive chemicals.

Historic perspective on the isolation of marine biotoxins

Although the effects of marine toxins have been known for hundreds of years, the toxic principles involved were not discovered until the 20th century. The identification and characterization has been a lengthy process for some toxins. For instance, in the late 19th century, reports describe paralytic shellfish poisoning (PSP) as a poisoning caused by the consumption of blue mussels [11], the toxic principles of which also occur in starfish [12], without the identity of toxic principles being revealed. Groundbreaking work was completed by Sommer and Meyer [13] to link this toxicity to the occurrence of micro-algae and to conceive an assay that has remained the reference tool to our days, the mouse bioassay for paralytic toxins. Onoue et al. [14] started work on the isolation of saxitoxin analogues as the toxic principles of PSP. The efforts were significantly advanced by Schantz et al. [15, 16]. However, it was not until 40 years after initial isolation efforts that the structure of saxitoxin was finally confirmed by Wong et al. [17]. The characterization process has been hampered for many toxins in a similar fashion due to the lack of compound mass for the studies. This lack can be understood from the fact that the organisms producing the toxin cannot always be cultured, and scientists thus rely on the natural occurrence of the compounds. In addition, the structure elucidation in early days was mostly based on chemical reaction of the compounds. The onset of more powerful non-destructive techniques such as nuclear magnetic resonance (NMR) has allowed the characterization of smaller quantities: while several hundreds of milligrams were required to characterize a toxin in the 1950/60s, nowadays 10–100 µg of compound may be sufficient to complete the structure elucidation of a novel compound. Thus, the discovery of domoic acid as a shellfish toxin was completed within weeks from the poisoning event [18]. More typically, it takes one to several years from the initial poisoning event to the identification of the chemical responsible for the toxic effect, e.g., for the identification of okadaic acid and azaspiracids [19, 20].

Chemical nature of marine biotoxins

This section describes the characteristics of a selected range of marine biotoxins to demonstrate the wide-ranging chemical diversity of these groups of compounds. From a natural products or biosynthesis point of view, the compounds described in this section belong to several classes including amino acids (domoic acid), alkaloids (saxitoxin) and polyketides (all others). Therefore, algal toxins are often referred to as small molecules. Thus, the selection of toxins excludes all compounds that are typically referred to as natural polymers (proteins, carbohydrates, nucleic acids). Indeed the molecular mass of phycotoxins typically ranges between 300 and 1500 Da; nevertheless, some compound groups such as palytoxins and maitotoxins are very sizeable molecules of 2677 and 3422 Da, respectively. Maitotoxin has been reported as the largest non-proteinaceous natural toxin. The chemical nature and molecular size classification distinguish phycotoxins from the very large group of venoms from snakes, spiders or cone snails which are typically very potent mixtures of proteinaceous toxins. Table 1 gives an overview of some characteristics of the compound groups discussed in the specific sections.

In addition to the above-mentioned difficulties in isolation of a toxin for its initial identification, it should be noted that one of the problems with natural compounds is the possible co-occurrence of isomers (compounds with the same molecular weight but slightly different structural arrangements) and analogues (compounds that derive from the same structural skeleton but have some structural difference leading to a different molecular weight). The term "analogue" is often used synonymously with the terms "metabolite" or "derivative" (see also section below, "common routes of metabolism"). While the framework of this chapter is too limited to exhaustively describe all known analogues of the toxin groups dealt with, we give some examples of the complexity of analogues for several groups in the specific section (e.g., saxitoxin, okadaic acid and pectenotoxins). All toxin groups have 10 or more analogues, often up to 30 or more.

Saxitoxins

Saxitoxin (STX)-group toxins are closely related compounds based on a tetrahydro purine skeleton. The basic character of the hydro purine group renders the molecule highly water soluble. More than 30 saxitoxins, mainly from marine dinoflagellates and shellfish that feed on toxic algae, have been identified [21–23], at least 18 have toxicological relevance (Fig. 2). They are mainly produced by dinoflagellates belonging to the genus *Alexandrium*, e.g., *A. tamarensis*, *A. minutum* (syn. *A. excavata*), *A. catenella*, *A. fraterculus*, *A. fundyense* and *A. cohorticula*. Also other dinoflagellates such as *Pyrodinium bahamense* and *Gymnodinium catenatum* have been identified as sources of STX-group toxins [21]. In addition, some analogues have been identified in some cyanobacteria which may occur in fresh and brackish waters.

STX analogues do not exhibit a strong ultraviolet (UV) absorbance or fluorescence. They are typically stable to heat treatment up to 100 °C. Different acid and base treatments will lead to various transformations. In particular, all C11-epimeric pairs (e.g., GTX2 and 3 or GTX1 and 4) will interconvert and equilibrate to a constant ratio at high pH. Similarly, carbamoyl and sulfocarbamoyl derivatives will convert to decarbamoyl (dc) analogues through cleavage of the carbamoyl-ester group at high pH (e.g., GTX2 or C1 to dc-GTX2 and GTX3 or C2 to dc-GTX3). Under acidic conditions, the carbamoylester is relatively stable but the sulfate ester will be cleaved to convert sulfocarbamoyl groups into carbamoyl groups (e.g., C1 to GTX2 and C2 to GTX3). These transformations may only occur partially when shellfish tissues or human tissues or fluids contaminated with STXs are exposed to these conditions, as biological tissues typically buffer the pH. Since conversion reactions can result in a several fold increase in toxicity, a potential danger of these toxins was suggested [24]. To

Table 1. Characteristics of marine biotoxins: chemical formula, molecular weights, UV-absorption maxima, acidity constants and lipophilicity

Toxin	Chemical class	Formula	Molar weight	UV [nm]	pKa$_{1,2,3,4}$	Lipophilicity
Saxitoxin (STX)	Tetrahydro-purine alkaloid	$C_{10}H_{17}N_7O_4$	299	n/a	8.1, 11.5	Hydrophilic
Domoic acid (DA)	Cyclic amino acid, 3 carboxy groups	$C_{15}H_{21}NO_6$	311	242	2.1, 3.7, 5.0, 9.8	Hydrophilic
Okadaic acid (OA)	Polyether, spiro-keto assembly	$C_{44}H_{68}O_{13}$	804	n/a	4.9[§]	Lipophilic
Azaspiracid (AZA)	Polyether, second amine, 3-spiro-ring	$C_{47}H_{71}NO_{12}$	841	n/a	5.8[§]	Lipophilic
Palytoxin (PlTX)[*]	Polyether, 2 amide & a primary amine	$C_{129}H_{223}N_3O_{54}$	2677	263, 233	n/rep	Amphiphilic
Pectenotoxin-2 (PTX2)	Polyether, ester macrocycle	$C_{47}H_{70}O_{14}$	858	235	n/a[§]	Lipophilic
Gymnodimine	Cyclic imine, macrocycle	$C_{32}H_{45}NO_4$	507	n/a	n/rep	Lipophilic
Prorocentrolide	Cyclic imine, lactone macrocycle	$C_{56}H_{85}NO_{13}$	979	n/rep	n/rep	Lipophilic
13-Desmethyl Spirolide C	Cyclic imine, macrocycle	$C_{41}H_{61}NO_7$	691	n/a	n/rep	Lipophilic
Yessotoxin (YTX)	Ladder-shaped polyether	$C_{55}H_{82}O_{21}S_2$	1140	230	n/rep, 6.9[§]	Amphiphilic
Brevetoxin (BTX)-B	Ladder-shaped polyether	$C_{50}H_{70}O_{14}$	894	208	n/a	Lipophilic
Gambierol (Gb)	Ladder-shaped polyether	$C_{43}H_{64}O_{11}$	757	n/rep	n/a	Lipophilic
P-Ciguatoxin (CTX)-4B	Ladder-shaped polyether	$C_{60}H_{85}O_{16}$	1061	223	n/a	Lipophilic
Maitotoxin	Polyether, four fused ring systems	$C_{164}H_{256}O_{68}S_2Na_2$	3422	230	n/rep	Amphiphilic

[*] Palytoxin from *Palythoa toxica*

[§] Fux and Hess (unpublished observations) determined chromatographically (for YTX the pKa$_1$ was too low to be determined chromatographically, pKa$_2$ is given).

n/a, not applicable; n/rep, not reported

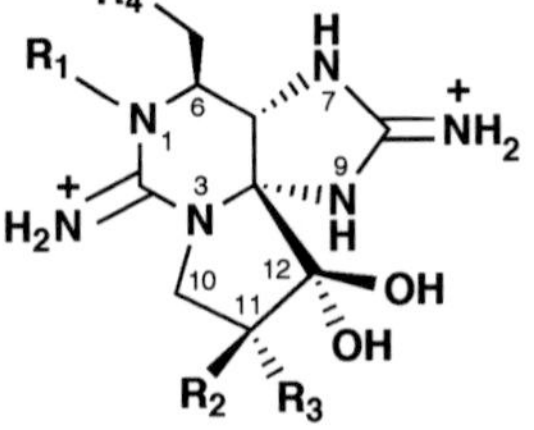

R_1	R_2	R_3	R_4	Toxin
H	H	H	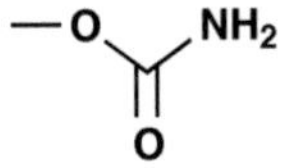	STX
H	H	OSO_3^-		GTX2
H	OSO_3^-	H		GTX3
OH	H	H		NEO
OH	H	OSO_3^-		GTX1
OH	OSO_3^-	H		GTX4
H	H	H	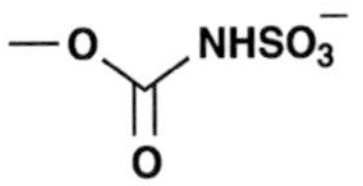	GTX5 (B1)
H	H	OSO_3^-		C1
H	OSO_3^-	H		C2
OH	H	H		GTX6 (B2)
OH	H	OSO_3^-		C3
OH	OSO_3^-	H		C4
H	H	H		dc-STX
H	H	OSO_3^-		dc-GTX2
H	OSO_3^-	H		dc-GTX3
OH	H	H		dc-NEO
OH	H	OSO_3^-		dc-GTX1
OH	OSO_3^-	H		dc-GTX4

Figure 2. Saxitoxins.

examine this phenomenon experimentally, B1 (GTX5) was incubated at conditions simulating the human stomach and analyzed by the mouse bioassay. After 5-h incubation at 37 °C, a twofold increase of toxicity corresponding to 9% conversion of toxin was observed in the artificial gastric juice at pH 1.1 and no apparent increase of toxicity in rat gastric juice at pH 2.2 [25].

The marine organisms most often affected are mussels and oysters, but also puffer fish and marine snails (e.g., abalone) have been reported to accumulate dangerous concentrations. The hydrophilic character of the compounds may partially explain the relatively rapid depuration of these toxins from mussels.

This rapid depuration complicates the regulatory surveillance for these toxins, which is therefore usually complemented by observations of the algae responsible for *in situ* production.

Complex toxin profiles, possible conversions and lack of reference materials have led most countries to maintain the mouse bioassay introduced by Sommer and Meyer [13] and validated as AOAC method (959.08) [26]. This assay can be used for the quantitation of levels above 350–400 µg/kg. Alternative methods have been proposed based on chromatography and fluorescence detection by Oshima [27], and Lawrence et al. [28], the latter also being officially validated as AOAC method (2005.06) [29]. These HPLC methods are technically challenging, time consuming and depend on a continuous supply of a large number of toxin standards as reference compounds. Due to the hydrophilic character of STXs, their complete chromatographic separation proved difficult until the introduction of hydrophilic interaction chromatography by Dell'Aversano et al. [30]. Also, the physicochemical determination of STXs has relatively high quantification limits, which are slightly lower than or similar to the detection limits of the mouse bioassay for complex toxin profiles.

Domoic acid group
Domoic acid (DA) is a small cyclic amino acid (311 Da), with three carboxylic acid groups (Fig. 3). These groups are responsible for its solubility in water and its relatively high polarity, resulting in early elution in reverse-phase chromatography [31]. The acid constants (pKa) of the three carboxylic acids and the cyclic amino group have been determined using NMR techniques by Walter et al. [32] (Tab. 1). Although numerous isomers and several analogues have been reported [33–38], so far only DA and its C5-diastereomer have been

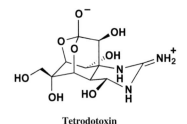

Domoic acid

Tetrodotoxin

Figure 3. Small water-soluble toxins: domoic acid (DA) and tetrodotoxin (TTX).

shown to be of toxicological relevance [39]. DA transforms into its diastereo-mer through heat or long-term storage [40] and analysis has focused on determination of the sum of these two isomers as best estimate of the total toxicity. A conjugated double bond in the aliphatic side chain allows detection of DA by UV absorbance and both UV and MS detection are commonly used for the physicochemical determination of DA [41]. The conjugated double bond also leads to light sensitivity and is the cause of radical-mediated oxidative metab-olism. As a contaminant in shellfish tissues, DA is heat stable and cooking does not typically destroy the toxin. However, protein coagulation leads to retraction of the tissues and DA as a water-soluble compound may be trans-ferred significantly to cooking fluids [42]. Its stability under various condi-tions has been studied, and storage of raw or autoclaved tissues only resulted in ca. 50% degradation of the toxin after 5 months [43].

Domoic acid has been reported in a wide variety of seafoods, including mussels, scallops and anchovies. Due to the common occurrence of its source organism (the diatom *Pseudo-nitzschia* spp.), DA is spread worldwide. Thanks to the lightly diarrheic properties caused by the macro-alga *Chondria armata* (of which DA is the active ingredient), it has been used in Japan as anti-worm-ing agent (reviewed in [39]). However, the severe poisoning in 1987 in Canada of over 100 people following consumption of mussels, including 3 fatalities, stopped this practice. The water-soluble character also results in relatively rapid depuration from shellfish (similar to STX), and regulatory surveillance is complemented by screening of shellfish production waters for *Pseudo-nitzschia* to allow early warning in an attempt to prevent human poisoning.

Azaspiracid group
Azaspiracid (AZA1) is an intermediately sized polyether toxin (841 Da, Fig. 4). The chemistry, ecology and toxicology of AZAs have been extensive-

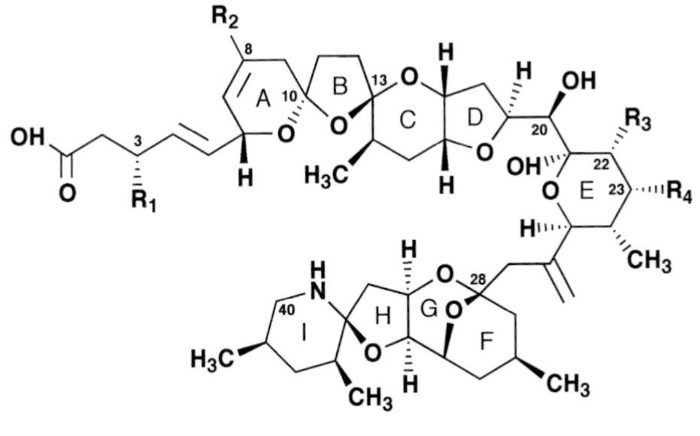

Azaspiracids

Figure 4. Azaspiracids: AZA1 ($R_{1,2,4}$ = H; R_3 = CH$_3$), AZA2 ($R_{1,4}$ = H; $R_{2,3}$ = CH$_3$). The initial structure proposed by Satake et al. [20] was corrected by Nicolaou et al. [51, 52]. The corrected structure is shown.

ly reviewed by Twiner et al. [44]. Although its geographical distribution was initially believed to be restricted to Europe, recent work has also demonstrated the compound in shellfish from North Africa, and in Canadian waters [44, 45]. AZA2 has recently also been identified in the sponge *Echinoclathria* sp., collected from Japanese waters, indicating that its producers occur worldwide [46]. However, so far poisoning directly attributed to AZA has only been reported from Europe, either due to environmental conditions not being appropriate for the producer to reach seafood in other locations, or due to the predominant screening for marine biotoxins with the mouse bioassay, an intrinsically unspecific method of detection of toxins. Also, the symptoms of AZA in human poisoning events are similar to diarrheic shellfish poisoning (DSP) from okadaic acid group compounds, and may therefore not always be followed up with further investigation. The mouse bioassay, initially introduced by Yasumoto et al. [19], for the detection of DSP toxins, also detects AZAs at similar levels [47].

Chemically, AZA is characterized by a cyclic amine group, a carboxylic acid and a unique tri-spiro ring assembly. Similar to okadaic acid, it is likely that the acid-labile character of the compound is related to the spiro-keto assembly (rings A, B and C in Fig. 4) [48]. Contrarily to okadaic acid, AZAs are also labile to strong bases, i.e., their destruction can be completed in methanolic solution through treatment with NaOH for 10 min at 76 °C. The mechanism for this reaction remains to be clarified. Due to the absence of conjugated double bonds or aromatic rings, the molecule has no chromophore or specific UV absorbance above 200 nm; therefore, physicochemical determination is mostly based on separation by liquid chromatography (LC) followed by detection using mass spectrometry (MS). An initial proposal of the chemical structure was made by Satake et al. [20], but a correction was made after chemical synthesis by Nicolaou et al. [49–52]. Approximately 20 analogues have been reported to occur naturally in shellfish [53]. However, only two of these, AZA1 and AZA2, have been reported to be produced by the previously unknown dinoflagellate *Azadinium spinosum* [54, 55]. Due to the minuscule nature of the causative organism (<20 μm), it cannot be easily identified using light microscopy and had only been discovered 12 years after the first poisoning event that was attributed to this toxin group [56]. The metabolism of AZA1 and AZA2 in mussels is presumed to follow an oxidative path at C3 and C23 and the methyl group at C22. Following the initial observation by Hess et al. [57] of increased AZA concentrations after heat treatment of AZA-contaminated mussel tissues, McCarron et al. [58] postulated that a carboxylic acid located at C22 is a product of such metabolism and that heat treatment leads to decarboxylation and further analogues of AZAs. In shellfish it is anticipated that the decarboxylation happens spontaneously over time. There are no reports on mammalian metabolism of AZAs. From the lipophilic nature of AZAs (Fux and Hess, unpublished observations), it is presumed that AZAs can pass the intestinal barrier, if they are sufficiently bioavailable. Stomach simulation experiments by Rehmann et al. [53] and Alfonso et al. [48] suggest that there may be limited bioavailability due to the lipophilic character of AZA1; however, further *in vivo* studies will be required to clarify such behavior. Initial evaluation of the compounds using intraperitoneal (i.p.) injection in mouse bioassays suggests that the hydroxyl analogues are less toxic than the parent compounds [59]. Further structure-activity studies by Ito et al. [60] showed that a synthetic stereoisomer of AZA1 (C_{1-20} epi-AZA1) was three to four times less toxic than AZA1, and that a variety of smaller epitopes did not induce any effect similar to AZA1, thus suggesting that the entire skeleton is required to effectively interact with the biological target.

Okadaic acid group
Okadaic acid (OA) was originally found in the sponge *Halichondria okadaii* [1] but was only identified by Yasumoto et al. [19] as a shellfish contaminant following a series of poisoning events in 1976 (Fig. 5). In 1980, Yasumoto et al. [61] clearly demonstrated that DSP was associated with blooms of *Dinophysis fortii*, a dinoflagellate in which the authors also isolated an ana-

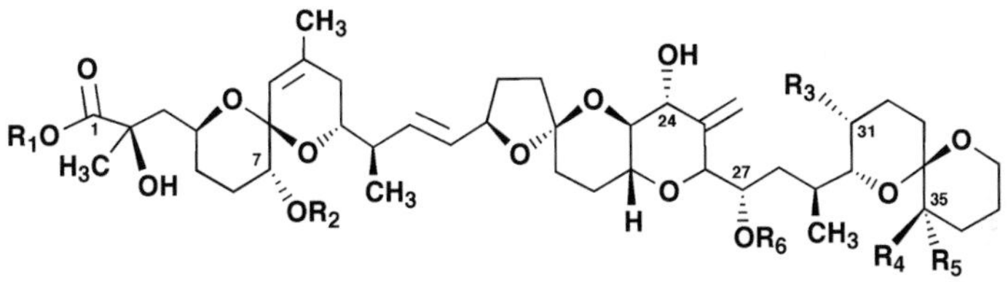

Toxin	R_1	R_2	R_3	R_4	R_5	R_6
OA	H	H	CH_3	H	H	H
DTX1	H	H	CH_3	CH_3	H	H
DTX2	H	H	H	H	CH_3	H
DTX3	H	acyl	as parent	as parent	as parent	H
Diol-ester	diol	H/acyl	as parent	as parent	as parent	H
DTX4	diol-ester	H	as parent	as parent	as parent	H
DTX5	diol-ester	H	as parent	as parent	as parent	H
27-*O*-acyl	H	H	CH_3	H	H	acyl

Figure 5. Okadaic acid (OA) and dinophysistoxin (DTX) derivatives; stereochemistry at C31 and C35 was clarified by Larsen et al. [313]. OA, DTX1 and DTX2 are the parent compounds independently produced by micro-algae. All other compounds listed are derivatives of these three, either identified in algae or in shellfish. DTX3-type compounds are ester derivatives (acyl group at C7–OH) of OA, DTX1 or DTX2 that have only been found in shellfish so far. Diol esters, DTX4 and DTX5 are derivatives of either OA, DTX1 or DTX2 detected in algae (but some recently in shellfish as well). The 27-*O*-acyl derivative has so far only been identified in a sponge.

logue of OA, dinophysistoxin-1 (DTX1). The same compound class was rapidly found as the causative agents of DSP in Europe [62]. Dinophysistoxin-2 (DTX2) has been discovered as a third main analogue by Hu et al. [63], explaining shellfish toxicity found in Irish mussels. OA and DTXs are produced by a variety of different dinoflagellates from the *Dinophysis* and *Prorocentrum* genera, including *D. acuta* and *D. acuminata*, as well as *P. lima* and *P. belizeanum*. Although the toxins of the OA group have been mainly reported from Japan and Europe, recent evidence in the gulf of Mexico demonstrates that *Dinophysis* in these regions may also produce the same compounds under appropriate environmental conditions [64]. Therefore, a global distribution of these toxins is now widely accepted and monitoring should occur during shellfish production.

Chemically, OA is one of the many polyether toxins among the phycotoxins (Fig. 5). Its structure is characterized by a carboxylic acid group and three spiro-keto ring assemblies, one which connects a five with a six-membered ring. OA, DTX1 and DTX2 withstand a wide pH range from mildly acidic to strongly basic, e.g., no degradation is found for up to 40 min at 76 °C in 0.3 M methanolic NaOH solution. Treatment with strong mineral acids, e.g., HCl, leads to rapid degradation: OA and DTX1 are completely destroyed within 20 min at 76 °C of 0.3 M methanolic HCl, even in the presence of shellfish matrix in the extract. However, without the addition of acid, the compounds are rather stable to heat. Also, recent work on stomach simulation experiments in the author's laboratory suggests that the food itself has a buffering capacity on the acid and the toxins may not be destroyed significantly in the gastric juice. In normal cooking procedures the toxins are not destroyed, although the coagulation of proteins in shellfish tissues may lead to redistribution within the organs of shellfish and some toxins may be released into the cooking fluids [65].

Different types of esters of OA and DTXs have been reported. In algae (so far mainly *P. lima* and *P. belizeanum*), esters of allylic diols with the carboxylic acid at C1 of OA and DTXs have been reported [63, 66, 67]; these esters were named DTX4, DTX5, etc. When the algae enter shellfish through natural filter-feeding, it is believed that these esters are rapidly degraded [68]. The shellfish then further metabolize OA and its analogues to form esters of OA and DTXs with fatty acids (at the C7–OH group). These esters were initially identified for DTX1 as shellfish derivatives [69] and their toxicity has been described to be similar to the parent compounds, although the onset appears later in the i.p. mouse model [70]. A further fatty acid ester of DTX1 at the C27–OH group has been reported in a sponge [71], and most recently, Torgersen et al. [72] also reported mixed esters of diols (at the C1 carboxyl end) and fatty acids (at the C7–OH position) in shellfish, suggesting that partial degradation and simultaneous metabolism may co-occur during digestion of algae by shellfish. The multitude of compounds potentially present in shellfish (free toxins, diol esters and their derivatives, fatty acids and mixtures of diol and fatty acid esters) leads to difficulty in determining the complete toxin content in shellfish samples. This complexity has added to the difficulties in estimating the potency of these toxins and evaluation of their risk. The ester bond has not shown any degradation in long-term stability studies in the authors' laboratory; however, fatty acids have been reported to oxidize easily if they contain double bonds. Any of the esters discussed above (either at the C1–carboxyl or at the C7–OH) may be quantitatively cleaved through treatment with strong base, e.g., 0.3 M methanolic NaOH at 76 °C for 10–40 min; this characteristic, in combination with the stability of the parent compounds (OA, DTX1 and DTX2) to base treatment, has been extensively used to quantitatively determine the equivalent of parent compound present in any given shellfish sample [73].

A recent review of recorded poisoning events suggests that esters of OA and DTXs have very similar toxicity to the parent compounds in human poisoning [74]. OA and DTX1 are considered to be of approximately equal toxicity when injected i.p. into mice, while DTX2 has been reported to have only ~50–60% of the toxicity of OA [75], both by i.p. injection into mice and by assessment of their inhibitory character towards phosphoprotein phosphatases (see section "Mechanism of action of ocadaic acid and related compounds" below).

Pectenotoxin group
Pectenotoxins (PTXs, Fig. 6) are produced by *Dinophysis*, one of the main producers of OA and analogues. Pectenotoxin-2 (PTX2) is the main compound produced by *Dinophysis*. For this reason, PTXs were initially associated with diarrheic poisoning; however, subsequent studies clearly demonstrated that PTXs have a distinct mechanism of action that differs from that of OA and analogues (see section "Mechanism of action of pectenotoxins" below). PTXs are a group of polyethers with molecular weights similar to the OA and AZA groups, and PTXs also have two spiro-ketal ring assemblies. Contrarily to OA and AZA, active forms of PTXs represent a macrocyclic intramolecular ester and do not possess a free carboxylic acid group (Fig. 6). Thus, PTX2 behaves chromatographically like a neutral compound of high lipophilicity (Fux and Hess, unpublished observations). A comprehensive review of the occurrence, chemistry and shellfish metabolism of PTX analogues is given by Miles [76]. We describe here several analogues that exemplify the three main routes of metabolism in shellfish. In the Japanese scallop (*Patinopecten yessoensis*), PTX2 is successively metabolized to PTX1, PTX3 and finally PTX6 [77]. In all these analogues the macrocycle is maintained, which means their lipophilicity is only slightly altered. In contrast, in mussels (*Mytilus edulis*), PTX2 is metabolized to a seco-acid (PTX2sa), in which the macrocycle is opened [78]. This ring opening is clearly related to a loss in the bioactivity, as PTX2sa shows no activity when injected i.p. in mice. A further route of metabolism in mussels is the esterification of PTX2sa with fatty acids to yield PTX2sa fatty acid esters [79]. Although the toxicity of these compounds has not yet been evaluated, it is anticipated that it is relatively reduced as the parent PTX2sa already does not show any toxicity. Ito et al. [80], also showed evidence for a reduced oral tox-

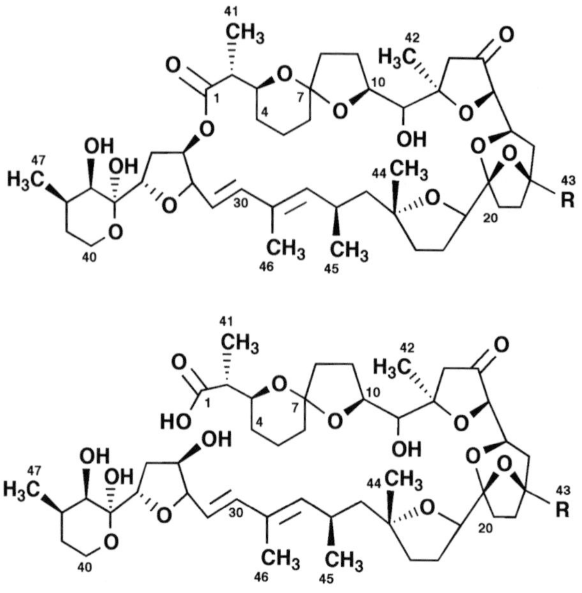

Figure 6. Pectenotoxins. The complete macrocyclic ester of the PTX2 structure (and its derivatives) is shown in the top panel while the bottom-figure depicts the structure of the hydrolyzed seco-acid (sa) compound (PTX2sa), where the macrocycle is opened. C_7, configuration at position C7.

Toxin	R (position 43)	C_7
PTX1	CH_2OH	7R
PTX2	CH_3	7R
PTX3	CHO	7R
PTX4	CH_2OH	7S
PTX6	COOH	7R
PTX7	COOH	7S
PTX2sa	CH_3	7R
7-epi-PTX2sa	CH_3	7S

icity of PTX6, compared to PTX2, thereby suggesting that the main issue with pectenotoxins would be the presence of still non-metabolized PTX2. It is not clear whether such remaining PTX2 is bioavailable (due to its high lipophilicity it may not be effectively liberated during human digestion of shellfish tissues) or whether it withstands human digestive conditions. PTX2 has been shown to be rather labile, even under lightly acidic or lightly basic conditions and very rapid metabolism to non-toxic seco acids is likely if the compound is effectively liberated during digestion.

Yessotoxin group

Yessotoxin (YTX) and analogues are also polycyclic ether compounds; special characteristics consist of the 11 contiguously transfused ether rings, an unsaturated side chain and two sulfate ester groups (Fig. 7). The contiguously transfused rings make YTX and analogues chemical relatives of brevetoxins and ciguatoxins; this structural characteristic has also led to the classification of ladder-shaped polyethers. Although this rigid structure constitutes a rather unpolar part of the molecule, YTX is considered of intermediate lipophilicity, as it also features two sulfate ester groups. The biogenetic origin, its chemistry, synthesis and structure-activity relationships of analogues have been recently reviewed by Hess and Aasen [81].

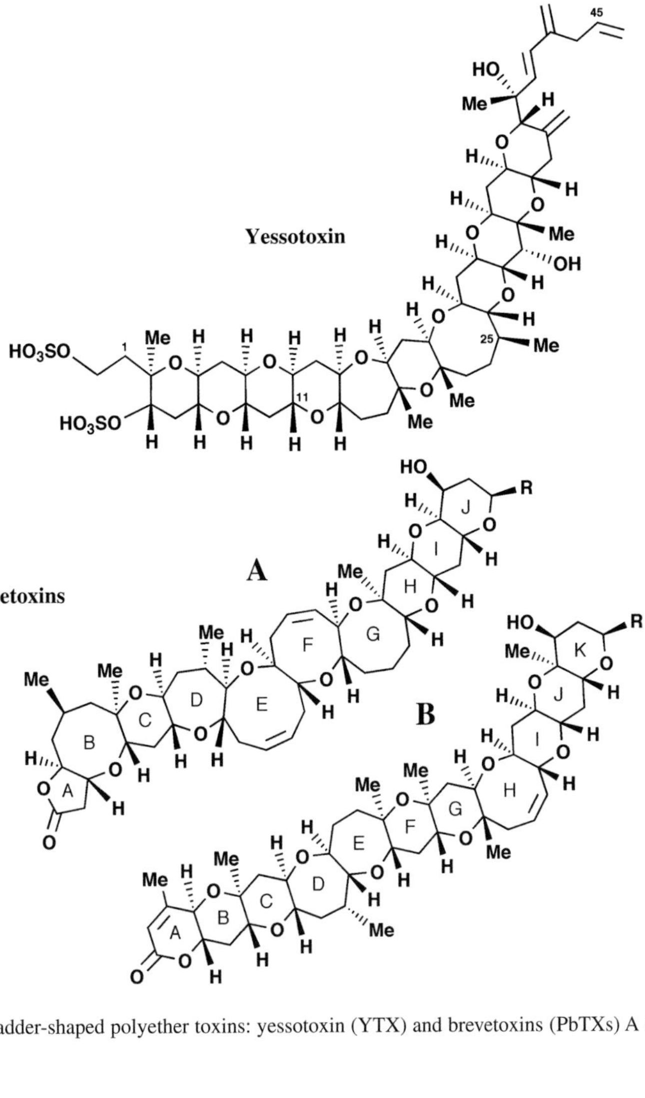

Figure 7. Ladder-shaped polyether toxins: yessotoxin (YTX) and brevetoxins (PbTXs) A and B.

YTX was first isolated from the digestive glands of scallops *Patinopecten yessoensis* in Japan [82]. Because of its discovery through the mouse bioassay originally developed for the detection of DSP [19], and due to its frequent co-occurrence with truly diarrheic toxins, YTX was initially mis-classified as one of the DSP toxins. Later, it was shown that YTX does not cause diarrheic effects when administered orally to mice [83–85]. Yessotoxin and its analogues are produced by the dinoflagellate algae *Protoceratium reticulatum* [86–89], *Lingulodinium polyedrum* [90] and, as recently reported, also by *Gonyaulax spinifera* [91]. Since the initial discovery of YTX, several more analogues of YTXs have been discovered in many parts of the world including Japan, Norway, Italy, Scotland and Chile [92]. Over the last few years, this toxin group has been shown to contain a large number of analogues, including 45-hydroxy-YTX, carboxy-YTX, 1-desulfo-YTX, homo-YTX, 45-hydroxy-homo-YTX, carboxyhomo-YTX, heptanor-41-oxo-YTX, heptanor-41-oxo-homo-YTX, trinor-YTX, adriatoxin, (44-*R,S*)-44,55-dihydroxy-YTX, and 9-methyl-YTXs [93]. Miles et al. [94] have described numerous analogues of YTX in *P. reticulatum*.

Although different toxicities have been reported for YTX itself when using different mouse strains (e.g., [82, 83]), crude estimates of relative toxicities can be obtained when using the same strain of mice for comparison of analogues, preferably in parallel. In this way, it is clear that YTX and homo-YTX have approximately the same toxicity [95], and that all other analogues have lesser toxicity than YTX, with hydroxyl and carboxy derivatives being approximately five times less toxic than the parent compounds. Some derivatives such as the trihydroxylated amides of 41-a-homo-YTX and the 1,3-enone isomer of heptanor-41-oxo-YTX have not shown any toxicity by i.p. injection into mice at levels >5000 µg/kg body weight [96, 97].

Another major pharmacological phenomenon directly related to the chemical structure is the large difference observed between toxicity of YTX in mice injected i.p. and those orally exposed to YTX [83]. This study showed that two out of three mice died when injected with a dose of 0.75 mg YTX/kg body weight, and three of three mice died when injected with a dose of 1 mg YTX/kg body weight, while all mice survived when exposed orally to a dose of 10 mg/kg. Similar observations were made by Munday and coworkers (quoted in [21]). The difference in i.p. and oral toxicity of YTX is probably related to low YTX absorption in the gastrointestinal tract. While the solubility of YTX in water facilitates bioavailability of YTX, it is probably also the reason for very short residence time in the gastrointestinal tract, thus diminishing overall absorption. The large differences in toxicity between YTX and its oxidized analogues 45-hydroxy-YTX and carboxy-YTX are likely to be related to the further increase in water solubility. A different approach to determining the relationship between structure and activity was taken by Ferrari et al. [98], where different YTX analogues were dosed onto cultured cells. The authors obtained different toxic equivalence factors with the 45-hydroxy and the 55-carboxy analogues being ~20–50 times less toxic. These differences could be related to the more complex toxicology in live animals or to differences in the standards used.

Palytoxin group

With a continuous chain of 115 carbons, palytoxin (PlTX) is one of the largest polyether-type phycotoxins (Fig. 8). The many hydroxyl groups in the molecule characterize it as a polyol and together with the amine and amide groups are responsible for its hydrophilicity. The long carbon chain constitutes a lipophilic part. Thus, PlTX has a mixed hydrophilic and lipophilic character that also results in soap-like behavior at larger concentrations in aqueous solutions. The structure of PlTX was clarified in 1981 [99–101]. Recent reviews demonstrate that there is a lack of understanding on possible origins of PlTX and related compounds [102, 103]. While the compound was originally reported from the coelenterate zoanthids *Palythoa toxica* [6] and *Palythoa tuberculosa* [104], it is now clear that some micro-algae (*Ostreopsis siamensis* [105], *Ostreopsis ovata* [106] and *Ostreopsis mascarenensis* [107]) also produce PlTX and a number of related compounds. Symbiotic micro-organisms have been postulated as the true source of PlTX [108, 109] and bacterial involvement is still not excluded [110]. This toxin group was traditionally associated with fish poisoning and aerosol problems in the tropics. More recently, *Ostreopsis* spp. as well as PlTX and related compounds were also found in Southern Europe (Spain, Italy and Greece), mostly causing problems to people bathing at beaches on the Italian coast of Genoa [111], and by mouse assays of shellfish from Greece [112].

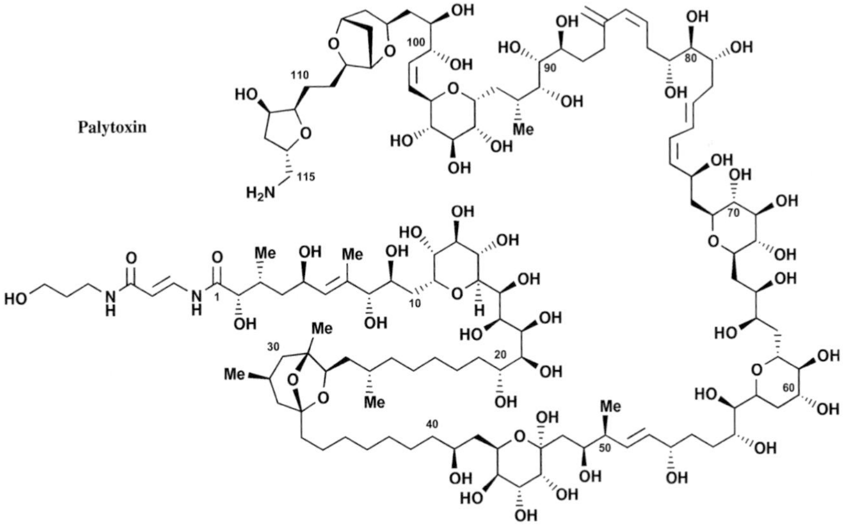

Figure 8. Palytoxin (PlTX).

Cyclic imines

Several compound groups have been found in this category: gymnodimines, spirolides, pinnatoxins and pteriatoxins, pinnaic acids and halichlorines, prorocentrolides and symbio-imines [67, 113–116]. A selection of chemical structures for some of these groups are shown in Figure 9. A common structural feature of all these compound groups is the hexa- or heptacyclic imine ring, which is believed to contribute substantially to the bioactivity of these compounds. Using spirolides as an example, the opening of this ring has been related to loss of bioactivity [117]. However, this is not the only contributing factor as intricate stereochemical features may also play important roles, as demonstrated by McCauley et al. [118]. They were able to show that natural (+)-pinnatoxin A was very toxic, while synthetic (–)-pinnatoxin A was non-toxic. The unique neurotoxicity of cyclic imines is visible in mice following i.p. injection of the toxin, which leads to rapid death within minutes; this feature has led to grouping cyclic imines together as "fast-acting toxins". Due to the structural variety of the group, it is difficult to give physicochemical details in the frame

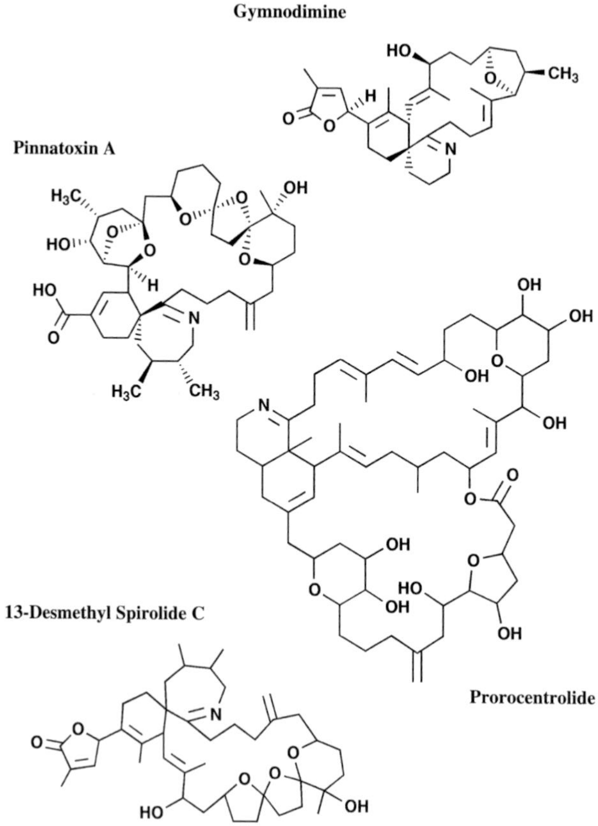

Figure 9. Cyclic imines.

of this chapter. Recent reviews give an overview of the chemistry and toxicology of these groups [119–121].

Brevetoxin group

Brevetoxins are a group of polyether toxins produced by the dinoflagellate *Karenia brevis*, and they also belong to the class of ladder-shaped polyethers, such as yessotoxin and ciguatoxin. Two types of abbreviations have been used (BTX and PbTX), sometimes leading to confusion. There are two basic skeletons (Fig. 7), a type-A skeleton, with 10 fused polyether rings, and a type-B skeleton with 11 fused polyether rings. BTX-A group compounds include the analogues PbTX-1, -7 and -10, while BTX-B compounds include PbTX-2, -3, -5, -6 and -9. The structure of PbTX-4 has never been confirmed, and PbTX-8 is an artifact from extraction procedures during the preparative isolation of brevetoxins [122]. *K. brevis* had undergone a number of name changes and was previously referred to as *Gymnodinium brevis*, *Gymnodinium breve* and *Ptychodiscus brevis*, the latter name leading to the abbreviation PbTX. Interestingly, another *Karenia* species, *K. mikimotoi*, produces a related ladder-shaped polyether toxin, gymnocin [123]. PbTX-2 (= BTX-B) is the main analogue produced by *K. brevis* and tends to be the main analogue found in seawater during *K. brevis* blooms; however, it is rapidly transformed into the ten times more toxic PbTX-3 (dihydro-PbTX-2), which is the main constituent in marine aerosols [124]. Brevetoxins had initially been only reported from U.S. and the Mexican gulf, but have subsequently also been found in New Zealand waters. Although the illness is known since the mid 19th century, full structure elucidation was only possible during the 1980s [125–127]. In Florida, *K. brevis* is known as a red tide organism, and the effects of the algae are threefold: aerosol exposure leading to skin damage and respiratory problems as well as accumulation in seafood leading to neurotoxic shellfish poisoning (NSP) (see sections below). While the brevetoxins produced by algae are very lipophilic compounds, some metabolites in shellfish have a slightly more hydrophilic character, due to the biotransformation to cysteine conjugates [128, 129]. Abraham et al. [130] have recently reported more polar metabolites from marine aerosols, in which the A-ring is opened, leading most likely to a reduced toxicity if the same structure activity relationship applies as found by Rein et al. [131]. Bourdelais et al. [132], have isolated an interesting compound from *K. brevis*, namely brevenal. This compound is potentially a biosynthetic precursor to brevetoxins but has been shown to completely inhibit PbTX action on Na^+ channels by competitive binding and is not toxic to fish. Dechraoui et al. [133] have studied the binding of analogues of this group to voltage-gated Na^+ channels, further contributing to the knowledge on the relative toxicity of analogues.

Ciguatera-related toxins

The toxins related to ciguatera fish poisoning comprise multiple groups. Although okadaic acid, palytoxin and other compounds have been implicated in some cases of ciguatera, we focus here on those toxins that are part of the ciguatera complex that have not been described previously. Ciguatoxins (CTXs), gambierol and maitotoxin (MTX) are three groups of compounds among the toxic metabolites produced by *Gambierdiscus toxicus*, the main dinoflagellate responsible for contamination of fish by ciguatera toxins (Fig. 10). MTX is amphiphilic and is thus soluble in water, methanol and dimethyl sulfoxide. It is relatively stable in alkaline but not in acidic conditions [134]. MTX as polyhydroxy polyether with two sulfate ester groups is amongst the more hydrophilic polyethers, does not migrate up the food web, and is restricted to herbivorous fish (and potentially other grazing organisms). Gambierol and CTXs are more lipophilic polyethers and thus will persist and move up the food chain more easily to predatory (piscivorous) fish. The CTX analogue shown in Figure 10 is P-CTX-4B, one of the primary compounds produced by *G. toxicus* in the pacific. It appears to be a precursor to P-CTX-1 from moray eel [135, 136], which is the major constituent in most piscivorous fish in the Pacific, frequently contributing >90% to the overall toxic equivalents [137, 138]. A number of additional, often minor, analogues were isolated from the Indian, Pacific and Caribbean oceans [135, 136, 138–142]. The very low doses, which may already cause problems to consumers, result in challenges of ultra-trace detection in the range of 0.1 µg/kg to several µg/kg.

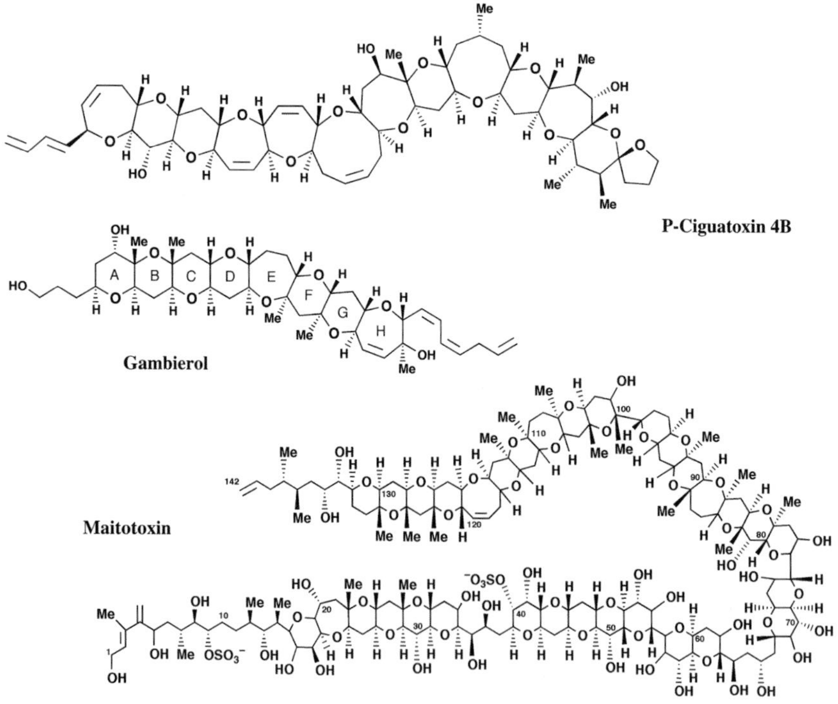

Figure 10. Ciguatera-related toxins: pacific (P-) ciguatoxin (CTX) 4B (P-CTX-4B), gambierol and maitotoxin (MTX).

For this reason, there are few methods available for the detection of these toxins, and worldwide, there are only few groups capable of analyzing CTXs, mainly located in Canada, US, Japan and Australia [143].

Preference of *G. toxicus* for warm water temperatures was demonstrated through correlation of sea surface temperatures with the occurrence of the organism [144]. Thus, CTXs are currently restricted to tropical and subtropical latitudes; however, distribution may well increase through rising sea surface temperatures in many areas. They are globally distributed across the Indian, Pacific and Caribbean oceans. A recent review by Dickey [143] describes difficulties in the analysis and diagnosis of this complex illness. The organism *G. toxicus* was discovered by Yasumoto et al. [145] and first described by Adachi and Fukuyo [146].

Common routes of metabolism of marine toxins

For a number of lipophilic shellfish toxins like PTXs, OA, DTXs, PbTXs, and spirolides, fatty acid ester derivatives have been reported to occur in shellfish tissue [69, 79, 129, 147]. However, until now no such esters have been reported for yessotoxins (YTXs) (although more than 80 different analogs of YTX have been reported so far [94]) or for AZAs [53]. In return, YTXs have shown hydroxy, dihydroxy and carboxy analogs, as discovered for AZAs [53, 93, 95, 148]. In respect to formation of analogs, AZAs show some similarities to YTXs and it is thus possible that more AZA analogues will be discovered in the future. Furanoside analogues have been reported for YTXs [149], and cysteine conjugates for brevetoxins [128]. Therefore, it is likely that further metabolites will still be discovered for several toxin groups; however, it should also be noted that many isolation efforts have been directed by bioactivity screening using either mouse bioassays or, more recently, cytotoxicity or functional assays. This approach facilitates the discovery of toxicologically relevant analogues, whereas a purely chemical structure-based approach, e.g., by LC-MS or ELISA methodology tends to discover all related chemical structures, irrespective of their toxicological relevance. It is arguable if one or the other approach should be favored; certainly the combination of approaches has allowed for the clarification of metabolism in fish or shellfish of many algal toxins and for such exciting discoveries as the brevenal antagonist of brevetoxins produced in the alga itself.

Mechanisms of action of phycotoxins

Our knowledge and understanding of the molecular mechanisms of action of the different marine biotoxins vary widely. In some cases, available data allow an appropriate comprehension of the events triggered by toxins and the description of the molecular bases of effects detected in living organisms. In

other instances, the picture is barely sketched, and many aspects remain undetermined. Our outline of the mechanisms of action of marine biotoxins is
organized taking these differences into account. When we describe the toxins
whose molecular mechanisms of action are not yet established our presentation is aimed at summarizing the most relevant findings about individual
groups, with regards to their possible toxicological implications. Any association between effective concentrations/doses used *in vitro* and found *in vivo* is
taken into account, if available. In mechanistic terms, particular attention is
given to the molecular events triggered by lower toxin concentrations, imply-
ing high affinity binding to their primary molecular targets (receptors).

Molecular mechanisms of phycotoxins acting through binding to ion channels and other ion transfer systems

The better characterized mechanisms of action involve several groups of biotoxins whose recognized primary molecular targets are proteins involved in the
movement of ions that are located at the level of the plasma membrane.

Biotoxins altering ion transport mechanisms in sensitive cells at the level of
plasma membrane, perturb primarily, but not exclusively, the normal functioning of neuronal and other excitable tissues. The biotoxins considered in this
section comprise components classified in different chemical groups, including saxitoxins (and tetrodotoxin), brevetoxins, ciguatera toxins (ciguatoxins,
maitotoxin, gambierol), palytoxins, domoic acid and cyclic imines.

The primary molecular targets (receptors) of these toxins and/or their mechanism of action differ, depending on individual components, and a certain level
of complexity is apparent, as a consequence of the primary event caused by
individual toxins. Many basic biological processes, in fact, depend on the
maintenance of specific ion gradients across the plasma membrane. Thus, an
alteration of the intracellular concentration of one ion can trigger a secondary
change in the intracellular concentrations of other ions in the course of the
molecular events triggered by the interaction of a toxin with its receptor. A
schematic representation of toxin receptors and their mechanisms of action are
reported in Figures 11 and 12.

Mechanism of action of saxitoxins
The voltage-gated sodium channel (VGNC, Fig. 11A) is the recognized receptor of both saxitoxins (STXs, Fig. 2) and tetrodotoxin (TTX, Fig. 3). Before
we consider the functional consequences of toxin interaction with the VGNC,
we briefly outline the molecular organization and general functioning of these
membrane proteins, which are also the target of other groups of algal biotoxins. Furthermore, the VGNC is a prototype for membrane proteins functioning
as ion channels, and some description of this channel will be useful in analyzing the mechanism of action of groups of marine biotoxins that affect the functioning of other ion channels (see below).

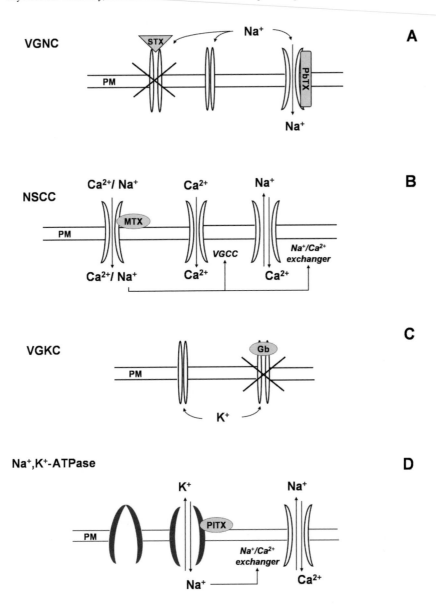

Figure 11. Schematic representation of the molecular mechanisms of action of saxitoxins, brevetoxins, ciguatoxins, maitotoxin, gambierol, palytoxins. (A) Mechanism of action of saxitoxin (STX) and brevetoxins (PbTXs), exerted by binding to voltage-gated sodium channels (VGNC). (B) Mechanism of action of maitotoxin (MTX) by binding to non-selective cation channels (NSCC). In the case of membrane depolarization caused by sodium entry, a secondary increase of intracellular Ca^{2+} concentrations would be induced by opening of voltage-gated calcium channels (VGCC), and some Na^+/Ca^{2+} exchangers. (C) Mechanism of action of gambierol (Gb) by binding to voltage-gated potassium channels (VGKC). (D) Mechanism of action of palytoxin (PlTX) by binding to Na^+,K^+-ATPase: sodium entry determines a secondary increase of intracellular Ca^{2+} concentrations, due to the activity of Na^+/Ca^{2+} exchangers. PM, plasma membrane. See text for details.

The VGNC is a large family of plasma membrane proteins that are expressed primarily in excitable cells (reviewed in [150]). The functional channel consists of an oligomer comprising one large α subunit and one or two smaller β subunits. The α subunit is endowed with both the voltage-sensing function and the ion-transporting structures, whereas the β subunits have roles in the modulation of functional properties and subcellular location of the α subunits.

The structure of α subunits comprises four homologous domains that are formed by six transmembrane segments (S1–S6). Segment S4 is primarily involved in voltage sensing, whereas segments S5 and S6 are involved in the formation of the ion channel itself. The transmembrane segments of the four domains are connected by loops of the polypeptide chain that are mostly exposed to the aqueous environment at the two sides of the plasma membrane. The long loop connecting segments S5 and S6 includes a portion that is inserted within the membrane itself and the arrangement of the loops from the four domains of the VGNC forms the pore that controls the passage of the ion through the channel. The changes in the ion concentration inside the cell are the basis of the voltage sensing by segment S4, which undergoes a conformational change. This change results in the opening of the pore and the entry of sodium ions into the cell, leading to membrane depolarization and the response of excitable cells.

The VGNC is the target of many neurotoxins, interacting with different sites on the channel protein. STXs and TTX have different chemical structures and belong to separate toxin groups, but share their mechanism of action because they both interact with site 1 of the VGNC, which undergoes essentially the same structural change. Site 1 is shaped by a short portion of the amino acid stretches connecting the S5 and S6 transmembrane segments, giving rise to a cavity that accomodates the toxin. The interaction of one STX molecule (and of TTX) with the site 1 of the α subunit in the sodium channel [151] essentially plugs the channel at the level of the pore, as originally proposed by Hille [152], thereby blocking its ion conductance [153]. The loss of sodium conductance in excitable cells then prevents membrane depolarization and the transmission of the action potential, representing the molecular basis of the toxic effects of STXs. As a consequence of VGNC blockade, a progressive loss of neuromuscular function ensues.

Although the binding of STXs and the consequent blocking of the ionic flux is recognized as the mechanistic basis of the symptoms recorded in humans intoxicated by these toxins, the possibility that other ion fluxes might be affected by STXs, either directly or indirectly, should be borne in mind. The significant homologies among channels for different cations [150], in fact, could be the basis for other biological effects of this class of toxins. For instance, the action of STX on potassium and calcium channels has been reported [154, 155], but the effective doses in those molecular systems are three to four orders of magnitude higher (10^{-6}–10^{-5} M) than those affecting VGNC (10^{-10}–10^{-8} M), and the observed effect could be explained by a lower affinity interaction of STXs with these channels. Thus, the toxicological relevance of the effects exerted by high STX concentrations through binding to channels other than the VGNC *in vivo* is questionable.

Finally, it has long been recognized that STXs can bind to soluble proteins, such as saxiphilin (reviewed in [156]), and this could add an additional set of molecular responses induced in sensitive systems.

Mechanism of action of brevetoxins and ciguatoxins
The VGNC is the primary molecular target of other phycotoxins, such as brevetoxins (PbTXs) and some ciguatoxins (CTXs), that cause the opening of the ion pore and sodium entry into the cells. These algal toxins interact with site 5 on the VGNC, leading to changes in the gating properties of the channel (Fig. 11A). Site 5 comprises sequences of the transmembrane segments S5 and S6, and the binding region of PbTXs would essentially span the entire transmembrane segments [150].

The components classified among ciguatera-related toxins include an heterogeneous array of natural compounds produced by *Gambierdiscus toxicus*, possessing distinct chemical properties (see section "Ciguatera-related toxins" above). Among the toxins produced by this algal species, only CTXs appear to selectively target the VGNC [157], whereas maitotoxin (MTX) and gambierol have separate molecular targets (see below).

The binding of toxins to the site 5 of the VGNC determines an increase in the activation threshold to more negative membrane potentials and blocks the inactivation of voltage of the VGNC, leading to enhancement of the sodium entry into the cell. The increased membrane permeability to sodium initially determines excitatory cellular responses (including release of neurotransmitters at some synapses), but loss of cell excitability eventually ensues, leading to paralysis [158, 159].

Mechanism of action of maitotoxin
Although the ingestion of food contaminated with MTX and gambierol has resulted in some symptoms of ciguatera in humans, providing the basis to include these compounds among ciguatera toxins [158, 159], the primary molecular mechanisms of action of MTX and gambierol do not appear to involve their interaction with VGNC (Fig. 11B and C).

The mechanism of action of MTX has long been recognized to involve increased calcium entry into cells, lending support to the conclusion that MTX acts through binding to the plasma membrane calcium channels, resulting in channel opening and enhanced calcium influx (reviewed in [160, 161]). In some systems, however, MTX has been shown to induce both sodium and calcium entry into cells [162], supporting the conclusion that the toxin would actually target a non-selective cation channel [163–165], as depicted in Figure 11B. The increased intracellular sodium concentrations, resulting from the opening of the non-selective cation channel, might then determine membrane depolarization and secondary increases in intracellular Ca^{2+} concentrations, due to opening of voltage-dependent calcium channels, or some Na^+/Ca^{2+} exchangers [161].

In any case, the increase in intracellular calcium concentrations is considered the major event in the mechanism of action of MTX, and the proximal cause of effects observed in biological systems exposed to this toxin. The increase in intracellular Ca^{2+} concentrations detected in cells exposed to MTX is several-fold [164, 165], and the ion reaches levels that are known to trigger specific calcium-dependent responses (reviewed in [160]), such as neurotransmitter secretion and contraction in excitable tissues [166, 167], stimulation of hormone secretion [168, 169], increased metabolism of phosphoinositides [170–172] and activation of protein kinases [172, 173]. The toxicological relevance of some of these responses *in vivo*, however, remains to be established.

Although MTX has been a useful pharmacological tool in investigations probing Ca^{2+}-dependent cellular processes, a better characterization of molecular responses to MTX is needed to fully understand its mode of action and the molecular bases of the effects exerted in living animals. In particular, MTX is a potent cytotoxic agent [173–175], and exposure of biological systems to this compound is expected to result in disruption of cellular functioning and tissue damage.

Mechanism of action of gambierol

Only a few studies have been carried out on the molecular mechanism of action of gambierol, focusing the attention to the effects that this compound might exert on ion movement across the plasma membrane. The most recent data obtained by the patch clamp technique in different cellular systems have shown that voltage-gated potassium channels (VGKC) are blocked by gambierol with an IC_{50} in the $10^{-9}–10^{-8}$ M range [176, 177]. In those studies, VGNC were found to be insensitive to gambierol concentrations three to four orders of magnitude higher ($10^{-6}–10^{-5}$ M) than the IC_{50} measured for gambierol inhibition of VGKC [176, 177]. VGNC could be targeted by gambierol at concentration ranges higher than 10–100 µM [178]. This effect on VGNC has been explained as a secondary event induced by the membrane depolarization and lowering of the action potential threshold following the proximal blockade of VGKC exerted by the toxin [177]. The possibility of low affinity binding of high gambierol concentrations to ion channels other than VGKC *in vivo* can not be excluded at the moment, although any toxicological relevance of the effects exerted by high gambierol concentrations through binding to VGNC *in vivo* is uncertain.

As opposed to other toxins produced by *G. toxicus*, gambierol does not appear to be cytotoxic up to a 50 nM concentration, although it induces a stress response in affected cells [179].

Based on available information, the VGKC appears the relevant target of gambierol in living animals (Fig. 11C), and the blockade of potassium efflux in sensitive cells would be the proximal event leading to some of the symptoms recorded in humans intoxicated by food contaminated by this toxin, such as disturbances of taste and pain [158, 159, 176].

Mechanism of action of palytoxins

The Na^+,K^+-ATPase is the recognized receptor of palytoxin (PlTX) (Fig. 11D). The binding of PlTX to the N-terminal segment of the α subunit of the Na^+,K^+-ATPase, located on the extracellular portion of the molecule, converts the ion pump into a non-selective cation channel [180–182]. The details of the interaction between the toxin and its receptor have not been fully characterized, but its occurrence has been exploited for an extensive description of molecular features of the Na^+,K^+-ATPase and its functioning [183–187].

The identification of the Na^+,K^+-ATPase as the receptor of PlTXs stemmed from the pioneering studies by Habermann, showing that K^+ efflux was induced as an early response of erythrocytes exposed to picomolar concentrations of PlTX [188], and was fully established by demonstrating that PlTX-dependent ionic fluxes are induced upon expression of the Na^+,K^+-ATPase in yeast [189], and transmembrane cation fluxes are induced by PlTX in a cell-free system when *in vitro* synthesized Na^+,K^+-ATPase is incorporated in artificial membranes [190].

Plasma membrane proteins involved in ion transport, other than the Na^+,K^+-ATPase, have been proposed to contribute to molecular responses induced by PlTX in some sensitive systems. These include some non-selective cation channels [191], whose characterization has remained elusive so far. Moreover, VGNC and calcium channels have also been indicated as primary targets of PlTX [191, 192]. Although the contribution of these molecules to the effects exerted by PlTX in excitable cells may not be excluded at the moment, a large body of evidence would indicate that the Na^+ influx and K^+ efflux through the Na^+,K^+-ATPase should be the most relevant and proximal events in the mechanism of action of PlTXs.

Taking into consideration that the Na^+,K^+-ATPase is ubiquitous in animals, the sensitivity of both excitable and non-excitable cells to palytoxins is expected. In mechanistic terms, several events can be induced by the potassium efflux and sodium entry into the cell, resulting in membrane depolarization (Fig. 11D). The available data indicate a high level of complexity in the array of molecular and functional alterations caused by PlTX *in vitro* and *in vivo*, as outlined below.

In the first instance, sodium-dependent transport of calcium ions across the plasma membrane would be triggered, mostly by the involvement of Na^+/Ca^{2+} exchangers [191, 193, 194]. The increased intracellular Ca^{2+} concentrations would then trigger other Ca^{2+}-induced responses, such as muscle contraction and, in the heart, arrhythmias [181, 182, 191, 193, 195]. The lowering of intracellular pH, due to Na^+ efflux through Na^+/H^+ exchangers, could be another secondary event triggered by PlTXs [196–198].

The metabolism of eicosanoids is also affected by PlTX, by enhancing the production and release of prostaglandins in many biological systems

[199–201]. The increased release of prostaglandins from the endothelium and smooth muscle cells determines norepinephrine release and contraction of the rabbit aortas [202].

Other molecular processes have been shown to contribute to cellular responses to PlTX. A possible role of PlTX in carcinogenesis was originally proposed based on indications of some effect as a tumor promoter [199, 203]. This early observation led to investigations aimed at understanding the molecular mechanism responsible for that effect, and studies were primarily devoted to ascertaining whether the toxin could alter protein kinases involved in the control of cell proliferation, such as extracellular signal-regulated kinases (ERK) and the c-Jun-NH$_2$-terminal protein kinases (JNK) [204]. The major conclusions of those studies are that altered ion fluxes through the Na$^+$,K$^+$-ATPase induced by PlTX determine the activation of some ERK and JNK isoforms by different mechanisms, including increased prostaglandin production, the activation of pathways responsible for phosphorylation of ERK and JNK, respectively, and the inhibition of ERK dephosphorylation (reviewed in [205]).

In contrast to the experiments showing the tumor-promoting effect of PlTX, cytolysis has been found in several systems exposed to this toxin [180, 188, 206]. An altered Na$^+$,K$^+$-ATPase is recognized as the proximal cause of cytolysis, indicating that altered ion homeostasis and osmotic stress are involved in the process [180, 188, 206]. However, cytolysis can not represent the simple outcome of cell swelling accompanying altered Na$^+$ and K$^+$ fluxes in cells exposed to PlTX, because the cytolytic response is delayed compared to potassium efflux from the cells [188].

In conclusion, only some of the many molecular and functional effects of PlTX found in experimental systems can be integrated in a coherent picture providing a mechanistic explanation of the toxic responses observed in intact animals, and some of the effects detected in cellular systems most likely reflect cell-specific responses, under controlled experimental conditions. Still, the large body of evidence shows a complex array of events that are secondary to PlTX binding to Na$^+$,K$^+$-ATPase and conversion of the pump to a nonspecific ion channel.

Mechanism of action of domoic acid

The mechanism of action of domoic acid (DA) involves toxin binding to non-N-methyl-D-aspartate (non-NMDA) glutamate receptors (Fig. 12). Glutamate is one of the major neurotransmitters in the brain [207], and its importance in normal functioning of the central nervous system has been a primary drive for the extensive investigations on the mechanism of action of DA.

DA binds to non-NMDA receptors in several regions of the central nervous system, and the effects ensue from a coordinated and synergistic action of receptors functioning at the two sides of the synapse, resulting in altered neurotransmission (see [39, 208, 209] for excellent recent reviews). Non-NMDA receptors include α-amino-3-hydroxy-5-methyl-4-isoxazolepropionate (AMPA)

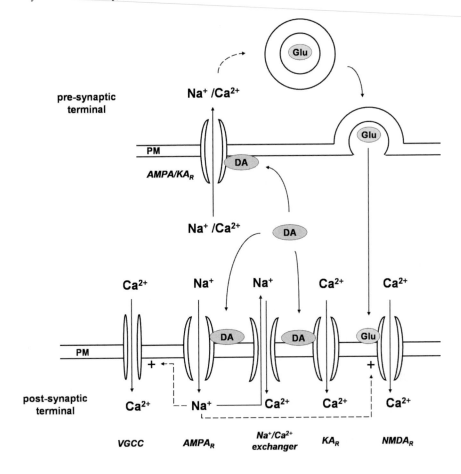

Figure 12. Schematic representation of the molecular mechanisms of action of domoic acid (DA). Mechanism of action of DA by binding to AMPA (AMPA$_R$) and kainate (KA$_R$) receptors. Glu, glutamate; NMDA$_R$, NMDA receptor; PM, plasma membrane; VGCC, voltage-gated calcium channels. See text for details.

and kainate receptors, which represent ligand-dependent ion channels, and the binding of DA determines the opening of the channels [210, 211]. When DA binds to AMPA channels, influx of Na$^+$ into the cell occurs, whereas influx of extracellular Ca^{2+} ions into the cell is induced by DA binding to kainate receptors [210, 211]. The molecular mechanism of action of DA, however, may not be reduced to these two receptor systems, because other ion channels and receptors are recognized to participate in the response induced by the toxin [39, 208]. In particular, DA also induces the influx of extracellular Ca^{2+} through voltage-gated calcium channels [212, 213], and by reverse action of Na$^+$/Ca^{2+} exchangers [213]. In both cases, the effect would follow Na$^+$ influx through AMPA receptor and membrane depolarization [213]. Furthermore,

NMDA receptors could contribute to the processes leading to increased intracellular Ca^{2+} concentrations in affected cells, as NMDA receptors would be activated by glutamate released from the synapsis, following DA binding to pre-synaptic AMPA/kainate receptors [214–218].

The mechanism of action of DA would then involve a primary stimulation of influx of Na^+ and Ca^{2+} ions in neurons, as a consequence of DA binding to post-synaptic AMPA and kainate receptors (Fig. 12). The membrane depolarization would then enhance the influx of extracellular Ca^{2+} ions through voltage-gated calcium channels [212, 213] and NMDA receptors [214–218]. The calcium conductance of NMDA receptors would be caused by the binding of glutamate released from nerve endings, following a reduction of the voltage-dependent Mg^{2+} block of NMDA receptors [217, 218]. The glutamate secretion, in turn, would be induced by the pre-synaptic action of DA, but the molecular details of this response have not been fully clarified, and different proposals have been put forth [39, 208]. The increased intracellular Na^+ concentrations would also stimulate an influx of extracellular Ca^{2+} ions through Na^+/Ca^{2+} exchangers (Fig. 12). The combination of the molecular transducers of DA response would lead to an overall increase in intracellular Ca^{2+} concentrations, which would trigger Ca^{2+}-dependent responses [39, 208, 209].

The action of glutamate receptors under normal conditions would contribute to coordinated neurotransmission among neurons in the central nervous system. The desensitization of receptors that contributes to normal glutamate-based neurotransmission is impaired in receptors bound to DA [39, 211, 219], and this condition then results in unrestrained signaling of DA-bound receptors, leading to Ca^{2+} overload in cells exposed to the toxin [39, 211]. The prolonged calcium load then determines a loss in the regulatory mechanisms of cell functions involving controlled intracellular calcium homeostasis, leading to cell damage and overt neurotoxicity, which represent the major effects of DA *in vitro* and *in vivo* [39, 208, 209, 211, 217, 220–224]. Thus, DA in the brain would determine a sustained signaling through glutamate receptors in some neurons, leading to altered neurological and behavioral activities, which are apparent in the symptoms recorded in humans and animals that have been poisoned by this toxin (see section "Amnesic shellfish poisoning" below).

Mechanism of action of cyclic imines
The components of this group of algal toxins share several structural features that have been the basis of the hypothesis that they might have a common mechanism of action [120]. The investigation on the molecular effects of cyclic imines, however, has been very limited so far, and therefore it seems premature to make any firm proposal about their mechanism of action. Within this constraint, the few available data on spirolides would suggest that these toxins exert their effects through alteration of ion conductance at the level of the plasma membrane (primarily Ca^{2+}), acting on some acetylcholine receptors [225]. The increased frequency in the detection of this class of compounds in

shellfish indicates the need for greater research efforts to characterize their mechanism(s) of action.

Mechanism of action of okadaic acid and related compounds

It has long been recognized that okadaic acid (OA) and related compounds bind and inhibit serine/threonine phosphoprotein phosphatases (PPases), and, among them, the 2A isoform (PP2A) shows a particularly high affinity for the toxin [226, 227]. The mechanism of action of OA and related compounds, therefore, involves the inhibition of PPases, leading to stabilization of the phosphorylated states of proteins that are substrate of OA-sensitive enzymes (Fig. 13).

The phosphorylation of amino acids in proteins is a widespread process through which the functioning of individual proteins is controlled in eukaryotic cells, so that different activities are usually associated with the phosphorylation pattern of individual proteins, and the functional states existing under defined conditions in biological systems may be more than the simple active/inactive opposition [228–230]. Although hundreds of PPases are believed to be expressed in eukaryotes [231], the inhibition of only some isoforms of PPases (primarily PP1 and PP2A) by OA has dramatic consequences, because these isoforms are responsible for the dephosphorylation of many enzymes and regulatory proteins in living systems [232]. The original study of Haystead et al. [233] provided the clear demonstration that, in OA-treated cells, OA

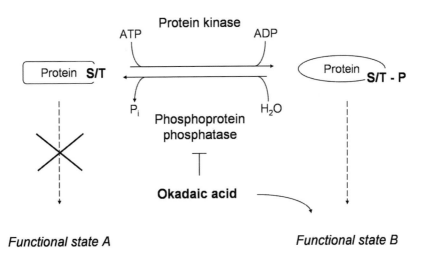

Figure 13. Schematic representation of the mechanism of action of okadaic acid (OA). The phosphorylation reaction has been referred to a serine/threonine residue (S/T) of the protein, in a reaction involving ATP, as the phosphate donor, and ADP as the product. The dephosphorylation reaction is a hydrolysis, leading to release of orthophosphate (P_i).

leads to increased levels of phosphorylated proteins and altered cell functioning and, indeed, a simple literature search reveals that the phosphorylation
states of cellular proteins are frequently affected by exposure of biological systems to OA. This toxin, therefore, can disrupt the molecular mechanisms controlling functions in biological systems. Many examples regarding single regulatory pathways could be described, but only two general phenomena are discussed, as they refer to the two major responses found in animals exposed to
OA.

The tumor-promoting effect of OA and related compounds has been described in two models of two-stage carcinogenesis [234, 235]. Taking into consideration that cell proliferation is stimulated by protein phosphorylation cascades [204], the stabilization of phosphorylated forms of key regulatory proteins, as a consequence of inhibition of PPases due to OA, could represent a
molecular explanation for the tumor-promoting effect of this toxin in some
biological systems.

OA, however, does not represent a carcinogen on its own [234, 235], and its
tumor-promoting effects have been observed in systems that were subjected to
tumor initiation by exposure to a chemical carcinogen, before being challenged with OA [234, 235], in keeping with the general process of two-stage
carcinogenesis [236]. In turn, the evidence obtained in many systems *in vitro*
and *in vivo*, indicates that cells exposed to OA do not respond by a stimulation
of cell proliferation, but the toxin actually induces cell death (reviewed in
[237]). The death response induced by OA has been observed with both normal and transformed cells, and the disruption of several regulatory pathways
due to inhibition of PPases in cells exposed to OA can explain the death
responses reported in literature. The disruption of proper cell functioning and
cell death is actually considered the molecular basis of the diarrhea that represents the major symptom of animals and humans poisoned by OA and related
toxins (see below).

In vitro studies have shown that OA does not significantly affect ion currents in intestinal cell monolayers and in stripped rabbit colonic mucosa, but
it attenuates the cellular response to secretagogues, such as forskolin and car-
bachol, supporting the conclusion that OA does not act as a secretagogue in
the intestine [238]. The analysis of OA effect on transepithelial electrical
resistance showed that the toxin significantly decreased the resistance of cell
monolayers, lending support to the notion that it disrupts the barrier function
of intestinal cells and increases paracellular permeability [238]. E-cadherin is
the protein responsible for cell-cell adhesion of intestinal epithelia [239], and
the destruction of E-cadherin has been described in epithelial cells exposed to
OA [240], indicating that cell disposal of the E-cadherin system would contribute to increased paracellular permeability of intestinal epithelial cells. The
observation that OA decreases transepithelial electrical resistance without
any measurable effect on ion currents of intestinal tissue has been confirmed
in an animal study [241], providing convincing evidence that the mechanism
by which OA induces diarrhea in animals includes sub-mucosal fluid collec-

tion in the intestine, followed by its flowing into the intestine through the paracellular pathway of the epithelium and its secretion into the intestinal lumen [241].

Mechanism of action of yessotoxins and azaspiracids

The chemistry (see above) and toxicity of these two groups of compounds are quite different. Animal studies have shown that azaspiracids (AZAs) are toxic by both i.p. injection and the oral route [44, 242], and the oral toxicity of AZAs has been confirmed in humans [242]. A different picture is available for yesso-toxins (YTXs), which are toxic when injected i.p. in the mouse, while only limited alterations have been recorded after oral administration [83–85, 243]. A recent study has shown that only little gastrointestinal absorption of YTX occurs, as low (10^{-9}–10^{-8} M) toxin concentrations have been detected in the blood of mice that received comparatively large doses of the compound orally [243]. In line with the low toxicity of YTX found in animal studies, no episodes of human intoxications have been linked to ingestion of shellfish contaminated with this group of compounds so far, and the acute toxicity of YTXs remains a matter of debate.

The precise mechanisms by which AZAs and YTXs trigger their effects in biological systems are undetermined at the moment, although many studies have been carried out by different groups, using primarily cultured cells. The difficulties in extrapolating the results obtained *in vitro* with regard to their toxicological relevance *in vivo* should then be borne in mind. In the account that follows, therefore, the attention is focused on the molecular events that have been recorded in experimental systems by the use of toxin concentrations up to 10^{-8} M, which are compatible with exposure upon ingestion of food contaminated with AZAs and YTXs, based on the toxin levels found in animal tissues after oral administration of the compounds [242, 243]. For reviews reporting the molecular effects detected *in vitro* by exposing cells to high (10^{-7}–10^{-6} M) AZA and YTX concentrations, the reader is referred to some recent reviews [244–246].

A cytotoxic effect of 10^{-9} and 10^{-8} M AZA1 (Fig. 4) has been described in a variety of cellular systems [247–250]. In some of those model systems, alterations of F-actin-based cytoskeletal structures have been found upon cell treatment with nanomolar concentrations of AZA1 [247, 248], and the effects of the toxin on cytoskeletal structures showed some degree of cell specificity [248, 249]. Furthermore, AZA1 was found to alter cell adhesion [248, 249], and to induce the accumulation of a fragmented form of E-cadherin, termed ECRA$_{100}$ [249]. AZA1 treatment of primary cultured neurons has been shown to cause increased nuclear levels of phosphorylated (active) JNK, and an inhibitor of JNK could prevent the cytotoxic effect of AZA1 in that experimental system [251]. Thus, the cytotoxic effect of AZA1 could be brought about by an array of molecular events, whose mechanistic links remain to be defined.

In a different line of investigation, the analysis of the effects of AZA1 on the transcription profiles of T lymphocytes has shown that a 24-h exposure of these cells to 10 nM AZA1 affects the expression of several genes, including a coordinated up-regulation of those coding for enzymes involved in cholesterol and fatty acid synthetic pathways [252]. At the moment, it is unclear how the various effects found *in vitro* can be linked to the observed toxic effects *in vivo*.

Turning to the molecular effects elicited by YTX (Fig. 7) in cultured cells, three major responses triggered by toxin concentrations up to 10^{-8} M have been reported. Some of those effects have been observed only in some cell lines, indicating a certain degree of cell specificity in the responses elicited by YTX in sensitive systems. The induction of cell death as the most prominent effect of YTX has been observed with cell lines of different histological types and is detected 1–2 days after addition of 10^{-10}–10^{-8} M YTX to cell cultures [253–257], suggesting that a general alteration would be induced by YTX in sensitive lines, leading to cell death. The increase in intracellular Ca^{2+} concentrations is another effect triggered within minutes of YTX addition to some cells, due to the opening of voltage-sensitive calcium channels [246]. The increase is limited, leading to less than doubling of the intracellular Ca^{2+} concentrations, and in primary cultures of neuronal cells it is induced by YTX concentrations that are about 10^{-8} M [255]. In other systems, YTX concentrations higher than 10^{-7} M were needed to elicit the same kind of response [246]. The functional consequences of the very limited increase in intracellular Ca^{2+} concentrations elicited by YTX are presently undetermined, and experiments carried out in two different systems have shown that it should not be involved in the induction of cell death by YTX [255, 257].

Another molecular effect elicited by YTX is the disruption of the E-cadherin system in epithelial cells [258–260]. The effect is induced by very low YTX concentrations (10^{-10}–10^{-9} M) and is detected by the accumulation of a 100-kDa fragment of E-cadherin (ECRA$_{100}$), that has lost the intracellular C-terminal domain of the protein [259]. YTX does not enhance E-cadherin degradation per se, but interferes with the normal turnover of the plasma membrane protein, preventing endocytosis and complete disposal of the protein fragment produced after the initial proteolytic attack, and leading to accumulation of proteolytic fragments in vescicular structures in the proximity of the plasma membrane [260]. Taking into consideration that the half-life of E-cadherin was about 8 h in both control and YTX-treated cells, the detection of ECRA$_{100}$ at levels comparable to those of the intact protein 16–20 h after YTX addition to cultured cells indicates that the blockade of endocytosis by the toxin should be a rapid and early response of sensitive cells [260]. Interestingly, decreased levels of a proteolytic fragment of E-cadherin lacking the intracellular domain of the protein have also been found in the colon of mice after oral administration of YTX [261], indicating that YTX can decrease the disposal of E-cadherin both *in vitro* and *in vivo*.

Notwithstanding the recognized differences between AZAs and YTXs, the experimental findings described above reveal that similar effects can be triggered by low concentrations (10^{-10}–10^{-9} M) of AZA1 and YTXs in the same cell line. Among the molecular responses induced by AZAs and YTXs described so far, cell death appears ubiquitous, whereas disruption of the F-actin cytoskeleton and the inhibition of endocytosis of membrane proteins appear cell specific. In the case of the effects exerted on E-cadherin, the knowledge on the molecular details pinpoints the fact that the effect of AZA1 was undistinguishable from that induced by YTX in epithelial cells [249]. Thus, it has been proposed that AZAs and YTXs might share their molecular mechanism(s) of action in some target cells and/or biological settings [249].

The extensive structural features distinguishing AZAs from YTXs make the possibility that the two classes of compounds share the same receptor unlikely, although it can not be excluded at the moment. In turn, two different molecular mechanisms of action of AZAs and YTXs could converge toward some shared effectors that could mediate common responses with identical endpoints, and cross-talks would then occur at multiple levels, as has been found in the case of other algal toxins [179]. This working hypothesis is presented in Figure 14, where AZAs and YTXs are considered to induce their effects by interacting with different receptors, thereby triggering responses through the involvement of distinct sets of effectors. The two pathways would include, however, mechanistic links between some effectors, either directly or indirectly. In this hypothetical model, for instance, the effects exerted by both AZAs and YTXs on the E-cadherin system would converge on the inhibition of a key endocytic step, and could occur through several pathways. The most direct pathways for AZAs and YTXs in our model would include steps 1, 3, 12, and 6, 7, 12, respectively (Fig. 14). Alternatives would be possible, however, through disruption of the F-actin cytoskeleton, as a consequence of converging mechanisms to effector $E_{AZA/YTX}$, and the subsequent steps 10 and 13 (Fig. 14). This latter pathway, however, would represent a cell-specific alternative, as cell treatment with pectenotoxin-6, which disrupts the F-actin cytoskeleton (see below), does not lead to accumulation of the $ECRA_{100}$ fragment of E-cadherin [262], indicating that a general alteration of actin cytoskeleton may not be sufficient to cause the effect on E-cadherin. A third possible mechanism would incorporate the recent evidence that AZA1 induces the accumulation of early endosomes in the proximity of the plasma membrane [263]. These should be the vescicles accumulating $ECRA_{100}$ in YTX-treated cells [260], and we recently observed that AZA1 inhibits endocytosis of plasma membrane proteins (Bellocci et al., in preparation). In this third mechanism, AZA1 and YTX would bring about their response through the common effector $E_{AZA/YTX}$, and steps 11 and 14 (Fig. 14). Interestingly, the alteration of proteins involved in snRNP functioning and mRNA maturation could be another response shared by AZA1 and YTX [263, 264], a possibility that has been embedded in the model of Figure 14.

Similar considerations could be put forward about the death responses, which would result from multiple cellular events, such as the disruption of cel-

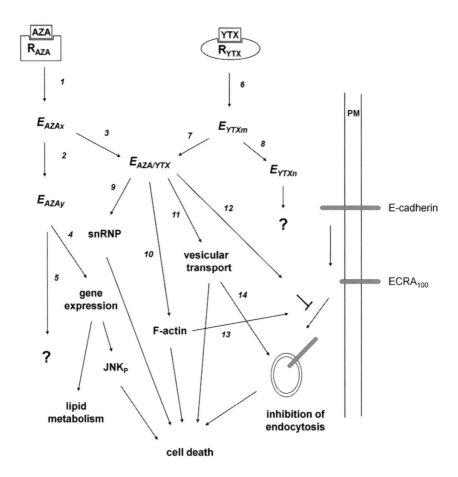

Figure 14. Hypothetical model of the cross-talks between the mechanisms of action of azaspiracids (AZAs) and yessotoxins (YTXs). The subcellular location of the AZA and YTX receptors (R_{AZA} and R_{YTX}), as well as the number and mechanistic links between effectors of the pathways ($E_{AZAx,y}$ and $E_{YTXm,n}$) are entirely speculative. Some steps of the different pathways have been numbered. PM, plasma membrane. See text for explanation.

lular ultrastructures (cytoskeleton) and processes (endocytosis and mRNA maturation), including cell-specific events. The redundancy in signaling pathways, as hypothesized in the schematic model of Figure 14, is common in transduction systems in eukaryotes, and could contribute to cell-specific responses to AZAs and YTXs.

We wish to stress the hypothetical nature of the pathways reported in Figure 14, and remark that the similarity among some molecular responses elicited by AZAs and YTXs could be exploited for studies on cross-talks between distinct mechanisms of action of algal toxins.

Mechanism of action of pectenotoxins

Few data are available on the toxicity of pectenotoxins (PTXs, Fig. 6), indicating that this group of compounds is less toxic when administered by the oral route, as opposed to i.p. injection [265]. It has been hypothesized that this difference would stem from low absorbance of these toxins in the gastrointestinal tract. Chromatographic studies by Fux and Hess (unpublished observations) confirm the nonpolar character of PTX2, the primary algal metabolite, which may result in low bioavailability in the intestinal tract, and studies by Miles et al. [78] clearly demonstrate rapid transformation of PTX2 into inactive PTX2-seco acid in aqueous systems. However, *in vivo* data on absorption and toxicokinetics of PTXs are lacking.

Taking into consideration these limitations, it is recognized that PTXs interact with F-actin, leading to alterations in the ultrastructure and functioning of the cellular cytoskeleton. Initial evidence suggesting that F-actin might be a target of PTXs stemmed from the histopathological damages found in the liver of mice injected with PTX1, which resembled those induced by phalloidin [266]. The observation that PTX1 disrupts stress fibers then provided the first direct indication that PTXs alter F-actin [267]. This observation was later confirmed with PTX2 [268], leading to the conclusion that PTXs cause actin depolymerization [269–272].

More recently, detailed crystallographic analysis of the interaction between PTX2 and actin has shown that the toxin and actin form a 1:1 complex [273]. F-actin is composed of two helices containing polymers of non-covalently bound actin monomers, and PTX2 could interfere with polymerization by associating with actin monomers at a site that is close to the "inner" filament axis, inhibiting the lateral subunit interactions critical for filament assembly [273]. PTXs have been shown to induce cell death in many cell lines, in a wide concentration range ($10^{-9}-10^{-6}$ M), through multiple mechanisms [274–282], and F-actin depolymerization induced by PTX2 appears the causative event leading to cell death [276].

Shellfish poisoning

The route of human exposure to phycotoxins is most often oral, through ingestion of food contaminated with toxins. In some instances, however, living systems may become exposed to phycotoxins through other routes, as in the case of breathing aerosols containing toxins and/or direct skin contact with toxins. In this section, we summarize the major symptoms of and, whenever available, possible remedies for the most relevant poisonings that may occur in humans exposed to phycotoxins, independently of the routes of toxin entry into the body. The poisonings have been classified mostly on the basis of recorded symptoms, and our description follows the existing classification.

Paralytic shellfish poisoning (PSP)

Saxitoxins (STXs) are the causative agents of this poisoning, which results from ingestion of contaminated shellfish [283, 284]. The same kind of poisoning is due to ingestion of tetrodotoxin (TTX), as a consequence of eating raw meat from puffer fish. The gonads and liver of the puffer fish can accumulate bacterial TTX as a consequence of its feeding behavior: if the puffer fish viscera are not carefully dissected from the rest of the meat, this meat can become contaminated and cause poisoning when ingested [285].

PSP has been recorded worldwide, and its symptoms are experienced within 30 minutes from ingestion of contaminated seafood, related to the severity of the poisoning [284]. Mild symptoms include altered perception (burning or tingling sensation and numbness of the lips, that can spread to the face and neck), headache, dizziness and nausea. More severe symptoms include incoherent speech, a progression of altered perception to arms and legs, a progressive loss in the coordination of limbs, and general weakness. Respiratory difficulty is a late symptom, as a consequence of muscular paralysis progressing in the whole body, and death may be the outcome of PSP by respiratory paralysis [284]. The blockade of ion conductance due to binding of STX to the voltage-gated sodium channel (VGNC) is the mechanistic basis of the symptoms of PSP (Fig. 11A).

Artificial respiration has been the most appropriate remedy for PSP so far, as patients subjected to mechanical intervention have a high probability of a full and rapid recovery [283, 286].

Neurotoxic shellfish poisoning (NSP)

Brevetoxins (PbTXs) are the causative agents of this poisoning, which may occur after both inhaling aerosol containing the toxins or as a consequence of eating contaminated seafood. When poisoning is through the respiratory tract, the exposure usually occurs on or near the waters where a bloom of PbTX producers has developed. NSP has been recorded primarily in the southeastern coast of the United States, the Gulf of Mexico, and New Zealand [283, 284, 287].

The symptoms due to contaminated shellfish appear minutes/hours after its ingestion, and are more severe than those found when contaminated aerosol is involved. In the former case, symptoms are both gastrointestinal (nausea, diarrhea, and abdominal pain) and neurological (circumoral paresthesia and hot/cold temperature reversal). In more severe cases, the muscular system may be affected (altered heart contractions, convulsions, and respiratory difficulties). Death from NSP has never been reported in humans, and symptoms resolve within a few days after exposure to the toxins [283, 284].

When exposure to PbTXs is through contaminated aerosols, symptoms involve primarily conjunctival irritation, copious catarrhal exudates, rhinorrhea, nonproductive cough, and bronchoconstriction [288–291]. In the normal population, these symptoms are usually reversed by leaving the beach area or entering an air-conditioned area [291]. The molecular mechanism at the basis of brevetoxin poisoning is related to the increased ion conductance that these compounds induce on interacting with, and opening, the VGNC (see Fig. 11A). Thus, an initial phase of increased neurotransmission (firing of action potentials and release of acetylcholine at muscular endplates) and muscular contraction is followed by a progressive inhibitory action [283].

No specific therapy is available for NSP, but some of the effects of PbTXs can be reversed by infusion with hyperosmotic solutions [292]. The finding that brevenal is an antagonist of PbTX action [132] opens interesting perspectives for the therapeutic use of drugs counteracting the effects of these natural toxins.

Amnesic shellfish poisoning (ASP)

The symptoms due to eating domoic acid (DA)-contaminated shellfish appear within the first few hours after ingestion, and in more severe cases may persist for months [39, 208, 209, 220, 293]. Initial symptoms affect the gastrointestinal tract, with nausea, vomiting, abdominal cramps and diarrhea. These are followed by headache and other neurological symptoms that often result in disturbances of memory, an effect that has led to the naming of this type of shellfish poisoning. The most severe cases may result in death [39, 208, 209, 220, 293].

The neurological symptoms of ASP have been shown to evolve in the weeks (months) following poisoning, and anterograde memory disturbances can be accompanied by confusion, disorientation, peripheral nerve damage and changes in memory threshold [220, 293, 294]. Postmortem histopathological analysis of the brain in an individual who had suffered ASP, and whose death was unrelated to the poisoning, showed atrophy of the hippocampus [220, 293].

Overall, the symptoms of ASP are related to damage of structures of the nervous system, which can be fully explained by unrestrained post-synaptic activity and neuronal toxicity induced by DA stimulation of non-NMDA glutamate receptors (Fig. 12). Because of the agonistic properties of DA in this receptor system, the toxic effects of this algal toxin can be antagonized by glutamate receptor antagonists *in vitro* and *in vivo* [216, 222, 295–297].

Diarrheic shellfish poisoning (DSP)

The contamination of seafood by okadaic acid (OA) and related compounds is very common in European and Asia-Pacific Countries [283]. The symptoms of DSP appear within 1 h after ingestion of contaminated seafood, and affect the gastrointestinal tract, producing nausea, vomiting, abdominal cramps and diarrhea [283]. The symptoms do not last long and usually disappear within a few days. No death has been recorded due to DSP. No long-term effects have been described in humans, although experiments in animal systems have recorded a tumor-promoting effect of OA in two-stage carcinogenesis models [234, 235]. In those cases, the effect depended on protocols of toxin administration involving repeated dosing at least twice per week over periods of several months [234, 235]. The conditions of those studies do not appear to be easily comparable to human intake of OA and related compounds, and a study aimed at probing whether residual levels of OA in shellfish might increase the risk of cancer among regular shellfish consumers has yielded inconclusive results [298].

The mechanism of action of OA and the molecular events detected in biological systems exposed to this toxin provide a clear explanation of the DSP symptoms (Fig. 13). Taking into consideration, however, the vast array of molecular responses elicited by this group of compounds, through alteration of regulatory pathways in the cells, further investigations are needed to better clarify possible long-term effects of exposure to OA. When gastrointestinal symptoms of DSP are severe, their treatment is symptomatic, e.g., rehydration.

Ciguatera

Globally, ciguatera is probably one of the most frequent poisonings with estimates reaching from 50 000 to 500 000 events per annum [299]. This poisoning is caused by eating fishes in tropical marine areas, and the toxins responsible for this poisoning are components produced by *G. toxicus* (see sections above) that are accumulated in fish through the food chain. A vast literature exists on ciguatera, and the reader is referred to some excellent reviews for detailed descriptions [158, 159, 283].

As toxins possessing different chemical properties and mechanisms of action have been involved in ciguatera, a discussion of this poisoning in humans demands some attention to specific issues related to toxin groups and the molecular bases of their effects. Furthermore, despite the increasing understanding of the multiple processes set in motion by ciguatoxins (CTXs), maitotoxin (MTX) and gambierol, there are still significant uncertainties about the specific contribution given by each group of toxins. Based on this consideration, we first describe the most relevant symptoms of ciguatera, and then discuss the possible cause-effect relationships that have been proposed for individual toxin groups.

Ample spectra of symptoms have been recorded for ciguatera, with a manifestation that starts within hours after the ingestion of contaminated food, often resolves within 1 week, but may last up to some years. Furthermore a higher susceptibility to ciguatera toxins has been observed in both humans [300] and animals [175, 301] that had experienced previous exposure to these toxins. The symptoms are both gastrointestinal and neurological, with nausea, diarrhea and vomiting representing early signs of poisoning, accompanied by neurological symptoms, such as numbness and circumoral paresthesia, inversion of thermal sensations ("dry ice sensation"), and metallic taste. In severe cases, paresthesia may progress to other parts of the body, accompanied by difficulties in breathing, and death may ensue due to respiratory paralysis, heart dysrythmias or cerebral edema [158, 159, 283].

Although any attempt to link the different symptoms of ciguatera to any specific group of toxins should be considered an oversimplification at the moment, some preliminary indication can be made on the basis of available knowledge on molecular mechanisms of action of CTXs, MTX and gambierol. It is recognized, for instance, that many symptoms of ciguatera are similar to those found in NSP, and they are most likely due to the effect of CTXs, by opening the VGNC, whereby the increased sodium conductance would lead to increased neurotransmission, followed by a progressive inhibitory action. MTX, however, could contribute to increased neurotransmission with regard to muscle contraction, and the symptoms of heart dysrythmias. MTX also causes extensive cell damage in animal studies, and has a potent cytotoxic effect in cultured cells, and could therefore contribute to neurotoxic symptoms [173–175]. The role of gambierol in ciguatera is less clear, but its impairment of VGKC functioning in taste buds [176] suggests that it might have a role in the taste disturbances that have been recorded. MTX does not move up the marine food chain (probably related to its solubility in water) and its contribution to ciguatera-poisoning is more likely when the poisoning arises from the consumption of herbivorous fish.

No specific therapy has been proposed for ciguatera so far, and its treatment remains symptomatic. In particular, intravenous infusion of mannitol has been used, the protective effect of which has been attributed to the inhibition of edema formation in several tissues [302]. In keeping with the shared mechanism of action of brevetoxins and ciguatoxins, brevenal has been reported to inhibit ciguatoxin-induced neurotoxic effects and might represent an appropriate therapeutic tool [303].

Palytoxin poisoning

The potential of palytoxins (PlTXs) to cause human poisonings is a matter of discussion [304]. On the one hand, human illness and even fatal cases have been linked to PlTXs that could have entered the human body as a consequence of eating contaminated food [304], or through small skin injuries [305]. On the other hand, hundreds of human cases have been reported in coastal areas of some Mediterranean countries (Italy, France, Greece and Spain) in recent years, and have been linked to blooms of algae producing PlTXs (*Ostreopsis* species [8, 9, 111, 306]). Although a formal proof that PlTXs were responsible for those human cases is still lacking, circumstantial evidence would suggest that this could be the case, because intoxications involved people residing at or close to the coastal areas where the harmful algal blooms (HABs) were taking place, and PlTXs were found in the *Ostreopsis* algae present in those coastal areas, supporting the proposal that the PlTXs present in the aerosols were the causative agents of those intoxications [8, 9].

The symptoms of PlTX poisoning are to be considered within these constraints, and can be differentiated based on the proposed route of entry into the body. When intoxication was apparent following ingestion of contaminated food [304], gastrointestinal symptoms (nausea, vomiting, diarrhea) have been recorded, together with neurological disturbances (circumoral paresthesia and paresthesia of the extremities, muscle spasms and pain, respiratory problems), and death has been observed in a few instances. Tissue damage has been documented in several cases, suggesting a cytotoxic effect of PlTXs in these tissues [180, 188, 206].

In many cases, the presence of other toxins contaminating the ingested food, and/or a lack of knowledge regarding the toxins present in the materials have led to uncertainties about the actual involvement of PlTXs in the recorded cases [304], although PlTXs have been found in seafood in coastal areas where blooms of *Ostreopsis* algae were ongoing.

When PlTX exposure was attributed to toxic aerosols, in turn, the mucosae were primarily affected, and symptoms included conjunctivitis, respiratory distress, rhinorrhea, cough and fever [8, 9]. The symptoms of PlTX poisoning through contact, in turn, were both local (swelling and paresthesia around the site of injury) and systemic (dizziness, weakness, myalgia, irregularities of the ECG and indications of rhabdomyolysis), indicating that PlTX or its analogues were absorbed into the blood stream through the skin injuries [305].

Some of the recorded symptoms of PlTX poisoning, particularly the neurological ones, can be explained by alterations of ion conductance in excitable cells. The clarification of the molecular bases of the recorded symptoms, however, is far from being complete.

As in the case of ciguatera poisoning, no specific therapy exists for palytoxin poisoning, and the treatment of suspected poisoning has been symptomatic, including the intravenous infusion of mannitol [307].

Azaspiracid poisoning

The symptoms of azaspiracid (AZA) poisoning in humans are very similar to those described for DSP, including nausea, vomiting, abdominal cramps and diarrhea, which disappear within a few days after the ingestion of contaminated shellfish [242]. As in the case of OA responses (see above), the gastrointestinal effects of AZAs, including the destruction of intestinal epithelia [308], might be explained by the alterations they induce in cytoskeletal structures and the E-cadherin system, with disruption of cell-cell and cell-matrix interactions, as well as perturbation of the intestinal barrier function [247–249].

An animal study aimed at probing the carcinogenic potential of AZAs [309] has provided limited information on this issue, and more data are needed to consider a possible carcinogenic risk posed to humans by exposure to AZAs.

Uncertainties existing on the risks posed by some phycotoxins

We are not aware of cases of human intoxication that can be attributed with certainty to ingestion of food contaminated with either YTXs, or PTXs, or cyclic imines. Animal studies aimed at characterizing the toxicity of these three groups of compounds have shown that symptoms of acute toxicity can be detected only after oral administration of high doses (in the mg/kg range) [121, 265, 310]. Thus, the inclusion of YTXs, PTXs, and cyclic imines among toxins that can pose risks to the consumer through ingestion of contaminated seafood is debated.

The many facets of the ongoing discussions are not described here, although it seems appropriate to call attention to a few items that indicate the need for further studies on the mechanisms of action and toxicity of those compounds.

YTXs, for instance, are cytotoxic at the very low concentrations (nanomolar) that can be found in animals after oral administration. Furthermore, YTX has been shown to inhibit the endocytosis of E-cadherin *in vitro* and this could occur also *in vivo* (see above). Taking into consideration that proteins located at the level of the plasma membrane comprise hormone and neurotransmitter receptors, ion channels and pumps, transporters, adhesion proteins, etc., that are often involved in the control of relevant cellular and biological functions (see for instance [311]), the possibility that low YTX concentrations might alter endocytosis (and phagocytosis) *in vivo* should be evaluated [312].

The molecular mechanism of action of PTXs has been well characterized in cultured cells, but it is not clear whether effective doses of this group of compounds can exist *in vivo* after ingestion of contaminated food.

Final remarks

The information on chemistry, mechanism of action and toxicity of phycotoxins has accumulated rapidly over the last few years, but many relevant aspects remain to be characterized.

It should be noted that most of the toxins discussed above are rather chemically complex molecules, and chemical synthesis is typically not a viable route to obtaining large amounts of these compounds for extensive studies. In most cases, chemical synthesis is used to clarify the structure, and to establish basic structure-activity relationships; however, preparative isolation still plays a major role in the supply of large amounts of compounds for analytical method development, routine analysis and toxicological evaluation. Preparative isolation is also difficult due to the difficulty in separating chemically closely related analogues, and poor yields in the preparative separation and purification of trace analytes (ng/kg to mg/kg range). In addition, the algae responsible for the biosynthesis of a toxin are not always known from the beginning, are sometimes not (easily) culturable and may only grow slowly or produce little toxin in culture. Thus, isolation often relies on natural occurrence, which is most often poorly predictable and involves monitoring with unspecific techniques, such as animal assays. Therefore, the knowledge on these toxins remains limited and requires further studies.

There are many gaps in the knowledge of marine toxins, beginning with their poorly understood biological and ecological roles (chemical defense, intercellular signaling or storage?). Also the biosynthetic routes to the compounds have virtually not been explored. The many remaining gaps in the chemical behavior of phycotoxins can be categorized into the following areas: physical constants (log P_{ow}, pKa, thermal stability, etc.), chemical behavior in different pH environments and reactivity in biological systems (toxicokinetics).

Our understanding of the molecular events induced by several phycotoxin groups in different biological systems, mostly in cultured cells, is steadily increasing, and the molecular details of the mechanisms by which algal toxins trigger their effects have been remarkably characterized in a few cases. Still, many relevant features of the series of molecular events triggered by phycotoxins are not known yet, and investigations in this area are needed for a deeper understanding of their modes of action. Within this frame, the recognition that phycotoxins are increasingly used as research tools for the characterization of basic biological processes will attract the interest of researchers. The characterization of the molecular targets of those toxins for which they are not discovered may lead to the discovery of novel targets, which will most likely lead to new therapies and remedies for diseases unrelated to phycotoxin poisoning.

Moreover, the toxicity of phycotoxins, particularly in the case of their acute effects, has been characterized for many groups of compounds, but significant gaps remain, with particular regard to long-term toxicity, the possible toxicity of repeated ingestion of low doses of toxins, and the combined toxicity of mixtures of toxins belonging to different chemical groups (that often co-occur in the same naturally contaminated seafood).

The lack of the pure toxins and the poor understanding of the reactivity results in many delays in method development and validation, and in poor understanding of their toxicity. However, the authors are confident that rising awareness of the potential of marine toxins in biotechnology and medicine will contribute to the rapidly increasing knowledge on these interesting compounds.

Many exciting challenges await the investigators in the field of phycotoxins.

References

1 Tachibana K, Scheuer PJ, Tsukitani Y, Kikuchi H, Van Engen D, Clardy J, Gopichand Y, Schmitz FJ (1981) Okadaic acid, a cytotoxic polyether from two marine sponges of the genus *Halichondria. J Am Chem Soc* 103: 2469–2471
2 Takemoto T, Daigo K (1958) Constituents of *Chondria armata. Chem Pharm Bull* 6: 578–580
3 Daigo K (1959) Constituents of *Chondria armata*. I. Detection of the anthelmintic constituents. *Yakugaku Zasshi* 79: 350–353
4 Daigo K (1959) Constituents of *Chondria armata*. II. Isolation of an anthelmintic constituent.

Yakugaku Zasshi 79: 353–356

5 Takemoto T, Daigo K (1960) Über die Inhaltsstoffe von *Chondria armata* und ihre pharmakologische Wirkung. *Arch Pharm* 293: 627–633

6 Moore RE, Scheuer PJ (1971) Palytoxin: A new marine toxin from a coelenterate. *Science* 172: 495–498

7 Hallegraeff GM (2004) Harmful algal blooms: A global overview. In: GM Hallegraeff, DM Anderson, AD Cembella (eds): *Manual on Harmful Marine Microalgae*, 2nd edn. UNESCO, Paris, 25–49

8 Gallitelli M, Ungaro N, Addante LM, Gentiloni N, Sabbà C (2005) Respiratory illness as a reaction to tropical algal blooms occurring in a temperate climate. *J Am Med Assoc* 293: 2599–2600

9 Durando P, Ansaldi F, Oreste P, Moscatelli P, Marensi L, Grillo C, Gasparini R, Icardi G (2007) Collaborative Group for the Ligurian Syndromic Algal Surveillance. *Eur Surveill* 12: E070607.1

10 Worm B, Barbier EB, Beaumont N, Duffy JE, Folke C, Halpern BS, Jackson JB, Lotze HK, Micheli F, Palumbi SR, Sala E, Selkoe KA, Stachowicz JJ, Watson R (2006) Impact of biodiversity loss on ocean ecosystem services. *Science* 314: 787–790

11 Virchow R (1885) Über die Vergiftungen durch Miesmuscheln in Wilhelmshaven. *Berl Klin Wochenschr* 48: 1–2

12 Wolff M (1887) Ueber das erneute Vorkommen von giftigen Miessmuscheln in Wilhelmshaven. *Virchows Arch* 110: 376–380

13 Sommer H, Meyer KF (1937) Paralytic shellfish poisoning. *AMA Arch Path* 24: 560–598

14 Onoue Y, Noguchi T, Maruyama J, Hashimoto K, Seto H (1931) Properties of two toxins newly isolated from oysters. *J Agric Food Chem* 2: 420–423

15 Schantz EJ, Mold JD, Stanger DW, Shavel J, Riel FJ, Bowden JP, Lynch JM, Wyler RS, Riegel B, Sommer H (1957) Paralytic shellfish poison. VI. A procedure for the isolation and purification of the poison from toxic clam and mussel tissue. *J Am Chem Soc* 79: 5230–5235

16 Schantz EJ, McFarren EF, Schafer ML, Lewis KH (1958) Purified shellfish poison for bioassay standardization. *J Assoc Off Anal Chem* 41: 160–168

17 Wong JL, Oesterlin R, Rapoport H (1971) The structure of saxitoxin. *J Am Chem Soc* 93: 1238–1239

18 Quilliam MA, Wright JLC (1989) The amnesic shellfish poisoning mystery. *Anal Chem* 61: 1053–1060

19 Yasumoto T, Oshima Y, Yamaguchi M (1978) Occurrence of a new type of shellfish poisoning in the Tohoku district. *Bull Jpn Soc Sci Fish* 44: 1249–1255

20 Satake M, Ofuji K, Naoki H, James KJ, Furey A, McMahon T, Silke J, Yasumoto T (1998) Azaspiracid, a new marine toxin having unique spiro ring assemblies, isolated from Irish mussels, *Mytilus edulis*. *J Am Chem Soc* 120: 9967–9968

21 FAO. Report of the Joint FAO/IOC/WHO *ad hoc* Expert Consultation on Biotoxins in Bivalve Molluscs, Oslo, Norway, Sept. 26–30, 2004. Available at: ftp://ftp.fao.org/es/esn/food/biotoxin_report_en.pdf (accessed 5 June 2009)

22 Dell'Aversano C, Eaglesham GK, Quilliam MA (2004) Analysis of cyanobacterial toxins by hydrophilic interaction liquid chromatography-mass spectrometry. *J Chromatogr A* 1028: 155–164

23 Dell'Aversano C, Walter JA, Burton IW, Stirling DJ, Fattorusso E, Quilliam MA (2008) Isolation and structure elucidation of new and unusual saxitoxin analogues from mussels. *J Nat Prod* 71: 1518–1523

24 Hall S, Reichaedt PB (1984) Cryptic paralytic shellfish toxins. In: EP Regalis (ed.): *Seafood Toxins*. American Chemical Society, Washington DC, 113–123

25 Harada T, Oshima Y, Yasumoto T (1984) Assessment of potential activation of gonyautoxin V in the stomach of mice and rats. *Toxicon* 22: 476–478

26 Association of Official Analytical Chemists (2005) Offial Method 959.08. Paralytic shellfish poison, biological method. In: *AOAC Official Methods of Analysis*, 18th edn., AOAC Gaithersburg, USA, 79–80

27 Oshima Y (1995) Postcolumn derivatization liquid chromatographic method for paralytic shellfish toxins. *J AOAC Int* 78: 528–532

28 Lawrence JF, Niedzwiadek B, Menard C (2004) Quantitative determination of paralytic shellfish poisoning toxins in shellfish using prechromatographic oxidation and liquid chromatography with fluorescence detection: Interlaboratory study. *J AOAC Int* 87: 83–100

29 Association of Official Analytical Chemists (2005) Off. Method 2005.06. Quantitative determina-

tion of paralytic shellfish poisoning toxins in shellfish using prechromatographic oxidation and liquid chromatography with fluorescence detection. In: *AOAC Official Methods of Analysis*, 18th edn., AOAC, Gaithersburg, USA, 81–82

30 Dell'Aversano C, Hess P, Quilliam MA (2005) Hydrophilic interaction liquid chromatography-mass spectrometry for the analysis of paralytic shellfish poisoning (PSP) toxins. *J Chromatogr A* 1081: 190–201

31 Quilliam MA, Hess P, Dell'Aversano C (2001) Recent developments in the analysis of phycotoxins by liquid chromatography – mass spectrometry. In: WJ De Koe, RA Samson, HP Van Egmond, J Gilbert, M Sabino (eds): *Mycotoxins and Phycotoxins in Perspective at the Turn of the Millenium*, W.J. de Koe, Wageningen, 383–391

32 Walter JA, Leek DM, Falk M (1992) NMR study of the protonation of domoic acid. *Can J Chem* 70: 1156–1161

33 Maeda M, Kodama T, Tanaka T, Yoshizumi H, Takemoto T, Nomoto K, Fujita T (1986) Structures of isodomoic acids A, B and C, novel insecticidal amino acids from the red alga *Chondria armata*. *Chem Pharm Bull* 34: 4892–4895

34 Maeda M, Kodama T, Tanaka T, Yoshizumi H, Takemoto T, Nomoto K, Fujita T (1987) Structures of domoilactone A and B, novel amino acids from the red alga, *Chondria armata*. *Tetrahedron Lett* 28: 633–636

35 Wright JLC, Falk M, McInnes AG, Walter JA (1990) Identification of isodomoic acid D and two new geometrical isomers of domoic acid in toxic mussels. *Can J Chem* 68: 22–25

36 Walter JA, Falk M, Wright JLC (1994) Chemistry of the shellfish toxin domoic acid: Characterization of related compounds. *Can J Chem* 72: 430–436

37 Zaman L, Arakawa O, Shimosu A, Onoue Y, Nishio S, Shida Y, Noguchi T (1997) Two new isomers of domoic acid from a red alga, *Chondria armata*. *Toxicon* 35: 205–212

38 Holland PT, Selwood AI, Mountford DO, Wilkins AL, McNabb P, Rhodes LL, Doucette GJ, Mikulski CM, King KL (2005) Isodomoic acid C, an unusual amnesic shellfish poisoning toxin from *Pseudo-nitzschia australis*. *Chem Res Toxicol* 18: 814–816

39 Ramsdell JS (2007) The molecular and integrative basis to domoic acid toxicity. In: LM Botana (ed.): *Chemistry and Pharmacology of Marine Toxins*, Blackwell Publishing, Oxford, 223–250

40 Quilliam MA, Xie M, Hardstaff WR (1995) A rapid extraction and cleanup procedure for the liquid chromatographic determination of domoic acid in unsalted seafood. *J AOAC Int* 78: 543–554

41 Hess P, Morris S, Stobo LA, Brown NA, McEvoy JDG, Kennedy G, Young PB, Slattery D, McGovern E, McMahon T, Gallacher S (2005) LC-UV and LC-MS methods for the determination of domoic acid. *TrAC – Trends Anal Chem* 24: 358–367

42 McCarron P, Hess P (2006) Tissue distribution and effects of heat treatments on the content of domoic acid in blue mussels, *Mytilus edulis*. *Toxicon* 47: 473–479

43 McCarron P, Burrell S, Hess P (2007) Effect of addition of antibiotics and an antioxidant, on the stability of tissue reference materials for domoic acid, the amnesic shellfish poison. *Anal Bioanal Chem* 387: 2495–2502

44 Twiner MJ, Rehmann N, Hess P, Doucette GJ (2008) Azaspiracid shellfish poisoning: A review on the ecology, chemistry, toxicology and human health impacts. *Marine Drugs* 6: 39–74

45 Taleb H, Vale P, Amanhir R, Benhadouch A, Sagou R, Chafik A (2006) First detection of azaspiracids in North West Africa. *J Shell Res* 25: 1067–1071

46 Ueoka R, Ito A, Izumikawa M, Maeda S, Takagi M, Shin-ya K, Yoshida M, van Zoest RWM, Matsunaga S (2009) Isolation of azaspiracid-2 from a marine sponge *Echinoclathria* sp. as a potent cytotoxin. *Toxicon* 53: 680–684

47 Hess P, Butter T, Petersen A, Silke J, McMahon T (2009) Performance of the EU harmonised mouse bioassay for lipophilic toxins for the detection of azaspiracids in naturally contaminated mussel (*Mytilus edulis*) hepatopancreas tissue homogenates characterised by liquid chromatography coupled to tandem mass spectrometry. *Toxicon* 53: 713–722

48 Alfonso C, Rehmann N, Hess P, Alfonso A, Wandscheer C, Abuin M, Vale C, Otero P, Vieytes M, Botana LM (2008) Evaluation of various pH and temperature conditions on the stability of azaspiracids, and their importance in preparative isolation and toxicological studies. *Anal Chem* 80: 9672–9680

49 Nicolaou K, Chen D, Li Y, Qian W, Ling T, Vyskocil S, Koftis T, Govindasamy M, Uesaka N (2003) Total synthesis of the proposed azaspiracid-1 structure, part 2: Coupling of the C1–C20, C21–C27, and C28–C40 fragments and completion of the synthesis. *Angew Chem* 42: 3649–3653

50 Nicolaou K, Li Y, Uesaka N, Koftis T, Vyskocil S, Ling T, Govindasamy M, Qian W, Bernal F,

Chen D (2003) Total synthesis of the proposed azaspiracid-1 structure, part 1: Construction of the enantiomerically pure C1–C20, C21–C27, and C28–C40 fragments. *Angew Chem* 42: 3643–3648

51 Nicolaou KC, Vyskocil S, Koftis TV, Yamada YM, Ling T, Chen D, Tang W, Petrovic G, Frederick M, Li Y, Satake M (2004) Structural revision and total synthesis of azaspiracid-1, part 1: Intelligence gathering and tentaive proposal. *Angew Chem Int Ed* 116: 4412–4418

52 Nicolaou KC, Koftis T, Vyskocil S, Petrovic G, Ling T, Yamada YM, Tang W, Frederick M (2004) Structural revision and total synthesis of azaspiracid-1, part 2: Definition of the ABCD domain and total synthesis. *Angew Chem Int Ed* 116: 4418–4424

53 Rehmann N, Hess P, Quilliam MA (2008) Discovery of new analogs of the marine biotoxin azaspiracid in blue mussels (*Mytilus edulis*) by ultra performance liquid chromatography–tandem mass spectrometry. *Rapid Commun Mass Spectrom* 22: 549–558

54 Krock B, Tillmann U, John U, Cembella AD (2009) Characterization of azaspiracids in plankton size-fractions and isolation of an azaspiracid-producing dinoflagellate from the North Sea. *Harmful Algae* 8: 254–263

55 Tillmann U, Elbrachter M, Krock B, John U, Cembella A (2009) *Azadinium spinosum gen. et sp nov* (Dinophyceae) identified as a primary producer of azaspiracid toxins. *Eur J Phycol* 44: 63–79

56 McMahon T, Silke J (1996) Winter toxicity of unknown aetiology in mussels. *Harmful Algal News* 14: 2

57 Hess P, Nguyen L, Aasen J, Keogh M, Kilcoyne J, McCarron P, Aune T (2005) Tissue distribution, effects of cooking and parameters affecting the extraction of azaspiracids from mussels, *Mytilus edulis*, prior to analysis by liquid chromatography coupled to mass spectrometry. *Toxicon* 46: 62–71

58 McCarron P, Kilcoyne J, Miles CO, Hess P (2009) Formation of azaspiracids-3, -4, -6, and -9 *via* decarboxylation of carboxyazaspiracid metabolites from shellfish. *J Agric Food Chem* 57: 160–169

59 Ofuji K, Satake M, McMahon T, James KJ, Naoki H, Oshima Y, Yasumoto T (2001) Structures of azaspiracid analogs, azaspiracid-4 and azaspiracid-5, causative toxins of azaspiracid poisoning in Europe. *Biosci Biotechnol Biochem* 65: 740–742

60 Ito E, Frederick MO, Koftis TV, Tang W, Petrovic G, Ling T, Nicolaou KC (2006) Structure toxicity relationships of synthetic azaspiracid-1 and analogs in mice. *Harmful Algae* 5: 586–591

61 Yasumoto T, Oshima Y, Sugarawa W, Fukuyo Y, Oguri H, Igarashi T, Fujita N (1980) Identification of *Dinophysis fortii* as the causative organism of diarrhetic shellfish poisoning. *Bull Jpn Soc Sci Fish* 46: 1405–1411

62 Kumagai M, Yanagi T, Murata M, Yasumoto T, Kat M, Lassus P, Rodriguez-Vazquez JA (1986) Okadaic acid as the causative toxin of diarrhetic shellfish poisoning in Europe. *Agric Biol Chem* 50: 2853–2857

63 Hu T, Doyle J, Jackson D, Marr J, Nixon E, Pleasance S, Quilliam MA, Walter JA, Wright JLC (1992) Isolation of a new diarrhetic shellfish poison from Irish mussels. *J Chem Soc Chem Commun* 39–41

64 Swanson K, Villareal T, Campbell L (2008) The 2008 DSP event along the Texas coast: Detection and observations. Poster presentation at the 122nd AOAC Annual Meeting and Exposition, 21–25 September 2008, Dallas, TX

65 McCarron P, Kilcoyne J, Hess P (2008) Effects of cooking and heat treatment on concentration and tissue distribution of okadaic acid and dinophysistoxin-2 in mussels (*Mytilus edulis*). *Toxicon* 51: 1081–1089

66 Yasumoto T, Murata M, Lee JS, Torigoe K (1989) Polyether toxins produced by dinoflagellates. In: S Natori, K Hashimoto, Y Ueno (eds): *Mycotoxins and Phycotoxins '88*, Elsevier, Amsterdam, 375–382

67 Hu TM, Curtis JM, Oshima Y, Quilliam MA, Walter JA, Watsonwright WM, Wright JLC (1995) Spirolide-B and spirolides-D, 2 novel macrocycles isolated from the digestive glands of shellfish. *J Chem Soc Chem Comm* 2159–2161

68 Vale P (2007) Chemistry of diarrhetic shellfish poisoning toxins. In: LM Botana (ed.): *Chemistry and Pharmacology of Marine Toxins*, Blackwell Publishing, Oxford, 211–221

69 Yasumoto T, Murata M, Oshima Y, Sano M (1985) Diarrhetic shellfish toxins. *Tetrahedron* 41: 1019–1025

70 Yanagi T, Murata M, Torigoe K, Yasumoto T (1989) Biological activities of semisynthetic analogs of dinophysistoxin-3, the major diarrhetic shellfish toxin. *Agric Biol Chem* 53: 525–529

71 Britton R, Roberge M, Brown C, van Soest R, Andersen RJ (2003) New okadaic acid analogues

from the marine sponge *Merriamum oxeato* and their effect on mitosis. *J Nat Prod* 66, 838–843

72 Torgersen T, Miles CO, Rundberget T, Wilkins AL (2008) New esters of okadaic acid in seawater and blue mussels (*Mytilus edulis*). *J Agric Food Chem* 56: 9628–9635

73 Lee JS, Igarashi T, Fraga S, Dahl E, Hovgaard P, Yasumoto T (1989) Determination of diarrhetic shellfish toxins in various dinoflagellate species. *J Appl Physiol* 1: 147–152

74 EFSA (2008) Marine biotoxins in shellfish – Okadaic acid and analogues, Scientific Opinion of the Panel on Contaminants in the Food Chain. *EFSA J* 589: 1–62

75 Aune T, Larsen S, Aasen J, Rehmann N, Satake M, Hess P (2007) Relative toxicity of dinophysistoxin-2 (DTX-2) compared with okadaic acid, based on acute intraperitoneal toxicity in mice. *Toxicon* 49: 1–7

76 Miles CO (2007) Pectenotoxins. In: LM Botana (ed.): *Chemistry and Pharmacology of Marine Toxins*, Blackwell Publishing, Oxford, 159–186

77 Suzuki T, Igarashi T, Ichimi K, Watai M, Suzuki M, Ogiso E, Yasumoto T (2005) Kinetics of diarrhetic shellfish poisoning toxins, okadaic acid, dinophysistoxin-1, pectenotoxin-6 and yessotoxin in scallops *Patinopecten yessoensis*. *Fish Sci* 71: 948–955

78 Miles CO, Wilkins AL, Munday R, Dines MH, Hawkes AD, Briggs LR, Sandvik M, Jensen DJ, Cooney JM, Holland PT, Quilliam MA, MacKenzie AL, Beuzenberg V, Towers NR (2004) Isolation of pectenotoxin-2 from *Dinophysis acuta* and its conversion to pectenotoxin-2 seco acid, and preliminary assessment of their acute toxicities. *Toxicon* 43: 1–9

79 Wilkins AL, Rehmann N, Torgersen T, Rundberget T, Keogh M, Petersen D, Hess P, Rise F, Miles CO (2006) Identification of fatty acid esters of pectenotoxin-2 seco acid in blue mussels (*Mytilus edulis*) from Ireland. *J Agric Food Chem* 54: 5672–5678

80 Ito E, Suzuki T, Oshima Y, Yasumoto T (2008) Studies of diarrhetic activity on pectenotoxin-6 in the mouse and rat. *Toxicon* 51: 707–716

81 Hess P, Aasen JB (2007) Chemistry, origins and distribution of yessotoxin and its analogues. In: LM Botana (ed.): *Chemistry and Pharmacology of Marine Toxins*, Blackwell Publishing, Oxford, 187–202

82 Murata M, Kumagai M, Lee JS, Yasumoto T (1987) Isolation and structure of yessotoxin, a novel polyether compound implicated in diarrhetic shellfish poisoning. *Tetrahedron Lett* 28: 5869–5872

83 Aune T, Sorby R, Yasumoto T, Ramstad H, Landsverk T (2002) Comparison of oral and intraperitoneal toxicity of yessotoxin towards mice. *Toxicon* 40: 77–82

84 Tubaro A, Sosa S, Carbonatto M, Altinier G, Vita F, Melato M, Satake M, Yasumoto T (2003) Oral and intraperitoneal acute toxicity studies of yessotoxin and homoyessotoxins in mice. *Toxicon* 41: 783–792

85 Tubaro A, Sosa S, Altinier G, Soranzo MR, Satake M, Della Loggia R, Yasumoto T (2004) Short-term oral toxicity of homoyessotoxins, yessotoxin and okadaic acid in mice. *Toxicon* 43: 439–445

86 Ciminiello P, Dell'Aversano C, Fattorusso E, Forino M, Magno S, Guerrini F, Pistocchi R, Boni L (2003) Complex yessotoxins profile in *Protoceratium reticulatum* from north-western Adriatic sea revealed by LC-MS analysis. *Toxicon* 42: 7–14

87 Samdal IA, Naustvoll LJ, Olseng CD, Briggs LR, Miles CO (2004) Use of ELISA to identify *Protoceratium reticulatum* as a source of yessotoxin in Norway. *Toxicon* 44: 75–82

88 Satake M, MacKenzie L, Yasumoto T (1997) Identification of *Protoceratium reticulatum* as the biogenetic origin of yessotoxin. *Nat Toxins* 5: 164–167

89 Satake M, Ichimura T, Sekiguchi K, Yoshimatsu S, Oshima Y (1999) Confirmation of yessotoxin and 45,46,47-trinoryessotoxin production by *Protoceratium reticulatum* collected in Japan. *Nat Toxins* 7: 147–150

90 Draisci R, Ferretti E, Palleschi L, Marchiafava C, Poletti R, Milandri A, Ceredi A, Pompei M (1999) High levels of yessotoxin in mussels and presence of yessotoxin and homoyessotoxin in dinoflagellates of the Adriatic Sea. *Toxicon* 37: 1187–1193

91 Rhodes L, McNabb P, de Salas M, Briggs L, Beuzenberg V, Gladstone M (2006) Yessotoxin production by *Gonyaulax spinifera*. *Harmful Algae* 5: 148–155

92 Draisci R, Lucentini L, Mascioni A (2000) Pectenotoxins and yessotoxins: Chemistry, toxicology, pharmacology, and analysis. In: Botana, LM (ed.): *Seafood and Freshwater Toxins: Pharmacology, Physiology, and Detection*, Marcel Dekker, New York, 289–324

93 Finch S, Wilkins A. Hawkes A, Jensen D, MacKenzie L, Beuzenberg V, Quilliam M, Olseng C, Samdal I, Aasen J, Selwood AI, Cooney JM, Sandvik M, Miles CO (2005) Isolation and identification of (44-*R,S*)-44,55,dihydroxyyessotoxin from *Protoceratium reticulatum*, and its occurrence in extracts of shellfish from New Zealand, Norway and Canada *Toxicon* 46: 160–170

94 Miles CO, Samdal IA, Aasen JAB, Jensen DJ, Quilliam M, Petersen D, Briggs LM, Wilkins AL, Rise F, Cooney JM, MacKenzie AL (2005) Evidence of numerous analogs of yessotoxin in *Protoceratium reticulatum*. *Harmful Algae* 4: 1075–1091

95 Satake M, Tubaro A, Lee JS, Yasumoto T (1997) Two new analogs of yessotoxin, homoyessotoxin and 4,5-hydroxyhomoyessotoxin, isolated from mussels of the Adriatic Sea. *Nat Toxins* 5: 107–110

96 Miles CO, Wilkins AL, Jensen DJ, Cooney JM, Quilliam MA, Aasen J, Mackenzie AL (2004) Isolation of 41a-homoyessotoxin and the identification of 9-methyl-41a-homoyessotoxin and nor-ring A-yessotoxin from *Protoceratium reticulatum*. *Chem Res Toxicol* 17: 1414–1422

97 Miles CO, Wilkins AL, Hawkes AD, Selwood AI, Jensen DJ, Munday R, Cooney, JM, Beuzenberg V (2005) Polyhydroxylated amide analogs of yessotoxin from *Protoceratium reticulatum*. *Toxicon* 45: 61–71

98 Ferrari S, Ciminiello P, Dell'Aversano C, Forino M, Malaguti C, Tubaro A, Poletti R, Yasumoto T, Fattorusso E, Rossini GP (2004) Structure-activity relationships of yessotoxins in cultured cells. *Chem Res Toxicol* 17: 1251–1257

99 Moore RE, Bartolini G (1981) Structure of palytoxin. *J Am Chem Soc* 103: 2491–2494

100 Uemura D, Ueda K, Hirata Y, Naoki H, Iwashita T (1981) Further studies on palytoxin.1. *Tetrahedron Lett* 22: 1909–1912

101 Uemura D, Ueda K, Hirata Y, Naoki H, Iwashita T (1981) Further studies on palytoxin. 2. Structure of palytoxin. *Tetrahedron Lett* 22: 2781–2784

102 Katikou P (2008) Palytoxin and analogues: Ecobiology and origin, chemistry, metabolism, and chemical analysis. In: LM Botana (ed.): *Seafood and Freshwater Toxins – Pharmacology, Physiology and Detection*, CRC Press, Taylor & Francis Group, Boca Raton, FL, 631–663

103 Kita M, Uemura D (2008) Diverse chemical structures and bioactivities of marine toxins: Palytoxin and symbiodinolide. In: LM Botana (ed.): *Seafood and Freshwater Toxins – Pharmacology, Physiology and Detection*, CRC Press, Taylor & Francis Group, Boca Raton, FL, 665–674

104 Kimura S, Hashimoto Y, Yamazato K (1972) Toxicity of the zoanthid *Palythoa tuberculosa*. *Toxicon* 10: 611–617

105 Onuma Y, Satake M, Ukena T, Roux J, Chanteau S, Rasolofonirira N, Ratsimaloto M, Naoki H, Yasumoto T (1999) Identification of putative palytoxin as the cause of clupeotoxism. *Toxicon* 37: 55–65

106 Penna A, Vila M, Fraga S, Giacobbe MG, Andreoni F, Riobo P, Vernesi C (2005) Characterization of *Ostreopsis* and *Coolia* (Dinophyceae) isolates in the western Mediterranean sea based on morphology, toxicity and internal transcribed spacer 5.8S rDNA sequences. *J Phycol* 41: 212–225

107 Lenoir S, Ten-Hage L, Turquet J, Quod JP, Bernard C, Hennion MC (2004) First evidence of palytoxin analogues from an *Ostreopsis mascarenensis* (Dinophyceae) benthic bloom in Southwestern Indian Ocean. *J Phycol* 40: 1042–1051

108 Moore RE, Bartolini G, Barchi J, Bothnerby AA, Dadok J, Ford J (1982) Absolute stereochemistry of palytoxin. *J Am Chem Soc* 104: 3776–3779

109 Uemura D, Hirata Y, Iwashita T, Naoki H (1985) Studies on palytoxins. *Tetrahedron* 41: 1007–1017

110 Frolova GM, Kuznetsova TA, Mikhailov VV, Elyakov GB (2000) An enzyme linked immunosorbent assay for detecting palytoxin-producing bacteria. *Bioorg Khim* 26: 315–320

111 Ciminiello P, Dell'Aversano C, Fattorusso E, Forino M, Tartaglione L, Grillo C, Melchiorre N (2008) Putative palytoxin and its new analogue, ovatoxin-a, in *Ostreopsis ovata* collected along the Ligurian coasts during the 2006 toxic outbreak. *J Am Soc Mass Spectrom* 19: 111–120

112 Aligizaki K, Katikou P, Nikolaidis G, Panou A (2008) First episode of shellfish contamination by palytoxin-like compounds from *Ostreopsis* species (Aegean Sea, Greece). *Toxicon* 51: 418–427

113 Uemura D, Chou T, Haino T, Nagatsu A, Fukuzawa S, Zheng S, Chen H (1995) Pinnatoxin A: A toxic amphoteric macrocycle from the Okinawan bivalve *Pinna muricata*. *J Am Chem Soc* 117: 1155–1156

114 Takada N, Umemura N, Suenaga K, Uemura D (2001) Structural determination of pteriatoxins A, B and C, extremely potent toxins from the bivalve *Pteria penguin*. *Tetrahedron Lett* 42: 3495–3497

115 Lu CK, Lee GH, Huang R, Chou HN (2001) Spiro-prorocentrimine, a novel macrocyclic lactone from a benthic *Prorocentrum* sp of Taiwan. *Tetrahedron Lett* 42: 1713–1716

116 Seki T, Satake M, MacKenzie L, Kaspar HF, Yasumoto T (1995) Gymnodimine, a new marine

toxin of unprecedented structure isolated from New Zealand oysters and the dinoflagellate, *Gymnodinium* sp. *Tetrahedron Lett* 36: 7093–7096

117 Hu TM, Curtis JM, Walter JA, Wright JLC (1996) Characterization of biologically inactive spirolides E and F: Identification of the spirolide pharmacophore. *Tetrahedron Lett* 37: 7671–7674

118 McCauley JA, Nagasawa K, Lander PA, Mischke SG, Semones MA, Kishi Y (1998) Total synthesis of pinnatoxin A. *J Am Chem Soc* 120: 7647–7648

119 Molgo J, Girard E, Benoit E (2007) Cyclic imines: An insight into this emerging group of bioactive marine toxins. In: LM Botana (ed.): *Phycotoxins, Chemistry and Biochemistry*, Blackwell Publishing, Oxford, 319–335

120 Cembella AD, Krock B (2008) Cyclic imine toxins: Chemistry, biogeography, biosynthesis and pharmacology. In: LM Botana (ed.): *Seafood and Freshwater Toxins, Pharmacology, Physiology and Detection*, Taylor & Francis Ltd, Boca Raton, FL, 561–580

121 Munday R (2008) Toxicology of cyclic imines: Gymnodimine, spirolides, pinnatoxins, pteriatoxins, prorocentrolide, spiro-prorocentrimine and symbioimines. In: LM Botana (ed.): *Seafood and Freshwater Toxins, Pharmacology, Physiology and Detection*, Taylor & Francis Ltd, Boca Raton, FL, 581–594

122 Baden DG, Bourdelais AJ, Jacocks H, Michelliza S, Naar J (2005) Natural and derivative brevetoxins: Historical background, multiplicity, and effects. *Environ Health Perspect* 113: 621–625

123 Satake M, Shoji M, Oshima Y, Naoki H, Fujita T, Yasumoto T (2002) Gymnocin-A, a cytotoxic polyether from the notorious red tide dinoflagellate, *Gymnodinium mikimotoi*. *Tetrahedron Lett* 43: 5829–5832

124 Pierce RH, Henry MS, Blum PC, Hamel SL, Kirkpatrick B, Cheng YS, Zhou Y, Irvin CM, Naar J, Weidner A, Fleming LE, Backer LC, Baden DG (2005) Brevetoxin composition in water and marine aerosol along a Florida beach: Assessing potential human exposure to marine biotoxins. *Harmful Algae* 4: 965–972

125 Alam M, Sanduja R, Hossain MB, van der Helm D (1982) *Gymnodinium breve* toxins. I. Isolation and X-ray structure of *O,O*-dipropyl (E)-2-(1-methyl-2-oxopropylidene)phosphorohydrazidothioate (E)-oxime from the red tide dinoflagellate *Gymnodinium breve*. *J Am Chem Soc* 104: 5232–5234

126 Lin YY, Risk M, Ray SM, van Engen D, Clardy J, Golik J, James JC, Nakanishi K (1981) Isolation and structure of brevetoxin B from the "red tide" dinoflagellate *Ptychodiscus brevis* (*Gymnodinium breve*). *J Am Chem Soc* 103: 6773–6775

127 Shimizu Y, Chou HN, Bando H, van Duyne G, Clardy JC (1986) Structure of brevetoxin A (GB-1 toxin), the most potent toxin in the Florida red tide organism *Gymnodinium breve* (*Ptychodiscus brevis*). *J Am Chem Soc* 108: 515–516

128 Plakas SM, Wang ZH, El Said KR, Jester ELE, Granade HR, Flewelling L, Scott P, Dickey RW (2004) Brevetoxin metabolism and elimination in the Eastern oyster (*Crassostrea virginica*) after controlled exposures to *Karenia brevis*. *Toxicon* 44: 677–685

129 Wang Z, Plakas SM, El Said KR, Jester ELE, Granade HR, Dickey RW (2004) LC/MS analysis of brevetoxin metabolites in the Eastern oyster (*Crassostrea virginica*). *Toxicon* 43: 455–465

130 Abraham A, Plakas SM, Wang ZH, Jester ELE, El Said KR, Granade HR, Henry MS, Blum PC, Pierce RH, Dickey RW (2006) Characterization of polar brevetoxin derivatives isolated from *Karenia brevis* cultures and natural blooms. *Toxicon* 48: 104–115

131 Rein KS, Lynn B, Gawley RE, Baden DG (1994) Brevetoxin B: Chemical modifications, synaptosome binding, toxicity, and an unexpected conformational effect. *J Org Chem* 59: 2107–2113

132 Bourdelais AJ, Campbell S, Jacocks H, Naar J, Wright J, Carsi J, Baden DG (2004) Brevenal is a natural inhibitor of brevetoxin action in sodium channel receptor binding assays. *Cell Mol Neurobiol* 24: 553–563

133 Dechraoui MYB, Wacksman JJ, Ramsdell JS (2006) Species selective resistance of cardiac muscle voltage gated sodium channels: Characterization of brevetoxin and ciguatoxin binding sites in rats and fish. *Toxicon* 48: 702–712

134 Murata M, Yasumoto T (2000) The structure elucidation and biological activities of high molecular weight algal toxins: Maitotoxin, prymnesins and zooxanthellatoxins. *Nat Prod Rep* 17: 293–314

135 Murata M, Legrand AM, Ishibashi Y, Yasumoto T (1989) Structures of ciguatoxin and its congener. *J Am Chem Soc* 111: 8929–8931

136 Murata M, Legrand AM, Ishibashi Y, Fukui M, Yasumoto T (1990) Structures and configurations

of ciguatoxin from the moray eel *Gymnothorax javanicus* and its likely precursor from the dinoflagellate *Gambierdiscus toxicus*. *J Am Chem Soc* 112: 4380–4386

137 Legrand AM, Fukui M, Cruchet P, Yasumoto T (1992) Progress on chemical knowledge of ciguatoxins. *Bull Soc Pathol Exot* 85: 467–469

138 Lewis RJ, Sellin M, Poli MA, Norton RS, MacLeod JK, Sheil MM (1991) Purification and characterization of ciguatoxins from moray eel (*Lycodontis javanicus*, Muraenidae). *Toxicon* 29: 1115–1127

139 Poli MA, Lewis RJ, Dickey RJ, Musser SM, Buckner CA, Carpenter LG (1997) Identification of Caribbean ciguatoxins as the cause of an outbreak of fish poisoning among U.S. soldiers in Haiti. *Toxicon* 35: 733–741

140 Satake M, Murata M, Yasumoto T (1993) The structure of CTX3C, a ciguatoxin congener isolated from cultured *Gambierdiscus toxicus*. *Tetrahedron Lett* 34: 1975–1978

141 Satake M, Morohashi A, Oguri H, Oishi T, Hirama M, Harada N, Yasumoto T (1997) The absolute configuration of ciguatoxin. *J Am Chem Soc* 119: 11325–11326

142 Satake M, Fukui M, Legrand AM, Cruchet P, Yasumoto T (1998) Isolation and structures of new ciguatoxin analogs, 2,3-dihydroxyCTX3C and 51-hydroxyCTX3C, accumulated in tropical reef fish. *Tetrahedron Lett* 39: 1197–1198

143 Dickey RW (2008) Ciguatera toxins: Chemistry, toxicology and detection. In: LM Botana (ed.): *Seafood and Freshwater Toxins – Pharmacology, Physiology and Detection*, CRC Press, Taylor & Francis Group, Boca Raton, FL, 479–500

144 Chateau-Degat ML, Chinain M, Cerf N, Gingras S, Hubert B, Dewailly E (2005) Seawater temperature, *Gambierdiscus* spp. variability and incidence of ciguatera poisoning in French Polynesia. *Harmful Algae* 4: 1053–1062

145 Yasumoto T, Nakajima I, Bagnis R, Adachi R (1977) Finding of a dinoflagellate as a likely culprit of ciguatera. *Bull Jap Soc Sci Fish* 43: 1021–1026

146 Adachi R, Fukuyo Y (1979) The thecal structure of a toxic marine dinoflagellate *Gambierdiscus toxicus gen. et spec. nov.* collected in a ciguatera-endemic area. *Bull Jap Soc Sci Fish* 45: 67–71

147 Aasen JAB, Hardstaff W, Aune T, Quilliam M (2006) Discovery of fatty acid ester metabolites of spirolide toxins in mussels from Norway using liquid chromatography/tandem mass spectrometry. *Rapid Commun Mass Spectrom* 20: 1531–1537

148 Ciminiello P, Fattorusso E, Forino M, Poletti R, Viviani R (2000) Structure determination of carboxyhomoyessotoxin, a new yessotoxin analogue isolated from Adriatic mussels. *Chem Res Toxicol* 13: 770–774

149 Miles CO, Wilkins AL, Selwood AI, Hawkes AD, Jensen DJ, Cooney JM, Beuzenberg V, MacKenzie AL (2006) Isolation of yessotoxin 32-*O*-[β-L-arabinofuranosyl-(5′→1″)-β-L-arabinofuranoside] from *Protoceratium reticulatum*. *Toxicon* 47: 510–516

150 Castèle S, Catterall WA (2000) Molecular mechanisms of neurotoxin action on voltage-gated sodium channels. *Biochimie* 82: 883–892

151 Hartshorne RP, Catterall WA (1984) The sodium channel from rat brain. Purification and subunit composition. *J Biol Chem* 259: 1667–1675

152 Hille B (1975) The receptor for tetrodotoxin and saxitoxin: A structural hypothesis. *Biophys J* 15: 615–619

153 Hille B (1968) Pharmacological modifications of the sodium channels of frog nerves. *J Gen Physiol* 51: 199–219

154 Wang J, Salata JJ, Bennett PB (2003) Saxitoxin is a gating modifier of hERG K$^+$ channels. *J Gen Physiol* 121: 583–598

155 Su Z, Sheets M, Hishida H, Li F, Barry WH (2004) Saxitoxin blocks L-type I_{Ca}. *J Pharmacol Exp Ther* 308: 324–329

156 Llewellyn LE (2006) Saxitoxin, a toxic marine natural product that targets a multitude of receptors. *Nat Prod Rep* 23: 200–222

157 Lombert A, Bidard JN, Lazdunski M (1987) Ciguatoxins and brevetoxins share a common receptor site on the neuronal voltage-dependent Na$^+$ channel. *FEBS Lett* 219: 355–357

158 Randall JE (1958) A review of ciguatera, tropical fish poisoning, with a tentative explanation of its cause. *Bull Mar Sci Gulf Carib* 8: 236–267

159 Terao K (2000) Ciguatera toxins: Toxinology. In: LM Botana (ed.): *Seafood and Freshwater Toxins*, Marcel Dekker, New York, 449–472

160 Gusovsky F, Daly JL (1990) Maitotoxin: A unique pharmacological tool for research on calcium-dependent mechanisms. *Biochem Pharmacol* 39: 1633–1639

161 Trevino CL, Escobar L, Vaca L, Morales-Tlalpan V, Ocampo AY, Darszon A (2008) Maitotoxin: A unique pharmacological tool for elucidating Ca^{2+}-dependent mechanisms. In: LM Botana (ed.): *Seafood and Freshwater Toxins, Pharmacology, Physiology and Detection*, Taylor & Francis Ltd, Boca Raton, FL, 503–516

162 Morales-Tlalpan V, Vaca L (2002) Modulation of the maitotoxin response by intracellular and extracellular cations. *Toxicon* 40: 493–500

163 Dietl P, Völkl H (1994) Maitotoxin activates a nonselective cation channel and stimulates Ca^{2+} entry in MDCK renal epithelial cells. *Mol Pharmacol* 45: 300–305

164 Estacion M, Nguyen HB, Gargus JJ (1996) Calcium is permeable through a maitotoxin-activated nonselective cation channel in mouse L cells. *Am J Physiol* 270: C1145-C1152

165 Leech CA, Habner JF (1997) Insulinotropic glucagon-like peptide-1-mediated activation of nonselective cation currents in insulinoma cells is mimicked by maitotoxin. *J Biol Chem* 272: 17987–17993

166 Ohizumi Y, Yasumoto T (1983) Contraction and increase in tissue calcium content induced by maitotoxin, the most potent known marine toxin, in intestinal smooth muscle. *Br J Pharmacol* 79: 3–5

167 Takahashi M, Tatsumi M, Ohizumi Y, Yasumoto T (1983) Ca^{2+} channel activating function of maitotoxin, the most potent marine toxin known, in clonal rat pheochromocytoma cells. *J Biol Chem* 258: 10944–10949

168 Schettini G, Koike K, Login IS, Judd AM, Cronin MJ, Yasumoto T, MacLeod RM (1984) Maitotoxin stimulates hormonal release and calcium influx in rat anterior pituitary cells *in vitro*. *Am J Physiol* 247: E520–E525

169 Holz GG, Leech CA, Habener JF (2000) Insulinotropic toxins as molecular probes for analysis of glucagon-like peptide-1 receptor-mediated signal transduction in pancreatic β-cells. *Biochimie* 82: 915–926

170 Gusovsky F, Daly JW, Yasumoto T, Rojas E (1988) Differential effects of maitotoxin on ATP secretion and on phosphoinositide breakdown in rat pheochromocytoma cells. *FEBS Lett* 233: 139–142

171 Choi OH, Gusovsky F, Yasumoto T, Daly JW (1990) Maitotoxin: Effects on calcium channels, phosphoinositide breakdown, and arachidonate release in pheochromocytoma PC12 cells. *Mol Pharmacol* 37: 222–230

172 Gusovsky F, Yasumoto T, Daly JW (1989) Calcium-dependent effects of maitotoxin on phosphoinositide breakdown and on cyclic AMP accumulation in PC12 and NCB-20 cells. *Mol Pharmacol* 36: 44–53

173 Malaguti C, Yasumoto T, Rossini GP (1999) Transient Ca^{2+}-dependent activation of ERK1 and ERK2 in cytotoxic responses induced by maitotoxin in breast cancer cells. *FEBS Lett* 458: 137–140

174 Kobayashi M, Kondo S, Yasumoto T, Ohizumi Y (1986) Cardiotoxic effects of maitotoxin, a principal toxin of seafood poisoning, on guinea pig and rat cardiac muscle. *J Pharmacol Exp Ther* 238: 1077–1083

175 Terao K, Ito E, Sakamaki Y, Igarashi K, Yokoyama A, Yasumoto T (1988) Histopathological studies of experimental marine toxin poisoning. II. The acute effects of maitotoxin on the stomach, heart, and lymphoid tissues in mice and rats. *Toxicon* 26: 395–402

176 Ghiaroni V, Sasaki M, Fuwa H, Rossini GP, Scalera G, Yasumoto T, Pietra P, Bigiani A (2005) Inhibition of voltage-gated potassium currents by gambierol in mouse taste cells. *Toxicol Sci* 85: 657–665

177 Cuypers E, Abdel-Mottaleb Y, Kopljar I, Rainier JD, Raes AL, Snyders DJ, Tytgat J (2008) Gambierol, a toxin produced by the dinoflagellate *Gambierdiscus toxicus*, is a potent blocker of voltage-gated potassium channels. *Toxicon* 51: 974–983

178 Louzao MC, Cagide E, Vieytes MR, Sasaki M, Fuwa H, Yasumoto T, Botana LM (2006) The sodium channel of human excitable cells is a target for gambierol. *Cell Physiol Biochem* 17: 257–268

179 Sala GL, Ronzitti G, Sasaki M, Fuwa H, Yasumoto T, Bigiani A, Rossini GP (2009) Proteomic analysis reveals multiple patterns of response in cells exposed to a toxin mixture. *Chem Res Toxicol* 22: 1077–1085

180 Habermann E, Chhatwal GS (1982) Ouabain inhibits the increase due to palytoxin of cationic permeability of erythrocytes. *Naunyn-Schmeideberg's Arch Pharmacol* 319: 101–107

181 Muramatsu I, Nishio M, Kigoshi S, Uemura D (1988) Single ionic channels induced by palytox-

in in guinea-pig ventricular myocytes. *Br J Pharmacol* 93: 811–816

182 Ikeda M, Mitani K, Ito K (1988) Palytoxin induces a nonselective cation channel in single ventricular cells of rat. *Naunyn-Schmeideberg's Arch Pharmacol* 337: 591–593

183 Artigas P, Gadsby DC (2003) Na⁺/K⁺-pump ligands modulate gating of palytoxin-induced ion
channels. *Proc Natl Acad Sci USA* 100: 501–505

184 Artigas P, Gadsby DC (2004) Large diameter of palytoxin-induced the Na/K pump channels and
modulation of palytoxin interaction by Na/K pump ligands. *J Gen Physiol* 123: 357–376

185 Artigas P, Gadsby DC (2006) Ouabain affinity determining residues lie close to the Na/K pump
ion pathway. *Proc Natl Acad Sci USA* 103: 12613–12618

186 Reyes N, Gadsby DC (2006) Ion permeation through the Na⁺/K⁺-ATPase. *Nature* 443: 470–474

187 Takeuchi A, Reyes N, Artigas P, Gadsby DC (2008) The ion pathway through the opened Na⁺,K⁺-
ATPase pump. *Nature* 456: 413–416

188 Habermann E, Ahnert-Hilger G, Chhatwal GS, Beress L (1981) Delayed haemolytic action of
palytoxin. General characteristics. *Biochim Biophys Acta* 649: 481–486

189 Redondo J, Fiedler B, Scheiner-Bobis G (1996) Palytoxin-induced Na⁺ influx into yeast cells
expressing the mammalian sodium pump is due to the formation of a channel within the enzyme.
Mol Pharmacol 49: 49–57

190 Hirsh JK, Wu CH (1997) Palytoxin-induced single-channel currents from the sodium pump synthesized by *in vitro* expression. *Toxicon* 35: 169–176

191 Frelin C, van Renterghem C (1995) Palytoxin. Recent electrophysiological and pharmacological
evidence for several mechanisms of action. *Gen Pharmacol* 26: 33–37

192 Sauviat MP (1989) Effect of palytoxin on the calcium current and the mechanical activity of frog
heart muscle. *Br J Pharmacol* 98: 773–780

193 Kockskämper J, Ahmmed GU, Zima AV, Sheehan KA, Glitsch HG, Blater LA (2004) Palytoxin
disrupts cardiac excitation-contraction coupling through interactions with P-type ion pumps. *Am
J Cell Physiol* 287: C527–C538

194 Vale C, Alfonso A, Suñol C, Vieytes MR, Botana LM (2006) Modulation of calcium entry and
glutamate release in cultured cerebellar granule cells by palytoxin. *J Neurosci Res* 83: 1393–1406

195 Ito K, Karaki H, Urakawa N (1977) The mode of contractile action of palytoxin on vascular
smooth muscle. *Eur J Pharmacol* 46: 9–14

196 Frelin C, Vigne P, Breittmayer JP (1990) Palytoxin acidifies chick cardiac cells and activates the
Na⁺/H⁺ antiporter. *FEBS Lett* 264: 63–66

197 Yoshizumi M, Houchi H, Ishimura Y, Masuda Y, Morita K, Oka M (1991) Mechanism of palytoxin-induced Na⁺ influx into cultured bovine adrenal chromaffin cells: Possible involvement of
Na⁺/H⁺ exchange system. *Neurosci Lett* 130: 103–106

198 Monroe JJ, Tashjan AH Jr (1996) Palytoxin modulates cytosolic pH in human osteoblast-like
Saos-2 cells *via* an interaction with Na⁺-K⁺-ATPase. *Am J Physiol* 270: C1277-C1283

199 Levine L, Fujiki H (1985) Stimulation of arachidonic acid metabolism by different types of tumor
promoters. *Carcinogenesis* 6: 1631–1634

200 Lazzaro M, Tshjian AH Jr, Fujiki H, Levine L (1987) Palytoxin: An extraordinary potent stimu-
lator of prostaglandin production and bone resorption in cultured mouse clavariae. *Endocrinology*
120: 1338–1345

201 Miura D, Kobayashi M, Kakiuchi S, Kasahara Y, Kondo S (2006) Enhancement of transformed
foci and induction of prostaglandins in Balb/c 3 T3 cells by palytoxin: *In vitro* model reproduces
carcinogenic responses in animal models regarding the inhibitory effect of indomethacin and
reversal of indomethacin's effect by exogenous prostaglandins. *Toxicol Sci* 89: 154–163

202 Nagase H, Karaki H (1987) Palytoxin-induced contraction and release of prostaglandins and
norepinepfrine in the aorta. *J Pharmacol Exp Ther* 242: 1120–1125

203 Fujiki H, Suganuma M, Nakayasu M, Hakii H, Horiuchi T, Takayama S, Sugimura T (1986)
Palytoxin is a non-12-*O*-tetradecanoylphorbol-13-acetate type tumor promoter in two-stage
mouse skin carcinogenesis. *Carcinogenesis* 7: 707–710

204 Katz M, Amit I, Yarden Y (2007) Regulation of MAPKs by growth factors and receptor tyrosine
kinases. *Biochim Biophys Acta* 1773: 1161–1176

205 Wattenberg EV (2007) Palytoxin: Exploiting a novel skin tumor promoter to explore signal transduction and carcinogenesis. *Am J Cell Physiol* 292: C24–C32

206 Bellocci M, Ronzitti G, Milandri A, Melchiorre N, Grillo C, Poletti R, Yasumoto T, Rossini GP
(2008) A cytolytic assay for the measurement of palytoxin based on a cultured monolayer cell
line. *Anal Biochem* 374: 48–55

207 Meldrum BS (2000) Glutamate as a neurotransmitter in the brain: Review of physiology and pathology. *J Nutr* 130: 1007S–1015S

208 Pulido OM (2008) Domoic acid toxicologic pathology: A review. *Mar Drugs* 6: 180–219

209 Doucette DA, Tasker RA (2008) Domoic acid: Detection methods, pharmacology, and toxicology. In: LM Botana (ed.): *Seafood and Freshwater Toxins, Pharmacology, Physiology and Detection*, Taylor & Francis Ltd, Boca Raton, FL, 397–429

210 Ozawa S, Kamiya H, Tsuzuki K (1998) Glutamate receptors in the mammalian central nervous system. *Prog Neurobiol* 54: 581–618

211 Lerma J, Paternain AV, Rodríguez-Moreno A, López-García J (2001) Molecular Physiology of kainate receptors. *Physiol Rev* 81: 971–998

212 Xi D, Ramsdell JS (1996) Glutamate receptors and calcium entry mechanisms for domoic acid in hippocampal neurons. *NeuroReport* 26: 1115–1120

213 Berman FW, LePage KT, Murray TF (2002) Domoic acid neurotoxicity in cultured cerebellar granule neurons is controlled by the NMDA receptor Ca^{2+} influx pathway. *Brain Res* 924: 20–29

214 Brown JA, Njjar MS (1995) The release of glutamate and aspartate from rat brain synaptosomes in response to domoic acid (amnesic shellfish toxin) and kainic acid. *Mol Cell Biochem* 151: 49–54

215 Malva JO, Carvalho AP, Carvalho CM (1996) Domoic acid induces the release of glutamate in the rat hippocampal CA3 sub-region. *NeuroReport* 7: 1330–1334

216 Berman FW, Murray TF (1997) Domoic acid neurotoxicity in cultured crebellar granule neurons is mediated predominantly by NMDA receptors that are activated as a consequence of excitatory amino acid release. *J Neurochem* 69: 693–703

217 Novelli A, Kispert J, Fernández-Sánchez MT, Torreblanca A, Zitko V (1992) Domoic acid-containing toxic mussels produce neurotoxicity in neuronal cultures through a synergism between excitatory amino acids. *Brain Res* 577: 41–48

218 Berman FW, Murray TF (1996) Characterization of glutamate toxicity in cultured rat cerebellar granule neurons at reduced temperature. *J Biochem Toxicol* 11: 111–119

219 Bowie D, Lange GD (2002) Functional stoichiometry of glutamate receptor desensitization. *J Neurosci* 22: 3392–3403

220 Teitelbaum JS, Zatorre RJ, Carpenter S, Gendron D, Evans AC, Gjedde A, Cashman NR (1990) Neurologic sequelae of domoic acid intoxication due to the ingestion of contaminated mussels. *N Engl J Med* 322: 1781–1787

221 Cendes F, Andermann F, Carpenter S, Zatorre RJ, Cashman NR (1995) Temporal lobe epilepsy caused by domoic acid intoxication: Evidence for glutamate receptor-mediated excitotoxicity in humans. *Ann Neurol* 37: 123–126

222 Tasker RA, Strain SM, Drejer J (1996) Selective reduction in domoic acid toxicity *in vivo* by a novel non-*N*-methyl-D-aspartate receptor antagonist. *Can J Physiol Pharmacol* 74: 1047–1054

223 Jakobsen B, Tasker A, Zimmer J (2002) Domoic acid neurotoxicity in hippocampal slice cultures. *Amino Acids* 23: 37–44

224 Giordano G, White CC, Mohar I, Kavanagh TJ, Costa LG (2007) Glutathione levels modulate domoic acid induced apoptosis in mouse cerebellar granule cells. *Toxicol Sci* 100: 433–444

225 Gill S, Murphy M, Clausen J, Richard D, Quilliam M, MacKinnon S, LaBlanc P, Mueller R, Pulido O (2003) Neural injury biomarkers of novel shellfish toxins, spirolides: A pilot study using immunochemical and transcriptional analysis. *NeuroToxicology* 24: 593–604

226 Bialojan C, Takai A (1988) Inhibitory effect of a marine sponge toxin, okadaic acid, on protein phosphatases. *Biochem J* 256: 283–290

227 Takai A, Mieskes G (1991) Inhibitory effect of okadaic acid on the *p*-nitrophenyl phosphate phosphatase activity of protein phosphatases. *Biochem J* 275: 233–239

228 Krebs EG (1985) The phosphorylation of proteins: A major mechanism for biological regulation. *Biochem Soc Trans* 13: 813–820

229 Roach PJ (1991) Multisite and hierarchal protein phosphorylation. *J Biol Chem* 266: 14139–14142

230 Kholodenko BN (2006) Cell-signalling dynamics in time and space. *Nat Rev Mol Cell Biol* 7: 165–176

231 Hunter T (1995) Protein kinases and phosphatases: The yin and yang of protein phosphorylation and signaling. *Cell* 80: 225–236

232 Tolstykh T, Lee J, Vafai S, Stock JB (2000) Carboxyl methylation regulates phosphoprotein phosphatase 2A by controlling the association of regulatory B subunits. *EMBO J* 19: 5682–5691

233 Haystead TA, Sim ATR, Carling D, Honnor RC, Tsukitani Y, Cohen P, Hardie DG (1989) Effects of the tumor promoter okadaic acid on intracellular protein phosphorylation and metabolism. *Nature* 337: 78–81

234 Suganuma M, Fujiki H, Suguri H, Yoshizawa S, Hirota M, Nakayasu M, Ojika M, Wakamatsu K, Yamada K, Sugimura T (1988) Okadaic acid: An additional non-phorbol-12-tetradecanoate-13-acetate-type tumor promoter. *Proc Natl Acad Sci USA* 85: 1768–1771

235 Suganuma M, Tatematsu M, Yatsunami J, Yoshizawa S, Okabe S, Uemura D, Fujiki H (1992) An alternative theory of tissue specificity by tumor promotion of okadaic acid in glandular stomach of SD rats. *Carcinogenesis* 13: 1841–1845

236 Berenblum I, Haran-Ghera N (1955) The significance of the sequence of initiating and promoting actions in the process of skin carcinogenesis in mouse. *Br J Cancer* 3: 268–271

237 Rossini GP (2000) Neoplastic activity of DSP toxins: The effects of okadaic acid and related compounds on cell proliferation: Tumor promotion or induction of apoptosis? In: LM Botana, (ed.): *Seafood and Freshwater Toxins*, Marcel Dekker, New York, 257–288

238 Tripuraneni J, Koutsoris A, Pestic L, De Lanerolle P, Hect G (1997) The toxin of diarrhetic shellfish poisoning, okadaic acid, increases intestinal epithelial paracellular permeability. *Gastroenterology* 112: 100–108

239 Nollet F, Kools P, van Roy F (2000) Phylogenetic analysis of the cadherin superfamily allows identification of six major subfamilies besides several solitary members. *J Mol Biol* 299: 551–572

240 Malaguti C, Rossini GP (2002) Recovery of cellular E-cadherin precedes replenishment of estrogen receptor and estrogen-dependent proliferation of breast cancer cells rescued from a death stimulus. *J Cell Physiol* 192: 171–181

241 Hosokawa M, Tsukada H, Saitou T, Kodama M, Onomura M, Nakamura H, Fukuda K, Seino Y (1998) Effects of okadaic acid on rat colon. *Dig Dis Sci* 43: 2526–2535

242 EFSA (2008) Marine biotoxins in shellfish – Azaspiracid group, Scientific Opinion of the Panel on Contaminants in the Food chain *EFSA J* 723: 1–52

243 Tubaro A, Giangaspero A, Ardizzone M, Soranzo MR, Vita F, Yasumoto T, Maucher JM, Ramsdell JS, Sosa S (2008) Ultrastructural damage to heart tissue from repeated oral exposure to yessotoxin resolves in 3 months. *Toxicon* 51: 1225–1235

244 Rossini GP, Ronzitti G, Callegari F (2006) The modes of action of yessotoxin and the toxic responses of cellular systems. In: F Goudey-Perrière, E Benoit, M Goyffon, P Marchot (eds): *Toxines et Cancer*, Lavoisier, Paris, 67–76

245 Paz B, Daranas AH, Norte M, Riobó P, Franco JM, Fernández JJ (2008) Yessotoxins, a group of marine polyether toxins: An overview. *Mar Drugs* 6: 73–102

246 Alfonso A, Alfonso C (2008) Pharmacology and mechanism of action: Biological detection. In: LM Botana (ed.): *Seafood and Freshwater Toxins, Pharmacology, Physiology and Detection*, Taylor & Francis Ltd, Boca Raton, FL, 315–327

247 Twiner MJ, Hess P, Bottein Dechraoui MY, McMahon T, Samons MS, Satake M, Yasumoto T, Ramsdell JS, Doucette GJ (2005) Cytotoxic and cytoskeletal effects of azaspiracid-1 on mammalian cell lines. *Toxicon* 45: 891–900

248 Vilariño N, Nicolaou KC, Frederick MO, Cagide E, Ares IR, Louzao MC, Vieytes MR, Botana LM (2006) Cell growth inhibition and actin cytoskeleton disorganization induced by azaspiracid-1 structure-activity studies. *Chem Res Toxicol* 19: 1459–1466

249 Ronzitti G, Hess P, Rehmann N, Rossini GP (2007) Azaspiracid-1 alters the E-cadherin pool in epithelial cells. *Toxicol Sci* 95: 427–435

250 Vale C, Nicolaou KC, Frederick MO, Gómez-Limia B, Alfonso A, Vieytes MR, Botana LM (2007) Effects of azaspiracid-1, a potent cytotoxic agent, on primary neuronal cultures. A structure-activity relationship study. *J Med Chem* 50: 356–363

251 Vale C, Gómez-Limia B, Nicolaou KC, Frederick MO, Vieytes MR, Botana LM (2007) The c-Jun-N-terminal kinase is involved in the neurotoxic effect of azaspiracid-1. *Cell Physiol Biochem* 20: 957–966

252 Twiner MJ, Ryan JC, Morey JS, van Dolah FM, Hess P, McMahon T, Doucette GJ (2008) Transcriptional profiling and inhibition of cholesterol biosynthesis in human T lymphocyte cells by the marine toxin azaspiracid. *Genomics* 91: 289–300

253 Leira F, Alvarez C, Vieites JM, Vieytes MR, Botana LM (2002) Characterization of distinct apoptotic changes induced by okadaic acid and yessotoxin in the BE(2)-M17 neuroblastoma cell line. *Toxicol in Vitro* 16: 23–31

254 Malaguti C, Ciminiello P, Fattorusso E, Rossini GP (2002) Caspase activation and death induced by yessotoxin in HeLa cells. *Toxicol in Vitro* 16: 357–363

255 Pérez-Gomez A, Ferrero-Gutierrez A, Novelli A, Franco JM, Paz B, Fernández-Sánchez MT (2006) Potent neurotoxic action of the shellfish biotoxin yessotoxin on cultured crebellar neurons. *Toxicol Sci* 90: 168–177

256 Malagoli D, Marchesini E, Ottaviani E (2006) Lysosomal as target of yessotoxin in invertebrate and vertebrate cells. *Toxicol Lett* 167: 75–83

257 Dell'Ovo V, Bandi E, Coslovich T, Florio C, Sciancalepore M, Decorti G, Sosa S, Lorenzon P, Yasumoto T, Tubaro A (2008) *In vitro* effects of yessotoxin on a primary culture of rat cardiomyocytes. *Toxicol Sci* 106: 392–399

258 Pierotti S, Malaguti C, Milandri A, Poletti R, Rossini GP (2003) Functional assay to measure yessotoxins in contaminated mussel samples. *Anal Biochem* 312: 208–216

259 Ronzitti G, Callegari F, Malaguti C, Rossini GP (2004) Selective disruption of the E-cadherin-catenin system by an algal toxin. *Br J Cancer* 90: 1100–1107

260 Callegari F, Rossini GP (2008) Yessotoxin inhibits the complete degradation of E-cadherin. *Toxicology* 244: 133–144

261 Callegari F, Sosa S, Ferrari S, Soranzo MR, Pierotti S, Yasumoto T, Tubaro A, Rossini GP (2006) Oral administration of yessotoxin stabilizes E-cadherin in mouse colon. *Toxicology* 227: 145–155

262 Callegari F, Ronzitti G, Ferrari S, Rossini GP (2004) Yessotoxins alter the molecular structures of cell-cell adhesion in cultured cells. In: K Henshilwood, B Deegan, T McMahon, C Cusack, S Keaveney, J Silke, M O'Cinneide, D Lyions, P Hess (eds): *Molluscan Shellfish Safety*, Proceedings of the 5th International Conference on Molluscan Shellfish Safety; Galway, 407–413

263 Kellman R, Schaffner CAM, Grønset TA, Satake M, Ziegler M, Fladmark KE (2009) Proteomic response of human neuroblastoma cells to azaspiracid-1. *J Proteomics* 72: 695–707

264 Young C, Truman P, Boucher M, Keyzers RA, Northcote P, Jordan TW (2009) The algal metabolite yessotoxin affects heterogeneous nuclear ribonucleoproteins in HepG2 cells. *Proteomics* 9: 2529–2542

265 Munday R (2008) Toxicology of the pectenotoxins. In: LM Botana (ed.): *Seafood and Freshwater Toxins, Pharmacology, Physiology and Detection*, Taylor & Francis Ltd, Boca Raton, FL, 371–380

266 Terao K, Ito E, Yanagi T, Yasumoto T (1986) Histopathological studies on experimental marine toxin poisoning. 1. Ultrastructural changes in the small intestine and liver of suckling mice induced by dinophysistoxin-1 and pectenotoxin-1. *Toxicon* 24: 1141–1151

267 Zhou ZH, Komivama M, Terao K, Shimada Y (1994) Effects of pectenotoxin-1 on liver cells *in vitro*. *Nat Toxins* 2: 132–135

268 Spector I, Braet F, Shochet NR, Bubb MR (1999) New anti-actin drugs in the study of the organization and function of the actin cytoskeleton. *Microsc Res Tech* 47: 18–37

269 Hori M, Matsuura Y, Yoshimoto R, Ozaki H, Yasumoto T, Karaki H (1999) Actin depolymerizing action by marine toxin, pectenotoxin-2. *Nippon Yakurigaku Zasshi* 114: 225P–229P

270 Leira F, Cabado AG, Vieytes MR, Roman Y, Alfonso A, Botana LM, Yasumoto T, Malaguti C, Rossini GP (2002) The marine toxin pectenotoxin-6 induces *in vitro* depolymerization of F-actin in neuroblastoma cells. *Biochem Pharmacol* 63: 1979–1988

271 Ares IR, Louzao MC, Vieytes MR, Yasumoto T, Botana LM (2005) Actin cytoskeleton of rabbit intestinal cells is a target for potent marine phycotoxins. *J Exp Biol* 208: 4345–4354

272 Ares IR, Louzao MC, Espiña B, Vieytes MR, Miles CO, Yasumoto T, Botana LM (2007) Lactone ring of pectenotoxins: A key factor for their activity on cytoskeletal dynamics. *Cell Phys Biochem* 19: 283–292

273 Allingham JS, Miles CO, Rayment I (2007) A structural basis for regulation of actin polymerization by pectenotoxins. *J Mol Biol* 371: 959–970

274 Jung JH, Sim CJ, Lee CO (1995) Cytotoxic compounds from a two-sponge association. *J Nat Prod* 58: 1722–1726

275 Fladmark KE, Serres HM, Larsen NL, Yasumoto T, Aune T, Døskeland SO (1998) Sensitive detection of apoptogenic toxins in suspension cultures of rat and salmon hepatocytes. *Toxicon* 36: 1101–1114

276 Chae HD, Choi TS, Kim BM, Jung YJ, Shin DY (2005) Oocyte-based screening of cytokinesis inhibitors and identification of pectenotoxin-2 that induces Bim/Bax-mediated apoptosis in p53-

deficient tumors. *Oncogene* 24: 4813–4819

277 Shin DY, Kim GY, Kim ND, Jung JH, Kim SK, Kang HS, Choi YH (2008) Induction of apoptosis by pectenotoxin-2 is mediated with the induction of DR4/DR5, Egr-1 and NAG-1, activation of caspases and modulation of the Bcl-2 family in p53-deficient Hep3B hepatocellular carcinoma cells. *Oncol Rep* 19: 517–526

278 Kim MO, Moon DO, Kang SH, Heo MS, Choi YH, Jung JH, Lee JD, Kim GY (2008) Pectenotoxin-2 represses telomerase activity in human leukemia cells through suppression of hTERT gene expression and Akt-dependent hTERT phosphorylation. *FEBS Lett* 582: 3263–3269

279 Kim MO, Moon DO, Heo MS, Lee JD, Jung JH, Kim SK, Choi YH, Kim GY (2008) Pectenotoxin-2 abolishes constitutively activated NF-κB, leading to suppression of NF-κB related gene products and potentiation of apoptosis. *Cancer Lett* 271: 25–33

280 Moon DO, Kim MO, Kang SH, Lee KJ, Heo MS, Choi KS, Choi YH, Kim GY (2008) Induction of G(2)/M arrest, endoreduplication, and apoptosis by actin depolymerization agent pectenotoxin-2 in human leukemia cells, involving activation of ERK and JNK. *Biochem Pharmacol* 76: 312–321

281 Chae HD, Kim BM, Yun UJ, Shin DY (2008) Deregulation of Cdk2 causes Bim-mediated apoptosis in p53-deficient tumors following actin damage. *Oncogene* 27: 4115–4121

282 Canete E, Diogene J (2008) Comparative study of the use of neuroblastoma cells (Neuro-2a) and neuroblastomaxglioma hybrid cells (NG108-15) for the toxic effect quantification of marine toxins. *Toxicon* 52: 541–550

283 FAO (2004) Marine Biotoxins. FAO Food and Nutrition Paper 80. Food and Agriculture Organization, Rome

284 Gessner BD, McLaughlin JB (2008) Epidemiologic impact of toxic episodes: Neurotoxic toxins. In: LM Botana (ed.): *Seafood and Freshwater Toxins, Pharmacology, Physiology and Detection*, Taylor & Francis Ltd, Boca Raton, FL, 77–103

285 Hwang DF, Noguchi T (2007) Tetrodotoxin poisoning. *Adv Food Nutr Res* 52: 141–236

286 Gessner BD, Bell P, Doucette GJ, Moczydlowski E, Poli MA, van Dolah F, Hall S (1997) Hypertension and identification of toxin in human urine and serum following a cluster of mussel-associated paralytic shellfish poisoning outbreaks. *Toxicon* 35: 711–722

287 Ishida, H, Muramatsu, M, Kosuge, T, Tsuji, K (1996) Study on neurotoxic shellfish poisoning involving New Zealand shellfish *Crassostrea gigas*. In: T Yasumoto, Y Oshima, Y Fukuyo (eds): *Harmful and Toxic Algal Blooms*, Intergovernmental Oceanographic Commission of UNESCO, 491–494

288 Baden DG, Mende TJ, Bikhazi G, Leung I (1982) Bronchoconstriction caused by Florida red tide toxins. *Toxicon* 20: 929–932

289 Pierce R (1986) Red Tide (*Ptychodiscus brevis*) toxin aerosols: A review. *Toxicon* 24: 955–965

290 Fleming LE, Backer LC, Baden DG (2005) Overview of aerosolized Florida red tide toxins: Exposures and effects. *Environ Health Persp* 113: 618–620

291 Baden DG (1983) Marine foodborne dinoflagellate toxins. *Int Rev Cytol* 82: 99–150

292 Mattei C, Molgó J, Legrand AM, Benoit E (1999) Ciguatoxins and brevetoxins: Dissection of their neurobiological actions. *J Soc Biol* 193: 329–344

293 Perl TM, Bedard L, Kosatsky T, Hockin JC, Todd EC, Remis RS (1990) An outbreak of toxic encephalopathy caused by eating mussels contaminated with domoic acid. *N Engl J Med* 322: 1775–1780

294 Tasker RA, Connel BJ, Strain SM (1991) Pharmacology of systemically administered domoic acid in mice. *Can J Physiol Pharmacol* 69: 378–382

295 Jarrad LE, Meldrum BS (1993) Selective excitotoxic pathology in the rat hippocampus. *Neuropathol Appl Neurobiol* 19: 381–389

296 Larm JA, Beart PM, Cheung NS (1997) Neurotoxic domoic acid produces cytotoxicity *via* kainate- and AMPA-sensitive receptors in cultured cortical neurones. *Neurochem Int* 31: 677–682

297 Xi D, Peng YG, Ramsdell JS (1997) Domoic acid is a potent neurotoxin to neonatal rats. *Nat Toxins* 5: 74–79

298 Cordier S, Monfort C, Miossec L, Richardson S, Belin C (2000) Ecological analysis of digestive cancer mortality related to contamination by diarrhetic shellfish poisoning toxins along the coasts of France. *Environ Res* 84: 145–150

299 Fleming LE, Baden DG, Bean JA, Weisman RS, Blythe DG (1998) Seafood toxin diseases: Issues in epidemiology and community outreach. In: B Reguera, J Blanco, ML Fernandez, T Wyatt (eds): *Harmful Algae*, Xunta de Galicia and Intergovernmental Oceanographic Commission of

UNESCO, Paris, 245–248

300 Bagnis R, Kuberski T, Laugier S (1979) Clinical observations on 3009 cases of ciguatera (fish poisoning) in the South Pacific. *Am J Trop Med Hyg* 28: 1067–1073

301 Terao K, Ito E, Kakinuma Y, Igarashi K, Kobayashi M, Ohizumi Y, Yasumoto T (1989) Histopathological studies on experimental marine toxin poisoning. 4. Pathogenesis of experimental maitotoxin poisoning. *Toxicon* 27: 978–979

302 Blythe DG, De Sylva DP, Fleming LE, Ayyar RA, Baden DG, Shrank K (1992) Clinical experience with i.v. mannitol in the treatment of ciguatera. *Bull Soc Pathol Exot* 85: 425–426

303 Mattei C, Wen PJ, Nguyen-Huu TD, Alvarez M, Benoit E, Bourdelais AJ, Lewis RJ, Baden DG, Molgó J, Meunier FA (2008) Brevenal inhibits pacific ciguatoxin-1B-induced neurosecretion from bovine chromaffin cells. *PLoS ONE* 3: e3448.

304 Munday R (2008) Occurrence and toxicology of palytoxins. In: LM Botana (ed.): *Seafood and Freshwater Toxins, Pharmacology, Physiology and Detection*, Taylor & Francis Ltd, Boca Raton, FL, 693–713

305 Hoffmann K, Hermanns-Clausen M, Buhl C, Büchler MW, Schemmer P, Mebs D, Kauferstein S (2008) A case of palytoxin poisoning due to contact with zoantid corals through a skin injury. *Toxicon* 51: 1535–1537

306 Ciminiello P, Dell'Aversano C, Fattorusso E, Forino M, Magno GS, Tartaglione L, Grillo C, Melchiorre N (2006) The Genoa 2005 outbreak. Determination of putative palytoxin in Mediterranean *Ostreopsis ovata* by a new liquid chromatography tandem mass spectrometry method. *Anal Chem* 78: 6153–6159

307 Okano H, Masuoka H, Kamei S, Seko T, Koyabu S, Tsuneoka K, Tamai T, Ueda K, Nakazawa S, Sugawa M, Suzuki H, Watanabe M, Yatani R, Nakano T (1998) Rhabdomyolysis and myocardial damage induced by palytoxin, a toxin of blue humphead parrotfish. *Intern Med* 37: 330–333

308 Ito E, Satake M, Ofuji K, Kurita N, McMahon T, James K, Yasumoto T (2000) Multiple organ damage caused by a new toxin azaspiracid, isolated from mussels produced in Ireland. *Toxicon* 38: 917–930

309 Ito E, Satake M, Ofuji K, Higashi M, Harigaya K, McMahon T, Yasumoto T (2002) Chronic effects in mice caused by oral administration of sublethal doses of azaspiracid, a new marine toxin isolated from mussels. *Toxicon* 40: 193–203

310 EFSA (2009) Marine biotoxins in shellfish – Yessotoxin group, Scientific Opinion of the Panel on Contaminants in the Food chain. *EFSA J* 907: 1–62

311 Paolo S, Di Fiore PP (2006) Endocytosis conducts the cell signaling orchestra. *Cell* 124: 897–900

312 Orsi CF, Colombari B, Callegari F, Todaro AM, Ardizzoni A, Rossini GP, Blasi E, Peppoloni S (2009) Yessotoxin inhibits phagocytic activity of macrophages. *Toxicon, in press*

313 Larsen K, Petersen D, Wilkins AL, Samdal IA, Sandvik M, Rundberget T, Goldstone D, Arcus V, Hovgaard P, Rise F, Rehmann N, Hess P, Miles CO (2007) Clarification of the C-35 stereochemistries of dinophysistoxin-1 and dinophysistoxin-2, and its consequences for binding to protein phosphatase. *Chem Res Toxicol* 20: 868–875

Molecular, Clinical and Environmental Toxicology. Volume 2: Clinical Toxicology
Edited by A. Luch

Poisonous plants

Robert H. Poppenga

California Animal Health & Food Safety Laboratory System, Davis, CA, USA

Abstract. A large number of plants can cause adverse effects when ingested by animals or people. Plant toxicity is due to a wide diversity of chemical toxins that include alkaloids, glycosides, proteins and amino acids. There are several notable toxic plants for which a specific chemical responsible for toxicity has not been determined. There are many examples of species differences in terms of their sensitivity to intoxication from plants. Pets, such as dogs and cats, and people, especially children, are frequently exposed to the same toxic plants due to their shared environments. On the other hand, livestock are exposed to toxic plants that are rarely involved in human intoxications due to the unique environments in which they are kept. Fortunately, adverse effects often do not occur or are generally mild following most toxic plant ingestions and no therapeutic intervention is necessary. However, some plants are extremely toxic and ingestion of small amounts can cause rapid death. The diagnosis of plant intoxication can be challenging, especially in veterinary medicine where a history of exposure to a toxic plant is often lacking. Analytical tests are available to detect some plant toxins, although their diagnostic utility is often limited by test availability and timeliness of results. With a few notable exceptions, antidotes for plant toxins are not available. However, general supportive and symptomatic care often is sufficient to successfully treat a symptomatic patient.

Introduction

There is an overwhelming amount of information available concerning plants poisonous to humans, pets and livestock. As a result, no textbook chapter can comprehensively cover the topic. Several sources of information for human and animal exposures are recommended. For humans, *Goldfrank's Toxicologic Emergencies* [1], *Toxicity of Houseplants* [2] and *Critical Care Toxicology: Diagnosis and Management of the Critically Poisoned Patient* [3] are recommended. For animals, especially livestock, *Toxic Plants of North America* [4] is unsurpassed.

In general, the circumstances surrounding plant intoxications vary whether one is talking about people, pets or livestock. However, pets and children often share the same environment, so that the same plants are accessible to both. Lists of plants implicated in exposures or intoxications, with a few notable exceptions, are similar for children and pets and include common household plants such as those containing insoluble calcium oxalates [5, 6]. Livestock are often intoxicated by plants to which people and pets are not exposed due to their occurrence in pastures and rangelands. Livestock are also intoxicated as a result of people, unaware of the toxicity of a plant, intentionally giving them clippings from extremely toxic plants such as *Taxus* spp. or *Nerium oleander* [7, 8].

A number of unique factors contribute to the intoxication of livestock. Many toxic plants are not palatable, so livestock avoid their ingestion if other good quality forage is available [9]. Ingestion of toxic plants is much more likely during periods of forage scarcity such as during droughts. If pastures and ranges are not adequately managed toxic plants can proliferate to the point that non-toxic forage is scarce, forcing animals to eat the toxic plants [10]. Many plants toxic to livestock have variable toxicity depending on the stage of plant growth. Thus, pastures or rangelands can be safely utilized by livestock during certain times of the year when plant toxicity is low.

There can be significant differences among species in terms of susceptibility to intoxication, especially when discussing livestock. For example, sheep are able to tolerate much higher intakes of pyrrolizidine alkaloids (PAs) than cattle or horses [4]. This is due to the ability of rumen microbes of sheep to degrade PAs prior to absorption and to a decrease in formation of reactive pyrroles in the liver from absorbed PAs [11]. There are several notable small animal species differences in terms of susceptibility to intoxication as well (e.g., cats develop acute renal failure following consumption of lilies while dogs are unaffected). Alternatively, a number of poisonous plants affect people and animals in identical ways.

There are geographical differences with regard to the distribution of poisonous plants. Plants that are associated with intoxications in a particular geographical region are not found in other regions. However, a number of poisonous plants have been introduced into non-native areas and thrived to the point of presenting significant intoxication risks to people and animals [10, 12].

The widespread use of herbal preparations has increased the risk of herbal plant intoxication, especially in people [13]. Intoxication from herbal preparations is often due to misidentification or misuse of a particular herb. For example, the occurrence of a series of cases of progressive renal interstitial fibrosis was found to be due to ingestion of a weight loss product that mistakenly contained *Aristolochia fangchi* instead of *Stephania tetrandra* [14]. Although herbal preparations are used in veterinary medicine, no widespread intoxications of animals from their use have been reported. There are reports in the veterinary literature of intoxication due to the use of the volatile oils, pennyroyal oil and melaleuca oil and the dietary supplement, 5-hydroxytryptophan [15–17].

The goals of this chapter are to provide the reader with an understanding of the magnitude of plant intoxications in people and animals, an appreciation for which plants are most commonly implicated in plant intoxication, and approaches for the diagnosis and treatment of intoxications. In addition, a table has been included that provides a quick reference of clinical effects for a number of poisonous plants (Tab. 1). Scientific and common names are provided for the plants mentioned in the text; keep in mind that multiple common names are often given to the same plant (as provided in Tab. 1).

Table 1. Toxic plant information summary[*]

Latin name	Common names	Clinical signs	Toxin(s) and lethal doses
Abrus precatorius	Rosary pea, prayer bean, jequerity, precatory bean	Delayed 3 hours to 2 days; severe gastroenteritis, vomiting, hemorrhagic enteropathy, fluid loss; bleeding from retina and serous membranes is characteristic	Abrin (toxalbumin/lectin, 2 chains) in seeds; 0.5–2 seeds fatal to adult human
Abutilon hybridum	Chinese bellflower, flowering maple, parlor maple	Dermatitis, mild skin reactions; no oral toxicity reported	Unknown
Acalypha hispida	Chenille plant, red-hot cattail	Gastroenteritis, gastrointestinal inflammation; eye irritant	Euphorb latex (diterpene esters)
Aconitum spp.	Monk's-hood	Salivation within 10–20 minutes, then dryness of mouth, paresthesia beginning in extremities and spreading; then vomiting, violent diarrhea, hypothermia, hypotension, paralysis of skeletal musculature, intense pain, respiratory paralysis, cardiac failure and death	Aconitine, others (diterpene/ nor-diterpene alkaloids with alkylated amine); LD adult human is a few grams plant material
Acorus calamus	Sweet-flag	Rapid respiration, stupor, vomiting, bloody diarrhea, coma, hypocalcemic tetany; renal oxalosis unlikely to occur unless very large amounts are ingested	Soluble oxalates
Adonis spp.	Pheasant's eye	Vomiting, hyperkalemia, bradycardia, arrhythmias; sub-epidermal vesicant; not very toxic	Adonitoxin, 20 other cardenolides (cardiac glycosides); protoanemonin (vesicant irritant), extremely low amounts
Aechmea fasciata	Urn plant	Severe dermal and mucosal irritation, itching, burning, inflammation, possible blistering, hoarseness, salivation, vomiting	Insoluble calcium oxalate, proteolytic enzymes
Aesculus spp.	Horse-chestnut, buckeye	Vomiting, diarrhea; ataxia, muscle twitches, sluggishness or excitation	Aescin (saponin), unknown additional neurotoxin
Agapanthus orientalis	African blue lily, blue African lily	Conjunctivitis; oral irritation and ulceration, vomiting	Unknown; not likely to be fatal due to immediate oral discomfort

(continued on next page)

Table 1. (continued)

Latin name	Common names	Clinical signs	Toxin(s) and lethal doses
Ageratum spp.	Ageratum, floss-flower	Vomiting, ataxia, unconsciousness	Precocenes I and II, hepatotoxic chromenes
Aglaonema spp.	Chinese evergreen	Dermal and mucosal irritation, inflammation, hoarseness, salivation, vomiting; rarely oxaluria	Insoluble calcium oxalate; also soluble oxalates
Albizia julibrissin	Mimosa, silk-tree	Tremors, convulsions appear abruptly; seizures moderated by pyridoxine	5-Acetoxymethyl-3-hydroxy-4-methoxymethyl-2-methylpyridine (alkaloid)
Aleurites spp.	Tung oil tree	Vomiting, diarrhea; in eye, conjunctival hyperemia, punctate staining of cornea; by systemic absorption, pupillary dilatation, giddiness, delirium, convulsions	Tigliane-type phorbol esters
Allamanda catharctica	Yellow allamanda, Nani Ali'i, Flor de barbero	Conjunctivitis; irritation of oral mucosae, vomiting, diarrhea	Unknown strong irritant
Allium spp.	Garlic, onion	Contact allergens; Heinz body anemia (hemolytic) in canines	Tulipalins; *n*-propyl disulfide
Alocasia spp.	Elephant's ear	Severe dermal and mucosal irritation, inflammation, possible blistering, hoarseness, salivation, vomiting; if large amounts, dysphagia, respiratory compromise; severe pain in mouth, lips, throat, stomach; delirium and death in 6 hours	Calcium oxalate raphides and idioblasts; additional unknown toxin; small amounts root or leaf fatal to children
Aloe spp.	Candelabra aloe, octopus plant, torch plant, Barbados aloe, medicinal aloe	Abdominal pain, diarrhea; inhibition of gastric acid secretion; inhibition of water and electrolyte absorption from colon: potent cathartic	Barbaloin and other anthraquinone glycosides; small amount of leaf is purgative
Alstroemeria aurantica, hyb.	Peruvian lily, lily of the Incas	Strongly allergenic	Tulipalin A

(continued on next page)

Table 1. (continued)

Latin name	Common names	Clinical signs	Toxin(s) and lethal doses
Amaryllis spp.	Amaryllis	Persistent vomiting, diarrhea, salivation, hypotension, sedation, seizures; hepatic degeneration	Amaryllidaceae alkaloids
Ammi majus	Bishop's weed, Queen Anne's lace	Primary photosensitization	Furocoumarins
Amsinckia spp.	Fiddleneck, tarweed	Much delayed (weeks to months) anorexia, depression, rough pelage, diarrhea, emaciation, constipation, jaundice, hepatoencephalopathy, death	Pyrrolizidine alkaloids
Ananas comosus	Pineapple, pineapple tree	Oral and mucosal irritation, vomiting; allergen	Bromelin (digestive enzyme), calcium oxalate raphides, ethyl acrylate (skin sensitizer)
Anemone spp.	Anemone, Pasque flower, windflower, meadow anemone, crowfoot	Sub-epidermal vesicant; intense gastrointestinal irritation, abdominal pain, vomiting, diarrhea	Protoanemonin (related to cantharidin); saponins
Anthurium spp.	Flamingo flower	Severe dermal and mucosal irritation, inflammation, possible blistering, hoarseness, salivation, vomiting; if large amounts, dysphagia, airway obstruction, respiratory compromise; rapid respiration, stupor, hypocalcemic tetany; rarely renal oxalosis	Calcium oxalate raphides and idioblasts; also soluble oxalates
Apocynum cannabium	Dogbane, Indian hemp	Vomiting, diarrhea, cardiovascular collapse	Apocynamarin (cardioactive glycoside)
Arisaema triphyllum	Jack in the pulpit	Mucosal irritation, salivation, edema, vomiting	Insoluble calcium oxalates
Armoracia rusticana	Horseradish, red cole	Potent skin and eye irritant, vomiting; possible horse-radish syncope – vasodepressor mechanism initiated by direct irritation of the gastric or upper respiratory tract	Sinigrin (allyl glucosinolate)

(continued on next page)

Table 1. (continued)

Latin name	Common names	Clinical signs	Toxin(s) and lethal doses
Arnica montana	Arnica	Vomiting, diarrhea, bleeding, edema, respiratory stimulation, brief tachycardia, dyspnea, followed by cardiac paralysis, death; allergic contact dermatitis	Helenalin ester (sesquiterpene lactone with strong sulfhydryl cross-linking ability)
Artemisia absinthium	Wormwood, sagewort, sagebrush	Mucosal irritation and erythema, vomiting, diarrhea	Thujone (monoterpene) in essential oil
Arum maculatum	Lords-and-ladies, cuckoo pint, Adam-and-Eve	Severe dermal and mucosal irritation, inflammation, possible blistering, hoarseness, salivation, vomiting; if large amounts, dysphagia, airway obstruction, respiratory compromise; rapid respiration, stupor, hypocalcemic tetany, rarely renal oxalosis	Calcium oxalate raphides and idioblasts; also soluble oxalates
Asclepias spp.	Milkweed, butterfly weed	Vomiting, diarrhea, ataxia, weakness, dilated pupils, convulsions, respiratory paralysis, death	Cardenolides (cardioactive glycosides); 0.05–2.0% of body weight in plant material can be fatal
Atractylis gummifera	Mediterranean thistle	Strychnine-like convulsions	Atractyligenin, atractyloside and carboxyatractyloside
Atropa belladonna	Deadly nightshade	Tachycardia, dryness of mucous membranes, dilated pupils, excitation, confusion, hallucinations, frenzy, coma, respiratory paralysis, death	L-Hyoscyamine, scopolamine, atropine; 2–5 berries kill a child
Aucuba japonica	Aucuba, Japanese aucuba, Japanese laurel, spotted laurel	Vomiting, occasionally fever	Aucubin (triterpenoid saponins of the β-amyrin group)
Begonia semper-florens-cultorum	Wax begonia	No cases reported; dermal and mucosal irritation, inflammation, hoarseness, salivation, vomiting	Insoluble calcium oxalates, soluble oxalates
Begonia tuberhybrida	Tuberous begonia	Dermal and mucosal irritation, inflammation, hoarseness, salivation, vomiting	Insoluble calcium oxalates, soluble oxalates, cucurbitacin B

(continued on next page)

Table 1. (continued)

Latin name	Common names	Clinical signs	Toxin(s) and lethal doses
Berberis spp.	Barberry, pipperidge	Confusion, epistaxis, vomiting, diarrhea, renal irritation; high doses, primary respiratory arrest, hemorrhagic nephritis	Berberine (isoquinoline alkaloid)
Borago officinalis	Borage	Much delayed (weeks to months) anorexia, depression, rough pelage, diarrhea, emaciation, constipation, jaundice, hepatoencephalopathy, death	Pyrrolizidine alkaloids
Bowiea volubilis	Zulu potato, climbing onion	Vomiting, diarrhea, bradycardia, arrhythmias, conduction defects, hyperkalemia, seizures	Bufadienolide cardiotoxins: bovocide A, B, C and D, hellebrin
Brugmansia spp.	Angel's trumpet	Dilated pupils, oropharyngeal dryness, tachycardia, hypertension, fever, urinary retention, hallucination/violent agitation; persist up to 4 days; hyperactive deep tendon reflexes; grand mal seizures in 30%	Atropine, scopolamine, hyoscyamine; flowers can cause sudden flaccid paralysis and seizures in adult human
Brunfelsia calycina	Yesterday-today-and-tomorrow	Anxiety, excitation, persistent sneezing, vomiting, muscle tremors, worsening to ataxia, seizures, death within a few hours	Unknown
Bryonia spp.	Red bryony, white bryony	Drastic purgative, abdominal pain, bloody diarrhea, ataxia, renal inflammation, respiratory paralysis; dermal irritant, progressing to inflammation and blistering	Cucurbitacins (tetracyclic triterpenes); 6–8 berries fatal
Buxus sempervirens	Box, boxwood, common box	Vomiting, diarrhea, awkward gait, dyspnea, vocalization, ataxia, convulsions, respiratory failure, death	Buxine (cyclobuxine, pregnane alkaloids); 0.1 g/kg fatal to dogs; also tannins
Caesalpinia spp.	Bird-of-paradise	Delayed 30 minutes to several hours, profuse, persistent vomiting; later diarrhea; recovery within 24 hours	Seeds/pods contain tannins; child hospitalized after 5 pods
Caladium spp.	Caladium	Severe dermal and mucosal irritation, inflammation, possible blistering, hoarseness, salivation, vomiting; if large amounts, dysphagia, airway obstruction, respiratory compromise; rapid respiration, stupor rapid respiration, stupor, hypocalcemic tetany, rarely renal oxalosis	Calcium oxalate raphides and idioblasts; also soluble oxalates

(continued on next page)

Table 1. (continued)

Latin name	Common names	Clinical signs	Toxin(s) and lethal doses
Caltha palustris	Marsh-marigold, kingcup	Mucosal irritation, gastritis	Alkaloids, saponins, and very low level of protoanemonin
Cannabis sativa	Marijuana	Depression, excitation, dyspnea, muscle tremors, hallucination, aberrant behavior, subnormal temperature, sweating	Tetrahydrocannabinol
Capsicum annuum	Ornamental and cultivated peppers	Initial intense excitation followed by a period of insensitivity; vomiting, diarrhea; ocular erythema and tearing; irritant, carminative; may deplete nerve terminals of substance P	Capsaicin (70% of irritant capacity), less of dihydrocapsaicin, nor-dihydrocapsaicin, homocapsaicin, homodihydrocapsaicin
Caryota mitis	Fishtail palm	Oral and mucosal irritation, vomiting	Calcium oxalate raphides
Catharanthus rocus	Madagascar periwinkle	Depression, aggression, disturbed vision	Alkaloids throughout plant
Caulophyllum thalictroides	Blue cohosh	Vomiting, abdominal pain, circulatory collapse, ataxia, muscular weakness, respiratory paralysis, death	Lupin alkaloids (quinolizidine alkaloids) *N*-methyl cytisine
Cestrum diurnum	Day-blooming jessamine	Calcification of heart, liver, kidneys and lungs	1,25-Dihydroxycholecalciferol
Cestrum nocturnum	Night-blooming jessamine, Chinese inkberry	Chronic berry ingestion: diarrhea, vomiting, blood clots in stool; acute: salivation, collapse and death – gastroenteritis and congestion	Solanine alkaloids, nicotine, saponins, chlorogenic acid
Chelidonium majus	Greater celandine (bright yellow sap)	Vomiting, severe bloody diarrhea, hypovolemic shock	21 alkaloids (benzophenanthridine and protoberberine) with chelidonic acid
Chrysanthemum spp., hyb.	Chrysanthemum, marguerite, ox-eye daisy	Hypersensitivity, allergic contact dermatitis	Arteglasin A (sesquiterpene lactone) cross-links sulfhydryl groups of host proteins creating allergens
Cicuta spp.	Water hemlock, cowbane	Delayed 1 hour, burning pain of oral mucosa, abdominal pain, dizziness, vomiting, unconsciousness, frothing at the mouth, tonic-clonic convulsions, death	Cicutoxin (alkylating agent); one bite of chambered root-stock can be fatal; even bitten and spit out

(continued on next page)

Table 1. (continued)

Latin name	Common names	Clinical signs	Toxin(s) and lethal doses
Clematis spp.	Old man's beard, traveler's joy, virgin's bower	Sub-epidermal vesicant; intense gastrointestinal irritation, vomiting, diarrhea	Protoanemonin (related to cantharidin)
Clivia miniata	Kaffir lily	Delayed severe vomiting, salivation, diarrhea, perspiration, paralysis, collapse; central cholinesterase inhibition	Amaryllidaceae alkaloid lycorine, galanthamine; few grams fatal; insoluble calcium oxalates throughout plant
Cnidoscolus spp.	Nettle, stinging nettle, noseburn	Salivation, vomiting, arrhythmias, dyspnea, weakness, collapse	Acetylcholine, histamine in plant hairs
Codiaeum variegatum	Croton (ornamental)	Allergic contact dermatitis; oral irritation, vomiting	Low level phorbol diterpene esters
Colchicum autumnale	Meadow saffron, autumn crocus	Within 2–12 hours, abdominal pain, vomiting, diarrhea, dysphagia, paralysis, convulsions, hypovolemic shock, bone marrow depression in 4–5 days, death due to respiratory failure	Colchicine (antimitotic); 1.5–2 g plant material, 2–3 seeds or ½ flower fatal
Conium maculatum	Hemlock	Within 12 minutes, nervousness, trembling, progressing to ataxia, pupillary dilatation, bradycardia, paralysis, coma, respiratory paralysis, death	Coniine (piperidine alkaloid); 0.25–4% of body weight in green material can be fatal
Convallaria majalis	Lily-of-the-valley	Vomiting, abdominal pain, diarrhea, bradycardia, cardiac arrhythmias	Cardenolide cardiotoxins: primarily convallotoxin, convallamarin
Cornus spp.	Dogwood, dogberry, Cornelian cherry	No cases reported, dermal irritant	Cornin (= verbenalin, an iridioid) in leaves, has little toxicity
Corydalis spp.	Bulbous corydalis, golden corydalis, scrambled eggs, fitweed, fumitory	No case reported; early excitation, then depression, trembling and staggering, convulsions, frothing at the mouth, vomiting, dyspnea, diarrhea	Bulbocapnine and 20 other alkaloids
Crinum spp.	Crinum lily, spider lily, swamp lily	Rapid onset nausea, persistent vomiting, diarrhea, recovered in several hours	Lycorine, crinidine, bulbispermine, crinine, powelline, hippadine, other phenanthridine alkaloids

(continued on next page)

Table 1. (continued)

Latin name	Common names	Clinical signs	Toxin(s) and lethal doses
Crocus sativus	Saffron crocus, autumn crocus	Extensive bleeding from the skin, severe collapse, nephrotoxicity	Safranal (from protocrocin precursor, a tetraterpene glycoside); 5–10 g powdered stigmas (saffron) deadly
Crotalaria spp.	Crotalaria	Much delayed (weeks to months) anorexia, depression, rough pelage, diarrhea, emaciation, constipation, jaundice, hepatoencephalopathy, death	Pyrrolizidine alkaloids
Croton tiglium		Vomiting, diarrhea; in eye: conjunctival hyperemia, punctate staining of cornea; systemic effects: pupillary dilatation, delirium, convulsions	Crotin (toxalbumin); tigliane phorbol esters; few drops of sap can cause a reaction
Cryptanthus acaulis	Green earth star	Severe dermal and mucosal irritation, itching, burning, inflammation, possible blistering, hoarseness, salivation, vomiting	Insoluble calcium oxalates, proteolytic enzymes
Cycas spp.	Sago palm, leatherleaf palm, Japanese fern palm	Violent emesis, diarrhea, ataxia, seizures, coma, death; massive hepatic necrosis in dogs, hepatoencephalopathy; lower doses carcinogenic and teratogenic	Cycasin, neocycasin A and B, macrozamin; α-amino-β-ethyl-aminopropionic acid (BMAA); cycasin metabolite methylazoxy-methanol (MAM)
Cyclamen persicum	Persian violet, alpine violet, sowbread	Nausea, vomiting, diarrhea; if absorbed, convulsions and paralysis	Cyclamin (triterpenoid saponin); small pieces of tuber may cause convulsions
Cydonia spp.	Quince	No cases reported	Low levels cyanogenic glycosides
Cynoglossum officinale	Hound's-tongue	Much delayed (weeks to months) anorexia, depression, rough pelage, diarrhea, emaciation, constipation, icterus, hepatoencephalopathy, death	Pyrrolizidine alkaloids
Cytisus spp.	Broom	Vomiting, abdominal pain, circulatory collapse, cardiac arrhythmias, gradual paralysis, convulsions, respiratory paralysis, death	Sparteine (quinolizidine alkaloid)

(continued on next page)

Table 1. (continued)

Latin name	Common names	Clinical signs	Toxin(s) and lethal doses
Dahlia spp.	Dahlias	Dermatitis and slight photosensitization	Polyacetylene compounds in leaves
Daphne mezereum	Mezereon, spurge olive	Within a few hours, severe oral irritation, swelling of lips and face, salivation, hoarseness, dysphagia; severe abdominal pain, vomiting, bloody diarrhea, narcosis, muscle twitching; dermal exposure: erythema at 4–6 hours, pustules and blisters by 10 hours, take 2 days to disappear	Mezerein (daphnane diterpene ester); 2–3 fruits fatal; several flowers: week-long hospitalization
Datura stramonium	Jimsonweed, thorn-apple, moonflower	Excitation, tachycardia, confusion, dilated pupils, dry mouth, constipation, hallucinations, frenzy, coma, respiratory paralysis	L-hyoscyamine, scopolamine
Delphinium spp.	Larkspur	Uneasiness, vomiting, weakness, ataxia, paralysis, respiratory paralysis, death	Methyllycaconitine (MLA), other reversible nicotinic ACh receptor binders
Dicentra spp.	Bleeding heart, squirrel corn, Dutchman's breeches, staggerweed	Trembling, staggering, convulsions, frothing at the mouth, vomiting, dyspnea, diarrhea	Aporphine, bulbocapnine, proto-berberine, protopine (isoquinoline alkaloids)
Dieffenbachia spp.	Dieffenbachia, dumb cane	Severe dermal and mucosal irritation, inflammation, possible blistering, hoarseness, salivation, vomiting; if large amounts, dysphagia, airway obstruction, respiratory compromise; rapid respiration, stupor, hypocalcemic tetany, rarely renal oxalosis; in eye, corneal abrasion can take 3–4 weeks to heal	Calcium oxalate raphides, soluble oxalates; dumbcane (proteolytic enzyme)
Digitalis purpurea	Foxglove, common foxglove, long purples, dead men's fingers	Vomiting, diarrhea, lethargy, confusion, bradycardia, heart block, prolonged PR interval, inverted T waves, bigeminy, ventricular arrhythmias; hyperkalemia; ECG gradually normalizes over 1–2 weeks	Cardenolide cardiotoxins; desacetyl-digilanids A, B; glucogitaloxin; 10–20% hydrolyzed to digitoxin, gitoxin, gitalox-in; therapeutic index is steep; also con-tains saponins digitonin, gitonin, tigonin

(continued on next page)

Table 1. (continued)

Latin name	Common names	Clinical signs	Toxin(s) and lethal doses
Dioscorea batatas	Chinese yam, cinnamon vine	Dermal and mucosal irritant	Calcium oxalate raphides
Dracaena spp.	Corn plant	Vomiting (sometimes with blood), depression, ataxia, weakness, dilated pupils, tachycardia	Unknown
Dryopteris filix-mas	Male-fern	Local irritant, gastrointestinal irritation, abdominal pain; vision disturbances that may end in blindness	Filicin
Echium lycopsis	Purple viper's-bugloss, Patterson's curse, calamity Jane	Much delayed (weeks to months) anorexia, depression, rough pelage, diarrhea, emaciation, constipation, jaundice, hepatoencephalopathy, death	Pyrrolizidine alkaloids
Epipremnum aureum	Devil's ivy, ivy arum, pothos, Hunter's robe, taro vine	Dermal and mucosal irritation, inflammation, hoarseness, salivation, vomiting; if large amounts, dysphagia, airway obstruction, respiratory compromise; rapid respiration, stupor, hypocalcemic tetany; rarely renal oxalosis	Insoluble calcium oxalates, soluble oxalates
Equisetum spp.	Horsetail	Trembling, weakness	Palustrine; nicotine; thiaminase activity; probably requires chronic intake
Erythrina spp.	Coral bean, coral tree	Uneasiness, vomiting, weakness, ataxia, paralysis, respiratory paralysis, death	Isoquinoline alkaloids, reversible nicotinic ACh receptor binders
Erythronium spp.	Dog-tooth violet, trout lily, avalanche lily	Allergic contact dermatitis	Tulipalin A (>0.1%)
Eschscholzia californica	California poppy	Narcosis, muscular relaxation, depression of the central respiratory center, pin-point pupils, cyanosis, respiratory failure, death	Rhoeadine-type alkaloids, thebaine, papaverrubines, papaverine; small amounts compared to opium poppy
Eucalyptus spp.	Eucalyptus, blue gum, cider gum, silver dollar, Australian fever tree	Contact dermatitis; mucosal irritation and erythema, vomiting, diarrhea	Essential oil; cineole, α-pinene, linalool, α-terpenol, eudesmol, bicostol; citronellal; 30 g dried foliage can be lethal

(continued on next page)

Table 1. (continued)

Latin name	Common names	Clinical signs	Toxin(s) and lethal doses
Euonymus spp.	Euonymus, spindle	Delayed 8–15 hours: vomiting, severe diarrhea, fever, bradycardia, arrhythmias, asystole	Evonoside, evobioside, evomonoside (cardenolide cardiotoxins); evonine, neo-evonine, 4-deoxyevonine
Eupatorium rugosum	White snakeroot	Delayed 3–11 days; trembling, ataxia, weakness, severe repeated vomiting; constipation and thirst, acetone breath, prostration, delirium, coma, death	Tremetol/tremetone; 0.5–1.5% of body weight fatal; recovery rare, slow, can be incomplete
Euphorbia lactea	Candelabra cactus, false cactus, mottled spurge, dragon bones	Vomiting, diarrhea; in eye, conjunctival hyperemia, punctate staining of cornea; by systemic absorption, pupillary dilatation, giddiness, delirium, convulsions	Diterpene esters in milky sap (type not specified)
Euphorbia milii	Crown of thorns	Vomiting, diarrhea; in eye, conjunctival hyperemia, punctate staining of cornea; thorns tend to limit consumption/access	Hydroxyphorbol diterpene esters in milky sap (milliamines A-I); also triterpenes, flavonoids
Euphorbia myrisinites	Spurge, creeping spurge, donkeytail	Dermal blistering can take a week to heal; no ingestion data	Ingenane diterpene esters
Euphorbia pulcherrima	Poinsettia, Christmas star	Hot-house varieties: mucosal irritation and some vomiting; dermal hypersensitivity	Very little diterpene ester, considerable natural variability
Euphorbia resinifera	Euphorbium	Vomiting, diarrhea; in eye, conjunctival hyperemia, punctate staining of cornea; by systemic absorption, pupillary dilatation, giddiness, delirium, convulsions	Daphnane diterpene esters (resiniferatoxin); one of the most irritating euphorbs
Euphorbia tirucalli	Pencil tree, milkbush, Indian tree, rubber euphorbia, finger tree, naked lady	Vomiting, diarrhea; in eye, conjunctival hyperemia, punctate staining of cornea; by systemic absorption, pupillary dilatation, giddiness, delirium, convulsions	Phorbol diterpene esters
Euphorbia spp.	Spurges	Dermal and mucosal inflammation, swelling, vesicle formation; gastroenteritis, vomiting, abdominal pain, diarrhea; by systemic absorption, pupillary dilatation, giddiness, delirium, convulsions	Phorbol, daphnane and ingenane diterpene esters

(continued on next page)

Table 1. (continued)

Latin name	Common names	Clinical signs	Toxin(s) and lethal doses
Ficus benjamina	Weeping fig, Java willow, Benjamin tree, small-leaved rubber plant	Dermal contact urticaria, IgE mediated; vomiting	Allergen; irritant white sap
Fuchsia spp.	Fuchsia, lady's eardrops	Allergic reactions	Allergen
Galanthus nivalis	Snowdrop	Persistent vomiting, diarrhea, sedation, hypotension, seizures, hepatic degeneration	Lycorine (Amaryllidaceae alkaloid); galanthamine
Gelsemium sempervirens	Yellow jessamine, Carolina jessamine	Convulsions	Indolizidine alkaloids
Gloriosa superba	Gloriosa lily, glory lily, climbing lily	Within 2–12 hours, abdominal pain, profuse vomiting, diarrhea, dysphagia, oliguria or anuria; hypovolemic shock; bone marrow depression in 4–5 days; alopecia at 12 days; respiratory failure	Gloriosine and colchicine, both antimitotic; 7–11 mg fatal to adult human
Glycyrrhiza glabra	Licorice	Water retention, hypertension, congestive heart failure	Glycyrrhizin (triterpenoid saponin)
Gypsophila paniculata	Baby's breath	Dermal irritant and allergen; vomiting, diarrhea	Unknown
Haemanthus multiflorus	Blood lily, powderpuff lily	Salivation, vomiting, diarrhea, paralysis, collapse	Lycorine, chidanthine, hippeastrine, haemanthidine, haemultine
Hedera helix	English ivy, common ivy, Irish ivy	Single berry causes salivation, vomiting; large amount of leaves causes tachycardia, stupor, dilated pupils, convulsions	Hederasaponins B, C; rutin, caffeic acid, chlorogenic acid, α-hederin, emetine; falcarinol, falcarinone, didehydrofalcarinol (alkylating agents, irritants)
Heliotropium spp.	Heliotrope, potato weed	Much delayed (weeks to months) anorexia, depression, rough pelage, diarrhea, emaciation, constipation, jaundice, hepatoencephalopathy, death	Pyrrolizidine alkaloids

(continued on next page)

Table 1. (continued)

Latin name	Common names	Clinical signs	Toxin(s) and lethal doses
Helleborus spp.	Christmas rose, black hellebore	Intense vomiting, diarrhea, pupillary dilatation, bradycardia, prolonged P-R interval, idioventricular rhythm, bundle-branch block, ventricular fibrillation, asystole, hyperkalemia, hallucination	Hellebrin, other bufadienolide cardiotoxins; protoanemonin, ranunculin in foliage; helleborin (steroidal saponin)
Hemerocallis spp.	Day-lilies	Acute renal failure: vomiting, depression, anuria	Unknown toxin; only cats known to be affected
Hippeastrum aulicum	Lily of the palace, naked lady, amaryllis	Vomiting, salivation, some diarrhea, paralysis and central collapse	Lycorine (phenanthridine alkaloid), bulb
Hura crepitans	Sandbox tree, monkey pistol	Vomiting, diarrhea; in eye, conjunctival hyperemia, punctate staining of cornea; by systemic absorption, pupillary dilatation, giddiness, delirium, convulsions	Hurin (toxalbumin); daphnane diterpene esters
Hyacinthoides non-scripta	Bluebell	Choking, clammy skin, depression, attempted vomiting, weak, slow pulse, lowered temperature, bloody diarrhea	Glucosidase inhibitors: 2,5-dihydroxy-methyl-3,4-dihydroxypyrrolidine (DMDP); 1,4-dideoxy-1,4-imino-D-arabinitol (DAB)
Hyacinthus orientalis	Hyacinth, garden hyacinth, Dutch hyacinth	Vomiting, diarrhea, excessive salivation	Lycorine (phenanthridine alkaloids), bulb, less toxic than *Narcissus*
Hydrangea macrophylla	Hydrangea, hills of snow, French hydrangea, hortensia	Bloody diarrhea, gastroenteritis within a few hours; rapid recovery	Hydrangin (cyanogenic glycoside)
Hymenocallis spp.	Spider lily, crown-beauty, sea daffodil, basket flower, alligator lily	Very persistent vomiting, diarrhea	Lycorine (emetic) and tazettine (hypotensive) (phenanthridine alkaloids)
Hyoscyamus niger	Henbane	Excitation, tachycardia, dilated pupils, confusion, hallucinations, frenzy, coma, respiratory paralysis	L-Hyoscyamine, scopolamine

(continued on next page)

Table 1. (continued)

Latin name	Common names	Clinical signs	Toxin(s) and lethal doses
Hypericum spp.	St. John's wort, klamath weed	Primary photosensitization	Hypericin
Ilex spp.	Holly, yaupon, possum-haw	Abdominal pain, vomiting, diarrhea with more than 2 berries	Foliage: tannins, caffeine, triterpene compounds, theobromine, a hemolytic saponin, digitalis-like cardiotonic activity, a bis-nor-monoterpene
Ipomoea spp.	Morning glory, bindweed, pearly gates	Depression, dilated pupils, muscle tremors, ataxia, increased deep tendon reflexes, diarrhea, hypotension, hallucination	Indole alkaloids: D-lysergic acid amide, D-isolysergic acid amide, and elymoclavine are hallucinogenic; 200–300 seeds produce human hallucination
Iris spp.	Iris, crested iris, dwarf iris, flag, fleur-de-lis, blue flag, butterfly iris, poison flag, yellow iris	Vomiting, abdominal pain, bloody diarrhea, elevated body temperature, death	Iridin (irritant phenolic glycoside), myristic acid; triterpenes, benzoquinones (irisoquin)
Jatropha spp.	Physic nut, Berlandier nettlespurge	Vomiting, profuse, sometimes bloody diarrhea, ataxia	Curcin (toxalbumin); phorbol esters
Juniperus sabina	Savin	Profuse vomiting, diarrhea	Podophyllotoxins; sabinene, sabinyl acetate (terpene derivatives)
Kalanchoe spp.	Kalancho, Palm-Beach-bells, feltbush, velvet elephant ear, devil's backbone, lavender-scallops	Vomiting, diarrhea, ataxia, trembling, sudden death due to cardiac failure	Lanceotoxin A (cumulative bufadienolide cardiotoxins)
Kalmia spp.	Mountain laurel, dwarf laurel	Delayed about 1 hour, copious salivation, excitation, vomiting, perspiration, pin-point pupils, diarrhea, bradycardia, severe hypotension; conduction disturbances including atrioventricular block; weakness, ataxia, paralysis, coma, occasional seizures	Grayanotoxin I (cardioactive diterpenoid)

(continued on next page)

Table 1. (continued)

Latin name	Common names	Clinical signs	Toxin(s) and lethal doses
Karwinskia humboldtiana	Coyotilla, tullidora	Ascending posterior paresis	Karwinol A (neurotoxic polyphenol)
Laburnum anagyroides	Laburnum, golden chain tree	Delay 0.5–1 hour, salivation, sweating, centrally stimulated vomiting, persisting 1–2 days; delirium, excitation, tonic-clonic convulsions, respiratory paralysis, death	Cytisine (quinolizidine alkaloid); 23 pods fatal to adult human
Lantana camara	Lantana, shrub verbena, yellow sage, bunchberry	Gastrointestinal irritation, vomiting, diarrhea, weakness, ataxia, depression, cholestasis, hyperbilirubinemia, hepatic damage, lethargy, cyanosis, deep labored breathing, depressed tendon reflexes, photophobia, coma, death	Pentacyclic triterpenes lantadene A and B; unripe berries most toxic
Laurus nobilis	Laurel, bay laurel, sweet bay	Dermal irritation, vomiting, diarrhea	Unknown
Ledum palustre	Wild rosemary	Delayed 1 hour, copious salivation, excitation, vomiting, perspiration, pin-point pupils, diarrhea, bradycardia, severe hypotension; conduction disturbances including atrioventricular block; weakness, ataxia, paralysis, coma, occasional seizures	Grayanotoxin I (cardioactive diterpenoid); ledol, palustrol (sesquiterpene alcohols)
Leucothoe davisiae	Black laurel, mountain laurel	Delayed 1 hour, copious salivation, excitation, vomiting, perspiration, pin-point pupils, diarrhea, bradycardia, severe hypotension; conduction disturbances including atrioventricular block; weakness, ataxia, paralysis, coma, occasional seizures	Grayanotoxin I (cardioactive diterpenoid); ledol, palustrol (sesquiterpene alcohols)
Lilium spp., hyb.	Easter lily, star-gazer lily, tiger lily	Vomiting, depression, renal failure in cats	Unknown toxin; only known to affect cats
Ligustrum spp.	Privet, wax-leaf ligustrum	Abdominal pain, vomiting, watery diarrhea, rapid pulse	Unknown toxin in berries
Lobelia spp.	Lobelia, cardinal flower, blue lobelia	Salivation, vomiting, tachycardia, weakness, ataxia, depression, coma, death	Lobeline, nicotinic alkaloids

(continued on next page)

Table 1. (continued)

Latin name	Common names	Clinical signs	Toxin(s) and lethal doses
Lonicera spp.	Honeysuckle	Mild vomiting to no clinical signs, depending on species	Saponins; minimum 30 berries for clinical signs in adult human
Lophophora williamsii	Peyote, mescal, mescal button	Dilated pupils, vomiting, diarrhea, ataxia, hallucination	Mescaline
Lupinus spp.	Lupin, lupine, bluebonnet (not Texas bluebonnet)	Vomiting, abdominal pain, circulatory collapse, ataxia, muscular weakness, respiratory paralysis, death	Sparteine (quinolizidine alkaloid); 2 pods caused vomiting in adult human
Lycopersicon lycopersicum	Tomato	Delayed 4–9 hours, vomiting, severe diarrhea, possible fever and circulatory collapse; nausea and diarrhea lasting 3–6 days; hallucinations, apathy, restlessness, convulsions, visual disturbances; rarely fatal	Solanines in foliage; cholin esterase inhibition
Macadamia spp.	Macadamia nut	Depression, hyperthermia, weakness, hind-end stiffness; vomiting, tachycardia, tremors; in canines	Unknown toxin in nuts
Macrozamia spp.	Zamia	Violent emesis, diarrhea, ataxia, seizures, coma, death; massive hepatic necrosis in dogs; lower doses carcinogenic and teratogenic	Macrozamin, cycasin, neocycasins A, B; α-amino-β-ethylaminopropionic acid (BMAA); metabolite methylazoxy-methanol (MAM)
Mahonia spp.	Oregon grape, trailing Mahonia	Confusion, epistaxis, vomiting, diarrhea, renal irritation; high doses, primary respiratory arrest, hemorrhagic nephritis	Berberine (isoquinoline alkaloid)
Maianthemum bifolium	May lily	Gastrointestinal irritation, vomiting	Saponins
Melia azederach	Chinaberry, chinaberry tree	Within 2–4 hours, anorexia, vomiting, diarrhea, constipation, colic, ataxia, depression, convulsions, coma	Meliatoxins A1, A2, B1 (limonoid tetra-nor-terpenes); 5–6 fruits fatal to dog within 48 hours

(continued on next page)

Table 1. (continued)

Latin name	Common names	Clinical signs	Toxin(s) and lethal doses
Menziesia ferruginea	Mock azalea, rusty leaf	Delayed 1 hour, copious salivation, excitation, vomiting, perspiration, pin-point pupils, diarrhea, bradycardia, severe hypotension, conduction disturbances including atrio-ventricular block, weakness, ataxia, paralysis, coma, occasional seizures	Grayanotoxin I (cardioactive diterpenoid); ledol, palustrol (sesquiterpene alcohols)
Mirabilis jalapa	Four o'clock	Gastroenteritis, vomiting, abdominal pain, diarrhea	Unknown toxin in rootstocks and seeds
Monstera spp.	Ceriman, Swiss cheese plant, fruit-salad plant, split-leaf philodendron, Mexican breadfruit	Severe dermal and mucosal irritation, inflammation, possible blistering, hoarseness, salivation, vomiting; if large amounts, dysphagia, airway obstruction, respiratory compromise; rapid respiration, stupor, hypocalcemic tetany, rarely renal oxalosis	Calcium oxalate raphides and idioblasts; also soluble oxalates
Myristica fragrans	Nutmeg	Depression, aggression, hallucination	Myristicin
Nandina domestica	Nandina, heavenly bamboo	Vomiting, cyanosis, pale mucous membranes, bradycardia, seizures, respiratory failure	Cyanogenic glycosides
Narcissus spp.	Daffodil, trumpet narcissus, jonquil, pheasant's eye, tazette	Delayed persistent vomiting, salivation, diarrhea, sweating, sedation, hypotension, hepatic degeneration	Lycorine (Amaryllidaceae alkaloid), galanthamine; oxalate raphides, chelidonic acid (irritant)
Nephrolepis spp.	Boston fern, dwarf Boston fern, ladder fern, sword fern	Contact allergic dermatitis	Allergen
Nerium oleander	Oleander	Vomiting, diarrhea, bradycardia, arrhythmias, sudden death; Digibind® may be useful.	Oleandrin (cardenolide cardiac glyco-side), as little as 0.005% of animal's body weight in plant material can be fatal
Nicotiana spp.	Tobacco, tree tobacco (also consider cigarettes, chewing tobacco, etc.)	Vomiting, diarrhea, tremors; larger amount, circulatory collapse, shallow, rapid pulse, cold sweats, convulsions, loss of consciousness, cardiac arrest, respiratory paralysis	Nicotine; LD adult human 40–60 mg

(continued on next page)

Table 1. (continued)

Latin name	Common names	Clinical signs	Toxin(s) and lethal doses
Ornithogalum spp.	Star of Bethlehem, summer snowflake, dove's dung, nap-at-noon	Vomiting, diarrhea, hyperkalemia, bradycardia, heart block, arrhythmias	Convallotoxin; convalloside; other cardioactive glycosides (low levels); tulipalin A; calcium oxalate raphides
Oxalis spp.	Sorrel, wood sorrel	Rapid respiration, stupor, vomiting, bloody diarrhea, coma, hypocalcemic tetany; renal oxalosis is unlikely to occur unless very large amounts are ingested	Soluble oxalates throughout plant
Papaver somniferum	Opium poppy	Narcosis, muscular relaxation, central depression of respiration, pin-point pupils, cyanosis, respiratory failure, death	Morphine; narcotine; codeine; papaverine; thebaine
Papaver spp.	Poppies	Narcosis, muscular relaxation, depression of the central respiratory center, pin-point pupils, cyanosis, respiratory failure, death	Rhoeadine-type alkaloids, papa verrubines, thebaine, papaverine; very small amounts compared to opium poppy
Paris quadrifolia	Herb-Paris	Vomiting, diarrhea, pin-point pupils	Steroidal saponins throughout plant
Pelargonium spp.	Geranium, zonal geranium, ivy geranium	Allergic contact dermatitis	Geraniol, citronellol, linalool in essential oils (sensitizers)
Periploca graeca	Silk vine	Vomiting, diarrhea, bradycardia, arrhythmias, collapse, death	Cardioactive glycosides
Persea americana	Avocado	Non-infectious mastitis and agalactia in lactating animals; in larger amounts, cardiotoxic in some species	Persin [(Z, Z)-1-(acetyloxy)-2-hydroxy-12,15-heneicosadien-4-one]
Phaseolus vulgaris	Common bean	Severe hemorrhagic gastroenteropathy if not cooked; delayed 2–3 hours, vomiting, abdominal pain, diarrhea, circulatory collapse	Phasin (toxalbumin/lectin)
Philodendron spp.	Philodendron, sweetheart plant, panda plant, parlor ivy	Severe dermal and mucosal irritation, inflammation, possible blistering, hoarseness, salivation, vomiting; if	Calcium oxalate raphides and idioblasts; also soluble oxalates; 37 of 72 cat cases

(continued on next page)

Table 1. (continued)

Latin name	Common names	Clinical signs	Toxin(s) and lethal doses
		large amounts, dysphagia, airway obstruction, respiratory compromise; rapid respiration, stupor, hypocalcemic tetany, rarely renal oxalosis	reported were fatal
Phoradendron spp.	American mistletoe	Vomiting, diarrhea, cardiogenic shock, dyspnea, brady-cardia, behavioral changes	Phoratoxin (toxalbumin) in berries; hallucinogenic in humans
Physalis akekengi	Chinese lantern, winter cherry, Cape gooseberry	Vomiting, diarrhea; dermal irritation	Unknown
Phytolacca americana	Pokeweed, pokeberry, poke salad	Gastrointestinal irritation, vomiting, diarrhea saponins	Phytolaccatoxin, other triterpenoid
Pieris japonica	Pieris	Delayed 1 hour, copious salivation, excitation, vomiting, perspiration, diarrhea, bradycardia, severe hypotension, conduction disturbances including atrioventricular block, weakness, ataxia, paralysis, coma, occasional seizures	Grayanotoxin I (cardioactive diterpenoid)
Plumbago spp.	Cape plumbago, cape leadwort, Ceylon leadwort	Vomiting, gastritis, diarrhea	Plumbagin (quinone); vesicant irritant similar to cantharidin
Podophyllum spp.	May apple, mandrake	Vomiting, gastritis, severe diarrhea	Podophyllin group (lignan β-glycosides)
Polyscias spp.	Balfour aralia, dinner plate aralia, Ming aralia, geranium-leaf aralia, wild coffee, coffee tree	Tachycardia, stupor, dilated pupils, seizures	Falcarinone (alkylating agent, irritant); saponins
Polygonatum spp.	Solomon's-seal	Vomiting, diarrhea	Steroidal saponins; aglycone is diosgenin
Primula spp.	Primrose, German primrose, poison primrose	Dermal and mucosal hypersensitivity reactions can be mild to severe; liquefactive necrosis of the basal epidermal layer can occur	Primin (benzoquinone derivative), primetin (dihydroxyflavone)

(continued on next page)

Table 1. (continued)

Latin name	Common names	Clinical signs	Toxin(s) and lethal doses
Prunus armeniaca	Apricot	Vomiting (odor of bitter almonds), cyanosis, pale mucous membranes, bradycardia, seizures, respiratory failure	Amygdalin
Prunus domestica	Damson plum	Sublethal cyanide poisoning: see *P. armeniaca*	Amygdalin
Prunus dulcis var. *amara*	Bitter almond	Sublethal cyanide poisoning: see *P. armeniaca*	Amygdalin
Prunus laurocerasus	Cherry laurel	Vomiting (odor of bitter almonds), cyanosis, pale mucous membranes, bradycardia, seizures, respiratory failure, death	Prunasin; amygdalin
Prunus padus	Bird cherry	Sublethal cyanide poisoning: see *P. armeniaca*	Amygdalin
Prunus persica	Peach	Sublethal cyanide poisoning: see *P. armeniaca*	Amygdalin
Prunus serotina	Wild black cherry	see *P. laurocerasus*	Amygdalin
Pulsatilla spp.	Pulsatilla	Sub-epidermal vesicant; intense gastrointestinal irritation, abdominal pain, vomiting, diarrhea	Protoanemonin (lactone of γ-hydroxyvinylacrylic acid)
Pyracantha spp.	Firethorn	Gastrointestinal symptoms only	Non-cyanogenic vegetative organs, cyanogenic seeds (very low level)
Quercus spp.	Oak	Marked lack of appetite, diarrhea, hepatic injury, abdominal pain	Pyrogallol, tannins
Ranunculus spp.	Buttercup, meadow buttercup, crowfoot, lesser spearwort	Sub-epidermal vesicant; intense gastrointestinal irritation, abdominal pain, vomiting, diarrhea	Protoanemonin and ranunculin (related to cantharidin)
Raphanus rhaphinistrum	Wild radish	Gastroenteritis, liver and kidney disorders	Glucosinolates
Rhamnus spp.	Alder buckthorn	Mucosal irritation, vomiting, diarrhea; purgative	Glucofrangulin (anthracene glycoside)

(continued on next page)

Table 1. (continued)

Latin name	Common names	Clinical signs	Toxin(s) and lethal doses
Rheum rhabarbarum	Rhubarb, garden rhubarb, pie plant, water plant, wine plant	Immediate vomiting; occasionally jaundice, liver enlargement, renal insufficiency, albuminuria; no oxaluria	Anthraquinone cathartics; low level of soluble oxalate
Rhododendron spp.	Azaleas, rhododendrons	Delayed 1 hour, copious salivation, excitation, vomiting, perspiration, pupillary constriction, diarrhea, bradycardia, severe hypotension, conduction disturbances including atrioventricular block, weakness, ataxia, paralysis, coma, occasional seizures	Grayanotoxins I, II, III (cardioactive diterpenoids); not all species/hybrids toxic, great variability
Rhoeo spathacea	Oyster plant, boat lily, Moses in a boat	Oral and mucosal irritation; vomiting, abdominal pain; caused eye irritation in dogs that rolled in a bed of the plant	Unidentified irritant
Rhus spp.	Poison ivy, poison sumac, poison oak	Contact dermatitis in humans; no cases reported in animals	3-*n*-Pentadecylcatechol (sensitizer)
Ricinus communis	Castor bean plant	Delay 2–72 hours, dose dependent: vomiting, abdominal pain, bloody diarrhea, tenesmus, drowsiness, cyanosis, convulsions, circulatory collapse, renal failure, death	Ricin (toxalbumin, 2 chain); one seed can be fatal; 1 mg ricin/g seed; LD mouse, rat, dog ~1 g/kg; rabbit, 0.1 g/kg
Robinia pseudo-acacia	Black locust	Vomiting, abdominal pain, bloody diarrhea, tenesmus, drowsiness, cyanosis, convulsions, circulatory collapse, renal failure, death	Robin (toxalbumin/lectin); less toxic than abrin, ricin, phasin
Sambucus ebulus	Elder, red berried elder, dwarf elder, Danewort	Vomiting, diarrhea	Resinous substances
Schefflera spp.	Schefflera, umbrella tree, rubber tree, starleaf	Vomiting, copious diarrhea, ataxia, anorexia, leukopenia, tachycardia, stupor, dilated pupils, seizures	Soluble oxalates; falcarinol (alkylating agent, irritant)

(continued on next page)

Table 1. (continued)

Latin name	Common names	Clinical signs	Toxin(s) and lethal doses
Scilla spp.	Squill; starry hyacinth, autumn scilla, hyacinth scilla, Cuban lily, Peruvian jacinth, hyacinth of Peru, bluebell	Vomiting, diarrhea, bradycardia, arrhythmias, conduction defects, possible hyperkalemia, seizures; Ca^{2+}-binding agents decreased lethality	Proscillaridin A (bufadienolide cardiotoxin)
Senecio jacobaea	Common ragwort, tansy ragwort	Much delayed (weeks to months) anorexia, depression, rough pelage, diarrhea, emaciation, constipation, jaundice, hepatoencephalopathy, death	Jacobine plus five other pyrrolizidine alkaloids
Senecio spp.	Dusty miller, cineraria, Cape ivy, butterweed, German ivy, parlor ivy, water ivy, Natal ivy, wax vine, groundsel	Much delayed (weeks to months) anorexia, depression, rough hair coat, diarrhea, emaciation, constipation, jaundice, hepatoencephalopathy, death	Pyrrolizidine alkaloids
Sinapis spp.	White mustard, charlock	Acute gastroenteritis, pain, diarrhea	Glucosinolates
Solanum dulcamara	Bittersweet, woody nightshade, wild nightshade	Vomiting, dyspnea, hypothermia, tachycardia, respiratory failure, death	Variable major alkaloids: solanine, tomatine, solamarine, atropine, solasadine; 10 berries needed to produce signs and 200 to kill an adult human
Solanum nigrum	Black nightshade	Vomiting, dilated pupils, drowsiness, diarrhea; cholinesterase inhibition	Solasadine; solanine; only a few berries needed to produce clinical signs
Solanum pseudocapsicum	Jerusalem cherry, Christmas cherry, Natal cherry, winter cherry, ornamental pepper	Vomiting, dilated pupils, drowsiness; cholinesterase inhibition	Solanocapsine, solanocapsidine, solanine
Solanum tuberosum	Potato	Vomiting, diarrhea, fever, dilated pupils, tachycardia, dyspnea, weakness, hypotension, delirium, hallucination, stupor, coma; cholinesterase inhibition	Solanine; 0.035% critical level for human poisoning

(continued on next page)

Table 1. (continued)

Latin name	Common names	Clinical signs	Toxin(s) and lethal doses
Sophora spp.	Mescal bean, mountain laurel, frijolito, Eve's necklace	Salivation, vomiting, diarrhea; on forced exercise, trembling, stiff gait, falling and unconscious, followed by recovery; repeated cycles can occur; in a child, delirium was followed by sleep for 2–3 days	Nicotinic alkaloids (lupine-type); one seed, masticated, can be lethal; foliage at 1% body weight is toxic, 2% fatal
Sorbus spp.	Rowan, mountain ash, service tree, whitebeam	Minor gastroenteritis	Low levels amygdalin in seeds; parasorbic acid (local irritant)
Sparmannia africana	African hemp, indoor linden	Irritant, possible allergen	Unknown
Spathiphyllum spp.	Peace lily, white anthurium, spathe flower, snowflower, Mauna Loa	No cases reported; possible oral and mucosal irritation	Calcium oxalate raphides and idioblasts; also soluble oxalates
Symphytum officinale	Comfrey	Much delayed (weeks to months) anorexia, depression, rough pelage, diarrhea, emaciation, constipation, jaundice, hepatoencephalopathy, death	Pyrrolizidine alkaloids
Synadenium grantii	African milk bush	Eye irritation; delayed dermal irritation, blister formation; delayed oral and mucosal irritation; potentially vomiting, diarrhea	Tigliane-type diterpene esters (primary irritants, co-carcinogens)
Syngonium spp.	Goosefoot, nephthytis, African evergreen, arrowhead vine	Severe dermal and mucosal irritation, inflammation, possible blistering, hoarseness, salivation, vomiting; if large amounts, dysphagia, airway obstruction, respiratory compromise; rapid respiration, stupor, hypocalcemic tetany, rarely renal oxalosis	Calcium oxalate raphides and idioblasts; also soluble oxalates
Tagetes spp.	Marigold, African marigold, French marigold, bog marigold, Aztec marigold	Bloody diarrhea; primary photosensitization; allergen	Thiophene derivatives (polyacetylene irritants, phototoxic)

(continued on next page)

Table 1. (continued)

Latin name	Common names	Clinical signs	Toxin(s) and lethal doses
Tamus communis	Black bryony	Dermal and mucosal irritation, inflammation, possible blistering, hoarseness, salivation, vomiting, diarrhea; allergenic	Calcium oxalate raphides and idioblasts; traces of alkaloids; saponins; photosensitive phenanthrene derivatives
Taxus spp.	Yew, Japanese yew	Delayed 1 hour, dizziness, abdominal pain, coma, dilated pupils, shallow breathing, tachycardia; followed by bradycardia, decreased blood pressure, respiratory paralysis, diastolic arrest; or sudden death	Taxines; several bioflavonoids; cyanogenic glycoside not significant; several tablespoons to a handful of needles fatal
Tenacetum spp.	Common tansy	Severe gastroenteritis, rapid weak pulse, spasms, seizures, death	Tenacetin
Thamnosma texana	Dutchman's breeches	Primary photosensitization	Furocoumarins
Thevetia spp.	Yellow oleander, Mexican oleander	Vomiting, diarrhea, bradycardia, arrhythmias, collapse, sudden death. Digibind® may be useful.	Peruvoside (cardiac glycoside); 8–10 seeds to kill an adult human
Thuja occidentalis	White cedar	Strong local irritant, gastric bleeding, hepatic degeneration, renal damage, long-lasting tonic-clonic convulsions	Thujone (monoterpene)
Tillandsia cyanea	Pink quill	Severe dermal and mucosal irritation, itching, burning, inflammation, possible blistering, hoarseness, salivation, vomiting	Insoluble calcium oxalates, proteolytic enzymes
Tolmiea menziesii	Piggyback plant, pickaback plant, thousand-mothers, youth-on-age	Allergen	Unknown
Toxicodendron spp.	Poison ivy, poison oak, poison sumac	Dermal contact allergen in humans	Urushiol compounds (irritants)
Tragia spp.	Nettle, stinging nettle, noseburn	Salivation, vomiting, arrhythmias, dyspnea, weakness, collapse	Acetylcholine, histamine

(continued on next page)

Table 1. (continued)

Latin name	Common names	Clinical signs	Toxin(s) and lethal doses
Tulipa spp.	Tulip, garden tulip	Vomiting, salivation, heart palpitations, dyspnea, sweating; delayed dermatitis	Tuliposides A, B (convert to tulipalins A, B, lactone allergens); lectin that inhibits DNA synthesis
Urginea maritima	Sea onion	Vomiting, diarrhea, bradycardia, arrhythmias, seizures; Ca^{2+}-binding agents decreased lethality	Proscillaridin A (bufadienolide cardiotoxins)
Urtica spp.	Nettle, stinging nettle, noseburn	Salivation, vomiting, arrhythmias, dyspnea, weakness, collapse	Acetylcholine, histamine in plant hairs
Veratrum spp.	False hellebore, white hellebore	Salivation within minutes, then dryness of mouth, paresthesia beginning in extremities and spreading (like aconitine); vomiting, violent diarrhea, hypothermia, respiratory difficulties, arrhythmia, hypotension, collapse, respiratory paralysis and death; all can occur within 3 hours; prognosis poor; teratogenic: cyclops	Protoveratrines A, B (tetraesters); jerveratrum (furanopiperidines); steroidal alkaloids; 1–2 g dried root fatal in adult human
Vinca spp.	Periwinkle	Vomiting, collapse	Vincamine, vinblastine, vincristine (indole alkaloids)
Viscum album	European mistletoe	Local irritant, vomiting, diarrhea, hypotension	Viscotoxins; viscumin (toxalbumin)
Vitus spp.	Grapes, raisins	Acute renal failure: vomiting, depression, anuria	Unknown toxin; literature reports only in dogs, although anecdotally other animals might be affected
Vriesea fenestralis	Netted vriesea	Severe dermal and mucosal irritation, inflammation, possible blistering, hoarseness, salivation, vomiting	Insoluble calcium oxalate, proteolytic enzymes
Wisteria sinensis	Wisteria, Chinese kidney bean	Vomiting, gastroenteritis	Wisterin "sapotoxin"; lectins; 2 seeds cause vomiting/gastroenteritis in a child

(continued on next page)

Table 1. (continued)

Latin name	Common names	Clinical signs	Toxin(s) and lethal doses
Zantedeschia spp.	Calla lily	Severe dermal and mucosal irritation, inflammation, possible blistering, hoarseness, salivation, vomiting; if large amounts, dysphagia, airway obstruction, respiratory compromise; rapid respiration, stupor, hypocalcemic tetany, rarely renal oxalosis	Calcium oxalate raphides and idioblasts; also soluble oxalates; 1 spadix put a child in a 12 hour coma, recovered at 24 hours; can be fatal
Zephyranthes spp.	Zephyr lily, rain lily, fairy lily, fire lily	Nausea, vomiting, diarrhea (may be bloody) staggering, collapse, occasional death	Lycorine, haemanthamine
Zigadenus spp.	Death camas/camus	Salivation within minutes, then dryness of mouth, paresthesia beginning in extremities and spreading (like aconitine); vomiting, violent diarrhea, hypothermia, respiratory difficulties, arrhythmia, hypotension, collapse, respiratory paralysis and death; all can occur within 3 hours; prognosis poor	Zygadenine (steroidal alkaloids like those of *Veratrum*)

* Adapted from [82]; LD, lethal dosage.

General categories of plant toxins

There is no comprehensive and precise system for categorizing plant toxins. The classification scheme by Cheeke is perhaps as good as any and is based primarily on the chemical structure of the toxins [18].

One of the largest categories of plant toxins are the alkaloids. Alkaloids are compounds that contain nitrogen, usually in a heterocyclic ring. The nature of the heterocyclic ring serves to further categorize the toxins. Perhaps the most notable group of alkaloids is the pyrrolizidine alkaloids (PAs) whose nucleus consists of two five-membered rings. Several plant genera, including *Senecio* spp., *Amsinckia* spp., *Crotalaria* spp., *Echium* spp. and *Heliotropium* contain toxic PAs. Other important toxic alkaloids include the piperidine alkaloids found in *Conium maculatum* (poison hemlock), the pyridine alkaloids found in *Nicotiana* spp. (wild or cultivated tobacco, tree tobacco), indole alkaloids found in *Phalaris* spp. grasses and grasses infested with ergot (ergot alkaloids), quino-lizidine alkaloids found in *Lupinus* spp. (lupines), indolizidine alkaloids found in many *Astragalus* spp. (locoweeds) and *Swainsona* spp., tropane alkaloids found in *Datura* spp. (jimsonweed), and polycyclic diterpene alkaloids found in *Delphinium* spp. (larkspurs). Steroidal alkaloids include those found in *Solanum* spp. such as green tomatoes and potatoes, and nightshades and veratrum alka-loids found in *Veratrum californicum* and *Zigadenus* spp. (death camus).

Another group of plant toxins are glycosides (ethers that contain carbohy-drate and non-carbohydrate or aglycone moieties). Examples of glycosides include the cyanogenic glycosides found in numerous plants, which yield hydrocyanic acid when hydrolyzed; goitrogenic glycosides, called glucosino-lates, which are found in *Brassica* spp. (cabbage, kale) and are hydrolyzed by glucosinolases to form a variety of compounds such as isothiocyanates, nitriles and thiocyanates; coumarin glycosides found in *Melilotus* spp., which are con-verted by molds to dicoumarol; and steroid and triterpenoid glycosides which are further subdivided into cardiac glycosides found in various plant genera including *Digitalis* spp. and *Nerium oleander*, among others; and saponins. Additional glycosides include nitropropanol glycosides found in many *Astra-galus* spp., and which are metabolized to the toxins 3-nitropropanol in rumi-nants and 3-nitroproprionic acid in non-ruminants; vicine found in fava beans; calcinogenic glycosides found in *Cestrum diurnum* (day jessamine), *Solanum malacoxylon* (synonymous with *S. glaucophyllum* or waxyleaf nightshade) and *Trisetum flavescens* (yellow oatgrass) that contain an active metabolite of vita-min D (1,25-dihydroxycholecalciferol); carboxyatractyloside found in *Xanth-ium strumarium* (cocklebur); and isoflavones such as genistein, formononetin and coumestrol found in *Trifolium subterraneum* (subterranean clover) and *Glycine max* (soybeans) and which have estrogenic activity.

Plants also contain proteins, amino acids and amino acid derivatives that can cause adverse effects. Many legume seeds, potatoes and grains such as *Secale cereale* (rye) and *Triticosecale* x (triticale) contain trypsin inhibitors that can interfere with normal digestive processes and result in reduced growth. Another protein toxin is the enzyme thiaminase, found in *Pteridium aquilinum*, which can cause thiamine deficiency in some animals. Mimosine is a compound that is structurally similar to the amino acid tyrosine and is found in the tropical forage *Leucaena leucocephala*. Mimosine and its degradation product, 3-hydroxy-4(1*H*)-pyridone inhibits DNA and RNA synthesis; it also binds metals and is goitrogenic [4]. Amino acids containing selenium (selenoamino acids) are found in a variety of plants and can cause selenium intoxication in livestock.

Several toxic plant genera contain glycoproteins. Perhaps the most noteworthy glycoprotein is ricin which is found in *Ricinus communis* and which is considered to be a bioterror threat agent [19].

Metal-binding substances such as oxalates are found in some plant genera including *Rheum rhabarbarum* (rhubarb) and *Rumex* spp. (sorrel, curly dock). These plants contain soluble oxalates which, when absorbed, can combine with elements such as calcium and cause hypocalcemia. Insolulable oxalates are found in several common houseplants, such as *Philodendron* spp. and *Dieffenbachia* spp. (dumbcane). When plant tissue is disturbed *via* chewing, needle-like bodies are released, which penetrate mucus membranes and cause significant local irritation and inflammation [2].

Toxic phenolics constitute another category of plant toxins. Phenolics are compounds containing an aromatic ring with one or more hydroxyl groups. Hypericin is a phenolic found in *Hypericum perforatum* (St. John's Wort), a commonly used herb. Other phenolic plant toxins include gossypol, which is found in *Gossypium* (cottonseed), and tannins, which are found in *Quercus* spp. (oaks).

Terpenes and terpinoids are potential plant toxins that are derived from a 5-carbon isoprene unit. Terpenes are found in plant gums and resins. Resins can consist of a complex mixture of terpenes, including monoterpenes, sesquiterpenes, diterpene acids and phenolic compounds. Isocuppressic acid, a diterpene found in the needles of *Pinus* spp., is responsible for late-term abortions in cattle. It has been speculated that terpenes are responsible for adverse effects in cats following the dermal application of melaleuca (tea tree) oil [16].

Finally, there are a variety of miscellaneous plant toxins that are not easily categorized. Examples include fluoroacetate found in a number of toxic plants in Australia; cicutoxin, a potent neurotoxin found in *Cicuta* spp. (water hemlock); *n*-propyl disulfide found in *Allium* spp. such as onions and garlic and which is associated with red blood cell destruction and hemolysis in species such as cattle, dogs and cats; and nitrate, which can be accumulated by a number of plant species and intoxicate ruminants if sufficient concentrations are present in the plant tissue.

Incidence of intoxication

Data from one animal poison control center indicated that pet calls related to plant or mushroom exposures constituted 5.8% of the total calls to the center

[20]. The number of plant-related calls was relatively steady month-to-month with two small spikes occurring in December and April. The December spike was attributable to calls concerning pet exposure to *Euphorbia pulcherrima* (poinsettias), whereas the April spike was attributable to calls concerning exposure to *Lilium longiflora* (Easter lilies). Other plants for which calls were commonly made included *Rhododendron* (azalea), *Cycas revoluta* (sago palm), *Cannabis sativa* (marijuana), *Cyclamen* spp. (cyclamen), lilies of all varieties, and all varieties of oxalate-containing plants. Over 60% of the calls involved cats showing clinical signs after exposure to either lilies or oxalate-containing plants. Sago palm and marijuana associated calls were limited to dog exposures only.

The incidence of plants poisonings in livestock is harder to quantify. Based upon 1989 data, it was estimated that poisonous plants caused over $340 million annual loss to livestock producers in the 17 states in the western U.S. [21]. This figure only considered death losses; other losses due to lost grazing opportunities, additional feed costs, health care costs, losses due to poor productivity and culling costs were not considered.

The American Association of Poison Control Centers (AAPCC) Annual Report for 2007 indicated that 2.4% of calls received were related to plant exposures [5]. There were some differences in frequency of calls depending on age, with children ≤5 years being exposed more frequently than adults ≥19 years. Interestingly, plant exposures did not constitute one of the top 25 categories of toxicant exposure associated with fatalities. The top 10 categories of plant exposures in decreasing order were: unknown plants, *Spathipyllum* spp. (peace lily), *Phytolacca americana* (pokeweed), *Philodendron* spp., *E. pulcherrima* (poinsettia), *Toxicodendron radicans* (poison ivy), *Ilex* spp. (holly), cardiac glycoside-containing plants, *Taraxacum officinale* (dandelion plant), and cyanogenic plants.

Plants representative of the various plant toxins

Alkaloids

This is a diverse group of compounds that, as one might predict, has a variety of biological effects. Exposure to alkaloids can cause acute intoxication and rapid death or chronic intoxication associated with a slow, debilitating disease.

Conium alkaloids
Conium spp. (poison hemlock) are biennials that are found worldwide [4]. Only one species is found in the U.S. (*Conium maculatum*). The plants are found in "disturbed" or "waste" areas where the soil contains adequate moisture. Poison hemlock is perhaps one of the most well-known toxic plants, since it was believed to have been responsible for the death of Socrates [22].

Conium spp. contains a number of toxic piperidine alkaloids with coniine and γ-coniceine being among the most prevalent and toxic [10]. It is important to note that alkaloid concentrations and proportions can change significantly during plant growth [23]. γ-Coniceine is the predominant alkaloid during early vegetative growth and is believed to be the precursor for the other piperidine alkaloids [24]. Coniine is the predominant alkaloid during later growth and is primarily found in the seeds. γ-Coniceine is seven to eight times more toxic than coniine. Thus, the plant is particularly toxic in the spring during early growth and in the fall when re-growth from seeds can occur. The dried plant retains toxicity and livestock can be poisoned *via* ingestion of contaminated hay [25].

Conium alkaloids at sufficient doses cause an initial nicotinic receptor stimulation followed by non-depolarizing blockade of receptor activity within neuromuscular junctions and autonomic ganglia [10]. The teratogenic effects of *Conium* alkaloids are believed to be secondary to a reduction in fetal movement due to their neuromuscular effects [10].

Multiple species are susceptible to acute intoxication including cattle, swine, horses, goats, elk, turkeys, quail, geese and chickens, and people [10, 24, 26]. Clinical signs are fairly consistent among species and include initial central nervous system (CNS) stimulation, frequent urination and defecation, tachycardia, impaired vision in animals from nictitating membrane covering the eyes, muscular weakness, muscle fasiculations, ataxia, depression, recumbency, collapse and death due to respiratory paralysis.

As mentioned, ingestion of *Conium* alkaloids can also result in teratogenesis in a number of animal species. Naturally occurring cases have been reported in cattle and swine and have been experimentally produced in sheep, goats and swine [10, 24, 27, 28]. Teratogenic effects include arthrogyrposis, scoliosis, torticollis, and cleft palate. As with most teratogens, the occurrence of specific defects depends on when exposure occurs during pregnancy. For example, in cattle teratogenic effects occur if the dam is exposed to the alkaloids between days 40 and 70 of gestation. Cleft palate has been experimentally induced in goats following alkaloid exposure between days 35 and 41 of gestation.

Typically, there are no postmortem lesions in acutely intoxicated animals. A diagnosis is based upon a history of known exposure to the plant and detection of one or more alkaloids in gastrointestinal (GI) contents, liver, urine or blood. As with most toxic plants, the identification of plant material in the GI tract can assist with confirming exposure; this is especially useful in ruminant species where identifiable plant fragments are often found in the rumen.

Pyrrolizidine alkaloids

PA-containing plants are found worldwide and are potentially toxic to multiple animal species including horses, cattle, poultry and people [4]. PA-containing plants are largely restricted to three plant families: *Boraginaceae*, *Compositae* and *Leguminosae*. PA-containing plants in the *Boraginaceae* include *Amsinckia intermedia* (tarweed), *Borago officinalis* (borage), *Cyno-*

glossum officinale (hound's tongue), *Echium plantagineum* (echium), *Heliotropium europium* (heliotrope) and *Symphytum officinale* (comfrey). Borage and comfrey have been used in herbal preparations. *Senecio*, a large (over 1200 *Senecio* spp. worldwide) and widely distributed plant genus, is the primary PA-containing genus in the *Compositae*, while *Crotalaria* is the predominant PA-containing plant genus in the *Leguminosae*.

Multiple PAs have been chemically identified [4, 10]. PAs can be categorized as monoesters, non-cyclic diesters and cyclic diesters. Cyclic diesters such as jacobine and monocrotaline are considered to be the most toxic, while monoesters are the least toxic. Toxicity is dependent on the presence of a 1,2 double bond in the B ring of the pyrrolizidine base and branching within the ester group. Hepatoxic PAs are primarily esters of the bases retronecine and heliotridine, with the former being more toxic than the latter. PAs are stable in dried plants and ensiling does not lower PA concentrations appreciably [4].

There are significant species differences with regard to susceptibility to PA intoxication [4, 29]. For example, in cattle and horses, intakes of 5–10% of body weight on a dry matter basis of *Senecio jacobaea* or *S. vulgaris* is lethal, while sheep can tolerate and intake of several times their body weight of *S. jacobaea* [4]. The most likely explanations for the difference are detoxification of PAs in the rumen of sheep or decreased production or increased detoxification of toxic pyrroles in the liver [4]. Because sheep are relatively resistant to PA intoxication, they have been used to control moderate infestations of PA-containing plants [29]. In avian species, chickens and turkeys are highly sensitive to PAs, while Japanese quail are resistant [10].

In livestock, intoxication is most likely to occur from PA-contaminated hay or silage or from grazing in areas with substantial stands of a PA-containing plant and limited alternative forage. In people, intoxications are primarily a result of contamination of food grain with seeds from PA-containing plants or *via* use of PA-containing plants for medicinal purposes (e.g., borage or comfrey) [1].

PA toxicity is due to the bioactivation of PAs in the liver to highly reactive pyrroles [10]. Pyrroles are alkylating agents that react with multiple tissue constituents. Pyrroles cross-link DNA, resulting in an antimitotic effect, and covalently bind with nucleophiles such as glutathione and with proteins. Hepatotoxicity is primarily due to DNA cross-linking. Damage from pyrroles is not restricted to the liver, but effects on other organs can be dependent on which plant is ingested. For example, exposure to *Senecio* spp. primarily results in liver damage, while exposure to *Crotalaria* can cause significant damage to the lungs [4]. Pneumotoxicity is believed to depend on small quantities of long-lived pyrrole metabolites being absorbed by erythrocytes and delivered to the lungs [30].

Hepatocyte effects include cell swelling, megalocytosis, karyomegaly and necrosis [4, 31, 32]. In addition, there is bile duct proliferation, veno-occlusion and liver fibrosis. While acute liver damage can occur following exposure to large amounts of toxic PAs, the more typical scenario is slow and progressive loss of liver function as hepatocytes are lost and replaced by fibrosis. Typical clinical signs are due to a gradual loss of condition and liver failure. Liver failure results in complex pathophysiological effects that include hypoproteinemia and altered osmotic effects causing fluid shifts between blood and interstitial spaces and body cavities, hyperbilirubinemia causing icterus, anemia, and hyperammonemia leading to hepatic encephalopathy and susceptibility to photosensitization [4, 10, 33].

Common clinical signs in animals include ill thrift, depression, diarrhea, prolapsed rectum, ascites, photosensitization and abnormal behavior. In horses, neurological signs secondary to hepatic encephalopathy are manifested by "head pressing" and walking in straight lines irrespective of obstacles in their path [4, 10]. In people, the occurrence of specific clinical signs is dependent on whether acute, subacute or chronic intoxication occurs [30]. Signs associated with acute intoxication include abdominal pain, vomiting, ascites and hepatomegaly. Chronic intoxication is associated with weakness, fatigue and progressive ascites. In humans, approximately 20% of patients with acute intoxication die, 50% recover completely and the remainder develop signs consistent with hepatic veno-occlusive disease [1].

Diagnosis of intoxication can be problematic since clinical signs might not become evident until some time after exposure to PAs has ceased. Antemortem or postmortem assays for PAs or PA adducts in tissues and body fluids have not proven to be particularly useful for routine diagnostic use [30, 31, 34]. Postmortem lesions in the liver are highly suggestive of PA exposure and/or intoxication. Thus, confirmation of exposure through visual inspection of the environment and/or feedstuff of an animal for the presence of a PA-containing plant, possible assay for PAs in a feedstuff and the presence of consistent clinical signs, clinical chemistry abnormalities and/or liver lesions provides the basis for a diagnosis.

Because of the chronic nature of PA intoxication and extensive liver damage prior to a diagnosis, treatment of affected animals is often unrewarding [4, 10]. General supportive care including provision of a highly nutritious diet and avoidance of stress is indicated. A significant number of surviving animals or people have residual effects; animals often do not return to full productivity or fitness, while a substantial number of people develop chronic liver disease [1, 4, 10].

The ability of PAs to transfer into milk has been studied in people and animals [1, 4, 35]. Although PAs are found in milk, concentrations are low and are believed to be of relatively low hazard to nursing animals [4].

Teratogenic alkaloids

In addition to the alkaloids found in *Conium* spp., there are other plant alkaloids that cause teratogenic effects in animals [35]. Quinolizidine and piperidine alkaloids are found in various species of *Lupinus*. Those responsible for teratogenic effects include the quinolizidine alkaloid, anagyrine, and the piperidine alkaloids, ammodendrine and *N*-methyl ammodendrine [10]. Exposure of cattle to anagyrine during sensitive periods of gestation results in the occurrence of "crooked calf" disease, which is characterized by skeletal contracture-type defects such as arthrogyrposis with excessive limb flexure and malpositioning, malalignment and rotation of the limbs, scoliosis and torticollis in calves [4, 10]. Less commonly, cleft palate occurs. Anagyrine is believed to be teratogenic only to cattle. However, piperidine alkaloid-containing *Lupinus* spp. can cause similar teratogenic effects in both cattle and goats. The teratogenic effects following exposure to *Lupinus* spp. are very similar to those described following exposure to the piperidine-containing *Conium* spp. One hypothesis related to the cattle-specific effect of anagyrine suggested that cattle metabolize anagyrine to a complex piperidine alkaloid, which ultimately was responsible for teratogenicity [10]. However, this remains speculative.

Steroidal alkaloids found in *Veratrum* spp. cause rather unique teratogenic effects [4, 36]. Over 50 complex alkaloids have been identified in the plant genus. One group, the jervanines, are responsible for teratogenicity. More specifically, the steroidal alkaloids cyclopamine and jervine cause a congenital cyclopia or "monkey-faced" lamb syndrome in sheep [4, 35, 36]. This defect occurs when pregnant sheep are exposed to the alkaloids on day 14 of gestation, which is the blastocyst stage of development of the sheep embryo. Cyclopamine causes cyclopia by blocking Sonic hedgehog (Shh) signal transduction [37]. Other teratogenic defects such as limb abnormalities and tracheal stenosis occur in lambs whose dams are exposed between 28 and 33 days of gestation.

One effective way to avoid losses due to teratogenic plants is to prevent grazing during critical stages of gestation. For example, losses of lambs due to *Veratrum* spp. can be eliminated by not allowing pregnant sheep to graze pastures containing the plants during the first trimester of pregnancy [4]. It is important to point out that both *Lupinus* spp. and *Veratrum* spp. contain other toxins that can cause acute disease in livestock. These genera are good examples of the complex nature of the toxicity of many poisonous plants.

Tropane alkaloids

Tropane alkaloids are found in a number of plants including *Datura* spp., *Hyoscyamus* spp., *Atropa* spp., *Mandragona* spp., *Dubiosia* spp. and *Brugmansia* spp. They are also referred to as belladonna alkaloids and consist of atropine, hyoscyamine and scopolamine. *Datura stramonium* (Angel's trumpet, jimsonweed) is the most widespread of the tropane alkaloid-containing plants in the U.S.; intoxication is primarily reported in people using the plant for its hallucinogenic properties [1, 38, 39]. *D. stramonium* seeds contain the highest concentration of alkaloids (0.4%) followed by leaves and flowers (0.2%) [4]. Immature plants contain mostly scopolamine, whereas mature plants contain mostly hyoscyamine.

Tropane alkaloids are anticholinergics. As such they competitively block the binding of acetylcholine to cholinergic muscarinic receptors on postganglionic parasympathetic neurons, sympathetic postganglionic sweat gland receptors and receptors in cortical and subcortical regions of the brain.

Intoxication of people, especially juveniles looking for a hallucinogenic effect, occurs following consumption of seeds, smoking of leaves or flowers or ingestion of teas made from the plant [1]. The alkaloids are rapidly absorbed following ingestion and clinical signs of intoxication can occur as early as 5–10 minutes following ingestion of teas or within 1–3 hours following ingestion of seeds.

Clinical signs of intoxication in decreasing order of frequency include mydriasis, hyperreflexia, skin flushing, delirium, hallucinations, tachycardia and dry skin and membranes [1, 38, 39]. Signs that occur less frequently but are associated with serious complications include seizures, rhabdomyolysis, and respiratory and renal failure.

Typically a diagnosis of intoxication relies on obtaining a careful history and occurrence of an anti-cholinergic toxidrome. Analytical tests for the alkaloids are usually not available or performed. Treatment is primarily focused on controlling CNS signs, which often resolve following the administration of a benzodiazepine [1, 39]. The use of physostigmine, a cholinesterase inhibitor, has been recommended to help control CNS signs either alone or in combination with a benzodiazepine; its use is controversial due to potential accumulation of acetylcholine and resulting adverse effects [39]. Activated charcoal (AC) can bind tropane alkaloids and its use has been associated with reduced length of hospitalization. Other symptomatic and supportive care might be indicated.

Intoxication of animals can also occur following exposure to tropane alkaloids, although documented cases are scarce in the veterinary literature. The plants are generally not palatable, so exposure is most likely to occur following ingestion of contaminated hay. Clinical signs similar to those reported for people would be expected. In horses, signs of colic can occur as a result of intestinal ileus.

Glycosides

Cyanogenic glycosides

Plant species in several families are capable of cyanogenesis, i.e., production of cyanide-containing compounds [4]. However, many cyanogenic plants do not produce cyanide at concentrations that pose a threat to people or animals or are unable to maintain cyanogenesis throughout the year. The most widespread and hazardous cyanogenic plant species for livestock are found in the *Rosaceae* family and include *Prunus laurocerasus* (cherry laurel), *P. serotina* (black cherry) and *P. virginiana* (chokecherry). In people, cyanide exposure from plant sources is relatively uncommon, although it can occur *via* ingestion of seeds from *Malus pumila* (apple) or *Manihot esculenta* (cassava) [1]. Given the size and hardness of pits from cyanogenic plants such as apricots, peach-es, or cherries, cyanide exposure is unlikely from such sources, although the use of peach and apricot seeds as natural flavorings has become more popular with health food faddists [4]. Amygdalin, a cyanogenic glycoside derived from crushed apricot pits, has been sold as "laetrile", a purported cancer chemotherapeutic.

Cyanide in plants occurs primarily as O-β-glycosides of α-hydroxynitriles [4]. Approximately 24 cyanogenic glycosides are known to be synthesized by plants from amino acids. Specific cyanogenic glycoside occurrence among cyanogenic plants is variable. For example, amygdalin reportedly occurs only in *Rosaceae*, whereas prunasin occurs not only in *Rosaceae* but in non-*Rosaceae* plants such as *Eucalyptus* and *Sambucus* (elderberry) [4]. There is little to no free cyanide in plant tissues. Hydrolysis of cyanogenic glycosides to release free cyanide is required for toxicity; the cyanogenic glycosides themselves are not associated with intoxication. All plant parts have cyanogenic potential, although the concentrations of cyanogenic glycosides vary with plant tissue. Prunasin content of *P. virginiana* is 3.6%, 2.6% and 1.2% for buds, flowers and fruits, respectively [40]. The toxicity of cyanogenic glycosides is difficult to determine due to their diversity, varying rates of hydrolysis and rates of ingestion. However, plant tissues containing 200 ppm or greater of hydrogen cyanide (HCN) "potential" as determined by tests generating and measuring HCN from plant material are considered to be hazardous for ruminant livestock [4].

All animal species are susceptible to cyanide intoxication. However, ruminants are more susceptible to cyanogenic glycosides in plants because they are rapidly hydrolyzed in the rumen to free cyanide, which is readily absorbed. Interestingly, because of the rapid hydrolysis of cyanogenic glycosides within the GI tract, the toxicity of cyanogenic glycosides for ruminants is approximately equal to the toxicity from cyanide salts such as HCN [4].

Cyanide is eliminated from the body by multiple pathways. However, the major route of detoxification is *via* the conversion of cyanide to thiocyanate [4]. Rhodanese catalyzes the transfer of sulfane sulfur from a sulfur donor to cyanide to form thiocyanate, which is eliminated *via* the urine. The limiting factor in cyanide detoxification is the availability of sulfur donors; endogenous stores of sulfur are quickly depleted resulting in a slowing of cyanide inactivation.

Cyanide is an inhibitor of multiple enzymes including succinic acid dehydrogenase, superoxide dismutase, carbonic anhydrase and cytochrome oxidase [4, 41]. It is the inhibition of the latter enzyme that accounts for the toxicity of cyanide. Cyanide causes cell hypoxia by inhibiting cytochrome oxidase at the cytochrome a_3 portion of the electron transport chain. The combination of hydrogen ions with oxygen at the terminal end of the chain is inhibited, which results in lack of ATP formation and a failure of aerobic energy metabolism.

Exposure to toxic amounts of cyanide results in the onset of clinical signs within several minutes. In livestock intoxications, it is likely that an affected animal is found dead given the rapid progression of intoxication and lack of close observation. If clinical signs occur, they can include an initial apprehension and distress followed quickly by severe weakness, ataxia and rapid, labored breathing [4]. Animals become comatose and might be noted to have "paddling" convulsions prior to death. The entire course of intoxication might be as short as 10–15 minutes or up to 1 hour with lower, but still lethal doses. In people, signs and symptoms are consistent with progressive hypoxia and include headache, anxiety, agitation, confusion, lethargy, seizures, coma and death [1, 40]. In all species, venous blood can be bright red due to a high oxygen content as a result of the failure of cells to utilize oxygen. Typically, if an affected animal survives for an hour after the onset of clinical signs full recovery occurs due to the rapid metabolism of cyanide.

A diagnosis of cyanide intoxication relies on historical circumstances, consistent clinical signs and possibly a blood cyanide analysis [4, 40]. Unfortunately, given the rapid progression of cyanide intoxication, results from blood cyanide testing are rarely available quickly enough to guide therapy. In highly suspicious cases, initial therapy requires patient stabilization. This can include maintaining airway patency and providing ventilatory support and oxygenation. A cyanide antidote kit is available [40]. The kit contains amyl nitrite, sodium nitrite and sodium thiosulfate. The efficacy of nitrite is based upon the idea that methemoglobin, induced by nitrite, has a greater affinity for cyanide than cytochrome a_3. This restores cytochrome oxidase activity. The efficacy of nitrite might also relate to improved hepatic blood flow and nitric oxide formation [4]. Amyl nitrite can be inhaled, whereas sodium nitrite is given intravenously. Sodium thiosulfate serves as sulfur donor for rhodanese-mediated biotransformation to thiocyanate. In veterinary medicine, administration of the antidotes to livestock is rare since they are not typically seen quickly enough for the antidotes to be useful (i.e., the animal is either dead or significantly recovered by the time they are seen by a veterinarian).

Chronic exposure to cyanide from consumption of improperly processed cassava occasionally occurs in people and results in neurological manifestations [18, 42]. Parkinson-like disease, spastic paraparesis, sensory ataxia, optic atrophy and sensorineural hearing loss have been described in affected individuals. Elevated thiocyanate concentrations implicate cyanide as the etiology. Treatment involves the removal of cassava from the diet and the administration of vitamin B_{12} to treat a concomitant B_{12} deficiency. Chronic cyanide intoxication has not been confirmed in animals, although a disease syndrome of ataxia, cystitis and teratogenesis associated with the ingestion of sorghum has been described in horses [4, 43]. Hypothesized etiologies include plant-derived cyanide or nitriles, although limited experimental evidence does not support cyanide as the toxin [4].

Cardiac glycosides

There are a large number of plant species that contain cardiotoxins. Cardiac glycosides are a large group of compounds with substantial cardiotoxicity. Plant-derived cardiac glycosides are categorized as either cardenolides or bufadienolides [4]. They consist of an aglycone, chemically related to steroidal hormones, and one or more sugar molecules.

Cardiac glycoside ingestion is most commonly associated with acute disease, although chronic disease is associated with ingestion of bufadienolide-containing plants in South Africa [4, 44]. Some of the more commonly implicated plants causing acute intoxication in animals or people include *Digitalis* spp. (foxglove), *Nerium oleander* (oleander), and *Asclepias* spp. (milkweeds). Acute intoxication of animals from cardiac glycosides has been reported in North America, Australia and South Africa [33]. In veterinary medicine, ruminants are most commonly affected. Many cardiac glycoside-containing plants are unpalatable and are typically not eaten unless they are inadvertently incorporated into hay or silage or seeds contaminate grain-based feeds. Plants do not lose their toxicity when dried [4].

Cardiac glycosides inhibit sodium-potassium ATPase in cardiac muscle cells, enhance vagal nerve activity and reduce coronary blood flow through vasoconstriction [4, 45]. This results in cardiac arrhythmias, myocardial cell degeneration and necrosis and cardiac insufficiency.

In animals, acute intoxication is characterized by depression, a tendency of affected animals to stand with head bowed and abdomen tucked up, teeth grinding or groaning, tachycardia or bradycardia, heart block, dyspnea, ruminal atony, bloat, diarrhea, dehydration and posterior paresis [4]. Sudden death with few premonitory signs can occur. Acute renal failure is a common manifestation in camelids intoxicated by *Nerium oleander* [46]. In people, nausea, vomiting and abdominal pain typically occur first [1]. CNS signs can include lethargy, confusion and weakness. Cardiac effects can be manifested by the occurrence of nearly any type of cardiac dysrhythmia. Cardiac glycoside intoxication is strongly suspected in people when there is evidence of increased cardiac automaticity in combination with depressed conduction through the SA and AV nodes [1]. Bidirectional ventricular tachycardia is considered to be highly diagnostic.

A diagnosis in animals relies on a history of ingestion of a cardiotoxic plant and signs referable to cardiac dysfunction [7]. Assays for some cardiac glycosides are available. An immunoassay developed for the detection of digoxin also potentially cross-reacts with other cardiac glycosides such as oleandrin, thus giving a positive result [47]. More specific tissue or biological fluid assays have been developed for oleandrin [48].

Treatment of intoxicated patients consists of preventing further exposure to cardiac glycosides, appropriate GI decontamination, which most typically involves administration of AC (multiple doses of AC are warranted), close monitoring for the presence of cardiac dysrhythmias and, if present, appropriate pharmacological intervention, and general supportive care. Digoxin-specific antibody fragments, although specific for treating digoxin intoxication of people, appear to cross-react with at least some other cardiac glycosides [49]. Although expensive, such intervention might be warranted in animal intoxications depending on its economic value or the emotional attachment of the owner. Other potential antidotes such as atropine, isoproterenol, fructose-1,6-diphosphate, sodium bicarbonate, magnesium and phenytoin do not appear to be efficacious [50].

Proteins and amino acids

Bracken fern

Pteridium aquilinum (bracken fern) contains a type I thiaminase, which is found in the protein fraction of the plant tissues [4, 51]. The plant is common throughout the world and is perhaps best known for containing the carcinogenic compound, ptaquiloside. The carcinogenicity of the plant is of particular concern to people since *P. aquilinum* rhizomes and early plant growth (croziers or fiddlenecks) have been used as a human food source. In addition, milk from bracken-fed cows has been shown to be capable of inducing neoplasia in mice, rats and a calf following prolonged consumption [4].

P. aquilinum is an interesting toxic plant from the standpoint of the variety of disease syndromes associated with its consumption by people and animals. In addition to its carcinogenic potential (associated with esophageal and gastric cancers in people and bladder and intestinal cancers in cattle), ingestion of the plant for a sufficient length of time is associated with bone marrow aplasia and coagulopathy in cattle and progressive retinal degeneration in sheep [4, 51].

Thiamine deficiency due to the thiaminase has been reported, primarily in horses, although in theory other monogastrics can also be affected. Ruminants are unaffected because of sufficient endogenous production of thiamine. The thiaminase in the plant acts to competitively inhibit thiamine cofactor activity (type I thiaminase) as opposed to directly destroying thiamine (type II thiaminase) [4]. Ingestion of large amounts of *P. aquilinum* for a prolonged period of time is required to produce disease. Thiamine deficiency in horses is manifested by neurological signs that progress in severity over several days. Affected horses can be treated with thiamine and good nursing care as long as the disease has not progressed to the point of recumbency.

Selenosis

A variety of plants can accumulate potentially toxic concentrations of selenium in the form of selenoamino acids such as selenomethionine. Some plants require selenium for growth (obligate selenium accumulators) and are capable of accumulating selenium at much higher concentrations than are found in the surrounding soil. These plants [some *Astragalus* spp. (milk vetches), *Conopsis* spp. (golden weeds), *Xylorhiza* spp. (woody asters) and *Stanleya pinnata* (Prince's plume)] can accumulate up to 10 000 ppm selenium (dry matter). Other plants, encompassing a number of plant genera, are called secondary accumulators and can contain several hundred ppm selenium. Still other plants called passive accumulators typically have selenium concentrations from 5 to 50 ppm; some cereal grains such as wheat and forages such as alfalfa are considered passive selenium accumulators. Plants containing 5 ppm selenium or greater are considered to be hazardous to grazing animals [4]. Fortunately, the most hazardous selenium accumulators are typically not palatable.

Two disease syndromes (selenosis) have been described in animals consuming selenium-accumulating plants: an acute intoxication most commonly reported in sheep, and a chronic intoxication called "alkali" disease that affects other livestock species, especially horses [4, 52]. Chronic selenosis occurs more commonly than acute selenosis. Affected animals become stiff in their movements, depressed and lose body condition. Their hair coats are rough in appearance, mucous membranes are pale and there is marked weight and hair loss and cracking, growth deformation and eventual sloughing of hooves. The pathophysiology associated with chronic selenosis is due to the incorporation of selenium into proteins in place of sulfur with the subsequent disruption of disulfide linkages [4, 53]. In acute selenosis, selenium accumulates in and causes damage to heart, liver and kidneys.

Diagnosis of acute or chronic selenosis due to plant ingestion depends on a history of ingestion of a selenium-accumulating plant and direct measurement of selenium in plant, tissue, whole blood and hair samples. Treatment of affected animals primarily relies on removing the animal from the source of exposure and providing a protein-rich diet.

Ricin

Ricin is one of the more notable glycoprotein (or lectin) toxins found in plants due to its potential use as a bioterror agent [19]. Ricin is a water soluble tox-albumin found in *Ricinus communis* (castor bean) and is among the most toxic plant constituents identified. As little as 1 mg of ricin injected into a human is lethal [4, 19]. The plant is grown commercially for the oil contained in its seeds and is cultivated as an ornamental.

All animals (including man) are reportedly susceptible to intoxication. Documented cases in the veterinary literature have involved multiple livestock species, poultry, and waterfowl [4]. Additionally, cases have occurred in dogs [54, 55]. Ricin is particularly toxic when administered parenterally. Minimum lethal doses for mice and dogs following injection are 0.7–2.0 µg/kg and 1.0–1.75 µg/kg, respectively [19]. While still quite toxic when administered orally, toxicity is approximately a 1000-fold less than following parenteral administration. This is due to the relatively low bioavailability of ricin ($\leq 1\%$). The median lethal oral dose of ricin in mice is 30 mg/kg [19].

Intoxication is most often associated with ingestion of seeds. Oral lethal doses of seeds in animals range from 0.1 g/kg in horses to 14 g/kg in chickens [4]. Intoxication of children has been associated with ingestion of as few as one or two seeds. The toxicity of seeds is dependent on whether the seeds are swallowed intact or not; intact seeds are typically not digested and therefore do not release the toxin.

Ricin is a heterodimeric protein composed of an enzymatic A chain and a lectin B chain [56]. The chains are linked by a single disulfide bond. Systemically absorbed ricin binds to cells *via* the B chain, which facilitates internalization of the toxin [19, 56]. Once internalized, the B chain is removed by hydrolysis. Cellular toxicity is due to the A chain, which hydrolyzes an adenine from an *N*-glycosidic site on 28S rRNA. This prevents peptide elongation, inactivates eukaryotic 60S ribosomes, inhibits protein synthesis and, secondarily, DNA and RNA synthesis.

The onset of clinical signs following ricin exposure generally occurs within a few hours [19]. Signs include nausea, vomiting, severe watery and bloody diarrhea, severe abdominal pain, hypotension, weakness, trembling, anorexia, sweating and collapse. Cardiac, hematological, hepatic and renal damage often occur. Neurological signs such as seizures and coma can occur just prior to death. The most characteristic postmortem lesions are severe reddening, edema and necrosis of the stomach and small intestine.

A diagnosis is based upon a history of ingestion of *Ricinus* seeds, detection of seeds in vomitus or stool, occurrence of compatible clinical signs, and detection of ricin or ricinine in appropriate antemortem or postmortem samples [19, 54]. There is no antidote for ricin intoxication. Treatment relies primarily on symptomatic and supportive care [19].

Oxalates

A wide variety of plants contain soluble or insoluble oxalates that are potentially toxic. Intoxication of livestock following the ingestion of plants containing soluble oxalates (in the form of sodium or potassium oxalate) such as *Halogeton glomeratus* (halogeton) and *Sarcobatus vermicularis* (greasewood) is well documented [4]. In the U.S. the largest number of calls received by the AAPCC in 2007 concerning exposure of people to toxic plants, involved plants containing insoluble calcium oxalate crystals (*Spathiphyllum* spp. or peace lily among other names, *Philodendron* spp., *Caladium* spp., and *Epipremnum areum* or golden pathos among other common names) [5].

Oxalate intoxication of livestock most often occurs when sheep or cattle that are not adapted to the local environment are allowed to graze large amounts of *H. glomeratus* or *S. vermicularis* [4, 57]. Ingestion has to be sufficiently great to exceed the capacity of rumen microbes to detoxify the soluble oxalates. The susceptibility of ruminants to intoxication is lessened following adaptation to soluble oxalate-containing plants since an increased number of oxalate-degrading microbes are present in the rumen.

Soluble oxalates, once absorbed from the GI tract, rapidly combine with serum calcium and magnesium, resulting in hypocalcemia and hypomagnesemia [57]. Clinical signs include muscle tremors, tetany, weakness, collapse and death; the latter can occur within 12 hours of plant consumption. Animals surviving the acute effects of soluble oxalates subsequently develop kidney damage and failure as a result of precipitation of insoluble calcium oxalate in the renal tubules [4, 57].

A diagnosis relies on exposure to a plant containing soluble oxalates, occurrence of compatible clinical signs, detection of characteristic lesions in the kidneys, and, in some cases, measurement of oxalate concentrations in kidney tissue. Treatment of affected animals under typical range conditions is often not possible. When possible, treatment primarily focuses on administration of calcium gluconate and symptomatic and supportive care [4].

Ingestion of the aforementioned plants containing insoluble calcium oxalate crystals by people or pets can result in mechanical irritation to oral and pharyngeal mucous membranes as the crystals penetrate the membranes [57]. The concentration of calcium oxalate can be high; *Philodendron* species contain up to 0.7% oxalate. Local irritation, edema and dsyphagia are the most commonly reported clinical signs. The most serious consequence following exposure would be the occurrence of significant edema in the pharyngeal area that results in difficulty in breathing. Fortunately, although exposure to such plants is common, the occurrence of significant adverse effects requiring medical attention is uncommon. A diagnosis relies on evidence of exposure to a calcium oxalate-containing plant. Treatment is largely symptomatic and supportive.

Phenolic compounds

Quercus spp. (oaks) contain polyphenolic tannins that interact and denature proteins. Tannins are generally divided into two major groups, the condensed tannins and the hydrolysable tannins [4]. Condensed tannins pass through the GI tract unchanged and appear to have little toxicity. Hydrolysable tannins on the other hand are readily hydrolyzed by esterases in the GI tract to their constituent phenolics (e.g., gallic acid from gallotannins and ellagic acid from ellagotannins) and sugars. Gallic acid is further degraded to pyrogallol and other phenolics, which are then conjugated in the liver. Oaks vary considerably in terms of overall tannin content and proportions of condensed and hydrolysable tannins, although all oaks should be considered potentially toxic if ingested at sufficiently high amounts for at least several days [4, 10]. Interestingly, in moderation, oak foliage and acorns are considered to be valuable feedstuffs for livestock and wildlife [4].

It is hypothesized that tannin intoxication results when the liver is unable to adequately metabolize phenolic metabolites [4]. Phenolic metabolites are cytotoxic with most damage occurring at sites of highest concentration (i.e., liver and kidney). There appears to be significant variation as to sites of damage among species, although kidney is considered to be the most susceptible tissue to damage. In many animals, GI damage is also consistently found.

Oak intoxication is considered to be primarily a disease of cattle; sheep, goats and horses are rarely affected [4, 10]. Goats are able to utilize oak browse effectively and without adverse effects, even when it constitutes a major portion of their diet. Resistance is believed to be due to the presence of tannin-binding proteins in their saliva and lower GI tract [4]. There are reports in the veterinary literature of intoxication of a horse and a double-wattled cassowary following oak ingestion [58, 59].

Initial clinical signs in cattle include anorexia, lethargy, rumen stasis and constipation [4, 10]. These signs are followed by diarrhea (more or less bloody), dehydration, colic, subcutaneous edema of the neck, brisket, abdomen and perineum and increased frequency of urination. At this point, there is evidence of renal impairment and a metabolic acidosis: increased blood urea nitrogen and creatinine and altered electrolytes. Animals typically either die within a few days or become chronically debilitated as a result of persistent renal impairment.

A diagnosis typically relies on evidence of excessive consumption of oak buds, leaves or acorns and consistent postmortem renal lesions. Acorns, leaves or leaf fragments are often found in the rumen on postmortem examination; this confirms exposure in the absence of other evidence of plant ingestion. Detection of tannins in GI contents or liver can confirm exposure to oaks [59].

Treatment of cattle for renal failure is often problematic under typical management conditions. In circumstances that involve valuable animals, treatment is directed toward maintaining adequate hydration and urine production and correcting any electrolyte abnormalities. Prevention is the best approach. This involves limiting continued consumption of oak buds, leaves or acorns, providing 5–10% calcium hydroxide as a supplement or feeding alfalfa hay. Calcium hydroxide is believed to bind tannins forming insoluble tannin complexes [4].

Terpenes

A good example of intoxication from a terpene is that of late-term abortion in cattle associated with the ingestion of *Pinus ponderosa* (ponderosa pine) needles. The causative agent has been identified as isocupressic acid [60]. The toxin is also found in *Cupressus macrocarpa* and *Juniperus communis* (common juniper), although most reported problems follow ingestion of *P. ponderosa* [4]. Only cattle have been affected; goats, sheep and horses are not susceptible to intoxication.

Intoxication is characterized by late-term abortions in pregnant cattle following consumption of *P. ponderosa* needles [4, 10, 61]. Abortions can occur following a single exposure to the needles, but there is a greater chance of abortion if cows ingest needles over a several day period. Intoxications occur following the ingestion of either fresh green needles from trees or dry needles from the ground. The toxin, isocuppressic acid, is believed to reduce blood flow to the caruncular vascular bed, which stimulates the fetal parturition mechanism [10]. Abortions are characterized by weak uterine contractions, uterine bleeding, incomplete cervical dilatation, dystocia, birth of weak but viable calves, agalactia and retained fetal membranes. Cows are not directly affected by the toxin, but retained fetal membranes and associated metritis can cause illness.

A diagnosis of intoxication relies on a history of ingesting pine needles and the occurrence of late-term abortions. There is no specific treatment for exposed individuals. Antibiotic administration might be necessary in cows to avoid uterine infections secondary to retained fetal membranes.

Miscellaneous toxins

n-Propyl disulfide

Ingestion of *Allium* spp. has been associated with adverse effects in animals such as cattle, horses, dogs and cats [62–65]. Wild (*A. canadensis* and *A. validum*) and domesticated (*A. cepa*) onions, chives (*A. schoenoprasum*) and garlic (*A. sativum*) contain *n*-propyl disulfide and other sulfur containing compounds that can interfere with glucose-6-phosphate dehydrogenase in red blood cells [4]. Insufficient enzyme activity and reduced glutathione concentrations predispose hemoglobin and red blood cell membranes to oxidative injury. Oxidized hemoglobin precipitates to form Heinz bodies, which are subsequently removed by the spleen; this can result in anemia. The severity of Heinz body anemia varies with the species of animal, rate of ingestion and quantity ingested. In addition to Heinz body anemia, damage to red blood cell membranes can also result in hemolytic anemia. There are species differences with regard to susceptibility to intoxication from onions; goats and sheep are much less susceptible than cattle [4]. Cats are the most sensitive domestic animal species to hemoglobin oxidation. Interestingly, cats are susceptible to Heinz body formation following the ingestion of foods containing onion powder [66].

Intoxication of cattle most often occurs as a result of feeding cull or waste domestic onions; wild onion intoxication is rare [4]. Clinical signs reported in cattle include dark red to brown urine as a result of hemoglobinuria, pale mucous membranes, tachycardia, weak pulses, anemia, weakness and collapse. In the absence of known onion ingestion, a distinct odor of onions on the breath or from feces, urine or milk provides diagnostic evidence of exposure.

In people, the most likely scenario for the occurrence of adverse effects following ingestion of *Allium* spp. involves the use of garlic extract as an herbal supplement [67]. Side effects caused by use of garlic extracts include contact dermatitis, gastroenteritis, nausea and vomiting. Several constituents of garlic are known to have antiplatelet effects, which might increase the risk of bleeding in individuals who are concomitantly taking antiplatelet or anticoagulant agents [67].

Nitrate/nitrite

Nitrate (or more appropriately nitrite) intoxication is an economically important problem for ruminants that ingest plants that have accumulated toxic levels of nitrate [4]. Normally, plants absorb nitrate from the soil and utilize it to form plant proteins. Under certain circumstances such as drought with subsequent impairment of growth, a wide variety of plants can accumulate nitrate to potentially toxic concentrations. Many common weeds such as *Amaranthus* spp. (pigweeds) and *Sorghum halapense* (Johnson grass) and crop plants such as *Zea mays* (corn) and *Avena sativa* (oats) can potentially accumulate toxic concentrations of nitrate [4, 68].

Nitrate intoxication from plants occurs exclusively in ruminants as a result of the reduction of nitrate to nitrite in the reducing environment of the rumen. Nitrite is absorbed systemically and causes oxidation of hemoglobin to methemoglobin, which cannot transport oxygen. When 30–40% of the hemoglobin is converted to methemoglobin, clinical signs occur [4, 69]. Death generally results when methemoglobin levels reach 80%.

Typically, intoxicated animals are found dead due to the rapid progression of signs following ingestion of a toxic amount of nitrate. If noted, clinical signs include lethargy, weakness, muscular tremors, tachycardia, tachypnea or dyspnea, staggering and recumbency [4, 69]. Mucous membranes and blood can have a brownish discoloration due to methemoglobin formation.

A diagnosis of intoxication is confirmed by the measurement of nitrate and nitrite concentrations in fluids such as serum or aqueous humor. Additionally, measurement of nitrate concentrations in fresh forage or hay can assist with a diagnosis and help to prevent further losses (nitrate concentrations in plants in excess of 1% are potentially toxic) [4].

Treatment of affected animals includes the intravenous administration of a 1–2% aqueous solution of methylene blue at a rate of 1–2 mg/kg [4, 69]. As a reducing agent methylene blue converts methemoglobin to hemoglobin restoring normal oxygen transport. Affected animals should be handled with care to avoid worsening respiratory distress.

Examples of toxic plants with unidentified toxins

Lilies

Lilium longiflora (Easter lily), *L. tigrinum* (tiger lily), *L. hybridum* (Japanese show lily), *L. rubrum* (rubrum lily), numerous lily hybrids and *Hemerocallis* spp. (day lilies) are extremely toxic for cats [70]. The unidentified toxin or toxins in the plants cause acute renal failure through an unknown mechanism. The leaves and flowers are toxic and deaths of cats have been reported following ingestion of as few as two leaves [70, 71]. Nephrotoxicity has not been observed in rats, rabbits or dogs following ingestion of the plant. Clinical signs are secondary to renal failure and include vomiting, salivation, dehydration, depression and anorexia. Death is due to anuric renal failure. Moderate to severe, diffuse acute tubular cell necrosis is consistently noted on postmortem examination [70, 72].

A diagnosis of intoxication relies on evidence of plant ingestion and the occurrence of signs consistent with acute renal failure. Treatment consists of early GI decontamination and fluid therapy to maintain urine production and prevent dehydration. Once in anuric renal failure, peritoneal dialysis or hemo-dialysis are the only viable options. The presence of an intact basement mem-brane along renal tubules and mitotic figures suggest the ability of the kidney to recover if affected animals are kept alive for a sufficient length of time [70].

Grapes, raisins

Acute renal failure has been consistently reported in dogs following the con-sumption of grapes or raisins [73, 74]. The frequency of intoxication appears to be low, since many dogs are exposed to potentially toxic quantities of grapes or raisins and remain unaffected. The toxin or toxins have not been identified nor have factors that predispose individuals to intoxication. The clinical course, diagnosis and treatment approaches are similar to those discussed for cats following ingestion of lilies.

Macadamia nuts

Dogs have been intoxicated following the ingestion of as few as 2.4 g/kg of macadamia nuts (from *Macadamia integrifolia* or *M. tetraphylla*) [75]. Clini-cal signs generally occur within 12 hours of ingestion with recovery occurring within 48 hours; deaths have not been reported. The most common clinical sign is apparent weakness especially of the hind limbs. Depression, vomiting, ataxia and tremors have also been reported. The toxin responsible for intoxi-cation is unknown and only dogs are affected. Treatment consists of sympto-matic and supportive care.

Diagnosis of intoxication

The diagnosis of plant intoxication can be challenging especially in veterinary medicine where ingestion of plants is often not noted by animal owners and affected individuals cannot provide a history of exposure. Such circumstances might also apply to a young child ingesting a potentially toxic plant.

Given the number of plant toxins, there are relatively few specific tests that are available to confirm exposure to a specific plant. However, there are notable exceptions. For example, exposure to a plant containing a cyanogenic glycoside can potentially be confirmed by measurement of blood cyanide con-centrations. Unfortunately, even though a specific test might be available for antemortem or postmortem testing of biological samples, most tests are not quantitative. Even if a test could quantitate the amount of a toxin present in a sample, there are few diagnostic criteria available to interpret the significance of a quantitative result. The majority of diagnostic tests available can only be used to confirm exposure to a potentially toxic plant. In many situations involving an animal or a person who has possibly been exposed to a toxic plant and who is showing clinical signs, laboratory testing to confirm exposure is rarely available quickly enough to influence initial treatment interventions.

In veterinary medicine, postmortem confirmation of a toxic plant exposure can often result from the detection of identifiable plant fragments in the GI tract. This is especially true in ruminants who do not initially masticate forage to a great degree.

Pathological lesions can also be helpful in establishing a suspicion of plant intoxication. For example, certain cardiac lesions are highly suggestive of exposure to cardiotoxic plants such as *Nerium oleander*. As mentioned previously, characteristic liver lesions are associated with intoxication from PAs.

Treatment of intoxication

If an ingestion of a specific plant is known to have occurred and some estimate of the amount ingested is available, case assessment is relatively straightforward. However, an estimate of the toxicity of the plant needs to be made. As mentioned, at least in people, most toxic plant ingestions are benign and do not require any therapeutic intervention.

Once a determination is made that an animal or a person has been exposed to a toxic plant or is intoxicated, a general approach to case management should adhere to the following principles: (1) stabilize vital signs (this may include administration of an antidote if sufficient information concerning a specific toxicant exposure is immediately available), (2) obtain a history and clinically evaluate the patient, (3) prevent continued systemic absorption of the toxicant, (4) administer an antidote if indicated and available, (5) enhance elimination of absorbed toxicant, (6) provide symptomatic and supportive care, and (7) closely monitor the patient [76–78]. Obviously, each situation is unique and one or more of the steps may be eliminated. For example, there may not be an antidote for a given toxicant or a way to significantly enhance its elimination once systemically absorbed.

Discussion of specific approaches to stabilization of vital signs is beyond the scope of this chapter. Briefly, attention should be paid to maintaining a patent airway and providing adequate ventilation, maintaining cardiovascular function with attention to appropriate fluid and electrolyte administration, maintaining acid-base balance, controlling CNS signs such as seizures, and maintaining body temperature.

Gastrointestinal decontamination (GID) is a critical component of case management. Appropriate and timely decontamination may prevent the onset of clinical signs or significantly decrease the severity or shorten the course of intoxication. GID consists of three components: (1) gastric evacuation, (2) administration of an adsorbent, and (3) catharsis. Gastric evacuation *via* the induction of emesis or gastric lavage needs to be initiated as soon as possible after ingestion for maximum efficacy. Although there are possible exceptions, gastric evacuation should be attempted within 1–2 hours after ingestion if no contraindications are present [79, 80].

Realistically, the only adsorbent routinely used in veterinary or human medicine is AC. Although the adsorptive capacity of AC for most plant toxins has not been determined, their chemical nature suggests that AC should be effective. AC is available as a powder, an aqueous slurry or combined with cathartics such as sorbitol. AC given repeatedly is effective in interrupting enterohepatic recycling of a number of toxins and the continued presence of AC in the GI tract may allow the tract to serve as a sink for trapping toxin passing from the circulation into the intestines. There is little hazard to repeated administration of AC, although cathartics should be given only once. Timing of AC administration is important. In one study of the percent reduction of drug absorption following AC administration at various times after drug administration, there was a 51.7% reduction when AC was given at 30 minutes post-dosing, whereas AC given at 60 minutes and 180 minutes post-dosing resulted in a reduction of 38% and 21%, respectively [81].

Both saline (sodium sulfate or magnesium sulfate or citrate) and saccharide (sorbitol) cathartics are available for use. In theory, cathartics hasten the elimination of unabsorbed toxicant *via* the stools. In general, cathartics are safe, particularly if used only once. However, repeated administration of magnesium-containing cathartics can lead to hypermagnesemia manifested as hypotonia, altered mental status and respiratory failure. Also, repeated administration of sorbitol can cause fluid pooling in the GI tract, excessive fluid losses *via* the stool and severe dehydration.

Antidotes should be administered if indicated and available. However, with several exceptions, there are relatively few antidotes for plant toxins. The availability and use of antidotes can be region specific. For example, in the U.S., sodium nitrite and sodium thiosulfate is used to treat cyanide intoxication, whereas in Europe, 4-dimethyl-aminophenol is used in place of sodium nitrite, and hydroxycobalamine, a vitamin B_{12} precursor, is also used to treat acute and chronic cyanide intoxication [41]. Intoxication following ingestion of cardiac glycoside-containing plants can be treated with digoxin-specific antibody due to at least partial cross-reactivity among the glycosides, although higher doses might be necessary [1]. Unfortunately, due to the costs associated with some antidotes such as digoxin-specific antibody, veterinarians may not have ready access to all of those that are clinically useful. In addition, the logistics of treating livestock often precludes timely use of antidotes. Fortunately, many intoxicated patients will recover if attention is paid to appropriate symptomatic and supportive care.

References

1 Palmer M, Betz JM (2006) Plants. In: NE Flomenbaum, MA Howland, LR Goldfrank, NA Lewin, RS Hoffman, LS Nelson (eds): *Goldfrank's Toxicologic Emergencies*. McGraw Hill, New York, NY, 1577–1602

2 Spoerke Jr, DG, Smolinske SC (1990) *Toxicity of Houseplants*. CRC Press, Boca Raton, FL
3 Brent J, Phillips SD, Wallace KL, Donovan JW, Burkhart KK (2005) *Critical Care Toxicology: Diagnosis and Management of the Critically Poisoned Patient*. Elsevier Mosby, Philadelphia, PA
4 Burrows GE, Tyrl RJ (2001) *Toxic Plants of North America*. Iowa State University Press, Ames, IA
5 Bronstein AC, Spyker DA, Cantilena Jr, LR, Green JL, Rumack BH, Heard SE (2008) 2007 Annual Report of the American Association of Poison Control Centers' Data System (NPDS): 25th Annual Report. *Clin Toxicol* 46: 927–1057
6 Buck WB (1992) Top 25 generic agents involving dogs and cats managed by the National Animal Poison Control Center in 1992. In: JD Bonagura RW Kirk (eds): *Kirk's Current Veterinary Therapy XII: Small Animal Practice*. WB Saunders, Philadelphia, PA, 210
7 Galey FD, Holstedge DM, Plumlee KH, Tor E, Johnson B, Anderson ML, Blanchard PC, Brown F (1996) Diagnosis of oleander poisoning in livestock. *J Vet Diagn Invest* 8: 358–364
8 Alden CL, Fosnaugh CJ, Smith JB, Mohan R (1977) Japanese yew poisoning of large domestic animals in the Midwest. *J Am Vet Med Assoc* 170: 314–316
9 James LF (1988) Introduction. In: LF James, MH Ralphs, DB Nielson (eds): *The Ecology and Economic Impact of Poisonous Plants on Livestock Production*. Westview Press, Boulder, CO, 1–4
10 Panter KE, Gardner DR, Lee ST, Pfister JA, Ralphs MH, Stegelmeier BL, James LF (2007) Important poisonous plants of the United States. In: RC Gupta (ed.): *Veterinary Toxicology: Basic and Applied Principles*. Elsevier Academic Press, Amsterdam, 825–872
11 Bythe LL, Craig AM (1994) Role of the liver in detoxification of poisonous plants. *Vet Hum Toxicol* 36: 564–566
12 Knight AP (1988) Poisonous plants: Oleander poisoning. *Compend Food Animal* 10: 262–263
13 Hung OL, Lewin NA (2001) Herbal preparations. In: NE Flomenbaum, MA Howland, LR Goldfrank, NA Lewin, RS Hoffman, LS Nelson (eds): *Goldfrank's Toxicologic Emergencies*. McGraw Hill, New York, NY, 664–684
14 Debelle FD, Vanherweghem JL, Nortier JL (2008) Aristolochic acid nephropathy: A worldwide problem. *Kidney Int* 74: 158–169
15 Sudekum M, Poppenga RH, Raju N, Braselton WE Jr (1992) Pennyroyal oil toxicosis in a dog. *J Am Vet Med Assoc* 200: 817–818
16 Bischoff K, Guale F (1998) Australian tea tree (*Melaleuca alternifolia*) oil poisoning in three pure-bred cats. *J Vet Diagn Invest* 10: 208–210
17 Gwaltney-Brant SM, Albretsen JC, Khan SA (2000) 5-Hydroxytryptophan toxicosis in dogs: 21 cases (1989–1999) *J Am Vet Med Assoc* 216: 1937–1940
18 Cheeke PR (1998) *Natural Toxicants in Feeds, Forages and Poisonous Plants*. Interstate Publishers, Danville, IL
19 Audi J, Belson M, Patel M, Schier J, Osterloh J (2005) Ricin poisoning: A comprehensive review. *J Am Med Assoc* 294: 2342–2351
20 Hovda LR (2009) Toxin exposures in small animals. In: JD Bonagura, DC Twedt (eds): *Current Veterinary Therapy XIV*. Saunders Elsevier, St. Louis, MO, 92–94
21 Nielson DB, Rimbey NR, James LF (1988) Economic considerations of poisonous plants on livestock. In: LF James, MH Ralphs, DB Nielson (eds): *The Ecology and Economic Impact of Poisonous Plants on Livestock Production*. Westview Press, Boulder, CO, 5–15
22 Reynolds T (2005) Hemlock alkaloids from Socrates to poison aloes. *Phytochemistry* 66: 1399–1406
23 Vetter J (2004) Poison hemlock (*Conium maculatum* L.). *Food Chem Toxicol* 42: 1373–1382
24 Panter KE, Keeler RF (1988) The hemlocks: Poison hemlock (*Conium maculatum*) and water-hemlock (*Cicuta spp.*). In: LF James, MH Ralphs, DB Nielson (eds): *The Ecology and Economic Impact of Poisonous Plants on Livestock Production*. Westview Press, Boulder, CO, 207–225
25 Galey FD, Holstedge DM, Fisher EG (1992) Toxicosis in dairy cattle exposed to poison hemlock (*Conium maculatum*) in hay: Isolation of *Conium* alkaloids in plants, hay, and urine. *J Vet Diagn Invest* 4: 60–64
26 Jessup DA, Boermans HJ, Kock ND (1986) Toxicosis in tule elk caused by ingestion of poison hemlock. *J Am Vet Med Assoc* 189: 1173–1175
27 Edmonds LD, Selby LA, Case, AA (1972) Poisoning and congenital malformations associated with the consumption of poison hemlock by sows. *J Am Vet Med Assoc* 160: 1319–1324
28 Panter KE, Keeler RF, Buck WB (1985) Congenital skeletal malformations induced by maternal

ingestion of *Conium maculatum* (poison hemlock) in newborn pigs. *J Am Vet Med Assoc* 46: 2064–2066

29 Stegelmeier BL, Gardner DR, Davis TZ (2009) Livestock poisoning with pyrrolizidine alkaloid-containing plants (*Senecio, Crotalaria, Cynoglossum, Amsinckia, Heliotropium,* and *Echium* spp.). *Rangelands* 31: 35–37

30 Stewart MJ, Steenkamp V (2001) Pyrrolizidine poisoning: A neglected area in human toxicology. *Ther Drug Monit* 23: 698–708

31 Stegelmeier BL, Gardner DR, James LF, Molyneux RJ (1996) Pyrrole detection and the pathologic progression of *Cynoglossum officinale* (houndstongue) poisoning in horses. *J Vet Diagn Invest* 8: 81–90

32 Craig AM, Pearson EG, Meyer C, Schmitz JA (1991) Clinicopathologic studies of tansy ragwort toxicosis in ponies: Sequential serum and histopathologic changes. *Equine Vet Sci* 11: 261–371

33 Radostits OM, Gay CC, Hinchcliff KW, Constable PD (2007) *Veterinary Medicine: A Textbook of the Diseases of Cattle, Horses, Sheep, Pigs and Goats.* Saunders Elsevier, Edinburgh

34 Moore RE, Knottenbelt D, Matthews JB, Beynon RJ, Whitfield PD (2008) Biomarkers for ragwort poisoning in horses: Identification of protein targets. *BMC Vet Res* 4: 30–41

35 Shupe JL, James LF (1983) Teratogenic plants. *Vet Hum Toxicol* 25: 415–421

36 Knight AP (1989) *Veratrum californicum* poisoning. *Compendium* 11: 528–529

37 Incardona JP, Gaffield W, Lange Y, Cooney A, Pentchev PG, Liu S, Watson JA, Kapur RP, Roelink H (2000) Cyclopamine inhibition of sonic hedgehog signal transduction is not mediated through effects on cholesterol transport. *Dev Biol* 224: 440–452

38 Greene GS, Patterson SG, Warner E (1996) Ingestion of angel's trumpet: An increasingly common source of toxicity. *Southern Med J* 89: 365–369

39 Wiebe TH, Sigurdson ES, Katz LY (2008) Angel's trumpet (*Datura stramonium*) poisoning and delirium in adolescents in Winnipeg, Manitoba: Summer 2006. *Paediatr Child Health* 13: 193–196

40 Majak W, McDiarmid RE, Hall JW (1981) The cyanide potential of Saskatoon serviceberry (*Amelanchier alnifolia*) and chokecherry (*Prunus virginiana*). *Can J Anim Sci* 61: 681–686

41 Holstedge CP, Isom GE, Kirk MA (2006) Cyanide and hydrogen sulfide. In: NE Flomenbaum, MA Howland, LR Goldfrank, NA Lewin, RS Hoffman, LS Nelson (eds): *Goldfrank's Toxicologic Emergencies.* McGraw Hill, New York, NY, 1712–1724

42 Vetter J (2000) Plant cyanogenic glycosides. *Toxicon* 38: 11–36

43 Adams LG, Dollahite JW, Romane WM, Bullard TL, Bridges CH (1969) Cystitis and ataxia associated with sorghum ingestion by horses. *J Am Vet Med Assoc* 155: 518–524

44 Anderson LA, Joubert JP, Schultz RA, Kellerman TS, Pienaar BJ (1987) Experimental evidence that the active principle of the poisonous plant *Thesium lineatum* L.f. (*Santalaceae*) is a bufadienolide. *Onderstepoort J Vet Res* 54: 645–650

45 Baskin SI, Czerwinski SE, Anderson JB, Sebastian MM (2007) Cardiovascular toxicity. In: RC Gupta (ed.): *Veterinary Toxicology: Basic and Applied Principles.* Elsevier Academic Press, Amsterdam, 193–205

46 Kozikowski TA, Magdesian G, Puschner G (2009) Oleander intoxication in New World camelids: 12 cases (1995–2006). *J Am Vet Med Assoc* 235: 305–310

47 Jortani S, Helm RA, Valdes R Jr (1996) Inhibition of Na,K-ATPase by oleandrin and oleandrogenin, and their detection by digoxin immunoassays. *Clin Chem* 42: 1654–1658

48 Tor ER, Filigenzi MS, Puschner B (2005) Determination of oleandrin in tissues and biological fluids by liquid chromatography–electrospray tandem mass spectrometry. *J Agric Food Chem* 53: 4322–4325

49 Eddleston M, Rajapakse S, Rajakanthan, Jayalath S, Sjöström L, Santharaj W, Thenabadu PN, Sheriff MH, Warrell DA (2000) Anti-digoxin Fab fragments in cardiotoxicity induced by ingestion of yellow oleander: A randomised controlled trial. *Lancet* 355: 967–972

50 Roberts DM, Buckley NA (2006) Antidotes for acute cardenolide (cardiac glycoside) poisoning. *Cochrane Database Syst Rev* Oct 18; (4):CD005490

51 Vetter J (2009) A biological hazard of our age: Bracken fern [*Pteridium aquilinum* (L.) Kuhn]: A review. *Acta Vet Hung* 57: 183–196

52 Raisbeck MF, Dahl ER, Sanchez DA, Belden EL, O'Toole D (1993) Naturally occurring selenosis in Wyoming. *J Vet Diagn Invest* 5: 84–87

53 O'Toole D, Raisbeck MF (1995) Pathology of experimentally induced chronic selenosis (alkali disease) in yearling cattle. *J Vet Diagn Invest* 7: 364–373

54 Mouser P, Filigenzi MS, Puschner B, Johnson V, Miller MA, Hooser SB (2007) Fatal ricin toxi-cosis in a puppy confirmed by liquid chromatography/mass spectrometry when using ricine as a marker. *J Vet Diagn Invest* 19: 216–220

55 Albretson JC, Gwaltney-Brant SM, Khan SA (2000) Evaluation of castor bean toxicosis in dogs: 98 cases. *J Am Anim Hosp Assoc* 36: 229–233

56 Olsnes S, Kozlov JV (2001) Ricin. *Toxicon* 39: 1723–1728

57 Naude TW, Naidoo V (2007) Oxalates-containing plants. In: RC Gupta (ed.): *Veterinary Toxico-logy: Basic and Applied Principles*. Elsevier Academic Press, Amsterdam, 880–891

58 Anderson GA, Mount ME, Vrins AA, Ziemer EL (1983) Fatal acorn poisoning in a horse: Pathologic findings and diagnostic considerations. *J Am Vet Med Assoc* 182: 1105–1110

59 Kinde H (1988) A fatal case of oak poisoning in a double-wattled cassowary (*Casuarius casuar-ius*). *Avian Dis* 32: 849–851

60 Gardner DR, Molyneux RJ, James LF, Panter KE, Stegelmeier BL (1994) Ponderosa pine needle-induced abortion in beef cattle: Identification of isocupressic acid as the principal active com-pound. *J Agric Food Chem* 42: 756–761

61 James LF, Short RE, Panter KE, Molyneux RJ, Stuart LD, Bellows RA (1989) Pine needle abor-tion in cattle: A review and report of 1973–1984 research. *Cornell Vet* 79: 39–52

62 Verhoeff J, Hajer R, van den Ingh TSGAM (1985) Onion poisoning of young cattle. *Vet Rec* 117: 497–498

63 Pierce KR, Joyce JR, England RB, Jones LP (1972) Acute hemolytic anemia caused by wild onion poisoning in horses. *J Am Vet Med Assoc* 160: 323–327

64 Solter P, Scott R (1987) Onion ingestion and subsequent Heinz body anemia in a dog: A case report. *J Am Anim Hosp Assoc* 23: 544–546

65 Kobayashi K (1981) Onion poisoning in the cat. *Feline Prac* 11: 22–27

66 Robertson JE, Christopher MM, Rogers QR (1998) Heinz body formation in cats fed baby food containing onion powder. *J Am Vet Med Assoc* 8: 1260–1266

67 Hung OL, Lewin NA (2006) Herbal preparations. In: NE Flomenbaum, MA Howland, LR Goldfrank, NA Lewin, RS Hoffman, LS Nelson (eds): *Goldfrank's Toxicologic Emergencies*. McGraw Hill, New York, NY, 664–684

68 Pfister JA (1988) Nitrate intoxication of ruminant livestock. In: LF James, MH Ralphs, DB Nielson (eds): *The Ecology and Economic Impact of Poisonous Plants on Livestock Production*. Westview Press, Boulder, CO, 233–259

69 Nicholson SS (2007) Nitrate and nitrate-accumulating plants. In: RC Gupta (ed.): *Veterinary Toxicology: Basic and Applied Principles*. Elsevier Academic Press, Amsterdam, 876–879

70 Hall JO (2004) Lily. In: KH Plumlee (ed.): *Clinical Veterinary Toxicology*. Mosby, St. Louis, MO, 433–435

71 Rumbeiha WK, Francis JA, Fitzgerald SD, Nair MG, Holan K, Bugyei KA, Simmons H (2004) A comprehensive study of Easter lily poisoning in cats. *J Vet Diagn Invest* 16: 527–541

72 Langston CE (2002) Acute renal failure caused by lily ingestion in six cats. *J Am Vet Med Assoc* 220: 49–52

73 Morrow CM, Valli VE, Volmer PA, Eubig PA (2005) Canine renal pathology associated with grape or raisin ingestion: 10 cases. *J Vet Diagn Invest* 17: 223–231

74 Eubig PA, Brady MS, Gwaltney-Brant SM, Khan SA, Mazzaferro EM, Morrow CM (2005) Acute renal failure in dogs after the ingestion of grapes or raisins: A retrospective evaluation of 43 dogs (1992–2002) *J Vet Intern Med* 19: 663–674

75 Plumlee KH (2004) Macadamia nuts. In: KH Plumlee (ed.): *Clinical Veterinary Toxicology*. Mosby, St. Louis, MO, 435–436

76 Beasley VR, Dorman DC (1990) Management of toxicoses. In: VR Beasley (ed.): *Veterinary Clinics of North America*: *Toxicology of Selected Pesticides, Drugs, and Chemicals*. W.B. Saunders, Philadelphia, PA, 307–337

77 Flomenbaum NE, Goldfrank LR, Hoffman RS, Howland MA, Lewin NA, Nelson LS (2006) Principles of managing the poisoned or overdosed patient. In: NE Flomenbaum, MA Howland, LR Goldfrank, NA Lewin, RS Hoffman, LS Nelson (eds): *Goldfrank's Toxicologic Emergencies*. McGraw Hill, New York, NY, 42–50

78 Drellich S, Aldrich J (2006) Initial management of the acutely poisoned patient. In: ME Peterson, PA Talcott (eds): *Small Animal Toxicology*. Saunders Elsevier, St. Louis, MO, 45–59

79 Christophersen ABJ, Hoegberg LCG (2006) Techniques used to prevent gastrointestinal absorp-tion. In: NE Flomenbaum, MA Howland, LR Goldfrank, NA Lewin, RS Hoffman, LS Nelson

(eds): *Goldfrank's Toxicologic Emergencies*. McGraw Hill, New York, NY, 109–123

80 Peterson ME (2006) Toxicological decontamination. In: ME Peterson, PA Talcott (eds): *Small Animal Toxicology*. Saunders Elesevier, St. Louis, MO, 127–141

81 American Academy of Clinical Toxicology and European Association of Poisons Centres and Clinical Toxicologists (2005) Position paper: Single-dose activated charcoal. *Clin Toxicol* 43: 61–87

82 Barr AC (2004) Household and garden plants. In: ME Peterson, PA Talcott (eds): *Small Animal Toxicology*. Saunders Elsevier, St. Louis, MO, 345–410

Molecular, Clinical and Environmental Toxicology. Volume 2: Clinical Toxicology
Edited by A. Luch
© 2010 Birkhäuser Verlag/Switzerland

Toxic plants: a chemist's perspective

Bryan A. Hanson

Department of Chemistry and Biochemistry, DePauw University, Greencastle, IN, USA

Abstract. Chemistry has long been an integral part of toxicology, as the two fields originated in much the same way: the investigation of plants with interesting properties. In this chapter I review the role that chemistry has played in understanding toxic and medicinal plants. After some introductory remarks, three broad areas are addressed: the role of natural products in understanding plant taxonomy and evolution, recent developments in chemical synthesis, especially efforts to discover and efficiently synthesize novel structures based upon naturally occurring toxins, and finally, developments in the new field of systems toxicology, which seeks to integrate all aspects of an organism's response to toxic insult.

Introduction

"What the eyes perceive in herbs or stones or trees is not yet a remedy; the eyes see only the dross. But inside, under the dross, there the remedy lies hidden."
"Is not a mystery of nature concealed in every poison? What has God created that He did not bless with some great gift for the benefit of man?... In all things there is a poison, and there is nothing without a poison. It depends only upon the dose whether a poison is poison or not."

Paracelsus (1493–1541) [1, quoted in 2]

Natural products, the wide range of small molecules extracted from the dross of the biological realm, are the gift to which Paracelsus refers. Natural products are also known as secondary metabolites. They include molecules from plants, as well as those of bacterial, fungal, animal and marine origin. They have played a critical role in modern medicine – a medicine that saves someone from cancer is a poison to the cancer cell, but deliverance for the patient. Newman and Cragg at the National Cancer Institute in the United States have monitored the sources of new drugs over several decades [3]. Over the 25-year period from 1981 through mid-2006, 34% of candidate drug molecules were natural products or were made from natural products (only small molecules considered; vaccines and biologicals excluded). If one adds molecules prepared synthetically, but whose pharmacophores were inspired by natural products, the total is 51%. Among anticancer agents over the period from the 1940s to mid-2006, the numbers are even more impressive, 42 and 56%, respectively. Although few surveys have broken out plant-based substances from the entire spectrum of drug candidates, Butler has recently reported that of 225 natural product-derived drugs in various stages of development, 49% of them are of plant origin [4]. While individual pharmaceutical companies' interest in and emphasis on natural products has varied over the years, it is clear that natural products will continue to contribute significantly to drug discovery and development [5].

The number and diversity of these plant natural products are enormous [6]. These compounds represent investments by the plant in defense against herbivores such as insects and grazing animals, as well as infectious agents like fungi, bacteria, and viruses. In many cases, the compounds also serve communication functions. Defense is necessary due to the sessile lifestyle of plants; escape is not an option. Table 1 gives a sense of the number and variety of structures known. Further, in a plant, the synthesis of a particular molecule is not constant, but varies in a spatial and temporal manner. For instance, defensive compounds are often present in young leaves, but as the growing season progresses and the leaf matures, the type of compounds change. The type of tissue is also important. Reproductive organs such as seeds are frequently well-defended because of their importance to the survival of the organism, while fleshy fruits often have compounds designed to attract animals and ensure their dispersion (the seeds inside the fruit survive the gastrointestinal tract unharmed). Finally, it has recently become apparent that many compounds originally believed to be of plant origin are actually produced by endophytic fungi that live within the plant tissue [7–11]. This appears to be the case with some of our most important anticancer agents, taxol [12, 13], camptothecin [14, 15], and podophylum-derived compounds [16], as well as important herbal medicines like St. John's Wort [17] (Fig. 1).

Table 1. The diversity of natural products

Category		Number
Alkaloids		12 000
Cyanogenic glycosides		60
Phenylpropanoids (incl. tannins, anthocyanins, flavonoids, coumarins, lignans)		6000
Glucosinolates		100
Non-protein amino acids & miscellaneous amines		800
Polyacetylenes, alkylamides, fatty acids & waxes		1900
Terpenes		
C_{10} (monoterpenes)	2500	
C_{15} (sesquiterpenes)	5000	
C_{20} (diterpenes)	2500	
C_{30} (triterpenes)	5000	
C_{40} (tetraterpenes)	500	
	Total terpenes	15 500
	Grand total	43 560

Data adapted from Wink [35].

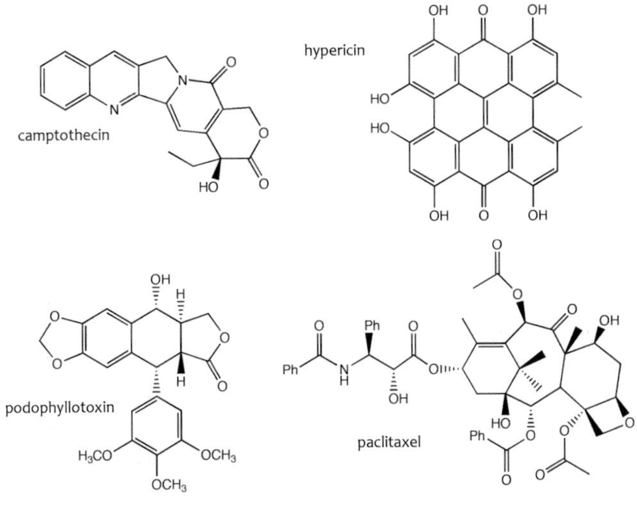

Figure 1. Some important natural products/toxins that are now known to be synthesized by endophytic fungi. Paclitaxel, podophyllotoxin and camptothecin are antitumor agents; hypericin is one component of St. John's Wort, an herb used for mild depression.

Considering their importance, their variety, and their complex role in biology, what then is the Chemist's Perspective on toxic plants? The Chemist's Perspective is very broad: there is significant overlap between the chemical viewpoint and toxicology, as well as pharmacology, pharmacognosy, medicinal chemistry, chemical synthesis, biosynthesis, ecology and alternative medicine. Plants are a rich source of useful materials and interesting scientific investigations. As there are many excellent resources on the toxicology of plants that consider the molecular action of particular molecules isolated from toxic plants [18–20], here I take a different approach. To provide the Chemist's Perspective, or at least one chemist's perspective, I take a more holistic look at the natural products found in toxic plants, and illustrate the connections between chemistry and other scientific disciplines.

Chemosystematics

Systematics is the science that attempts to reconstruct the evolutionary history of life, with the results presented in the form of a phylogeny or "tree of life". Most authorities place taxonomy, which specifically addresses classification issues, within the field of systematics, although not all agree [21]. In any case, humans have been keen observers of plant characteristics and utility throughout the full history of our species; we are all taxonomists whether we are conscious of it or not. Timothy Johns of McGill University makes a compelling argument that humans and plants coevolved in a process in which some plants were accepted as food, while others were found to be of medicinal value or outright deadly [22]. While the human brain gradually developed an increased capacity for observation and classification, sensory systems such as taste and olfaction, the liver's ability to detoxify an increasing range of xenobiotics and other physiological traits all evolved in a coordinated fashion. At some point, the human species was able to domesticate selected plants, in other words to select and manipulate plants for less toxicity. The invention of cooking, including the possible addition of acid or base, was another innovation to further detoxify plants by chemical and physical means.

The presence of specific chemical entities in plants, and their uneven distribution across the plant kingdom, did not escape early chemists. Morphine was isolated in 1805, long before its structure was correctly described in 1925 [23, 24]. During the 19th century, an increasing number of pure natural products were isolated, although, as with morphine, their structures were not known until much later (Tab. 2, Fig. 2). Structural studies had to wait for organic

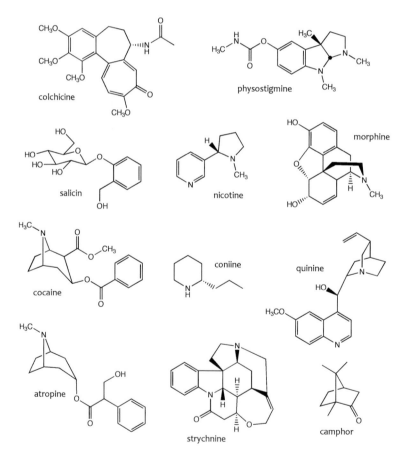

Figure 2. Natural products listed in Table 2.

Table 2. Early milestones in botanically derived toxins and medicinals

Compound	Botanical source	Category	Isolation	Correct structure	Synthesis
Morphine	*Papaver somniferum* (Papaveraceae)	alkaloid	1805 [23]	1925 [152]	1952 [153]
Strychnine	*Strychnos nux-vomica* (Loganiaceae)	alkaloid	1818 [154]	1946 [155]	1954 [156]
Quinine	*Cinchona* spp. (Rubiaceae)	alkaloid	1820 [157]	1918 [158]	1944 [159]
Colchicine	*Colchicum autumnale* (Liliaceae)	alkaloid	1820 [160]	1952 [161]	1961 [162]
Coniine	*Conium maculatum* (Apiaceae)	alkaloid	1826 [163]	1881 [164]	1889 [165]
Nicotine	*Nicotiana tabacum* (Solanaceae)	alkaloid	1828 [166]	1893 [167]	1904 [168]
Salicylic acid/salicin	*Salix* spp. (Salicaceae)	phenol	1830 [169]	1838 (salicin) [170]	1860 (salicylic acid) [171]; 1879 (salicin) [172]
Hyoscyamine/atropine	*Atropa belladonna* (Solanaceae)	alkaloid	1833 (atropine) [173]	1883 (atropine) [174]	1901 (atropine) [175]
Cocaine	*Erythroxylum coca* (Erythroxylaceae)	alkaloid	1860 [176]	1898 [177]	1898 [177]
Physostigmine	*Physostigma venenosum* (Fabaceae)	alkaloid	1864 [178]	1935 [59]	1935 [59]
Podophyllotoxin	*Podophyllum peltatum* (Berberidaceae)	lignan	1880 [179]	1951 [180]	1962 [181]
Camphor	*Cinnamomum camphora* (Lauraceae)	terpene	antiquity	1903 [182]	1903 [182]

Compounds that were described early are dominated by alkaloids, as they often readily crystallized as salts in pure form. An exception is coniine, whose free base is a liquid and which was the first alkaloid synthesized. The synthesis of several of these compounds was the subject of some dispute and drama. For quinine, see [57, 58]; for physostigmine, see [60]. In a number of cases, the synthesis of the compound was also the proof of structure.

chemistry to mature, as a modern understanding of bonding and structure did not coalesce until the latter half of that century. Significant improvements in laboratory methods and technology were also needed before structures could be confirmed. (The development of separation science, using paper chromatography, is one example.) Nevertheless, broad chemical classification of natural products and at least a partial description of properties was possible. Scientists began to realize that certain classes of chemicals were widely distributed, and others narrowly, in the plant kingdom as understood at that time. De Candolle published perhaps the earliest description of this sort, but well before any significant chemical understanding was available (1804) [25]. More chemically enlightened botanical surveys were not available until about 100 years later, with the work of Abbott (in 1896) [26] and Greshoff (in 1909) [27]. The latter coined the phrase "comparative phytochemistry" which was described as "the knowledge of the connection between the natural relationship of plants and their chemical composition". This definition set the stage for further development (see [28] for an excellent history of the field). Since that time, information about the chemical constituents of plants and their distribution continued to accumulate at ever increasing rates. The state of the art by the 1980s is exemplified by Harborne and Turner's "Plant Chemosystematics" [29]. Chapter 12, "Application of Chemistry at the Familial Level", describes surveys of various compound classes and maps them onto plant phylogenies popular at the time. One of the more broadly accepted phylogenies originated with Dahlgren [30]. Figure 3 shows his arrangement of plant superorders with the distribution of benzylisoquinoline alkaloids (BIAs) superimposed. This

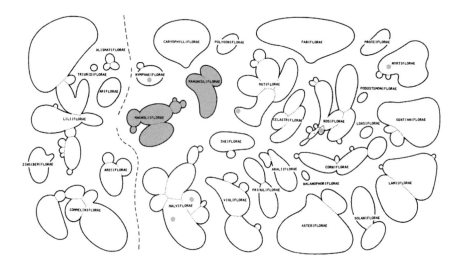

Figure 3. A Dahlgrenogram showing the distribution of benzylisoquinoline alkaloids (BIAs), as understood in 1980. Superorders known to produce BIAs are shown in gray. Adapted from Dahlgren [30] with permission of the publisher, Wiley-Blackwell.

alkaloid family consists of about 2500 different structures and includes important substances such as morphine, codeine and tubocurarine.

The entire landscape of chemosystematics changed dramatically, however,
in the 1980s with the biotechnology revolution. The ease and availability of
DNA sequencing, cloning and particularly the polymerase chain reaction
(PCR), changed the very nature of what was possible in two broad ways. First,
plant systematicists had entirely new information with which to construct a
phylogeny of plant families, as extensive sequences of chloroplast and mitochondrial DNA became available. These molecular phylogenies turned out to
be broadly similar to earlier phylogenies worked out based upon morphological details, reproductive strategies and chemical markers. However, a number
of classifications were changed, particularly at the family level. By 1998,
enough data was available to assemble a truly modern phylogeny of flowering
plants, and in 2003 a significant update was issued [31, 32]. Consider the following simple example which illustrates the significant changes that occurred
in thinking about the relationships between plants. For decades, at some point
in their science education, young students have typically learned that plants
can be divided into two main groups, the monocots and dicots (strictly, mono-
cotyledons and dicotyledons). This grouping followed the scientific thinking
common up until the late 1980s. Indeed, readers may remember learning that
monocots have parallel leaf veination, while dicots have a network of veins, or
that monocots have flower parts in multiples of three's. With the advent of
modern molecular phylogenetic methods, we now know that plants placed in
the monocots are indeed truly related to each other, because the molecular data
coincides with morphological and other data. Under scrutiny, however, the
dicots have not held up as a group, although a large portion of them are indeed
related and are now known as the eudicots, or true dicots [21, 33].

The second change made possible by biotechnology was that these tools
altered the way chemists could investigate the biosynthetic pathways leading
to natural products. Early approaches to biosynthesis studies involved detailed
tracking of molecular skeletons as they were gradually modified by the plant.
These approaches typically involved experiments in which isotopically labeled
simple precursor molecules were made available to the plant, such as acetate
ion labeled with ^{13}C at either carbon. Later, the natural products were isolated,
and the location of the isotopic labels investigated spectroscopically.
(Herbert's text [34] exemplifies this approach; but even earlier approaches
employed radioactive labels, with subsequent laborious chemical degradation.)
The steps employed by the plant to construct the molecule could then be
deduced. (Deducing the pathway was much easier if mutant strains could be
found or created that lacked certain enzymes along the biosynthetic route.
These individuals would accumulate the intermediate ahead of the missing
enzyme.) With the new biotechnology tools, one could investigate these
processes much more thoroughly and quickly by studying the enzymes that
carried out the transformations, rather than the products of those transformations. For example, once a particular enzyme had been identified as carrying

out a reaction of interest, the DNA sequence coding for that enzyme could be used to query databases for other species that possessed a similar or closely related enzyme. As genomic sequence data became available for more and more organisms, comparative studies over large numbers of plant species became possible. Alternatively, the DNA sequence could be used to create a probe for the mRNA coding for a particular enzyme in individual plants. A few examples of this strategy in action are discussed here, but for a full perspective of how biotechnology has changed the study of plants, please see the section on systems toxicology later in this chapter.

Phylogenies constructed prior to the widespread availability of sequence information had always reflected some curiosities in the distribution of natural products. It seemed unlikely that some complex molecular skeletons, which required a significant resource investment by the plants, would be isolated from apparently unrelated families. However, it was difficult to determine if these observations were real, or were due to mistakes in construction of the phylogenies, or perhaps due to incomplete information because an insufficient number of plant species had been studied in detail. As modern phylogenies became available, the occurrence of natural product families and the presence of particular molecular skeletons were mapped onto the new phylogenies. The results were fascinating. In certain plant families for which detailed data were available, it was clear that the presence of particular molecular skeletons was not evenly distributed. A good illustration comes from the laboratory of Michael Wink at University of Heidelberg [35]. Wink and coworkers examined the distribution of quinolizidine alkaloids and non-protein amino acids, two toxin classes common in the Fabaceae family (the legume or bean family). Figure 4 shows that the distribution of these two groups is not even across a number of representative species in this family, which contains about 18 000 species. This figure reveals another interesting finding, namely that species that contain quinolizidine alkaloids typically do not contain non-protein amino acids and *vice versa*; that is, the two categories do not overlap. Apparently, certain lineages have committed to the use of one toxin rather than the other, and resources are not wasted synthesizing both compound classes.

This uneven distribution of compounds could be explained in a number of ways. One could argue that at least some aspects of the distribution suffer from artifacts, such as chemical analyses that are too crude to detect low levels of compounds, or analyses that are not sufficiently selective and give false positives. Another possibility is that the compounds are not actually synthesized by the plants, but rather by endophytic fungi as previously discussed, and hence a plant phylogeny is irrelevant. However, if one assumes that these potential artifacts are fairly rare and that true errors are randomly distributed, then the observed distribution still begs for an explanation. Three explanations are consistent with a modern understanding of the mechanisms of evolution: the same enzymatic capacities have arisen several times independently (convergent evolution), or the genes for synthesizing both compound categories are present in

Quinolizidine Alkaloids   **Non-Protein Amino Acids**

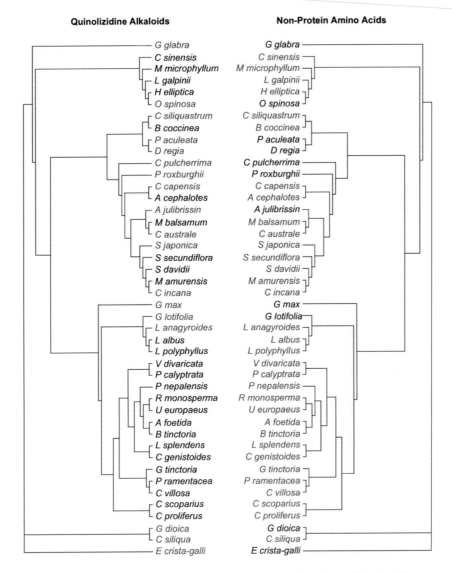

Figure 4. The distribution of quinolizidine alkaloids and non-protein amino acids in the Fabaceae. Bold names are species which contain the compounds, grey names are species in which the compounds are absent. After Wink [36]; based upon data deposited at the European Molecular Biology Laboratory.

all members of the Fabaceae but are turned off in certain taxa, or the genes have been lost in some taxa. Wink's work does not directly address this distinction, however, as his phylogenies are constructed using the sequence of the *rbc*L chloroplast gene, which reflects the overall evolution of the species, not the actual enzymes synthesizing the compounds studied [36].

   Workers in Peter Fachinni's laboratory at the University of Calgary have
pushed the analysis a step deeper in their study of the distribution of the BIAs
mentioned previously [37]. This group of compounds are found primarily in
the order Ranunculales but examples are known from other orders (see Fig. 5
for typical structures). A wide range of species were sampled for (S)-norco-
claurine synthase activity, the enzyme ultimately responsible for the synthesis
of all BIAs. Molecular phylogenies were constructed using the gene sequence
for the synthase along with the sequences for several other enzymes unique to
selected BIA subpathways. These data were compared with the distribution of
the alkaloids mapped onto a phylogeny constructed using chloroplast genes.
The results strongly suggest that the genes for the biosynthesis of BIAs are
present in a much wider range of plants than just those species from which the
alkaloids have been isolated. Hence, the hypothesis that genes for the synthesis of natural products are widespread but turned off in various taxa appears to
be strongly supported. In the case of the BIAs, the data suggest that the necessary genes originated prior to the origin of the eudicots; in other words, quite
early in the evolution of plants. These results (e.g., Fig. 4) can be compared to

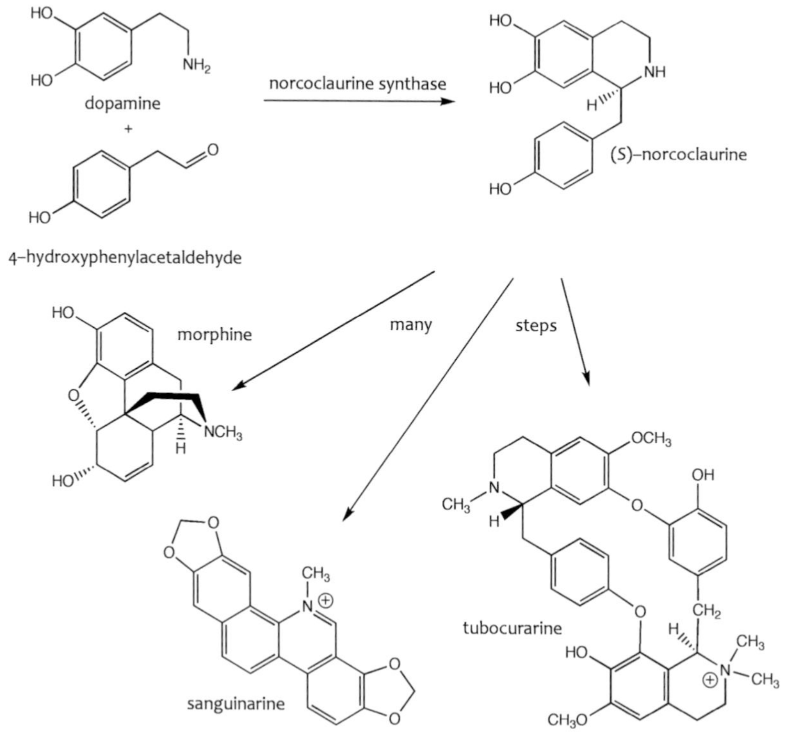

Figure 5. The synthesis of all benzylisoquinoline alkaloids (BIAs) begins with the action of norcoclaurine synthase, and leads to a wide variety of structural skeletons. Only a few examples are shown
here.

the Dahlgrenogram presented in Figure 3; clearly, modern analyses differ significantly in their very nature and certainly in their detail.

In contrast, an alternative scenario appears to operate in the case of the pyrrolizidine alkaloids (PAs), a diverse group of toxic substances. PAs are found in rather distantly related plant groups, including eudicots (families Asteraceae and Fabaceae) and monocots (family Orchidaceae). PAs have been implicated in cases of poisoning with herbal medicines (due to contamination [38–41]) and cause liver failure in livestock grazing on *Senecio* species (the ragworts and groundsels, family Asteraceae). PAs are activated in the liver, producing a metabolite that reacts with DNA to give a tumorigenic adduct [42, 43]. An early step in the synthesis of PAs is the conversion of the diamine putrescine to homospermidine, by transferring a C_4NH_2 chain from spermidine. This reaction is carried out by homospermidine synthase (HSS). Elaboration of homospermidine leads eventually to the necine base characteristic of PAs; additional steps add the diester-containing ring (Fig. 6). Work in the laboratories of Dietrich Ober and Thomas Hartmann at the Technical University of Braunschweig has revealed that HSS has likely arisen at least four separate times over evolutionary history [44]. This conclusion was reached by the analysis of amino acid sequences and genomic DNA of a number of species. It appears that the gene for a different enzyme, deoxyhypusine synthase, was duplicated, and the second copy underwent additional evolution

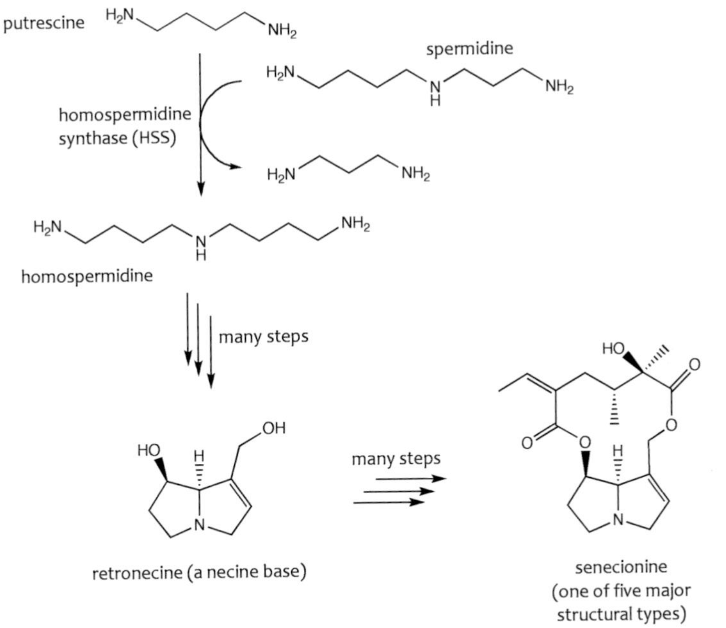

Figure 6. The biosynthesis of pyrrolizidine alkaloids begins with homospermidine synthase, and leads to a diverse array of toxic alkaloids.

to become HSS [45]. Deoxyhypusine synthase also transfers a C_4NH_2 chain from spermidine, but in this case the acceptor is a lysine side chain of a transcription factor. This is an example of convergent evolution by change of function after duplication. Other examples in which a no-longer-needed copy of a gene evolves to have a new function and eventually different product specificities and expression patterns are known from the terpene and flavonoid pathways [46].

In contrast to these more complex scenarios, there are some compound families which are narrowly distributed, suggesting that their biosynthetic pathways originated more recently. Perhaps the best example is that of the betalain pigments, which are found exclusively in the order Caryophyllales and serve as a reliable marker for this order [47, 48].

These examples demonstrate that there is a great deal to be learned from the distribution of natural products in light of modern molecular phylogenies. Unfortunately, the hope of systematicists that natural products would serve as simple taxonomic characters has proven to be too good to be true. They certainly can serve as useful markers, but a 'present/not present' interpretation is clearly a too-simple approach. The reality is that the study of natural products and the enzymes that produce them will enlighten systematics and the mechanisms of plant evolution greatly, but considerable investment will be needed to work out the details [28].

Chemical synthesis and structural diversity

The laboratory synthesis of natural toxins and medicinal substances has always been of great importance; it is the basis for the modern pharmaceutical industry. Typically, once the structure of a natural product has been described, there are always chemists ready to undertake its synthesis, although in one celebrated instance, these steps were reversed. In 1856, William Perkin undertook the synthesis of the critically important antimalarial quinine starting from aniline, even though he did not know the structure of quinine, which was not described until 1918. While this experiment was extraordinarily naïve in retrospect, Perkin did discover the compound mauveine, which launched the entire synthetic dye industry [49]. The synthesis of quinine was ultimately a much more difficult task, as it was not until 1944 that the synthesis was achieved (but not all agree about this, as described below).

"It is well worth looking at the proposition that chemical synthesis is an art form, needing no justification because it permits self-expression in its creators and produces aesthetic pleasure in those who examine its products."

J.W. Cornforth [50]

There are a number of reasons that chemists pursue synthesis. There are those who view the synthesis of complex molecules as a Mount Everest to be climbed or a chess game to be won [51–53]. Since the resulting synthetic schemes are generally long and complex, it is hard to argue that the process will lead to the preparation of large quantities of material for clinical or commercial use. Along the way, however, new reactions may be invented, which might be more efficient with regard to building up the skeleton or controlling stereochemistry, or which may be more environmentally friendly. The preparation of simpler analogs, often undertaken as an intermediate step in the synthesis of a more complex target compound, may lead to compounds that retain biological activity, which in turn gives insight into the pharmacophore and suggests other compounds to prepare.

Occasionally, the synthesis of a reported compound leads to the discovery of errors in the original structure, and to their correction [54]. And controversies arise from time to time. The synthesis of quinine, reported in 1944 [55], has been called into question with the publication of a stereoselective synthesis in 2001 [56]. The interesting story about who made what compound and when they made it has been analyzed in detail by Seeman [57] and reveals quite a bit about the science of total synthesis (see also the account by Kaufman and Rúveda [58]). Similarly, the synthesis of physostigmine, an ordeal poison used in traditional jurisprudence by certain African cultural groups, was achieved by African-American chemist Percy Julian working at a small college in rural America in 1935 [59]. This was an extraordinary achievement at the time, and all the more interesting because Julian completed the synthesis ahead of the very accomplished research group of Sir Robert Robinson at Oxford. In addition, Julian showed that Robinson had been wrong in some of his earlier publications. Addison Ault has provided a concise description of how Julian did it, and how Robinson was misled [60].

One of the most interesting debates in the field of synthesis is the issue of what molecules to make, and how to go about making them. A traditional approach favored by those who see synthesis as a chess game is to choose biologically active molecules that have high degrees of complexity or which have carbon skeletons that have not previously been made. (Funding is much easier to obtain for molecules which have biological activity of potential medical interest.) The chosen molecules are then synthesized by some combination of known reactions, or reactions which must be invented, often in very long sequences. This approach does not correspond to the needs of the pharmaceutical industry, where simpler molecules with high biological activity and good therapeutic profiles are mandatory, and shorter syntheses are critical. Consequently, a great deal of thought and strategy has gone into inventing alternative methods for choosing and making molecules, with the goal of minimizing the time necessary for discovering novel (i.e., patentable) active compounds which are easily made at reasonable cost.

Over the long haul Nature has provided a large fraction of our useful molecules, and the natural world continues to be a source of inspiration and ideas as discussed in the first section. However, it can be argued that most molecules with high biological activity, and which are present in modest quantities in their natural sources, were easy to discover and have already been exploited; hence, different approaches are needed to develop new drug candidates. One approach to thinking about this issue is to recognize that the potential structural diversity of small to medium-sized organic molecules is enormous, and can be described in a number of ways, some of which may lead us to new ideas. These descriptors include such things as connectivity, lipophilicity, topology, the functional groups present, chirality, flexibility and so forth. Collectively, these and other descriptors have been called the "chemical space" in which molecules exist [61]. The challenge in finding new useful molecules is then twofold: first, to describe this chemical space accurately, and second, to map the chemical space onto the corresponding biological-activity space in such a way that useful activity is found more quickly. One could argue that this is exactly what Nature has done through the process of evolution: sampling a wide swath of chemical space in search of a hit in biological-activity space. Biologically active natural products have been described as "evolutionarily selected", "prevalidated" or "privileged" by various authors.

This notion of chemical space and characterizing it is not really new; it is the basis for much of medicinal chemistry and rational drug design using quantitative structure-activity relationships (QSAR). However, the growth of publicly available databases has facilitated new approaches. Lipkus and colleagues at the Chemical Abstracts Service have analyzed their database of more than 24 million organic compounds described in the literature to measure their structural diversity [62]. Their results demonstrate that the number of known skeletons is actually quite limited and that most compounds are derivatives of these known skeletons, suggesting that true structural diversity is low (Bohacek has estimated the number of possible structures at 10^{60} [63]). Feher and Schmidt [64] have conducted a statistical analysis of the similarity of natural products, drugs on the market, and molecules made by combinatorial chemistry. (Combinatorial chemistry is the rapid, high-throughput assembly of modest size molecules from a set of building blocks in a somewhat randomly selected fashion. The result is a set – library – of molecules from which the active ones can hopefully be fished out by an appropriate assay.) They found that the chemical space explored by combinatorial chemistry appears to be significantly limited by the reactions typically employed in combinatorial work. In contrast, drugs in use and natural products cover a much greater volume of chemical space. Waldmann and colleagues at the Max Planck Institute of Molecular Physiology in Germany have carried out a similar structural classification of known natural products but have gone beyond mere description and used the results to design new drugs [65]. They have also reviewed recent approaches to describing chemical space [66]. Finally, researchers at Uppsala University and AstraZeneca have described ChemGPS-NP, whose name emphasizes the need to navigate within this chemical space [67]. All these studies reach the same general conclusion, namely that the information and diversity in natural product structures is underutilized relative to the full potential of chemical space.

As descriptions of chemical space have been refined, the questions of how this space relates to biological-activity space and which compounds to make has developed simultaneously [61, 68–71]. New approaches have been developed that consider, in principle, all (or at least more) of the possible chemical space, and which try to address a broad region of biological-activity space as well. These explorations have led to a number of interesting drug discovery strategies.

Foremost among these are investigations in which the principles and concepts of combinatorial chemistry are merged with the notion of using natural products directly as scaffolds, or as the inspiration for scaffolds [72]. The basic procedure is to begin with a natural product or perhaps a simplified version, and attach it to a resin for subsequent modifications by solid-phase synthesis. One then uses the existing functional groups to modify the structure, in effect adding a wide variety of "side chains" at several different sites. An alternative approach is to introduce the same building blocks, but with differing chirality. An example based upon the toxin galanthamine is shown in Figure 7 (the spelling in some publications is galantamine). Galanthamine is a selective and competitive acetylcholinesterase inhibitor found in the family Amarylidaceae [73], such as the bulb of the common daffodil (*Narcissus pseudonarcissus*). Developed from indigenous knowledge, it has recently become available for the treatment of Alzheimer's disease [74]. Shair and colleagues at Harvard have developed a library of compounds that are based upon a modified galan-

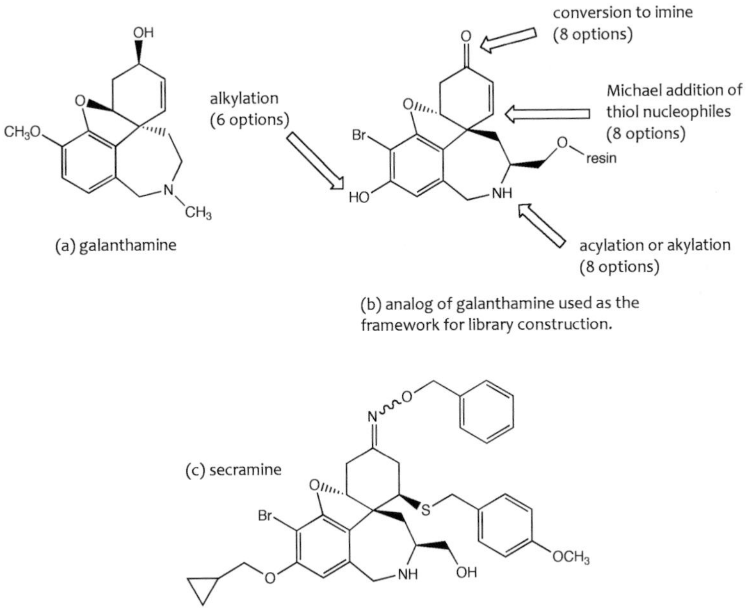

Figure 7. (a) Galanthamine; (b) strategy for construction of a library based upon galanthamine; (c) secramine, a structure isolated from the library with completely different biological activity.

thamine structure [75]. Beginning with an analog constructed on a solid resin, a variety of side chains were introduced in all possible combinations using the instrinsic reactivity of the analog's functional groups, leading to a library of 2527 different molecules (about 85% of the theoretical number). Screening of this library lead to the isolation of secramine (Fig. 7c), which is an inhibitor of protein trafficking, a biological activity completely unrelated to that of galanthamine. Many other examples employing a similar combinatorial approach have been reported [76, 77] and there is great promise for discovery of new structures with new activities.

Another approach to generating structural diversity takes advantage of the fact that many natural products are present as glycosides, that is, in combination (conjugation) with sugars. The function of these sugars is to increase the solubility of the often non-polar molecule (the aglycone) in the aqueous environment of the cell. The nature of these sugars, as well as their presence or absence, often has a large effect on their biological activity [78]. A typical and important example is that of digitoxin, derived from the Foxglove plant (*Digitalis purpurea,* Plantaginaceae), the subject of one of the earliest known clinical trials [79] (Fig. 8). Thorson and colleagues at the University of Wisconsin have developed several means of generating structural diversity by adding non-natural sugars to the aglycones, as well as methods for randomizing the sugars present using glycosyltransferases which are able to accept a variety of sugars as substrates (so-called promiscuous enzymes). Applying this approach to digitoxin, they created a library of 78 analogs by replacing the triose of digitoxin with a variety of monosaccharides, and varying the stereochemistry at the point of attachment [80]. The normal activity of digitoxin is to increase the force of heart-muscle contraction by inhibiting Na^+/K^+ ATPase activity. It also exhibits modest but non-specific cytotoxic effects on cancer cell lines. Bioassay of this library against various cancer cell lines led to the discovery of members with much more potent or selective cytotoxicity (but not both). Thorson has also created a library of 58 glycosides of the tubulin polymerization inhibitor colchicine (Fig. 2), a molecule that does not normally exist as a glycoside [81]. Once again, some members of this library exhibited greater potency or selectivity, and two members stabilized the structure of tubulin, the

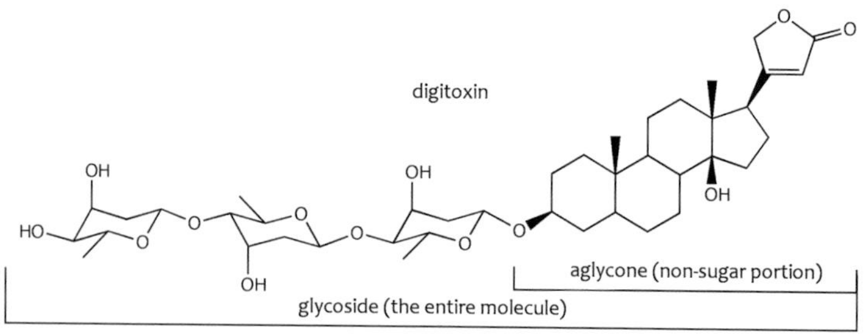

Figure 8. The structure of digitoxin, a glycoside that acts to increase the force of heart contraction.

opposite effect of colchicine. Digitoxin and colchicine are compounds from toxic plants, but the Thorson group has demonstrated the broad applicability of this approach with medicinal compounds from bacteria and fungi, and has shown that the enzymes involved can be engineered to great advantage [82–85].

"... I see no reason why we should not welcome enzymes and microbes as friends and colleagues. Since they work for even less than graduate students, perhaps we should at least acknowledge them..."

J.W. Cornforth [50]

In addition to strategies designed to create a greater diversity of chemical structures, scientists have sought to carry out the syntheses of naturally occurring compounds in more efficient ways, an approach that has benefited greatly from the developments in biotechnology described earlier [86]. One approach is to abandon traditional synthesis and develop cell cultures and other systems that produce the natural products of interest.

Several excellent examples exist; perhaps the most important is that of paclitaxel (trade name Taxol). This compound was one of several to be developed principally by Wall and Wani at Research Triangle Park [87]. Paclitaxel was first isolated from a thin layer of inner bark of the pacific yew tree (*Taxus brevifolia*, Taxaceae) in 1971. Its mode of action was unique at the time (tubulin stabilization [88]) and it was eventually marketed by Bristol-Meyers Squibb for the treatment of ovarian, breast and lung cancers. As its efficacy became apparent, problems quickly arose with the supply of the drug. Isolation from the tree was clearly untenable as it would create a considerable environmental disaster if pursued (one mature tree would produce about one dose) [89]. Subsequently, related species were found that produced paclitaxel or related structures, and these provided the supply necessary for clinical use. Even so, the compound is still quite expensive, about $ 300 000 per kilogram. Consequently, much effort has gone into studying the biosynthetic pathways leading to paclitaxel in the hopes of harnessing the enzymes. In addition, many investigators have worked on developing plant cell culture methods for the production of paclitaxel or a related molecule that can be converted to it in a cost-effective manner [90, 91]. Phyton Corporation produces paclitaxel in a 75 000-L fermentation/cell culture system. Current research is aimed at optimizing the cell culture conditions for initial growth, after which the cells are transferred to a different media that enhances the production of paclitaxel. The discovery that paclitaxel is apparently synthesized by an endophytic fungus (detailed earlier) has both complicated and simplified efforts. The important antimalarial artemisinin from *Artemisia annua* (Asteraceae) is currently going through much the same development cycle as paclitaxel [92].

A strategy that is both potentially very efficient and amenable to generating structural diversity is to genetically engineer microorganisms to carry out the syntheses [93]. In this so-called combinatorial biosynthesis, genes from a plant (possibly more than one) are moved into a different organism such as a bacterium or a yeast, and in combination with the native genes of that organism, they may be coaxed into synthesizing a desired product. The hope is that the heterologous system may be more practical in terms of the ease of culture and the production efficiency (Kayser and colleagues have reviewed a number of such investigations [94]). In addition to making the synthesis more efficient, such systems may be engineered to rearrange the order of genes and even combine genes from different organisms to produce novel structures, which may have novel mechanisms of action.

A good illustration of the first approach involves the BIAs discussed earlier. These compounds are synthesized in plants beginning with the action of norcoclaurine synthase, followed by a wide variety of additional enzymes depending upon the carbon skeleton found in a particular species (Fig. 5). Minami and Sato in Japan developed a two-organism, one-culture method for the efficient preparation of BIAs. These workers first prepared and cultured a transgenic *Escherichia coli* line with the plant genes for the synthesis of (*S*)-reticuline, a key branch point in the pathways leading to diverse BIAs. After a period of time, they added to the growing bacterial culture a transgenic *Saccharomyces cerevisiae* that contained additional genes for the transformation of reticuline into magnoflorine. In a second experiment, the added transgenic yeast contained the genes for the synthesis of scoulerine. These co-culture systems, containing transgenic plant genes carried in two different organisms, and supplemented by bacterial enzymes, were able to produce good quantities of structurally diverse alkaloids (Fig. 9) [95]. Both magnoflorine and scoulerine are of medicinal interest, but the success of this method opens the door to the synthesis of BIAs of even greater medical importance. A similar investigation has been reported by Hawkins and Smolke at the California

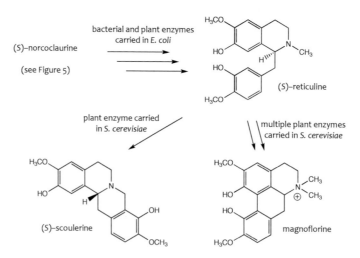

Figure 9. The Minami and Sato co-culture system for the preparation of benzylisoquinoline alkaloids (BIAs).

Institute of Technology using yeast cells containing plant and human enzymes [96]. This system was shown to synthesize a morphine precursor, in addition to sanguinarine/berberine skeletons.

A second and particularly ambitious example is the attempt by Verpoorte and colleagues to produce *Vinca* (*Catharanthus*) alkaloids in heterologous systems (Fig. 10) [97]. Vincristine and vinblastine are very important antineoplastic compounds and among the most structurally complex plant natural products known. They are produced in plants at extremely low levels, and cell culture methods have not been successful. Hence, there is great interest in a biotechnological solution. Unfortunately, the biosynthetic pathway involves at least 32 genes and 35 intermediates, along with 7 subcellular compartments (which is consistent with the structural complexity of the compounds). While portions of the pathways have been successfully transferred to *E. coli, S. cerevisiae* and *Nicotina tabacum*, efficient expression of the entire biosynthetic apparatus has not yet been achieved. However, McCoy and O'Connor at Harvard University have reported that seedlings and hairy root cultures of *Catharanthus roseus* are able to accept a wide variety of substituted tryptamine precursors and carry them through to compounds late in the biosynthetic sequence [98, 99].

The second broad approach, to generate novel structures by combining and re-ordering genes from several plants, has only recently begun to be explored. Polyketide synthases (PKS) are responsible for the synthesis of a wide range of interesting natural products. These modular enzyme complexes are able to build up a carbon chain from a variety of starting units, add multiple extender units, and modify the resulting structure by various combinations of cyclizations, reductions and dehydrations. Over evolutionary time, the individual genes in these complexes have been duplicated and subsequently modified, creating a set of tools that can accept different substrates, and be used in different orders for different results. In other words, Nature has been employing

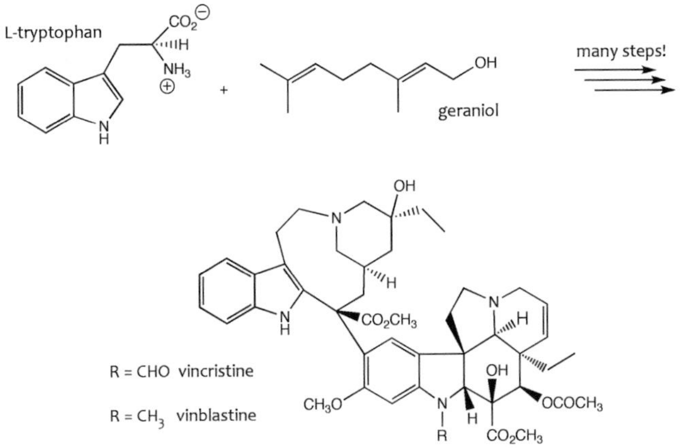

Figure 10. The biosynthesis of the *Vinca* alkaloids vincristine and vinblastine.

a sort of combinatorial biochemistry that humans have only recently recognized and tried to manipulate. The chemistry and genetic engineering of PKS
have been exploited for sometime in bacteria [100], but the plant enzymes have
only recently been cloned and put to use [101, 102]. By rearranging the order
of individual enzymes that carry out the cyclizations and other modifications,
new structures can be created. Some PKS are promiscuous as they will accept
a variety of starter units not found in Nature, which permits additional structural diversity. Figure 11 illustrates the overall process and structures of a few
important plant natural products generated by PKS.

Choosing a target for synthesis has clearly moved well beyond early moti-
vations. The means of synthesis have also changed significantly. The examples
described above demonstrate that the field of synthesis remains a very creative
and practical endeavor. While Nature has provided numerous useful drugs and
toxins, it is clear that creative chemists and molecular biologists will continue
to harness the tools that Nature has been using to create even more structural
variety and to do so by increasingly efficient means.

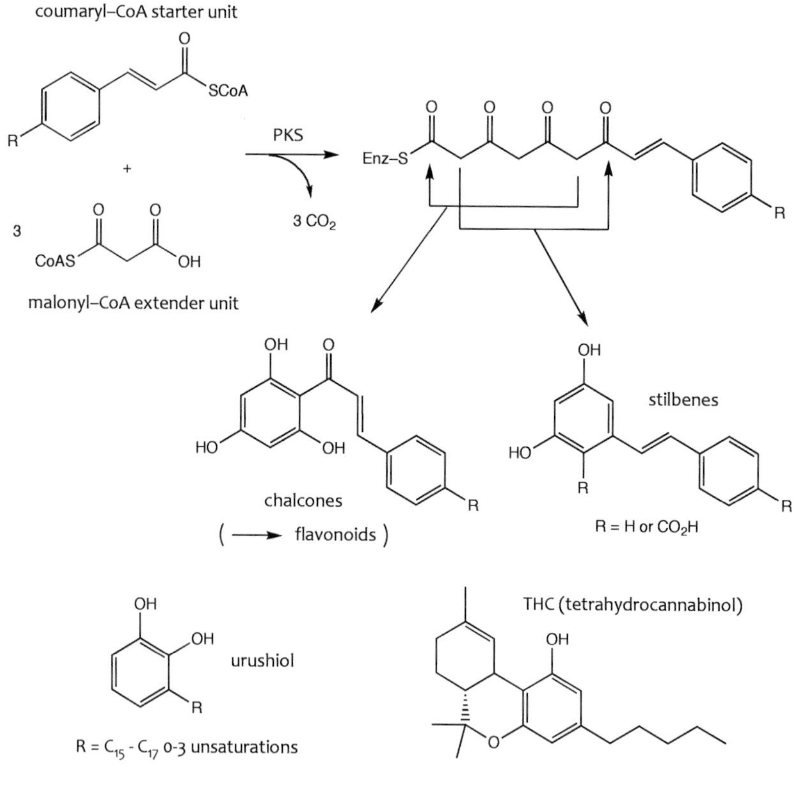

Figure 11. A typical plant biosynthetic pathway leading to polyketide intermediates, which can be
cyclized to give a variety of structures. PKS, polyketide synthase. THC (Δ^9-tetrahydrocannabinol) is
the active ingredient in marijuana. Urushiols are the active ingredients in poison ivy.

Systems toxicology

One of the most interesting recent developments bridging chemistry and biology is the development of systems biology, which seeks to integrate knowledge of the molecular workings of living organisms across several levels. Crick's "central dogma" is the unifying concept in molecular biology, which describes the flow of information in an organism, from DNA to RNA and finally to proteins [103]. The development of biotechnology led to an understanding of this information flow on a much grander scale within a single organism, and in a comparative fashion between organisms. Beginning with genomics (e.g., the human genome project), and later proteomics and transcriptomics, the available information has exploded in quantity and improved in quality. More recently, the field of metabolomics has made its debut – metabolomics studies the result of the flow of information out of the central dogma as well as its regulation – in other words, the identity and concentrations of all metabolites in an organism. Systems biology is an attempt to use all this information at once to study how the pieces function in an integrated fashion. Figure 12 illustrates the relationship between these concepts.

The systems biology approach can provide a great deal of information about an organism under normal conditions, but the greatest insight is derived by comparing this reference state to some sort of perturbed or stressed state. For instance, one might study the metabolism of carbohydrates by comparing growth under normal conditions to one in which a particular substrate is lacking or enhanced [104, 105]. Systems toxicology in particular is the study of organisms stressed by some sort of xenobiotic toxin, and has great potential in the pharmaceutical industry. Applications are being developed that use metabolomics to speed drug development by improving the preclinical screening process, the elucidation of metabolic pathways, and the determination of mechanisms of toxicity [106, 107]. Not surprisingly, there is also enormous interest in using these methods to develop diagnostic biomarkers for a wide variety of disease states, and in some cases molecular changes can be detected long before a disease makes its appearance *via* traditional clinical indications [108]. A good illustration of the strategy and potential of the systems toxicology approach is a study conducted by Nicholson's group at Imperial College London and colleagues at AstraZeneca [109]. These investigators studied the necrosis of liver tissue induced by methapyrilene in rats using a combination of gene expression analysis (transcriptomics), a comprehensive analysis of protein levels (proteomics) and NMR spectroscopy of urine and liver tissue samples (metabolomics). These methods were linked to more traditional histological analysis and revealed complex changes in the molecular systems that react to oxidative stress as well as those responsible for energy usage.

As with all applications of systems biology, one of the key challenges is the management of the flood of data that results from these complex studies. Several recent reviews have discussed the development of knowledge bases in

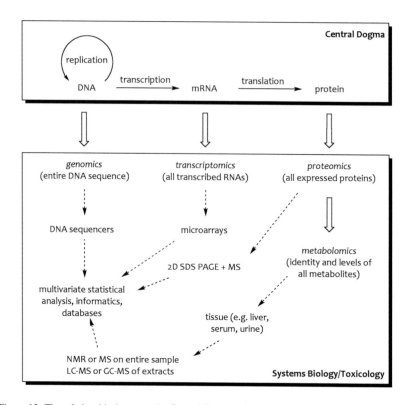

Figure 12. The relationship between the Central Dogma of molecular biology and systems biology concepts. Genomics is the study of the entire DNA sequence of an organism. Transcriptomics is the study of all transcribed mRNA sequences, normally a subset of the entire genome. Proteomics is the study of all expressed (and modified) proteins. Metabolomics is the study of all metabolites and their levels, which result from the action of the proteins through both enzymatic and regulatory activities. Each of these fields has associated techniques, which lead to large data sets that must be analyzed by appropriate statistical methods. MS, mass spectrometry; NMR, nuclear magnetic resonance; LC, liquid chromatography; GC, gas chromatography; SDS-PAGE, sodium dodecyl sulfate-polyacrylamide gel electrophoresis.

toxicology that endeavor to integrate the systems approach with more traditional types of toxicological studies [110, 111]. The development of the Chemical Effects in Biological Systems (CEBS) depository is one effort to organize data from a variety of experimental methods in a comprehensive manner so that the results can be mined for insights and compared across laboratories and organisms [112].

Systems toxicological studies of medicinal and toxic plants have only recently appeared in the literature. An area that has been a rich source of research programs are the traditional healing methods of China and India, known as Traditional Chinese Medicine (TCM) and ayurveda, respectively [113]. Both of these traditions are holistic healing paradigms that use a wide variety of individual herbs and especially mixtures of herbs. They are ideal candidates for the systems approach as the presence of multiple medicinal and toxic substances would be expected to have effects on a wide variety of organ systems. The broad and sometimes subtle effects produced by the phytomedicinal mixtures typical of these traditions are not easily identified or quantified by the usual drug discovery and development processes, which are strongly oriented toward single chemical entities [114]. In addition, the synergistic effects often claimed for herbal mixtures do not fit well with the Western paradigm for healing [115–117]. Several authors have pointed out that the systems approach is an excellent match for understanding the biological effects of these herbal mixtures, one that can provide a bridge between toxicology, molecular pharmacology and ethnopharmacology [118–125].

The most common systems toxicological studies involving plant extracts so far are transcriptomic studies using microarrays to measure changes in gene expression (i.e., mRNA expression levels). An early example demonstrating the power of the approach was the report by Watanabe et al. in 2001 [126] regarding the effect of herb *Ginkgo biloba* (Ginkgoaceae) on the cortex and hippocampus of mice. Ginkgo is an ancient Chinese herb used to treat a variety of cognitive deficits [127]. A number of the individual components of this herb are known to be biologically active as antioxidants and as platelet-activating factor antagonists [128–130]. The study analyzed ~12 000 mRNA transcripts and identified 10 genes that were up-regulated more than 3-fold in mice fed a supplement containing ginkgo. Functional annotation of these genes identified proteins with a role in neurotransmission, cell growth and neuroprotection. Another study involving brain function was designed by Wang et al. [131]. In this work, cerebral ischemia was induced in mice that had been maintained on various dosages of a standardized TCM herbal glycoside recipe, consisting of the compounds baicalein and dioscin (see Fig. 13 for structures of compounds mentioned in this section). These compounds are found in the Chinese herb *Scutellaria baicalensis* (Lamiaceae), which is one of the most important herbs in TCM. Microarray analysis of the hippocampus was coupled with measurements of spatial learning memory, measured by performance in a water maze. These authors found that the herbal treatment led to improved recovery from the ischemia (i.e., a better performance in the maze and a decreased infarct volume). Nine genes were observed to be up- or down-regulated by more than 1.8-fold in the two highest dosages of the herbal treatment. As with the previous study, the roles of these genes could reasonably be associated with improved learning and cognitive function; for instance, expression of the 5-hydroxytryptophan (serotonin) receptor decreased in a dose-dependent manner.

Phytoestrogens are plant compounds that mimic the effect of estrogen in humans. As a type of endocrine disruptor, they are of interest not only from a toxicological perspective, but also as potential treatments for estrogen-sensitive cancers. It is not surprising therefore that a number of researchers have examined the action of phytoestrogens using microarrays. A recent example is the study by several groups in Japan, who examined the effect of various phy-

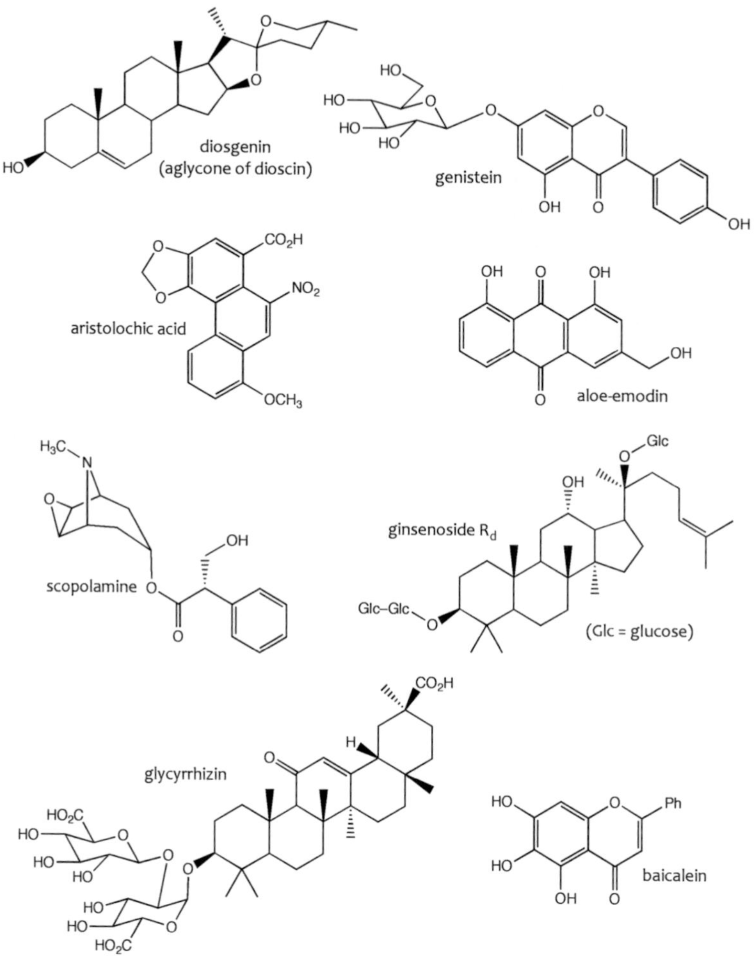

Figure 13. Structures of compounds mentioned in the section on systems toxicology.

toestrogens on human breast cancer cells [132]. Both pure phytochemicals (e.g., the isoflavone genistein) as well as extracts of soy beans (*Glycine max*, Fabaceae) were investigated using a custom microarray composed of genes known to be estrogen responsive. About 20 genes were identified that responded to the phytoestrogens differently than to estrogen. The majority of these genes have a known role in signal transduction in cancer. Another study using breast cancer cells was conducted by Dong and colleagues using extracts of licorice (*Glycyrrhiza glabra*, Fabaceae; licorice is also part of the TCM pharmacopeia) [133]. This extract promotes the growth of cancer cells due to certain components that activate the estrogen receptor. Analysis of the expression profiles allowed the authors to conclude that glycyrrhizin, the main triterpene in licorice, did not induce estrogen-responsive genes or cell proliferation.

Rather, it appears that a number of components acting in concert are responsible for the proliferation. As with the previous study, many genes associated with signaling are affected by the licorice extract. Endocrine disruptors are also known to affect development of the sexual organs *in utero*. Adachi et al. [134] demonstrated that neonatal exposure to genistein had a long-term effect on the expression of the estrogen and androgen receptors in mice testes, even though there were no morphological changes. Naciff and colleagues [135] at Proctor and Gamble also found that genistein had a significant transplacental effect on rat testes, and identified 23 genes that were up- or down-regulated by at least a factor of 1.5. At the highest dosages, 46 genes were significantly affected. The pattern observed for genistein was similar to an estrogen derivative as well as the important industrial toxin bisphenol A, suggesting that these compounds act in a similar fashion.

Several other transcriptomic studies of botanicals have been conducted. Hsieh and colleagues investigated *Scutellaria baicalensis*, mentioned above in a study of cognitive performance, regarding its role as an anti-inflammatory herb, another TCM-use for the plant [136]. Using human embryonic kidney cells, these researchers identified changes in expression of several genes associated with inflammatory and immune responses as the likely mechanism of action of the plant. Some of the same investigators reported a study of the rat hippocampus treated with scopolamine, a substance that induces memory impairment [137]. Key differences between treated and untreated rats involved genes related to the muscarinic receptors, and several others were genes associated with the development of Alzheimer's disease.

Proteomic studies have also been conducted on plants of toxic and medicinal interest, and not surprisingly plants from TCM have been the focus [138]. Two studies have been reported on the genus *Scutellaria*. Ong's group in Singapore studied *S. baicalensis* and its effect on proteins of the mouse liver [139]. At low doses no changes were observed, but at high doses, bile duct damage was observed along with changes in expression of proteins involved in triglyceride-rich particle processing, carbohydrate metabolism, cell signaling and xenobiotic transformation. The same group investigated *S. barbata* and its effect on human colon cancer cell lines [140]. A combined cell-cycle analysis and proteomic investigation revealed that the botanical extract induced cell death, apparently *via* changes in transcription factors and regulation of the cell cycle. Some members of the same group have studied the effect of rhubarb root (*Rheum palmatum*, Polygonaceae), also used in TCM, on human liver cancer cells [141]. Rhubarb contains bioactive anthroquinones such as aloe-emodin that are believed to be responsible for its biological action. The effect of rhubarb seemed to be mediated primarily by up-regulation of proteins involved in the oxidative stress response, which was confirmed by separate biochemical measurements. Other proteins whose expression varied significantly were those responsible for cell-cycle arrest and antimetastasis.

Cheng and colleagues in China studied the TCM material medica ShuangDan Decoction, which is a mixture of two herbs frequently used for myocardial infarction, angia and coronary heart disease [142]. Proteomic investigation of rat myocardium along with histological and biochemical studies revealed modulation of 23 proteins in ischemic hearts. These proteins generally fell into the categories of energy metabolism, oxidative stress response, and cytoskeleton maintenance. Wink and colleagues [143] investigated the influence of red clover (*Trifolium pratense*, Fabaceae), which contains large amounts of isoflavones, on both gene and protein expression in the liver of ovariectomized rats. They found that plasma lipid levels were differentially affected by the isoflavone treatments, and that genes affecting lipid metabolism and oxidative response were the main protein changes. Interestingly, compared to a limited number of changes in protein expression, there were quite a few changes in gene expression, involving not only lipid metabolism and oxidative responses, but also androgen/estrogen regulation and the metabolism of xenobiotics. Ginseng is another herb used extensively throughout Asia. Lee and colleagues in Korea have examined changes in the proteome of colon cancer cells as a result of treatment with ginsenoside R_d [144]. Significant changes were observed in proteins responsible for apoptosis, DNA replication and repair, protein synthesis and degradation, and mutagenesis. Although not an investigation of an animal model affected by a toxic/medicinal plant, as part of their overall investigation of *Vinca* alkaloids, Verpoorte and colleagues [145] have reported on the proteomics of cell suspension cultures of *Catharanthus roseus*. This study revealed some interesting insights into the biosynthesis of these alkaloids. Among other discoveries, the authors were able to identify two isoforms of strictosidine synthase, one of the key early enzymes in the biosynthetic pathway. This sort of study illustrates how the systems approach can also inform the taxonomic, biosynthetic and applied studies discussed earlier in this chapter.

Metabolomic studies of toxic and medicinal plants are just now beginning to appear in the literature. (There are a fairly large numbers of metabolomic-type studies on medicinal plants aimed at quality control and authentification. These are not discussed here as they do not directly deal with toxicology in organisms treated with the plants.) Chen et al. [146] studied the effect of aristolochic acid on rats. Aristolochic acid is a well-known nephrotoxin found in members of the family Aristolochiaceae. The acid and its derivatives have also been implicated as contaminants in various herbal mixtures, and cause serious problems such as acute renal failure and end-stage renal disease. These authors combined traditional histological examination with liquid chromatography–mass spectrometry (LC-MS) of urine using pattern recognition methods. Comparison of untreated rats with rats receiving pure aristolochic acid as well as a TCM preparation from the plant *Aristolochia manshuriensis* led to the discovery that metabolic pathways involving homocysteine and folate appeared to be activated, while those involving arachidonic acid were down-regulated. The authors concluded that these methods could be used as a rapid screening process for the detection of aristolochic acid ingestion. Chen and a different group of collaborators have also reported a metabolomic study of *Trypterygium wilfordii* (Celastraceae) using a similar approach [147]. This

TCM preparation is used to treat rheumatoid arthritis and other inflammatory conditions, but is known to have a number of undesirable side effects such as infertility and renal failure. Investigation of rat urine using GC- and LC-MS along with histological studies of the kidney, liver and testis revealed a time-dependent toxic effect at higher doses. Perturbations in metabolites related to energy status, amino acid processing and choline processing were observed. Other urinary metabolites observed suggested that the gut microflora populations were also affected by the extract.

There are several reports in the literature of metabolomic studies involving plants not considered to be toxic, but which are still of medicinal interest. Nicholson's lab has studied the widely consumed chamomile tea (*Matricaria recutita*, Asteraceae) in humans [148]. Using ^{1}H NMR spectroscopy to study metabolites in urine, these researchers identified non-trivial variations by gender and individual. In spite of these variations, however, they were able to identify increases in hippurate and glycine and decreases in creatinine as markers of chamomile tea ingestion; these changes in urinary metabolites were likely the result of changes in the gut microflora. Interestingly, these alterations persisted for 2 weeks after tea consumption was halted. Nicholson's lab has also reported two studies using ^{1}H NMR spectroscopic investigation of human plasma in subjects who had consumed soy isoflavones [149, 150]. These researchers identified clear differences in lipoprotein, amino acid and carbohydrate profiles resulting from the isoflavone consumption. As a final example, Ong's group mentioned earlier in connection with a proteomic study has also reported a metabolomic study on green tea consumption [151]. This comprehensive study combined GC-MS, LC-MS and ^{1}H NMR spectroscopic studies on human urine, and demonstrated significant changes in metabolites originating in energy and amino acid pathways immediately after ingestion of green tea.

Although really just beginning, systems toxicological studies such as the ones summarized here have tremendous potential. The reader has no doubt noticed that many different genes, proteins and metabolites are affected in a typical study. This is both the advantage and the weakness: holistic approaches are powerful but great effort must be expended to interpret the resulting data sets. It is likely that many researchers will gravitate to metabolomic studies, as these reflect the end result of changes in the transcriptome and proteome, and hence no speculation about what changes in a given mRNA level might ultimately mean is necessary. Metabolomics is also conceptually closest to traditional clinical chemical measurements, such as lipid panels, and as such may be more palatable to practicing clinicians.

Concluding remarks

The study of medicinal and toxic plants from any angle is fascinating, and motivates several disciplines. Although chemistry and toxicology began together, chemists have developed a uniquely molecular, historical and practical perspective on toxic plants. The Chemist's Perspective contributes both a supporting role, namely the practical synthesis of useful molecules, and an integrative role, one which connects phylogenetics to the biosynthesis of toxic molecules, and one which enables and bridges the different facets of systems toxicology.

Acknowledgments
This chapter is dedicated to the premier Costa Rican scientist Luis Diego Gómez, a good friend and my mentor in all things ethnobotanical. This project would not have been possible without the patience, support and encouragement of my wife Leslie. Special thanks go to Ms. Robin DiRocco for her excellent administrative support, and to the library staff at DePauw University, especially Ms. Mandy Henk. Their perseverance in locating yet another article for this project was invaluable. My son Keith A. Hanson made valuable suggestions on a draft.

References

1 Jacobi J (1979) *Paracelsus: Selected Writings*. Princeton University Press, Bollingen Series XXVIII, Princeton, NJ

2 Ball P (2006) *The Devil's Doctor: Paracelsus and the World of Renaissance Magic and Science*. Farrar, Straus and Giroux, New York, NY

3 Newman DJ, Cragg GM (2007) Natural products as sources of new drugs over the last 25 years. *J Nat Prod* 70: 461–477

4 Butler MS (2004) The role of natural product chemistry in drug discovery. *J Nat Prod* 67: 2141–2153

5 Harvey AL (2008) Natural products in drug discovery. *Drug Discov Today* 13: 894–901

6 Firn RD, Jones CG (2003) Natural products – A simple model to explain chemical diversity. *Nat Prod Rep* 20: 382–391

7 Gunatilaka AAL (2006) Natural products from plant-associated microorganisms: Distribution, structural diversity, bioactivity, and implications of their occurrence. *J Nat Prod* 69: 509–526

8 Guo B, Wang Y, Sun X, Tang K (2008) Bioactive natural products from endophytes: A review. *Appl Biochem Microbiol* 44: 136–142

9 Strobel G, Daisy B, Castillo U, Harper J (2004) Natural products from endophytic microorganisms. *J Nat Prod* 67: 257–268

10 Zhang HW, Song YC, Tan RX (2006) Biology and chemistry of endophytes. *Nat Prod Rep* 23: 753–771

11 Firáková S, Sturdíková M, Múcková M (2007) Bioactive secondary metabolites produced by microorganisms associated with plants. *Biologia* 62: 251–257

12 Shrestha K, Strobel GA, Shrivastava SP, Gewali MB (2001) Evidence for paclitaxel from three new endophytic fungi of Himalayan Yew of Nepal. *Planta Med* 67: 374–376

13 Stierle A, Strobel G, Stierle D, Grothaus P, Bignami G (1995) The search for a taxol-producing microorganism among the endophytic fungi of the Pacific yew, *Taxus-brevifolia*. *J Nat Prod* 58: 1315–1324

14 Rehman S, Shawl AS, Kour A, Andrabi R, Sudan P, Sultan P, Verma V, Qazi GN (2008) An endophytic *Neurospora* sp. from *Nothapodytes foetida* producing camptothecin. *Appl Biochem Microbiol* 44: 203–209

15 Kusari S, Zuhlke S, Spiteller M (2009) An endophytic fungus from *Camptotheca acuminata* that produces camptothecin and analogues. *J Nat Prod* 72: 2–7

16 Eyberger AL, Dondapati R, Porter JR (2006) Endophyte fungal isolates from *Podophyllum peltatum* produce podophyllotoxin. *J Nat Prod* 69: 1121–1124

17 Kusari S, Lamshoft M, Zühlke S, Spiteller M (2008) An endophytic fungus from *Hypericum perforatum* that produces hypericin. *J Nat Prod* 71: 159–162

18 Frohne D, Pfänder HJ (2005) *Poisonous Plants. A Handbook for Doctors, Pharmacists, Toxico-*

logists, Biologists and Veterinarians, 2nd edn. Timber Press, Portland, OR

19 Nelson LS, Shih RD, Balick MJ (2007) *Handbook of Poisonous and Injurious Plants*, 2nd edn. The New York Botanical Garden, Springer, New York, NY

20 Tracy TS, Kingston RL (2007) *Herbal Products: Toxicology and Clinical Pharmacology*, 2nd edn. Humana Press, Totowa, NJ

21 Simpson MG (2006) *Plant Systematics*. Elsevier Academic Press, Burlington, MA

22 Johns T (1990) *With Bitter Herbs They Shall Eat It: Chemical Ecology and the Origins of Human Diet and Medicine*. University of Arizona Press, Tucson, AZ

23 Sertürner FWA (1805) Darstellung der reinen Mohnsäure (Opiumsäure); nebst einer chemischen Unterschuchung des Opiums, mit vorzüglicher Hinsicht auf einen darin neu entdeckten Stoff. *J Pharm Ärzte Apoth Chem* 14: 47–93

24 Hesse M (2002) *Alkaloids: Nature's Curse or Blessing?* Wiley-VCH, Weinheim, Germany

25 De Candolle AP (1804) *Essai sur les propriétés des plantes, comparées avec leur formes extérieures et leur classification naturelle*. Méquignon, Paris

26 Abbott HC (1896) Certain chemical constituents of plants considered in relation to their morphology and evolution. *Botanical Gazette* 11: 270–272

27 Greshoff M (1909) *Phytochemical Investigations at Kew*. Bulletin of Miscellaneous Information, No. 10, 397–418

28 Reynolds T (2007) The evolution of chemosystematics. *Phytochemistry* 68: 2887–2895

29 Harborne JB, Turner BL (1984) *Plant Chemosystematics*. Academic Press, Orlando, FL

30 Dahlgren RMT (1980) A revised system of classification of the angiosperms. *Bot J Linn Soc* 80: 91–124

31 Bremer B, Bremer K, Chase MW, Reveal JL, Soltis DE, Soltis PS, Stevens PF, Anderberg AA, Fay MF, Goldblatt P, Judd WS, Kallersjo M (2003) An update of the Angiosperm phylogeny group classification for the orders and families of flowering plants: APG II. *Bot J Linn Soc* 141: 399–436

32 Stevens PF (2001) Angiosperm Phylogeny Website, Version 9, June 2008 (http://www.mobot.org/MOBOT/research/APWeb/)

33 Zomlefer W (1994) *Guide to Flowering Plant Families*. University of North Carolina Press, NC

34 Herbert RB (1981) *The Biosynthesis of Secondary Metabolites*. Chapman and Hall, London

35 Wink M (2003) Evolution of secondary metabolites from an ecological and molecular phylogenetic perspective. *Phytochemistry* 64: 3–19

36 Wink M, Mohamed GIA (2003) Evolution of chemical defense traits in the Leguminosae: Mapping of distribution patterns of secondary metabolites on a molecular phylogeny inferred from nucleotide sequences of the *rbc*L gene. *Biochem System Ecol* 31: 897–917

37 Liscombe DK, MacLeod BP, Loukanina N, Nandi OI, Facchini PJ (2005) Evidence for the monophyletic evolution of benzylisoquinoline alkaloid biosynthesis in angiosperms. *Phytochemistry* 66: 2500–2520

38 Fu PP, Xia QS, Chou MW, Lin G (2007) Detection, hepatotoxicity, and tumorigenicity of pyrrolizidine alkaloids in Chinese herbal plants and herbal dietary supplements. *J Food Drug Anal* 15: 400–415

39 Mei N, Guo L, Fu PP, Heflich RH, Chen T (2005) Mutagenicity of comfrey (*Symphytum officinale*) in rat liver. *Br J Cancer* 92: 873–875

40 Edgar JA, Roeder EL, Molyneux RJ (2002) Honey from plants containing pyrrolizidine alkaloids: A potential threat to health. *J Agric Food Chem* 50: 2719–2730

41 Steenkamp V, Stewart MJ, Zuckerman M (2000) Clinical and analytical aspects of pyrrolizidine poisoning caused by South African traditional medicines. *Ther Drug Monit* 22: 302–306

42 Fu PP, Xia QS, Lin G, Chou MW (2004) Pyrrolizidine alkaloids – Genotoxicity, metabolism enzymes, metabolic activation, and mechanisms. *Drug Metab Rev* 36: 1–55

43 Stegelmeier BL, Edgar JA, Colegate SM, Gardner DR, Schoch TK, Coulombe RA, Molyneux RJ (1999) Pyrrolizidine alkaloid plants, metabolism and toxicity. *J Nat Toxins* 8: 95–116

44 Reimann A, Nurhayati N, Backenköhler A, Ober D (2004) Repeated evolution of the pyrrolizidine alkaloid-mediated defense system in separate angiosperm lineages. *Plant Cell* 16: 2772–2784

45 Ober D, Harms R, Witte L, Hartmann T (2003) Molecular evolution by change of function – Alkaloid-specific homospermidine synthase retained all properties of deoxyhypusine synthase except binding the eIF5A precursor protein. *J Biol Chem* 278: 12805–12812

46 Ober D (2005) Seeing double: Gene duplication and diversification in plant secondary metabolism. *Trends Plant Sci* 10: 444–449

47 Stafford HA (1994) Anthocyanins and betalains – Evolution of the mutually exclusive pathways. *Plant Science* 101: 91–98

48 Clement JS, Mabry TJ, Wyler H, Drieding AS (1993) Chemical review and evolutionary significance of the betalains. In: TJ Mabry, HD Behnke (eds): *Caryophyllales: Evolution and Systematics*, Springer-Verlag, Berlin, 247–261

49 Garfield S (2001) *Mauve: How One Man Invented a Color that Changed the World*. W.W. Norton & Company, New York, NY

50 Cornforth JW (1994) The trouble with synthesis. *Aldrichim Acta* 27: 71–77

51 Nicolaou KC (2009) Inspirations, discoveries, and future perspectives in total synthesis. *J Org Chem* 74: 951–972

52 Nicolaou KC (2005) Joys of molecules. 1. Campaigns in total synthesis. *J Org Chem* 70: 7007–7027

53 Nicolaou KC (2005) Joys of molecules. 2. Endeavors in chemical biology and medicinal chemistry. *J Med Chem* 48: 5613–5638

54 Nicolaou KC, Snyder SA (2005) Chasing molecules that were never there: Misassigned natural products and the role of chemical synthesis in modern structure elucidation. *Angew Chem Int Ed* 44: 1012–1044

55 Woodward RB, Doering WE (1944) The total synthesis of quinine. *J Am Chem Soc* 66: 849

56 Stork G, Niu D, Fujimoto A, Koft ER, Balkovec JM, Tata JR, Dake GR (2001) The first stereoselective total synthesis of quinine. *J Am Chem Soc* 123: 3239–3242

57 Seeman JI (2007) The Woodward-Doering/Rabe-Kindler total synthesis of quinine: Setting the record straight. *Angew Chem Int Ed* 46: 1378–1413

58 Kaufman TS, Rúveda EA (2005) The quest for quinine: Those who won the battles and those who won the war. *Angew Chem Int Ed* 44: 854–885

59 Julian PL, Pikl J (1935) Studies in the indole series. IV. The synthesis of D,L-eserethole. *J Am Chem Soc* 57: 563–566

60 Ault A (2008) Percy Julian, Robert Robinson, and the identify of eserethole. *J Chem Educ* 85: 1524–1530

61 Dobson CM (2004) Chemical space and biology. *Nature* 432: 824–828

62 Lipkus AH, Yuan Q, Lucas KA, Funk SA, Bartelt WF, Schenck RJ, Trippe AJ (2008) Structural diversity of organic chemistry. A scaffold analysis of the CAS Registry. *J Org Chem* 73: 4443–4451

63 Bohacek RS, McMartin C, Guida WC (1996) The art and practice of structure-based drug design: A molecular modeling perspective. *Med Res Rev* 16: 3–50

64 Feher M, Schmidt JM (2003) Property distributions: Differences between drugs, natural products, and molecules from combinatorial chemistry. *J Chem Inform Comp Sci* 43: 218–227

65 Koch MA, Schuffenhauer A, Scheck M, Wetzel S, Casaulta M, Odermatt A, Ertl P, Waldmann H (2005) Charting biologically relevant chemical space: A structural classification of natural products (SCONP). *Proc Natl Acad Sci USA* 102: 17272–17277

66 Wetzel S, Schuffenhauer A, Roggo S, Ertl P, Waldmann H (2007) Cheminformatic analysis of natural products and their chemical space. *Chimia* 61: 355–360

67 Larsson J, Gottfries J, Muresan S, Backlund A (2007) ChemGPS-NP: Tuned for navigation in biologically relevant chemical space. *J Nat Prod* 70: 789–794

68 Clardy J, Walsh C (2004) Lessons from natural molecules. *Nature* 432: 829–837

69 Stockwell BR (2004) Exploring biology with small organic molecules. *Nature* 432: 846–854

70 Lipinski C, Hopkins A (2004) Navigating chemical space for biology and medicine. *Nature* 432: 855–861

71 Newman DJ (2008) Natural products as leads to potential drugs: An old process or the new hope for drug discovery? *J Med Chem* 51: 2589–2599

72 Kumar K, Waldmann H (2009) Synthesis of natural product inspired compound collections. *Angew Chem Int Ed* 48: 3224–3242

73 Marco-Contelles J, Carreiras MD, Rodríguez C, Villarroya M, García AG (2006) Synthesis and pharmacology of galantamine. *Chem Rev* 106: 116–133

74 Heinrich M, Teoh HL (2004) Galanthamine from snowdrop – The development of a modern drug against Alzheimer's disease from local Caucasian knowledge. *J Ethnopharmacol* 92: 147–162

75 Pelish HE, Westwood NJ, Feng Y, Kirchhausen T, Shair MD (2001) Use of biomimetic diversity-oriented synthesis to discover galanthamine-like molecules with biological properties beyond those of the natural product. *J Am Chem Soc* 123: 6740–6741

76 Breinbauer R, Manger M, Scheck M, Waldmann H (2002) Natural product guided compound library development. *Curr Med Chem* 9: 2129–2145

77 Abreu PM, Branco PS (2003) Natural product-like combinatorial libraries. *J Braz Chem Soc* 14: 675–712

78 Kren V, Martínková L (2001) Glycosides in medicine: The role of glycosidic residue in biological activity. *Curr Med Chem* 8: 1303–1328

79 Withering W (1785) *An account of the foxglove and some of its medical uses; with practical remarks on the dropsy, and some other diseases.* Swinney, Birmingham, UK

80 Langenhan JM, Peters NR, Guzei IA, Hoffmann M, Thorson JS (2005) Enhancing the anticancer properties of cardiac glycosides by neoglycorandomization. *Proc Natl Acad Sci USA* 102: 12305–12310

81 Ahmed A, Peters NR, Fitzgerald MK, Watson JA, Hoffmann FM, Thorson JS (2006) Colchicine glycorandomization influences cytotoxicity and mechanism of action. *J Am Chem Soc* 128: 14224–14225

82 Langenhan JM, Griffith BR, Thorson JS (2005) Neoglycorandomization and chemoenzymatic glycorandomization: Two complementary tools for natural product diversification. *J Nat Prod* 68: 1696–1711

83 Thorson JS, Hosted TJ, Jiang J, Biggins JB, Ahlert J (2001) Nature's carbohydrate chemists: The enzymatic glycosylation of bioactive bacterial metabolites. *Curr Org Chem* 5: 139–167

84 Williams GJ, Gantt RW, Thorson JS (2008) The impact of enzyme engineering upon natural product glycodiversification. *Curr Opin Chem Biol* 12: 556–564

85 Williams GJ, Zhang C, Thorson JS (2007) Expanding the promiscuity of a natural-product glycosyltransferase by directed evolution. *Nat Chem Biol* 3: 657–662

86 Oksman-Caldentey KM, Inzé D (2004) Plant cell factories in the post-genomic era: New ways to produce designer secondary metabolites. *Trends Plant Sci* 9: 433–440

87 Oberlies NH, Kroll DJ (2004) Camptothecin and taxol: Historic achievements in natural products research. *J Nat Prod* 67: 129–135

88 Jordan MA, Wilson L (2004) Microtubules as a target for anticancer drugs. *Nat Rev Cancer* 4: 253–265

89 Kingston DG, Newman DJ (2007) Taxoids: Cancer-fighting compounds from nature. *Curr Opin Drug Discov Devel* 10: 130–144

90 Frense D (2007) Taxanes: Perspectives for biotechnological production. *Appl Microbiol Biotechnol* 73: 1233–1240

91 Expósito O, Bonfill M, Moyano E, Onrubia M, Mirjalili MH, Cusidó RM, Palazón J (2009) Biotechnological production of taxol and related taxoids: Current state and prospects. *Anticancer Agents Med Chem* 9: 109–121

92 Covello PS (2008) Making artemisinin. *Phytochemistry* 69: 2881–2885

93 Chemler JA, Koffas MAG (2008) Metabolic engineering for plant natural product biosynthesis in microbes. *Curr Opin Biotechol* 19: 597–605

94 Julsing MK, Koulman A, Woerdenbag HJ, Quax WJ, Kayser O (2006) Combinatorial biosynthesis of medicinal plant secondary metabolites. *Biomol Eng* 23: 265–279

95 Minami H, Kim JS, Ikezawa N, Takemura T, Katayama T, Kumagai H, Sato F (2008) Microbial production of plant benzylisoquinoline alkaloids. *Proc Natl Acad Sci USA* 105: 7393–7398

96 Hawkins KM, Smolke CD (2008) Production of benzylisoquinoline alkaloids in *Saccharomyces cerevisiae*. *Nat Chem Biol* 4: 564–573

97 Van der Heijden R, Jacobs DI, Snoeijer W, Hallard D, Verpoorte R (2004) The *Catharanthus* alkaloids: Pharmacognosy and biotechnology. *Curr Med Chem* 11: 607–628

98 McCoy E, O'Connor SE (2006) Directed biosynthesis of alkaloid analogs in the medicinal plant *Catharanthus roseus*. *J Am Chem Soc* 128: 14276–14277

99 Bernhardt P, McCoy E, O'Connor SE (2007) Rapid identification of enzyme variants for reengineered alkaloid biosynthesis in periwinkle. *Chem Biol* 14: 888–897

100 Staunton J, Weissman KJ (2001) Polyketide biosynthesis: A millennium review. *Nat Prod Rep* 18: 380–416

101 Flores-Sanchez IJ, Verpoorte R (2009) Plant polyketide synthases: A fascinating group of enzymes. *Plant Physiol Biochem* 47: 167–174

102 Shi S, Morita H, Wanibuchi K, Mizuuchi Y, Noguchi H, Abe I (2008) Enzymatic synthesis of plant polyketides. *Curr Org Synth* 5: 250–266

103 Crick F (1970) Central dogma of molecular biology. *Nature* 227: 561–563

104 Ideker T, Thorsson V, Ranish JA, Christmas R, Buhler J, Eng JK, Bumgarner R, Goodlett DR, Aebersold R, Hood L (2001) Integrated genomic and proteomic analyses of a systematically perturbed metabolic network. *Science* 292: 929–934

105 Moxley JF, Jewett MC, Antoniewicz MR, Villas-Boas SG, Alper H, Wheeler RT, Tong L, Hinnebusch AG, Ideker T, Nielsen J, Stephanopoulos G (2009) Linking high-resolution metabolic flux phenotypes and trancriptional regulation in yeast modulated by the global regulator Gcn4p. *Proc Natl Acad Sci USA* 106: 6477–6482

106 Nicholson JK, Connelly J, Lindon JC, Holmes E (2002) Metabonomics: A platform for studying drug toxicity and gene function. *Nat Rev Drug Discov* 1: 153–161

107 Robertson DG, Reily MD, Baker JD (2007) Metabonomics in pharmaceutical discovery and development. *J Proteome Res* 6: 526–539

108 Ellis DI, Dunn WB, Griffin JL, Allwood JW, Goodacre R (2007) Metabolic fingerprinting as a diagnostic tool. *Pharmacogenomics* 8: 1243–1266

109 Craig A, Sidaway J, Holmes E, Orton T, Jackson D, Rowlinson R, Nickson J, Tonge R, Wilson I, Nicholson J (2006) Systems toxicology: Integrated genomic, proteomic and metabonomic analysis of methapyrilene induced hepatotoxicity in the rat. *J Proteome Res* 5: 1586–1601

110 Waters MD, Fostel JM (2004) Toxicogenomics and systems toxicology: Aims and prospects. *Nat Rev Genet* 5: 936–948

111 Waters MD, Olden K, Tennant RW (2003) Toxicogenomic approach for assessing toxicant-related disease. *Mutat Res* 544: 415–424

112 Xirasagar S, Gustafson SF, Huang CC, Pan Q, Fostel J, Boyer P, Merrick BA, Tomer KB, Chan DD, Yost KJ 3rd, Choi D, Xiao N, Stasiewicz S, Bushel P, Waters MD (2006) Chemical effects in biological systems (CEBS) object model for toxicology data, SysTox-OM: Design and application. *Bioinformatics* 22: 874–882

113 Patwardhan B, Warude D, Pushpangadan P, Bhatt N (2005) Ayurveda and traditional Chinese medicine: A comparative overview. *Evid Based Complement Alternat Med* 2: 465–473

114 Corson TW, Crews CM (2007) Molecular understanding and modern application of traditional medicines: Triumphs and trials. *Cell* 130: 769–774

115 Wagner H, Ulrich-Merzenich G (2009) Synergy research: Approaching a new generation of phytopharmaceuticals. *Phytomedicine* 16: 97–110

116 Williamson EM (2001) Synergy and other interactions in phytomedicines. *Phytomedicine* 8: 401–409

117 Ulrich-Merzenich G, Panek D, Zeitler H, Wagner H, Vetter H (2009) New perspectives for synergy research with the "omic" -technologies. *Phytomedicine* 16: 495–508

118 Verpoorte R, Choi YH, Kim HK (2005) Ethnopharmacology and systems biology: A perfect holistic match. *J Ethnopharmacol* 100: 53–56

119 Schmidt BM, Ribnicky DM, Lipsky PE, Raskin I (2007) Revisiting the ancient concept of botanical therapeutics. *Nat Chem Biol* 3: 360–366

120 Borisy AA, Elliott PJ, Hurst NW, Lee MS, Lehár J, Price ER, Serbedzija G, Zimmermann GR, Foley MA, Stockwell BR, Keith CT (2003) Systematic discovery of multicomponent therapeutics. *Proc Natl Acad Sci USA* 100: 7977–7982

121 Shyur LF, Yang NS (2008) Metabolomics for phytomedicine research and drug development. *Curr Opin Chem Biol* 12: 66–71

122 Heinrich M (2008) Ethnopharmacy and natural product research – Multidisciplinary opportunities for research in the metabolomic age. *Phytochem Lett* 1: 1–5

123 Urich-Merzenich G, Zeitler H, Jobst D, Panek D, Vetter H, Wagner H (2007) Application of the "-omic-" technologies in phytomedicine. *Phytomedicine* 14: 70–82

124 Wang M, Lamers R, Korthout H, van Nesselrooij JHJ, Witkamp RF, van der Heijden R, Voshol PJ, Havekes LM, Verpoorte R, van der Greef J (2005) Metabolomics in the context of systems biology: Bridging traditional Chinese medicine and molecular pharmacology. *Phytother Res* 19: 173–182

125 Kang YJ (2008) Herbogenomics: From traditional Chinese medicine to novel therapeutics. *Exp Biol Med* 233: 1059–1065

126 Watanabe CMH, Wolffram S, Ader P, Rimbach G, Packer L, Maguire JJ, Schultz PG, Gohil K (2001) The *in vivo* neuromodulatory effects of the herbal medicine *Ginkgo biloba*. *Proc Natl Acad Sci USA* 98: 6577–6580

127 May BH, Yang AWH, Zhang AL, Owens MD, Bennett L, Head R, Cobiac L, Li CG, Hugel H, Story DF, Xue CCL (2009) Chinese herbal medicine for mild cognitive impairment and age asso-

ciated memory impairment: A review of randomised controlled trials. *Biogerontology* 10: 109–123

128 Christen Y, Maixent JM (2002) What is *Ginkgo biloba* extract EGb 761? An overview – From molecular biology to clinical medicine. *Cell Mol Biol* 48: 601–611

129 Mahadevan S, Park Y (2008) Multifaceted therapeutic benefits of *Ginkgo biloba* L.: Chemistry, efficacy, safety, and uses. *J Food Sci* 73: R14–R19

130 Smith JV, Luo Y (2004) Studies on molecular mechanisms of *Ginkgo biloba* extract. *Appl Microbiol Biotechnol* 64: 465–472

131 Wang Z, Du QY, Wang FS, Liu ZR, Li BG, Wang AM, Wang YY (2004) Microarray analysis of gene expression on herbal glycoside recipes improving deficient ability of spatial learning memory in ischemic mice. *J Neurochem* 88: 1406–1415

132 Ise R, Han DH, Takahashi Y, Terasaka S, Inoue A, Tanji M, Kiyama R (2005) Expression profiling of the estrogen responsive genes in response to phytoestrogens using a customized DNA microarray. *FEBS Lett* 579: 1732–1740

133 Dong SJ, Inoue A, Zhu Y, Tanji M, Kiyama R (2007) Activation of rapid signaling pathways and the subsequent transcriptional regulation for the proliferation of breast cancer MCF-7 cells by the treatment with an extract of *Glycyrrhiza glabra* root. *Food Chem Toxicol* 45: 2470–2478

134 Adachi T, Ono Y, Koh KB, Takashima K, Tainaka H, Matsuno Y, Nakagawa S, Todaka E, Sakurai K, Fukata H, Iguchi T, Komiyama M, Mori C (2004) Long-term alteration of gene expression without morphological change in testis after neonatal exposure to genistein in mice: Toxicogenomic analysis using cDNA microarray. *Food Chem Toxicol* 42: 445–452

135 Naciff JM, Hess KA, Overmann GJ, Torontali SM, Carr GJ, Tiesman JP, Foertsch LM, Richardson BD, Martinez JE, Daston GP (2005) Gene expression changes induced in the testis by transplacental exposure to high and low doses of 17α-ethynyl estradiol, genistein, or bisphenol A. *Toxicol Sci* 86: 396–416

136 Chen CS, Chen NJ, Lin LW, Hsieh CC, Chen GW, Hsieh MT (2006) Effects of Scutellariae Radix on gene expression in HEK 293 cells using cDNA microarray. *J Ethnopharmacol* 105: 346–351

137 Hsieh MT, Hsieh CL, Lin LW, Wu CR, Huang GS (2003) Differential gene expression of scopolamine-treated rat hippocampus-application of cDNA microarray technology. *Life Sci* 73: 1007–1016

138 Cho WCS (2007) Application of proteomics in Chinese medicine research. *Am J Chinese Med* 35: 911–922

139 Ong ES, Len SM, Lee AC, Chui P, Chooi KF (2004) Proteomic analysis of mouse liver for the evaluation of effects of Scutellariae radix by liquid chromatography with tandem mass spectrometry. *Rapid Commun Mass Spectrom* 18: 2522–2530

140 Goh D, Lee YH, Ong ES (2005) Inhibitory effects of a chemically standardized extract from *Scutellaria barbata* in human colon cancer cell lines, LoVo. *J Agric Food Chem* 53: 8197–8204

141 Lu GD, Shen HM, Ong CN, Chung MC (2007) Anticancer effects of aloe-emodin on HepG2 cells: Cellular and proteomic studies. *Proteomics Clin Appl* 1: 410–419

142 Wang Y, Liu L, Hu CC, Cheng YY (2007) Effects of Salviae Mitiorrhizae and Cortex Moutan extract on the rat heart after myocardial infarction: A proteomic study. *Biochem Pharmacol* 74: 415–424

143 Pakalapati G, Li L, Gretz N, Koch E, Wink M (2009) Influence of red clover (*Trifolium pratense*) isoflavones on gene and protein expression profiles in liver of ovariectomized rats. *Phytomedicine* 16: 845–855

144 Lee SY, Kim GT, Roh SH, Song JS, Kim HJ, Hong SS, Kwon SW, Park JH (2009) Proteome changes related to the anti-cancer activity of HT29 cells by the treatment of ginsenoside R$_d$. *Pharmazie* 64: 242–247

145 Jacobs DI, Gaspari M, van der Greef J, van der Heijden R, Verpoorte R (2005) Proteome analysis of the medicinal plant *Catharanthus roseus*. *Planta* 221: 690–704

146 Chen MJ, Su MM, Zhao LP, Jiang J, Liu P, Cheng JY, Lai YJ, Liu YM, Jia W (2006) Metabonomic study of aristolochic acid-induced nephrotoxicity in rats. *J Proteome Res* 5: 995–1002

147 Chen MJ, Ni Y, Duan HQ, Qiu YP, Guo CY, Jiao Y, Shi HJ, Su MM, Jia W (2008) Mass spectrometry-based metabolic profiling of rat urine associated with general toxicity induced by the multiglycoside of *Tripterygium wilfordii* Hook. *Chem Res Toxicol* 21: 288–294

148 Wang YL, Tang HR, Nicholson JK, Hylands PJ, Sampson J, Holmes E (2005) A metabonomic

strategy for the detection of the metabolic effects of chamomile (*Matricaria recutita* L.) ingestion. *J Agric Food Chem* 53: 191–196

149 Solanky KS, Bailey NJ, Beckwith-Hall BM, Bingham S, Davis A, Holmes E, Nicholson JK, Cassidy A (2005) Biofluid ¹H NMR-based metabonomic techniques in nutrition research – Metabolic effects of dietary isoflavones in humans. *J Nutr Biochem* 16: 236–244

150 Solanky KS, Bailey NJ, Beckwith-Hall BM, Davis A, Bingham S, Holmes E, Nicholson JK, Cassidy A (2003) Application of biofluid ¹H nuclear magnetic resonance-based metabonomic techniques for the analysis of the biochemical effects of dietary isoflavones on human plasma profile. *Anal Biochem* 323: 197–204

151 Law WS, Huang PY, Ong ES, Ong CN, Li SFY, Pasikanti KK, Chan ECY (2008) Metabonomics investigation of human urine after ingestion of green tea with gas chromatography/mass spectrometry, liquid chromatography/mass spectrometry and ¹H NMR spectroscopy. *Rapid Commun Mass Spectrom* 22: 2436–2446

152 Gulland JM, Robinson R (1925) The constitution of codeine and thebaine. *Mem Proc Manch Lit Philos Soc* 69: 79–86

153 Gates M, Tschudi G (1952) The synthesis of morphine. *J Am Chem Soc* 78: 1380–1393

154 Pelletier PJ, Caventou JB (1818) Note sur un novel Alcali. *Annales de Chemie et de Physique* 104–105: 323–324

155 Openshaw HT, Robinson R (1946) Constitution of strychnine and the biogenetic relationship of strychnine and quinine. *Nature* 157: 438

156 Woodward RB, Cava MP, Ollis WD, Hunger A, Daeniker HU, Schenker K (1954) The total synthesis of strychnine. *J Am Chem Soc* 76: 4749–4751

157 Pelletier PJ, Caventou JB (1820) Rescherches chimiques sur les Quinquinas. *Annales de Chemie et de Physique* 15: 289–318

158 Rabe P, Kindler K (1918) Ueber die partielle Synthese des Chinins. *Ber Dtsch Chem Ges* 51: 466–467

159 Woodward RB, Doering, WE (1944) The total synthesis of quinine. *J Am Chem Soc* 66: 849

160 Pelletier PJ, Caventou JB (1820) Examen chimique de plusieurs végétaux de la famille des colchicées, et du principe actif qu'ils renferment (Cévadille (V*eratrum sabadilla*); hellébore blanc (*Veratrum album*); colchique commun (*Colchicum autumnale*)]. *Annales de Chemie et de Physique* 14: 69–83

161 King MV, De Vries JL, Pepinsky R (1952) An x-ray diffraction determination of the chemical structure of colchicine. *Acta Crystallogr B* 5: 437

162 Schreiber J, Leimgruber W, Pesaro M, Schudel P, Threlfall T, Eschenmoser A (1961) Synthese des colchicins. (Synthesis of colchicines.) *Helv Chim Acta* 65: 540–597

163 Giseke AL (1826) Ueber das wirksame Princip des Schierlings *Conium maculatum*. *Arch Apotheker-Vereins Nördl Teutschl* 20: 97–111

164 Hoffmann AW (1881) Einwirkung der Wärme auf die Ammoniumbasen. *Ber Dtsch Chem Ges* 14: 705–713

165 Ladenburg A (1889) Nachtrag zu der Mittheilung über die Synthese der activen Coniine. *Ber Dtsch Chem Ges* 22: 1403–1404

166 Posselt W, Reimann L (1828) Chemische Unterschungen des Tabaks und Darstellung des eigenthümlichen wirksamen Princips dieser Pflanze. *Geigers Magazin der Pharmacie* 24: 138–161

167 Pinner A (1893) Ueber Nicotin. Die Konstitution des Alkaloids. *Ber Dtsch Chem Ges* 26: 292–305

168 Pictet A, Rotschy A (1904) Synthese des Nicotins. *Ber Dtsch Chem Ges* 37: 1225–1235

169 Leroux H (1830) Analyse de l'écorce de saule et découverte de la salicine. *Journal de Chemie Médicale, de Pharmacie et de Toxicologie* 6: 340–342

170 Piria MR (1838) Sur la composition de la Salicine et sur quelques-unes de ses réactions. *Comptes Rendes* 6: 338

171 Kolbe H (1860) Ueber die Synthese der Salicylsäure. (Regarding the synthesis of salicylic acid.) *Liebigs Ann* 113: 125–127

172 Michael A (1879) On the synthesis of helicin and phenolglucoside. *Am Chem J* 1: 305–312

173 Geiger PL, Hesse H (1833) Darstellung des Atropins. *Liebigs Ann* 5: 43–81

174 Ladenburg A (1883) Die Constitution des Atropins. *Liebigs Ann* 217: 74–149

175 Willstätter R (1901) Conversion of tropidine into tropine. *Ber Dtsch Chem Ges* 34: 3163–3165

176 Niemann A (1860) Ueber eine neue organische Base in den Cocablättern. *Arch Pharm* 153: 129–155

177 Willstätter R, Müller W (1898) Ueber die Constitution des Ecgonins. *Ber Dtsch Chem Ges* 31: 2655–2669

178 Jobst J, Hesse O (1864) Ueber die Bohne von Calabar. (Regarding the bean from calabar.) *Liebigs Ann.* 129S: 115–121

179 Podwyssotski V (1880) Pharmakologische Studien über *Podophyllum peltatum. Arch Exp Pathol Pharmakol* 13: 29–52

180 Hartwell JL, Schrecker AW (1951) Components of Podophyllin. V. The Constitution of Podophyllotoxin. *J Am Chem Soc* 73: 2909–2916

181 Gensler WJ, Gatsonis CD (1962) Synthesis of Podophyllotoxin. *J Am Chem Soc* 84: 1748–1749

182 Komppa G (1903) Die vollständige Synthese de Camphersäure und Dehydrocamphersäure. *Ber Dtsch Chem Ges* 36: 4332–4335

Molecular, Clinical and Environmental Toxicology. Volume 2: Clinical Toxicology
Edited by A. Luch

High-molecular weight protein toxins of marine invertebrates and their elaborate modes of action

Daniel Butzke and Andreas Luch

Center for Alternatives to Animal Experiments (ZEBET), Federal Institute for Risk Assessment, Berlin, Germany

Abstract. High-molecular weight protein toxins significantly contribute to envenomations by certain marine invertebrates, e.g., jellyfish and fire corals. Toxic proteins frequently evolved from enzymes meant to be employed primarily for digestive purposes. The cellular interme- diates produced by such enzymatic activity, e.g., reactive oxygen species or lysophospho- lipids, rapidly and effectively mediate cell death by disrupting cellular integrity. Membrane integrity may also be disrupted by pore-forming toxins that do not exert inherent enzymatic activity. When targeted to specific pharmacologically relevant sites in tissues or cells of the natural enemy or prey, toxic enzymes or pore-forming toxins even may provoke fast and severe systemic reactions. Since toxin-encoding genes constitute "hot spots" of molecular evolution, continuous variation and acquirement of new pharmacological properties are guar- anteed. This also makes individual properties and specificities of complex proteinaceous ven- oms highly diverse and inconstant. In the present chapter we portray high-molecular weight constituents of venoms present in box jellyfish, sea anemones, sea hares, fire corals and the crown-of-thorns starfish. The focus lies on the latest achievements in the attempt to elucidate their molecular modes of action.

Introduction

Besides small bioactive molecules (peptides, polyketides, terpenes, etc.) high- molecular weight protein toxins (HMWPT) represent the multifunctional molecular "pocket knives" in Nature's "toxic toolbox". They not only carry a certain inherent "toxic principle" but also confer this principle to very specific and susceptible structures (acceptor sites) present in target tissues of suscepti- ble organisms. Upon arrival at tissue target sites, HMWPT can easily convert from a water-soluble to a membrane-bound or membrane-penetrating form by subtle modifications of their secondary, tertiary or quaternary structures. As with real pocket knives, momentarily advantageous functions are individually selectable from a wider repertoire that is on hold in the "standby" modus.

While structural variation of small non-proteinaceous biomolecules usually requires substantial genetic reorganization of the biosynthetic pathway(s) in charge (e.g., polyketide synthases, non-ribosomal synthetases), considerable variation of protein functionality may be achieved by simple introduction of only minor amino acid sequence alterations. Since protein toxins are employed in activities that ensure existence and well-being of the producing organism, i.e., feeding on prey and self-defense, structures are highly evolved and sophisticated in terms of efficiency and specificity toward the typical prey. However, the spectrum of accessible prey may vary depending on environmental conditions and thus the availability and storage of only single toxins with unique and narrow specificity clearly proves disadvantageous. Gene duplication has widely been a way out of this dilemma. Driven by unbalanced chromosomal recombination during meiosis, gene duplication facilitates the formation of gene families (paralogs) and thus represents a driving force for constant supply with weapons of new pharmacological properties by means of hidden evolution. Protein toxins therefore often emerge in a range of several isoforms, each of which confers remarkably unique pharmacological characteristics, that are all produced within the very same species. A well-known example of this "evolutionary strategy" is represented by phospholipase A_2 (PLA_2) enzymes present in snake venom and several marine invertebrates (cf. below). In addition to gene duplication, it has been shown that toxin-encoding genes often constitute "hot spots" of modification (i.e., evolution) within genomes. Sequence analysis of several snake venom PLA_2 genes revealed that "Darwinian-type accelerated substitutions" are widely manifest within protein-coding exons [1]. Similarly, during cloning of a highly cytotoxic L-amino acid oxidase (LAAO) from the "sea hare" *Aplysia punctata* a vast amount of slightly different DNA sequences presumably originating from copious paralogous genes emerged [2]. In direct comparison, however, the amino acid sequences varied only slightly among paralogs, arguing for an extremely narrow and well-concentrated selection pressure in this particular case.

The inherent biological potencies of HMWPT vary substantially, with botulinum neurotoxins (BoNT, ~150 kDa) produced from bacteria of the genus *Clostridium* at the very upper end, featuring a mouse intraperitoneal (i.p.) LD_{50} (lethal dosis 50%) of about 30 ng/kg [3]. On the other hand, according to present knowledge, the polyketide maitotoxin, which is produced by the dinoflagellate *Gambierdiscus* spp., represents the most potent biogenetically produced toxin among all compounds outside the protein or peptide domain. Its i.p. LD_{50} in mice has been determined at about the same range when compared to BoNT, i.e., 50 ng/kg [4]. The cytolytic protein toxins discussed in the remainder of this chapter exert mouse i.v. LD_{50} values in the range of micrograms per kilogram. This is well comparable to the toxicity level of snake venom components such as textilotoxin (1 μg/kg) and crotoxin (110 μg/kg) [5], or other important toxins like tetrodotoxin with 10 μg/kg [6].

In principle, the biological potencies of protein toxins correlate to their specific binding properties (specificity and affinity) at target cellular membranes [5], and – in the case of BoNT – to their ability to penetrate through the membrane and translocate into cell's interior [3]. Intrinsic enzymatic activities, such as phospholipid or peptide hydrolysis, often constitute the basic toxic mechanism exerted by protein toxins. Of course, these effects only contribute to acute local or systemic toxicities if toxins are capable of reaching the appropriate target tissues and structures in the body, e.g., the neuromuscular junctions. Moreover, the systemic impact of the toxin can be tremendous if susceptible target sites either encounter sustained levels of toxic mediators locally produced *via* enzymatic turnover of an abundant substrate (e.g., hydrogen peroxide from amino acids) or suffer from a sustained loss of essential physiological factors (e.g., SNAP25 through proteolytic cleavage by BoNT). Conversely, a rather local reaction at the application site may be inflicted when the proteinaceous toxin lacks systemically distributed targets. Here, local necrosis and inflammation would be the most obvious effects.

The marine biosphere harbors some of the most toxic small molecules (e.g., maitotoxin), and also gives rise to the most rapidly acting lethal factors (e.g., the lethal factor of box jellyfish). The pronounced efficiency of marine compounds is an essential prerequisite to simply overcome the diluting effects of the watery environment. On the other hand, rapid paralysis of potential prey prevents energy consuming pursuits in the aquatic space or damage to delicate structures of the predator (e.g., tentacles of jellyfish) caused by fiercely escaping attempts of the prey. By comparison, terrestrial venoms need to overcome the protecting integument of the target organism first. Thus, evolution of snakes, scorpions, insects and spiders produced elaborate means of penetration such as fangs, stings or claws. This terrestrial commonplace necessity applies only occasionally to the marine situation. For instance, the most sophisticated injection mechanism – the cnidarian nematocyst – has evolved in the aquatic environment. However, since many susceptible target structures of water organisms, such as gills or chemosensors, are in direct contact with the surroundings and thus easily accessible, marine venoms are often simply secreted. In some cases the toxic secretion can be spattered toward an attacker by means of a blowtube-like siphon. In other cases there is a simple release into the surrounding water. Even then, however, lethal concentrations may be reached. For instance, 0.5 µg of a 20 kDa sea anemone toxin per milliliter sea water is sufficient to kill non-symbiotic fish [7].

There are estimates that humans have actually only encountered a small fraction of relevant marine toxins. Many of these were discovered in the wake of extensive screening programs for new drugs leads from marine sources stimulated by successful identification of marine anticancer nucleosides in the 1950s [8]. On the other hand, divers, swimmers, fishermen and gourmets enjoying exotic and uncommon seafoods are likely of being particularly at risk of meeting with up-to-now unexpected further challenges from nature's "toxic toolbox".

The pore-forming cytolysins of box jellyfish and sea anemones

Toxins of jellyfish

Most likely due to their unrivalled ambivalent nature, jellyfish (medusae) have fascinated people for centuries [9]. These creatures feature an extremely delicate, fragile gelatinous body plan and their mode of locomotion by slow repulsion chiefly constrains them to passive drifting with ocean currents, or winds in the case of neustonic forms such as "bluebottles", also known as "Portu-guese Man-of-War" (*Physalia physalis*, Fig. 1). From a toxicologist's perspec-tive, some members of the phylum cnidaria, e.g., the cubozoan medusa *Chironex fleckeri* are considered among the most dangerous animals on earth [10]. Especially on hot days that are overcast but calm, these predatory inver-tebrates move into shallow subtropical waters along the Australian coastline to pursue small prawns and fish. Because of their translucent bodies the "quiet invasion of some popular swimming spots by *C. fleckeri* may go unnoticed" [10]. The medusae have a cubic or box-shaped bell that achieves dimensions of about 20 × 30 cm and leads to the name "box jellyfish". Embedded into this bell are four highly evolved sensory organs that contain numerous "eyes", vibration and motion sensors, and serve as a means of light-sensitive naviga-tion [11]. Adjacent to the bell are four "fleshy arms" (pedalia), attached with bundles of up to 15 translucent extensile tentacles that may stretch up to 3 m but can also be contracted to one quarter of their actual length. The tentacles form a deadly net covered with millions of "spring-loaded syringes" (nemato-cysts) which discharge a highly potent venom into the skin of any creature touching it by chance *via* a penetrating thread [10].

   When an unprotected swimmer blunders into this deadly net of a box jelly-fish he may be hit by some hundreds of thousands of micro-sized harpoon-like

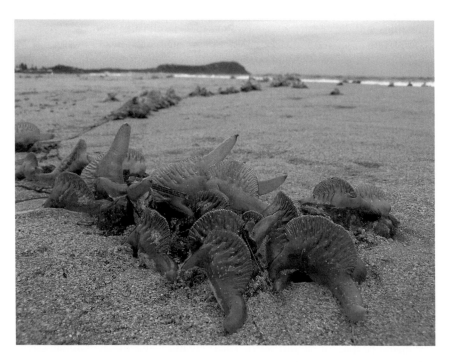

Figure 1. *Physalia physalis* ("bluebottle", also known as "Portuguese Man-of-War"); Systematics: cnidaria, hydrozoa, siphonophora (courtesy of Belinda G. Curley).

structures simultaneously, penetrating the epidermis by sharp tips. With an acceleration of about $40\,000 \times g$ (gravitation force) the venom filled threads are everted up to 1 mm into the dermis of the victim. Barbs at the basis of the threads are capable of attaching the nematocysts tightly onto the integument. In some jellyfish species, such as *C. fleckeri*, the nematocysts are anchored to the tentacles of the animal by flexible fibers that act like "grappling hooks" [10]. Through this mechanism the tentacles are pulled even closer to the victim resulting in much higher numbers of stinging cell batteries to be released into the dermis of the victim, maintaining a constantly growing envenomation [12].

It is vital for the delicately-build slow jellyfish to immobilize its fast-moving prey as rapid as possible to prevent serious structural damage to its soft tissues that may occur during fierce and uncoordinated attempts of the prey to escape from the scene. Therefore, the venoms of certain jellyfish species belong to the most rapid acting pharmacological mixtures of biogenic origin that have ever been characterized. When the toxic extract of about 50 000 nematocysts was injected into prawns immediate paralysis did occur [13]. This number of discharged nematocysts parallels a tentacle contact area of only about 33 mm^2 [14]. The toxic extract of approximately 35 000 nematocysts was sufficient to kill mice within 1–2 min when injected i.v. [13, 15, 16]. First rapid signs of systemic envenomation consist of respiration distress and convulsive muscular spasms. Since only local necrotic reaction was induced, much higher amounts of toxic extract (up to 45 times higher than the i.v. LD$_{50}$) were tolerated by mice when injected *via* the i.p., sub- (s.c.) or intracutaneous (i.c.) route [15].

In humans an excruciating pain is induced immediately after contact with the tentacles which are easily torn off the jellyfish and then adhere to the skin by the "grappling-hook" mechanism described above, thereby continuously discharging additional nematocysts. The pain constantly increases in mounting waves during the first 15 min and the victim may scream and become irrational. The concerned area of the skin exhibits clear signs of contact, i.e., multiple purple or brown colored lines featuring a pattern of transverse bars, reminiscent of a rope ladder. Edema, erythema and vesiculation soon follow und may persist for another 10 days. Areas of full-thickness necrosis leave behind permanent scars [17].

The severity of envenomation depends on both the size of the *C. fleckeri* specimen responsible and the area of contact. Amongst others, size dependency of the adverse reaction can be explained by variation of venom composition during ontogenesis. Distinct differences in venom constituents between mature and immature jellyfish have been reported in the related cubozoan species *Carukia barnesi*. Apparently, venom profiles strongly correlate to the types of prey, whether the jellyfish feeds on invertebrates or vertebrates [18]. In *C. fleckeri*, smaller specimens with a bell diameter of 5–7 cm rather induce painful local reactions. Larger jellyfish featuring a bell diameter wider than 15 cm may also induce extremely severe and systemic reactions [17], depending on the total length of tentacles attached to the skin of the victim. When 2–4 m of jellyfish tentacle tissue becomes attached to the body surface of a child, death is usually conceivable [19]. In adults, a total tentacle contact length of more than 6–7 m may be fatal [20]. In extreme cases, death is induced within minutes after contact with *C. fleckeri* due to combined cardiovascular and respiratory failure resulting in hypotension, apnea, and cardiac arrest. Yet the exact mechanisms underlying death in humans are not known with certainty [10].

As a result of more than four decades of biochemical, toxicological and pharmacological research, some HMWPT that may inflict the severe responses in jellyfish envenomation have been purified from several cubozoan species, although their modes of action remain ambiguous [21, 22]. Due to the following technical limitations, only few toxins could be isolated and characterized to date. Proteins considered to contribute to jellyfish' venom toxicity usually are unstable and exhibit a tendency to aggregate and to adhere to surfaces. Moreover, comparative studies have been hampered by huge variabilities in the sources of the crude venom (tentacle extracts, milked venom, nematocyst venom), in extraction methods, and analytical techniques applied. Please refer to the literature for an excellent illustration of the varying and occasionally contradictory results obtained in the attempts to characterize the venom of *C. fleckeri* by independent research groups [22].

However, a variety of bioactive proteins/protein aggregates have been isolated from *C. fleckeri* venom. The preparations differ in their molecular size and their patterns of biological activities exerted *in vivo* and *in vitro* (e.g., lethal/hemolytic; lethal/dermonecrotic, etc.). The results obtained *in vitro* may be imposed by the presence of different subunits in protein aggregates and/or the cellular models applied. The best characterized proteins among this variety belong to a group of labile basic proteins with apparent molecular sizes of 42–46 kDa. Proteins of this group exhibit potent hemolytic activity and represent the most abundant species present in nematocyst venom and tentacle extracts [22]. Several orthologous members of the protein family have been isolated and cloned from cubozoan species; i.e., CrTX-A and CrTX-B from *Carybdea rastoni*; CaTX-A, CaTX-B and CAH1 from *Carybdea alata*; CqTX-A from *Chiropsalmus quadrigatus* and CfTX-1 and CfTX-2 from *Chironex fleckeri*. The *in vivo* toxicity of the CrTXs from *C. rastoni* has been determined in mice [23]. The minimum i.v. lethal dose of purified CrTX-A in mice was less than 20 µg/kg. An i.p. injection of 100 µg/kg killed mice within 8 min; 0.1 µg CrTX-A i.p. caused skin inflammation in mice comparable to the reaction observed in humans stung by *C. rastoni*. Induction of hemolysis *in vitro* was demonstrated for all family members [23–27].

The cloned cDNAs of the toxins display no significant amino acid sequence homology to any other known and characterized protein family and thus represent a novel group of bioactive proteins [22, 25, 27]. Moreover, similar proteins are not encoded in the genomes of related cnidarian species (sea anemones/class anthozoa or sea firs/class hydrozoa), nor have they been isolated from other jellyfish (class scyphozoa). The lack of comparable and homologous sequences in related species suggests that the cubozoan toxin family may have evolved uniquely within this class of cnidaria [22].

Some structural features have been proposed through applying *in silico* analyses to protein toxins. According to these analyses α-helices and loop structures predominate at the N-terminal region, whereas the C terminus consists of β-strands and again loop structures [27]. Furthermore, the N-terminal portion is predicted to contain an amphiphilic helix and, adjacently, a common transmembrane-spanning region (TSR1) consisting of one or two hydrophobic α-helices. According to the proposed secondary structure, the cubozoan proteins may act as α-pore-forming toxins. Whether this alleged pore-forming capacity – that plausibly predisposes them to being hemolysins – takes responsibility for their lethal effects in mice has as yet not been clarified. When rat cardiomyocytes were treated with whole *C. fleckeri* venom *in vitro*, a sustained and irreversible cellular Ca^{2+} influx was first observed and then inhibited by nonspecific channel blocking lanthanum ions (La^{3+}), but not by verapamil [28]. Subsequent analysis by transmission electron microscopy confirmed the presence of pore-forming components in the venom. Whether this activity relies on specific properties of the proteins (rather than on unspecific precipitations triggered by cell culture medium) has still to be demonstrated *via* experiments using recombinant mutant proteins [29]. Similarly, specific interactions between protein toxins and membrane constituents of target cells require experimental proof.

The pore-forming capacity in cell membranes has also been demonstrated with nematocyst-derived venom from "bluebottles" (*Physalia physalis*, class hydrozoa, siphonophora, Fig. 1) [30]. The amount of assembled pores per unit of membrane area was shown to depend on the venom concentration characterized best by a hyperbolic function. The authors suggest that this form of dependency indicates the limiting role of a particular component (binding site) within the target membrane. Furthermore, the amount of venom necessary to induce pore formation varies among different cell types (excitable *versus* nonexcitable). Likewise, lysis efficiency induced by *P. physalis* toxin in target cells varies considerably [30]. The component of the venom most likely responsible for pore formation was isolated about 20 years ago [31]. Physalitoxin, a large heterotrimeric glycoprotein, is the major component found in *P. physalis* nematocyst venom that features a pronounced hemolytic capacity. Acute renal failure due to severe intravascular hemolysis and hemoglobinuria actually has been responsible for the death of a 4-year-old girl that had touched the tentacles of *P. physalis* [32, 33]. Unfortunately, the cloned cDNA and amino acid sequence of the protein toxin are still not available, thus hampering the precise and detailed elucidation of the structure-function relationship.

Toxins of sea anemones

Despite considerable efforts, the lethal principle of cubozoan venom has not yet been unequivocally identified. However, modern molecular biology and, in particular, the cloning and heterologous expression of alleged lethal proteins will eventually reveal the responsible factor(s). These techniques indeed have been employed with great success to elucidate the interactions of cytolytic protein toxins from sea anemones with target cell membranes, as briefly discussed in the remainder of this section. No less than 32 species of sea anemones have been reported to produce lethal cytolytic peptides and proteins [7], some exhibiting i.v. LD_{50} values as low as 35 μg/kg when injected into mice [34]. Presumably, however, due to a lower incidence of contact and a milder sting severity, the sedentary sea anemones – unlike their pelagic sibling taxons discussed above – have proven rather harmless to humans. Among the sea anemone's lethal proteins is a group of ~20 kDa pore-forming basic proteins whose cytolytic activity can be blocked by addition of sphingomyelin. The cDNAs of several members of this family, entitled actinoporins, have been cloned and the recombinant proteins have been functionally expressed in bacteria [7]. Determination of the three-dimensional structures of two family members in combination with site-directed mutagenesis studies revealed their elaborate structural organization that allows for target-specific pore formation in sphingomyelin-rich membranes.

The model cytolytic actinoporin is composed of a tightly folded β-sandwich core that is flanked on both sides by α-helices oriented perpendicular to each other. The N terminus including the upstream α-helix (amino acid residues 10–28) can undergo conformational changes without disturbing the structure of the central domain. Site-directed mutagenesis or gradual truncation of this amphiphilic portion of the molecule resulted in substantial decreases of its hemolytic activity, despite an unimpaired binding activity toward erythrocytes [35]. Upon removal of the entire N terminus, actinoporin completely lost its red blood cell lytic activity, demonstrating that this part of the protein actually is responsible for pore formation. The remaining sequence, however, was still capable of binding specifically to sphingomyelin. Located at the "bottom" of the β-sandwich, a patch of aromatic amino acids, together with some neutral residues, form a binding pocket for sphingomyelin. Site-directed mutagenesis highlighted the role of Trp112 for protein's initial contact with the membrane and the recognition of sphingomyelin [36]. Most intriguing, actinoporin-producing sea anemones incorporate sphingolipids other than sphingomyelin in their cell membranes, i.e., phosphonosphingolipids that differ in their phospholipid headgroups, thereby protecting themselves from the binding and cytolytic action of actinoporins.

Taken together, the above-mentioned data, along with additional insights on structure-function relationships, suggest a multi-step process in pore formation. The toxin first binds to the membrane *via* specific recognition of sphingomyelin by its aromatic binding pocket. The amphiphilic N-terminal segment comprising the upstream α-helix is then transferred to the lipid-water interface of the outer leaflet of the target membrane. When the amount of toxin bound to the membrane reaches sufficient levels, oligomerization of three to four monomers occurs and all of the N termini are concertedly pushed through the membrane to form an ion conductive pore with cation selectivity [36]. The remaining part of the protein, the β-sandwich core and the downstream α-helix, does not contribute to the physical structure of the pore but presumably is required to anchor the N terminus in the right orientation.

All actinoporins are highly cytotoxic by inducing lysis of a variety of cells, but certain cell types seem particularly susceptible. Isolated cardioventricular cells were demonstrated to be sensitive to the actinoporin family member EqtII at concentrations below 10^{-11} M (0.01 nM). Direct cardiotoxicity of EqtII at the isolated Langendorff heart has been proven in a detailed study, even at concentrations below 1 nM [37]. Perfusion with 10 nM EqtII lowered the coronary flow rate in a rat heart model by more than 90%, followed by arrhythmia and cardiac arrest. Although these acute adverse effects have not so far been described in humans, as a model for cytolytic protein toxins, actinoporins may eventually also help to uncover the deadly mode of action of the cubozoan nematocyst venom exerted in human victims (cf. above) [38].

Recycling of nematocysts

The data presented in this section clearly suggest that cnidarian nematocysts and their venom load are uniquely elaborate weapons. Coevolution of cnidarians and their predators resulted not only in the resistance against the venom of those animals that feed on cnidarians, but also in the means of recycling nematocysts from digested prey and subsequent storage of the fully functional weapons within specialized appendices ("cnidosacs") of the predator. Marine sea slugs (ophistobranchia) of the suborder of aeolidina are equipped with and protected by stolen nematocysts from cnidarian prey. The neustonic sea slug *Glaucus atlanticus*, for example, floats right under the surface of the open sea and feeds on "bluebottles" (*Physalia physalis*). This species is capable of recycling the strongly venomous nematocysts of its prey [39]. In Australia there were several reported incidents with children being stung while playing with the invertebrate slugs [40]. Besides adopting venomous organelles or accumulating low-molecular weight marine biotoxins, many species of marine snails are also endowed with means to produce their own toxins; snails belonging to the genus *Conus* that produce a wide range of toxic peptides represent famous examples. Other outstanding examples are "sea hares" that have been shrouded in legends for centuries (see next section).

A membrane disrupting oxidase from the multifunctional ink secretion of sea hares

"This hare doth cause terror in the sea; on land he is as the poor little hare, fearful and atrembling"

Olaus Magnus, 1555 [41]

Sea hares are marine snails (ophistobranchia, anaspidea) that populate various coastal habitats worldwide in great numbers. This fact is especially noteworthy, as these soft-tissued invertebrates lack any obvious defense mechanisms that would protect them against numerously emerging predators such as sea anemones, crustaceans and fish. Sea hares such as *Aplysia* spp. (Fig. 2) appear without a hard outer shell, have not lined their skin with adopted venomous nematocysts from cnidaria, nor have taken a shape that hides them from attention. However, in spite of their vulnerable appearance they can readily escape even if already engulfed by sea anemones (as documented in a video by Tom Nolen, NY, http://www.seaslugforum.net/showall.cfm?base=seahatac, see also [42]). The key of their success is the production of a multifunctional composite ink that can be spattered toward an attacker by means of a blowtube-like siphon. This composite ink consists of the secretions of two separate glands – the ink (purple or mantle) gland and the opaline gland – that are mixed within animal's mantle cavity just before ejection [43]. The antipredatory effects of the purple fluid have well been documented [44–46], and rely on the concerted action of several high- and low-molecular weight compounds that target various perceptive structures of the attacking animal. With regard to its com-

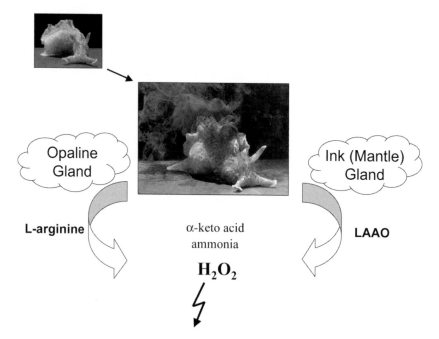

Figure 2. *Aplysia californica* ("sea hare"); Systematics: mollusca, opisthobranchia, anaspidea. The substrate of the aplysia ink enzyme LAAO (L-amino acid oxidase), L-arginine, is present at high concentrations in the secretion of the opaline gland. Just before ejection toward an attacker, the product of this gland is mixed with the one from the ink gland that contains the enzyme, eventually resulting in the formation of hydrogen peroxide (H_2O_2), ammonia, and the arginine-derived α-keto acid (courtesy of Genevieve "Genny" Anderson).

plex composition and multifunctionality, mollusc ink from sea hares (and cephalopods such as octopus, cuttlefish and squid) therefore equals other venoms produced by different groups of marine invertebrates [47, 48]. Apart from producing an ink deleterious to attackers, sea hares also accumulate marine biotoxins from their food, e.g., the strongly toxic non-ribosomal peptide dolastatin 10 from the cyanobacterium *Symploca* spp. VP642 [49]. These low-molecular weight toxins are stored predominantly in the skin and in digestive glands of the animal. The unpleasant "chemical" smell released by sea hares when touched and handled most likely results from the presence of brominated compounds secreted together with a mucous slime. It may have been this startling odor of the animals that made Pliny the Elder report nausea and vomiting being induced by sea hares immediately on the very first touch [9].

There have been rumors about the venomousness of sea hares for human health for centuries. It has been reported that ancient rulers routinely killed their political enemies with toxic extracts of these specimens [50]. In modern times, however, there have only been anecdotal reports of human poisoning after ingestion of sea hares, predominantly characterized by acute liver damage [51–53]. Although the causing agent has never been unequivocally revealed, it most likely consists mainly of various accumulated low-molecular weight biotoxins. In addition, HMWPT (e.g., enzymes) may also play a role in adverse reactions triggered by sea hare tissues and its secretions. For instance, the presence of an enzyme capable of disrupting cellular membranes of a wide range of human cells *in vitro* has been demonstrated in sea hare ink and eggs. This enzyme, an L-amino acid oxidase (LAAO) catalyzes oxidative deamination of the basic amino acids L-lysine and L-arginine. Products from this reaction are hydrogen peroxide (H_2O_2), ammonia and the corresponding α-keto acids (Fig. 2) [54, 55]. When added to cells in culture, the cytotoxic effects elicited by the enzyme occur rapidly. Within minutes the cell's metabolic activity is severely impaired, and after a few hours the plasma membrane integrity is lost and nucleic acids are degraded. This enzyme-induced cell death has been shown to be triggered by oxidative damage to cellular structures. It also became clear that the pathway functions independently of regular cellular apoptotic signaling. Thus, removal of enzymatically produced H_2O_2 by catalase rescued treated cells from demise, whereas caspase inhibitors such as zVAD did not show any beneficial effects on cellular survival. However, even if rescued by H_2O_2-scavenging catalase in first place, cells may eventually die due to consumption and subsequent shortage of essential amino acids in the media and the formation of toxic ammonia. This delayed cell death then occurs in a rather typical apoptotic, caspase-dependent manner [54, 55]. The amounts of H_2O_2 required to induce the observed effects in cells are extremely high. A concentration of $\geq 200\ \mu M\ H_2O_2$ in the cell culture medium was neccessary to mimic LAAO-induced effects. By contrast, at concentrations below $100\ \mu M\ H_2O_2$ the classical hallmarks of apoptosis could be observed [2, 54]. This agrees well with reports on the varying effects of H_2O_2 on key initiation and effector molecules of apoptosis, i.e., caspases. It has been shown that addition of H_2O_2 to cells at low concentrations ($50\ \mu M$) triggers apoptosis *via* activation of caspases; at higher concentrations, however, caspases become inhibited, and above 200 µM caspase activity is virtually nil [56].

The main substrate of the aplysia ink LAAO, L-arginine, is present at high concentrations in the secretion of its opaline gland. Just before ejection toward an attacker, the product of this gland is mixed with the one from the ink gland that contains the enzyme. It has been reported that incubation of the two components (enzyme and its substrate) at naturally occurring concentrations and conditions produces H_2O_2 levels in the millimolar range and also other reaction products within seconds [47, 48]. Therefore, the immediate effects observed *in vitro* can be substantiated and clearly recapitulate the situation given in the marine environment and *in vivo*. Elsewhere in the natural world, by employing reactive oxygen species, an attack can even be directed exactly against defined cellular structures of the predator. Thus, for several LAAOs present in snake venom (svLAAOs) a pinpoint interaction with cells by binding to specific acceptor sites at the plasma membrane could be demonstrated [57, 58]. However, the identity of the particular surface structures responsible for binding those snake venom enzymes has not been clarified yet. In the aplysia ink LAAO, the FAD binding site is preceded by a short stretch of positively charged amino acids interspersed with cysteine residues that are highly conserved among orthologs from other ink-producing sea hares. Upon release, this stretch becomes the uttermost part of the N terminus of the enzyme after processing of a signal sequence, and may structurally be qualified to mediate the binding to negatively charged acceptor domains in the cell membrane [2]. Given the extremely fast and high dilution effects in the natural habitat, local production of high amounts of H_2O_2 in the proximity of susceptible sites within target membranes seems perspicuous. For HMWPT, the importance of specific acceptor sites and structures as part of the cellular membranes of target cells has also been highlighted by another exemplary group of very effective venom compounds, the phospholipase A_2 (PLA_2) enzymes (see next section).

Cytotoxic phospholipases in marine invertebrates

Similar to the LAAOs discussed above, toxic PLA_2 enzymes are ubiquitous across all ranges of venomous snakes and significantly contribute to the pharmacological effects that result from a snake bite [58]. This class of HMWPT features a great structural, biochemical and functional variety while still sharing a common enzymatic route. In general, they catalyze the cleavage of glycerophospholipids (phosphoglycerides) such as phosphatidylcholine or -inositol. These lipids represent structural constituents of cellular membranes that originate from condensation of fatty acids with glycerol and a polar head group. PLA_2-mediated cleavage of its substrates generates lysophospholipids and free fatty acids, e.g., arachidonic acid. The latter molecule represents the physiological precursor of prostaglandins, thromboxanes and leukotrienes, all of which control a great variety of cellular functions including inflammation and pain.

The pharmacological effects of snake venom PLA_2 ($svPLA_2$) enzymes are numerous. They exhibit neuro-, myo- and cardiotoxicity, affect platelet aggregation and induce anticoagulation and hemolysis. Overall, these enzymes induce damage to several tissues and organs [59], although most toxic effects seem to depend only partly on their enzymatic activity. For instance, some of the most lethal neurotoxic $svPLA_2$ variants, i.e., taipoxin and textilotoxin, display only extremely low enzymatic activities [5]. Binding to specific high-affinity protein receptors (acceptors) or to lipid domains within the plasma membrane have been identified as the toxicologically crucial event [5, 58]. The binding specificity seems to be extremely variable among different $svPLA_2$ enzymes and constitutes the predominant factor in the particular pharmacological impact of the enzymes. It has been shown, for instance, that coagulation factor Xa is bound by potently anticoagulant $svPLA_2$ enzymes [60], whereas presynaptic membrane K^+ channels of peripheral nerves are predominantly targeted by neurotoxic β-bungarotoxin [61]. The so-called "pharmacological site" of the enzyme that is responsible for its high-affinity binding to the acceptors of specific cells has been shown to be structurally independent of the enzyme's active site, but sometimes overlaps with the latter [62]. Bioinformatic analysis of aligned $svPLA_2$ protein sequences, along with chemical modification studies, offered some valuable clues about conserved amino acid residues that may be involved in structurally forming certain subsets of this pharmacological site, such as the "anticoagulant site" [59, 63]. An unambiguous identification of the constituting residues, as has been achieved in the case of actinoporins (see above), however, has yet to be done.

Besides snake venoms, PLA_2 enzymes also have been found in several marine invertebrates like corals, crown-of-thorns starfish, sea cucumbers and sponges [64]. In particular, high levels of activity were demonstrated in crude extracts from the fire coral *Millepora* spp. and the stone coral *Pocillopora* spp. that are notorious for their capacity to induce skin irritation upon contact [65]. Fire corals, like jellyfish, belong to the phylum cnidaria and thus possess nematocysts that can fire miniature projectiles to penetrate the skin and inject their venom (cf. above). Although not being members of the group of "true corals", fire corals are important cohabitants of reef-building communities (class anthozoa) [66]. When unprotected human skin encounters the abundant and innocuous looking reef organism, an immediate burning sensation might be induced, ranging from mild to intense pain [67]. Within 1 day after contact a skin lesion may emerge that can progress toward erythematous urticarial wheals. It is unusual, however, for a fire coral sting to persist much beyond the acute painful phase [66].

Activity guided fractionation of the nematocyst venom from the Red Sea fire coral *Millepora platyphylla* yielded a 32.5 kDa protein factor that accounted for most of the crude extract's PLA_2 activity [68]. This protein, termed milleporin-1, also lysed human red blood cells at microgram per milliliter concentrations (maximum effect at 75 μg/mL). The hemolytic activity was greatly inhibited by addition of phosphatidylcholine – a finding that may suggest that the enzymatic activity of the protein directly relates to its hemolytic activity. Another protein similar to milleporin-1 was purified from a Caribbean relative, the fire coral *M. complanata* [69]. The hemolytic activity of this cnidarian PLA_2, however, could be inhibited by addition of cholesterol. Although not yet proven experimentally, the fire coral PLA_2 orthologs may be the molecular cause for the above-mentioned local skin reactions in response to a sting. Human divers and swimmers are regularly affected by fire coral stings. However, those organisms that actually should be stopped from touching (and devouring) the corals, e.g., the crown-of-thorns starfish portrayed below, have often evolved resistance to the fire coral's weapons.

A cell-intruding and hepatotoxic DNase from the crown-of-thorns starfish

The crown-of-thorns starfish *Acanthaster planci* is a very large (up to 60 cm in total diameter) invertebrate predator that feeds on corals [70]. It is infamous for its dramatic population explosions ("outbursts") that have regularly devastated coral reefs throughout the Indo-Pacific [71]. The starfish devours its prey by everting its stomach and imposing it on the coral surface [72]. The digestive enzymes are then released and break down the soft tissue of coral polyps, leaving the skeleton (made from calcium carbonate) intact [73]. Subsequently the enzymatically digested tissue is ingested *via* the imposed stomach surface. This type of food intake, i.e., external digestion of nutrient-rich soft parts, seems advantageous when feeding on animals such as corals and mussels armed with hard and defensive spines or shells [74]. A serious drawback, however, is the slowness of the process. Feeding crown-of-thorns starfishes have to remain motionless for hours exposing delicate body structures within tropical shallow waters where the predation pressure is extremely high [74]. For instance, here the animals need to cope with a fish bite frequency of about $150\,000/m^2$ per day [75].

To prevent fish and other attackers from "nibbling", the back of the starfish is covered with thousands of sharp thorn-like spines that also bring about the name "crown-of-thorns". The tips of these up to 28-mm-long structures are shaped like triangular spears [74]. One corner of the triangle features a razor-sharp edge that may aid in penetration of the attackers integument. Furthermore, the spines are covered with glandular tissue that is stripped off and remains in the wound after penetration [76]. The gland cells of this tissue produce a venom that contains several bioactive HMWPT, i.e., multiple hemolytic and myotoxic PLA_2 enzymes [77, 78], the anticoagulant peptide plancinin [79], and the plancitoxins I and II, shown to be lethally toxic in mice [80, 81]. When a swimmer is accidentally stung by these spines, severe pain, local swelling and redness occurs immediately [81, 82]. Although nausea and protracted vomiting may occur, the symptoms usually cease within few hours.

Among the toxic proteins present in the starfish venom, the plancitoxins I and II are most peculiar. Both purified protein toxins caused lethality in mice at an i.v. LD$_{50}$ of about 140 µg/kg [78]. Treated mice suffered from severe hepatotoxicity, i.e., enlargement and necrosis of hepatocytes, elevated serum levels of glutamic oxaloacetic transaminase (GOT) and glutamic pyruvic transaminase (GPT). Separation by gel electrophoresis and purification revealed that the 37 kDa proteins are composed of two subunits (10 and 27 kDa) linked by a disulfide bridge. Intriguingly, the amino acid sequence of plancitoxin I, deduced from the cloned cDNA, featured highest homology with mammalian DNase II (40–42%) [80]. Although this low grade of homology may not necessarily indicate functional accordance, plancitoxin I also shares two specific HxK motifs that together form the single active site in the mammalian enzyme [83]. In addition to active histidine residues, the mammalian enzyme requires N-glycosylation at several sites to exhibit nucleolytic activity [83]. By contrast, only one putative N-glycosylation site has been identified in the amino acid sequence of plancitoxin [84]. Whether or not the functional toxin is N-glycosylated has not yet been experimentally established. No dependency between the presence of sugar residues in the protein and its toxicity has been determined so far either.

Prompted by the molecular biology data mentioned above, the nuclease activity of plancitoxin was assayed. As proposed, the toxin was capable of digesting DNA *in vitro*. Its pH optimum of 7.2 is similar to physiological intracellular conditions, but deviates substantially from preferences known for all common DNase II isoforms. The latter are required for DNA "waste" removal and auxiliary apoptotic DNA fragmentation in higher eukaryotes, thereby being adapted to work in lysosomes at low pH values [83].

When rat liver cells were incubated with plancitoxin I, chromosomal DNA fragmentation was observed about 3 hours after addition of the toxin [81]. Treated cells died within 1 day apparently through caspase 3-independent apoptosis. Whether DNA fragmentation was instrumental in inducing cell death or rather a secondary effect of cell death-triggered nucleolytic processes remains to be clarified. In a confocal laser scanning microscopic study the authors describe the accumulation of plancitoxin I in the nuclei of treated cells. In order to accumulate within nuclei, the toxin needs to enter cells either by employing an active endocytotic internalization process or – much less likely – by simply penetrating the cellular membrane.

Some bacterial toxins such as the cytolethal distending toxins (Cdts) [85] share several peculiarities with plancitoxin. Three different monomers (CdtA, B, C), ranging from 20 to 30 kDa, may assemble to the fully active holotoxin capable of entering target cells by receptor-mediated endocytosis. Subsequently, CdtB is actively transported into the nucleus where it attacks chromosomal DNA, thus eventually causing cell cycle arrest and/or apoptosis [86]. Similar to plancitoxin, CdtB features position-specific homologies with mammalian DNase I and displays nucleolytic activity *in vitro* and *in vivo*. The cytotoxic activity of CdtB could be abolished by introducing point mutations at certain conserved amino acid residues localized within the active site and required for DNase activity [87]. Toxicity in cells was also completely inhibited under conditions that block fusion of early endosomes with downstream compartments, or upon disruption of the Golgi complex. Thus endocytotic transport across membranes toward the nucleus represents an indispensable process required for Cdt-mediated toxicity [88]. Whether the toxicity of plancitoxin actually depends on its DNase II activity and the way by which the toxin enters the cell, has yet to be determined. If the conclusions drawn by Shiomi and co-workers [80] on the toxic principle of plancitoxin are confirmed, this marine toxin would substantially broaden our understanding of the repertoires of enzymes employed in the marine world for defense or aggression.

Conclusion

HMWPT are widely produced in invertebrate animals. They have usually evolved from enzymes that are employed for digestive purposes. The products of this enzymatic activity, e.g., reactive oxygen species or lysophospholipids and free fatty acids, rapidly and effectively mediate adverse cell reactions by disrupting cellular integrity. Membrane integrity may also be more directly targeted by pore-forming toxins that actually lack enzymatic activity. In the natural world, the specific effects of complex venoms are highly diverse and inconstant. Nevertheless, up-to-date molecular biology techniques, particularly the cloning and mutational analyses of alleged lethal proteins, provide the tools to uncover the molecular basis for specific pharmacological signatures of individual toxins. Most importantly, research into the fundamental aspects of biogenic toxins will inevitably lead to the development of specific antidotes and causal therapies in the future.

References

1 Nakashima K, Nobuhisa I, Deshimaru M, Nakai M, Ogawa T, Shimohigashi Y, Fukumaki Y, Hattori M, Sakaki Y, Hattori S (1995) Accelerated evolution in the protein-coding regions is universal in crotalinae snake venom gland phospholipase A_2 isozyme genes. *Proc Natl Acad Sci USA* 92: 5605–5609

2 Butzke D (2003) APIT – The cytolytic toxin of ink from *Aplysia punctata*. PhD Thesis, Free University, Berlin, Germany (online available in German at: http://www.dart-europe.eu/full.php?id=55108)

3 Pearce LB, First ER, MacCallum RD, Gupta A (1997) Pharmacologic characterization of botulinum toxin for basic science and medicine. *Toxicon* 35: 1373–1412

4 Murata M, Naoki H, Matsunaga S, Satake M, Yasumoto T (1994) Structure and partial stereochemical assignments for maitotoxin, the most toxic and largest natural non-biopolymer. *J Am Chem Soc* 116: 7098–7107

5 Montecucco C, Gutierrez JM, Lomonte B (2008) Cellular pathology induced by snake venom phospholipase A_2 myotoxins and neurotoxins: Common aspects of their mechanisms of action. *Cell Mol Life Sci* 65: 2897–2912

6 Yotsu-Yamashita M, Urabe D, Asai M, Nishikawa T, Isobe M (2003) Biological activity of 8,11-dideoxytetrodotoxin: Lethality to mice and the inhibitory activity to cytotoxicity of ouabain and veratridine in mouse neuroblastoma cells, Neuro-2a. *Toxicon* 42: 557–560

7 Anderluh G, Maček P (2002) Cytolytic peptide and protein toxins from sea anemones (anthozoa: actiniaria). *Toxicon* 40: 111–124

8 Bergmann W, Feeney RJ (1951) Contribution to the studies of marine products. XXXII. The nucleosides of sponges. I. *J Org Chem* 16: 981–987

9 Bostock J, Riley HT (1855) *The Natural History. Pliny the Elder.* Taylor and Francis, London, UK (online available at: http://www.perseus.tufts.edu/cgi-bin/ptext?layout=;doc=Perseus%3Atext %3A1999.02.0137;query=toc;loc=7.24)

10 Tibballs J (2006) Australian venomous jellyfish, envenomation syndromes, toxins and therapy. *Toxicon* 48: 830–859

11 Gershwin LA, Dawes P (2008) Preliminary observations on the response of *Chironex fleckeri* (cnidaria: cubozoa: chirodropida) to different colors of light. *Biol Bull* 215: 57–62

12 Rifkin J, Endean R (1983) The structure and function of the nematocysts of *Chironex fleckeri* Southcott, 1956. *Cell Tissue Res* 233: 563–577

13 Endean R, Henderson L (1969) Further studies of toxic material from nematocysts of the cubomedusan *Chironex fleckeri* Southcott. *Toxicon* 7: 303–314

14 Barnes JH (1967) Extraction of cnidarian venom from living tentacle. In: FE Russell, PR Saunders (eds): *Animal Toxins*, Pergamon Press, Oxford, 115–129

15 Baxter EH, Marr AG, Lane WR (1968) Immunity to the venom of the sea wasp *Chironex fleckeri*. *Toxicon* 6: 45–50

16 Baxter EH, Marr AG (1969) Sea wasp (*Chironex fleckeri*) venom: Lethal, haemolytic and dermonecrotic properties. *Toxicon* 7: 195–210

17 Barnes JH (1960) Observations on jellyfish stingings in North Queensland. *Med J Aust* 47: 993–999

18 Underwood AH, Seymour JE (2007) Venom ontogeny, diet and morphology in *Carukia barnesi*, a species of Australian box jellyfish that causes Irukandji syndrome. *Toxicon* 49: 1073–1082

19 Sutherland SK (1983) *Australian Animal Toxins: The Creatures, Their Toxins, and Care of the Poisoned Patient.* Oxford University Press, Melbourne

20 Barnes JH (1966) Studies on three venomous cubomedusae. In: WJ Rees (ed.): *The Cnidaria and Their Evolution*, Academic Press, New York, 307–332

21 Brinkman D, Burnell J (2008) Partial purification of cytolytic venom proteins from the box jellyfish, *Chironex fleckeri*. *Toxicon* 51, 853–863.

22 Brinkman DL, Burnell JN (2009) Biochemical and molecular characterisation of cubozoan protein toxins. *Toxicon, in press*

23 Nagai H, Takuwa K, Nakao M, Ito E, Miyake M, Noda M, Nakajima T (2000) Novel proteinaceous toxins from the box jellyfish (sea wasp) *Carybdea rastoni*. *Biochem Biophys Res Commun* 275: 582–588

24 Nagai H, Takuwa K, Nakao M, Sakamoto B, Crow GL, Nakajima T (2000) Isolation and characterization of a novel protein toxin from the Hawaiian box jellyfish (sea wasp) *Carybdea alata*. *Biochem Biophys Res Commun* 275: 589–594

25 Nagai H, Takuwa-Kuroda K, Nakao M, Oshiro N, Iwanaga S, Nakajima T (2002) A novel protein toxin from the deadly box jellyfish (sea wasp, Habu-kurage) *Chiropsalmus quadrigatus*. *Biosci Biotechnol Biochem* 66: 97–102

26 Chung JJ, Ratnapala LA, Cooke IM, Yanagihara AA (2001) Partial purification and characterization of a hemolysin (CAH1) from Hawaiian box jellyfish (*Carybdea alata*) venom. *Toxicon* 39: 981–990

27 Brinkman D, Burnell J (2007) Identification, cloning and sequencing of two major venom proteins from the box jellyfish, *Chironex fleckeri*. *Toxicon* 50: 850–860

28 Bailey PM, Bakker AJ, Seymour JE, Wilce JA (2005) A functional comparison of the venom of three Australian jellyfish – *Chironex fleckeri, Chiropsalmus* sp., and *Carybdea xaymacana* – on cytosolic Ca^{2+}, haemolysis and *Artemia* sp. lethality. *Toxicon* 45: 233–242

29 Watanabe I, Nomura T, Tominaga T, Yamamoto K, Kohda C, Kawamura I, Mitsuyama M (2006) Dependence of the lethal effect of pore-forming haemolysins of Gram-positive bacteria on cytolytic activity. *J Med Microbiol* 55: 505–510

30 Edwards LP, Whitter E, Hessinger DA (2002) Apparent membrane pore-formation by Portuguese man-of-war (*Physalia physalis*) venom in intact cultured cells. *Toxicon* 40: 1299–1305

31 Hessinger DA (1988) Nematocyst venoms and toxins. In: DA Hessinger, HM Lenhoff (eds): *The Biology of Nematocysts,* Academic Press, San Diego, CA, 333–368

32 Guess HA, Saviteer PL, Morris CR (1982) Hemolysis and acute renal failure following a Portuguese man-of-war sting. *Pediatrics* 70: 979–981

33 Spelman FJ, Bowe EA, Watson CB, Klein EE (1982) Acute renal failure as a result of *Physalia physalis* sting. *South Med J* 70: 979

34 Maček P, Lebez D (1988) Isolation and characterization of three lethal and hemolytic toxins from the sea anemone *Actinia equina* L. *Toxicon* 26: 441–451

35 Anderluh G, Pungercar J, Krizaj I, Strukelj B, Gubensek F, Maček P (1997) N-terminal truncation mutagenesis of equinatoxin II, a pore-forming protein from the sea anemone *Actinia equina*. *Protein Eng* 10: 751–755

36 Kristan K, Viero G, Dalla Serra M, Maček P, Anderluh G (2009) Molecular mechanism of pore formation by actinoporins. *Toxicon, in press*

37 Bunc M, Drevensek G, Budihna M, Suput D (1999) Effects of equinatoxin II from *Actinia equina* (L.) on isolated rat heart: The role of direct cardiotoxic effects in equinatoxin II lethality. *Toxicon* 37: 109–123

38 Suput D (2009) *In vivo* effects of cnidarian toxins and venoms. *Toxicon, in press*

39 Thompson TE, Bennett I (1969) *Physalia* nematocysts: Utilized by mollusks for defense. *Science* 166: 1532–1533

40 Rudman WB (1998) *Glaucus atlanticus* Forster, 1777. Sea slug forum. Australian Museum, Sydney (online available at: http://www.seaslugforum.net/factsheet.cfm?base=glauatla, accessed 17 Juli 2009)

41 Carefoot TH (1987) *Aplysia*: Its biology and ecology. *Oceanogr Mar Biol Annu Rev* 25: 167–284

42 Nolen TG, Johnson PM (2001) Defensive inking in *Aplysia* spp.: Multiple episodes of ink secretion and the adaptive use of a limited chemical response. *J Exp Biol* 204: 1257–1268

43 Johnson PM, Kicklighter CE, Schmidt M, Kamio M, Yang H, Elkin D, Michel WC, Tai PC, Derby CD (2006) Packaging of chemicals in the defensive secretory glands of the sea hare *Aplysia californica. J Exp Biol* 209: 78–88

44 Kicklighter CE, Shabani S, Johnson PM, Derby CD (2005) Sea hares use novel antipredatory chemical defenses. *Curr Biol* 15: 549–554

45 Kicklighter CE, Derby CD (2006) Multiple components in ink of the sea hare *Aplysia californica* are aversive to the sea anemone *Anthopleura sola. J Exp Mar Biol Ecol* 334: 256–268

46 Nolen TG, Johnson PM, Kicklighter CE, Capo T (1995) Ink secretion by the marine snail *Aplysia californica* enhances its ability to escape from a natural predator. *J Comp Physiol A* 176: 239–254

47 Derby CD (2007) Escape by inking and secreting: Marine molluscs avoid predators through a rich array of chemicals and mechanisms. *Biol Bull* 213: 274–289

48 Derby CD, Kicklighter CE, Johnson PM, Zhang X (2007) Chemical composition of inks of diverse molluscs suggests convergent chemical defenses. *J Chem Ecol* 33: 1105–1113

49 Luesch H, Moore RE, Paul VJ, Mooberry SL, Corbett TH (2001) Isolation of dolastatin 10 from the marine cyanobacterium *Symploca* species VP642 and total stereochemistry and biological evaluation of its analogue symplostatin 1. *J Nat Prod* 64: 907–910

50 Halstead BW (1988) *Poisonous and Venomous Marine Animals of the World.* 2nd edn., Darwin Press, Princeton, NJ

51 Sakamoto Y, Nakajima T, Misawa S, Ishikawa H, Itoh Y, Nakashima T, Okanoue T, Kashima K, Tsuji T (1998) Acute liver damage with characteristic apoptotic hepatocytes by ingestion of *Aplysia kurodai*, a sea hare. *Intern Med* 37: 927–929

52 Hino K, Mitsui Y, Hirano Y (1994) Four cases of acute liver damage following the ingestion of a sea hare egg. *J Gastroenterol* 29: 679

53 Sorokin M (1988) Human poisoning by ingestion of a sea hare (*Dolabella auricularia*). *Toxicon* 26: 1095–1097

54 Butzke D, Machuy N, Thiede B, Hurwitz R, Goedert S, Rudel T (2004) Hydrogen peroxide produced by *Aplysia* ink toxin kills tumor cells independent of apoptosis *via* peroxiredoxin I sensitive pathways. *Cell Death Differ* 11: 608–617

55 Butzke D, Hurwitz R, Thiede B, Goedert S, Rudel T (2005) Cloning and biochemical characterization of APIT, a new L-amino acid oxidase from *Aplysia punctata. Toxicon* 46: 479–489

56 Hampton MB, Orrenius S (1997) Dual regulation of caspase activity by hydrogen peroxide: Implications for apoptosis. *FEBS Lett* 414: 552–556

57 Suhr SM, Kim DS (1996) Identification of the snake venom substance that induces apoptosis.

Biochem Biophys Res Commun 224: 134–139

58 Li R, Zhu S, Wu J, Wang W, Lu Q, Clemetson KJ (2008) L-Amino acid oxidase from *Naja atra* venom activates and binds to human platelets. *Acta Biochim Biophys Sin* 40: 19–26

59 Kini RM (2003) Excitement ahead: Structure, function and mechanism of snake venom phospholipase A$_2$ enzymes. *Toxicon* 42: 827–840

60 Stefansson S, Kini RM, Evans HJ (1990) The basic phospholipase A$_2$ from *Naja nigricollis* venom inhibits the prothrombinase complex by a novel nonenzymatic mechanism. *Biochemistry* 29: 7742–7746

61 Rowan EG (2001) What does β-bungarotoxin do at the neuromuscular junction? *Toxicon* 39: 107–118

62 Rosenberg P (1986) The relationship between enzymatic activity and pharmacological properties of phospholipases. In: JB Harris (ed.): *Natural Toxins,* Oxford University Press, Oxford, 129–147

63 Kini RM, Evans HJ (1987) Structure-function relationships of phospholipases. The anticoagulant region of phospholipases A$_2$. *J Biol Chem* 262: 14402–14407

64 Nevalainen TJ, Llewellyn LE, Benzie JAH (2001) Phospholipase A$_2$ in marine invertebrates. *Rapp Comm Int Explor Sci Mer Mediterr* 36: 202

65 Nevalainen TJ, Peuravuori HJ, Quinn RJ, Llewellyn LE, Benzie JAH, Fenner PJ, Winkel KD (2004) Phospholipase A$_2$ in cnidaria. *Comp Biochem Physiol B* 139: 731–735

66 Williamson JA, Fenner PJ, Burnett JW, Rifkin JF (1996) *Venomous and Poisonous Marine Animals: A Medical and Biological Handbook.* UNSW Press, Sydney

67 Bachand R (1983) Fire coral – The stingers. *Underwater Naturalist* 14: 12–15

68 Radwan FF, Aboul-Dahab HM (2004) Milleporin-1, a new phospholipase A$_2$ active protein from the fire coral *Millepora platyphylla* nematocysts. *Comp Biochem Physiol C Toxicol Pharmacol* 139: 267–272

69 Ibarra-Alvarado C, Garcia JA, Aguilar MB, Rojas A, Falcon A, Heimer de la Cotera EP (2007) Biochemical and pharmacological characterization of toxins obtained from the fire coral *Millepora complanata*. *Comp Biochem Physiol C Toxicol Pharmacol* 146: 511–518

70 Souter DW (2007) The ecology of individual specimens of *Acanthaster planci* in low density populations. PhD Thesis, University of Queensland, Australia (online available at: http://espace.library. uq.edu.au/view/UQ: 151707)

71 Vogler C, Benzie J, Lessios H, Barber P, Worheide G (2008) A threat to coral reefs multiplied? Four species of crown-of-thorns starfish. *Biol Lett* 4: 696–699

72 Brauer RW, Jordan MR, Barnes DJ (1970) Triggering of the stomach eversion reflex of *Acanthaster planci* by coral extracts. *Nature* 228: 344–346

73 Endean R (1973) Population explosion of *Acanthaster planci* and associated destruction of hermatypic corals in the Indo-West Pacific region. In: OA Jones, R Endean (eds): *Biology and Geology of Coral Reefs,* Academic Press, New York, 389–438

74 Motokawa T (1986) Morphology of spines and spine joint in the crown-of-thorns starfish *Acanthaster planci* (Echinodermata, Asteroida). *Zoomorphology* 106: 247–253

75 Carpenter RC (1986) Partitioning herbivory and its effects on coral reef algal communities. *Ecol Monogr* 56: 345–363

76 Mebs D (2000) *Gifttiere: Ein Handbuch für Biologen, Toxikologen, Ärzte und Apotheker.* 2nd edn., Wissenschaftliche Verlagsgesellschaft mbH, Stuttgart, 84–86

77 Mebs D (1991) A myotoxic phospholipase A$_2$ from the crown-of-thorns starfish *Acanthaster planci. Toxicon* 29: 289–293

78 Shiomi KA, Kazama A, Shimakura K, Nagashima Y (1998) Purification and properties of phospholipases A$_2$ from the crown-of-thorns starfish (*Acanthaster planci*) venom. *Toxicon* 36: 589–599

79 Karasudani I, Koyama T, Nakandakari S, Aniya Y (1996) Purification of anticoagulant factor from the spine venom of the crown-of-thorns starfish, *Acanthaster planci. Toxicon* 34: 871–879

80 Shiomi K, Midorikawa S, Ishida M, Nagashima Y, Nagai H (2004) Plancitoxins, lethal factors from the crown-of-thorns starfish *Acanthaster planci*, are deoxyribonucleases II. *Toxicon* 44: 499–506

81 Ota E, Nagashima Y, Shiomi K, Sakurai T, Kojima C, Waalkes MP, Himeno S (2006) Caspase-independent apoptosis induced in rat liver cells by plancitoxin I, the major lethal factor from the crown-of-thorns starfish *Acanthaster planci* venom. *Toxicon* 48: 1002–1010

82 Sato H, Tsuruta Y, Yamamoto Y, Asato Y, Taira K, Hagiwara K, Kayo S, Iwanaga S, Uezato H (2008) Case of skin injuries due to stings by crown-of-thorns starfish (*Acanthaster planci*). *J*

Dermatol 35: 162–167

83 Schäfer P, Cymerman IA, Bujnicki JM, Meiss G (2007) Human lysosomal DNase IIα contains two requisite PLD-signature (HxK) motifs: Evidence for a pseudodimeric structure of the active enzyme species. *Protein Sci* 16: 82–91

84 The UniProt Consortium (2008) The Universal Protein Resource (UniProtKB/Swiss-Prot Q75 WF2). *Nucleic Acids Res* 36: 190–195

85 Ohara M, Oswald E, Sugai M (2004) Cytolethal distending toxin: A bacterial bullet targeted to nucleus. *J Biochem* 136: 409–413

86 Thelestam M, Frisan T (2004) Cytolethal distending toxins. *Rev Physiol Biochem Pharmacol* 152: 111–133

87 Elwell CA, Dreyfus LA (2000) DNase I homologous residues in CdtB are critical for cytolethal distending toxin-mediated cell cycle arrest. *Mol Microbiol* 37: 952–963

88 Cortes-Bratti X, Chaves-Olarte E, Lagergard T, Thelestam M (2000) Cellular internalization of cytolethal distending toxin from *Haemophilus ducreyi*. *Infect Immun* 68: 6903–6911

Molecular, Clinical and Environmental Toxicology. Volume 2: Clinical Toxicology
Edited by A. Luch

Venomous animals: clinical toxinology

Julian White

Toxinology Department, Women's and Children's Hospital, North Adelaide, Australia

Abstract. Venomous animals occur in numerous phyla and present a great diversity of taxa, toxins, targets, clinical effects and outcomes. Venomous snakes are the most medically significant group globally and may injure >1.25 million humans annually, with up to 100 000 deaths and many more cases with long-term disability. Scorpion sting is the next most important cause of envenoming, but significant morbidity and even deaths occur following envenoming with a wide range of other venomous animals, including spiders, ticks, jellyfish, marine snails, octopuses and fish. Clinical effects vary with species and venom type, including local effects (pain, swelling, sweating, blistering, bleeding, necrosis), general effects (headache, vomiting, abdominal pain, hypertension, hypotension, cardiac arrhythmias and arrest, convulsions, collapse, shock) and specific systemic effects (paralytic neurotoxicity, neuroexcitatory neurotoxicity, myotoxicity, interference with coagulation, haemorrhagic activity, renal toxicity, cardiac toxicity). First aid varies with organism and envenoming type, but few effective first aid methods are recommended, while many inappropriate or frankly dangerous methods are in widespread use. For snakebite, immobilisation of the bitten limb, then the whole patient is the universal method, although pressure immobilisation bandaging is recommended for bites by non-necrotic or haemorrhagic species. Hot water immersion is the most universal method for painful marine stings. Medical treatment includes both general and specific measures, with antivenom being the principal tool in the latter category. However, antivenom is available only for a limited range of species, not for all dangerous species, is in short supply in some areas of highest need, and in many cases, is supported by historical precedent rather than modern controlled trials.

Introduction

Venom appears to have been a success story in evolution because venomous animals are found in such a range of taxa, but the success is muted since most animals remain non-venomous. Logically it follows that venom is not the answer to all life's challenges, so how does it benefit those animals that produce it? Venom appears to have two main functions; prey acquisition and processing, and defence against predators. The value mix between these two competing functions varies between animal groups, but for those venomous animals most likely to cause venomous harm to humans, notably snakes, scorpions, spiders, and jellyfish, prey acquisition seems to predominate. The honey bee, *Apis mellifera*, is the obvious exception, as the sting, with attached venom gland, is purely defensive, having no role in prey acquisition, but here it is not venom toxicity that affects humans, but venom allergy. So vast is the range and diversity of venomous life on earth that a single chapter cannot cover more than some key elements and groups, a caveat that readers should be cognisant of.

Epidemiology

For most venomous animals for much of the world, detailed statistics on the
number of humans bitten or stung, envenomed, or killed each year are unavailable. Published data are replete with conjecture, estimates, or guesstimates,
with variable validity. It is clear, however, that certain taxa of venomous animals cause significant morbidity and mortality amongst humans. Top of this
list are venomous snakes, with current estimates of >2.5 million cases and
around 100 000 deaths per year [1]. Subsequent analysis has indicated that
these estimates are likely on the high side, with low estimates nearer 1.2 million cases and 20 000 deaths annually [2] (Tab. 1). These figures hide the huge
toll of morbidity after snakebite, which affects far more cases than fatal outcomes, and often results in long-term suffering, and social and economic loss
[3]. That the snakebite toll is greatest in the rural tropics of the developing
world [4], where poverty, poor education and under-resourced health systems
combine to minimise effective care, is an ongoing tragedy of human existence,
made worse by the effects of natural disasters [5].

After snakebite, scorpion stings likely account for many medically significant
cases and incidence has been estimated as >1.2 million cases each year [6].
Mexico alone documents >200 000 cases requiring hospital care annually [6, 7].
In some regions scorpion stings are more frequent than snakebites; North Africa
is an example. Deaths are increasingly uncommon, perhaps as a result of
antivenom use plus higher standards of hospital care, but children remain at risk
[6–8].

Spiderbite is undoubtedly common [9], as are spiders [10], but most bites
are medically trivial and nearly all medically significant bites can be ascribed
to just a few groups of spiders: widow spiders (*Latrodectus*), recluse spiders
(*Loxosceles*), banana spiders (*Phoneutria*) and Australian funnel-web spiders
(*Atrax, Hadronyche*) [9, 11–13]. Deaths are rare.

Table 1. Summary of most recent published data on snakebite epidemiology globally [2]

Region	Envenoming		Deaths	
	Low estimate	High estimate	Low estimate	High estimate
Asia	237 379	1 184 550	15 385	57 636
Australasia	1099	1260	2	4
Caribbean	1098	8039	107	1161
Europe	3961	9902	48	128
Latin America	80 329	129 084	540	2298
North Africa and Middle East	3017	80 191	43	78
North America	2683	3858	5	7
Oceania	361	4635	227	516
Sub-Saharan Africa	90 622	419 639	3529	32 117
Total	420 549	1 841 158	19 886	93 945

Jellyfish encompass a vast range of species that share a common stinging mechanism, the cnidocil or nematocyst, an individual stinging cell that both makes and delivers venom [14, 15]. These cells can be numbered in the millions in the tentacles of large jellyfish, but while most species can induce local discomfort in humans, few can cause medically significant envenoming and almost none, lethal stings [14–16]. The clear exception, the Australo-Pacific box jellyfish (e.g., *Chironex fleckeri*), still occasionally kills humans, but in tiny numbers, almost unmeasurable compared to snakebite [14–18]. However, this threat has resulted in modified human behaviour in some at-risk regions, with consequent drops in rates of envenoming cases [19].

Stinging fish also will affect large numbers of humans, but while pain, however brief, can be severe, life is rarely at risk [15, 20].

Venomous animals: Taxonomy

Venomous animals are represented in 6 phyla, across 20 subphyla or classes, including multiple vertebrate taxa [21]. A detailed discussion of the taxonomy of venomous animals is beyond the scope of this chapter.

Venoms: A clinical overview

Venom can be defined as compounds or mixtures of toxins that are deleterious to another organism at a certain dosage [22]. Most venoms contain an array of toxins, usually with a diversity of actions. A single toxin can have multiple actions. For any single species of venomous animal, there will be a degree of variability in the composition of venom between individuals and even a single individual may have slight variations in venom composition over time [23–26]. Such variability can be seasonal or ontogenetic. The range of actions of toxins contained in a venom can reflect the variable types of prey that must be acquired, but may also reflect natural and rapid experimentation within populations of venomous animals [24, 25]. With such an array of toxins available, it might be expected that many would combine to cause toxicity in humans, but experience has shown that often clinical effects of significance can be attributed to just a few distinct toxins, or classes of toxins and it is these that are discussed further [27–29]. Venom classification is therefore considered below in terms of clinical effects in humans.

Neurotoxins

Paralysis

Paralytic neurotoxins are a recurring theme amongst venomous animals, being present in such diverse taxa as snakes, ticks, jellyfish, cone snails and octo-

Table 2. Major venomous animal groups commonly associated with neurotoxic paralysis [163]

Type of animal	Examples	Type of neurotoxin[#]
Elapid snakes	Kraits	Pre- and postsynaptic
	Coral snakes	Postsynaptic
	Mambas	Dendrotoxins and fasciculins
	Cobras (some)	Postsynaptic
	King cobra	Postsynaptic
	Selected Australian snakes; tiger snakes, taipans, rough scaled snake, death adders, copperheads	Pre- and postsynaptic
	Sea snakes	Postsynaptic
Viperid snakes	Mohave rattlesnake (some)	Presynaptic
	Neotropical rattlesnakes	Presynaptic
	Sri Lankan Russell's viper	Postsynaptic
Ticks	Paralysis ticks, *Ixodes* and *Dermacentor* spp.	Presynaptic
Cone shells	Variety of *Conus* spp.	Conotoxins
Octopusses	Blue ringed octopuses, *Hapalochlaena* spp.	Tetrodotoxin

[#] Definite, predominate or most likely major site of action/type of toxin in humans.

puses (Tab. 2). They are well characterised in snakes, where their primary site of action is the neuromuscular junction (Fig. 1), causing progressive flaccid paralysis, although the precise mechanism of action varies between toxins, often with multiple toxin types represented in a single venom [27–29]. The mode of action can be of great clinical relevance, affecting response to antivenom therapy. A number of other taxa possess paralytic neurotoxins, also causing flaccid paralysis, but their site and mode of action differ, again with clinical implications centred on duration of paralysis.

Excitation

Amongst invertebrate venomous animals, neuroexcitatory toxins predominate, especially amongst arthropods, but also amongst some marine animals, notably a few jellyfish species [21, 30]. The structure and mode of action varies amongst these toxins, but the prime clinical effect is generally similar, with rapid, sometimes extreme excitation of portions of the nervous system, most commonly autonomic stimulation resulting in a "catecholamine storm" effect, which can be rapidly lethal [31].

Myotoxins

Activated myotoxins induce myolysis and fall into two broad groups: the locally acting type and the systemically acting type, with the latter, in particular, able to cause potentially devastating and lethal effects as a result of secondary renal

1. Signal arrives at nerve cell ending (terminal axon) from brain
2. Neurotransmitter (ACh = Acetyl choline) is released from within nerve cell ending (terminal axon)
3. ACh leaves terminal axon and crosses the gap (synapse) to the muscle cell wall
4. The ACh binds to receptors (AChR) on the muscle cell wall, causing changes in the cell, resulting in muscle contraction
5. ACh is released from the receptor and broken down by an enzyme (ChEsterase)

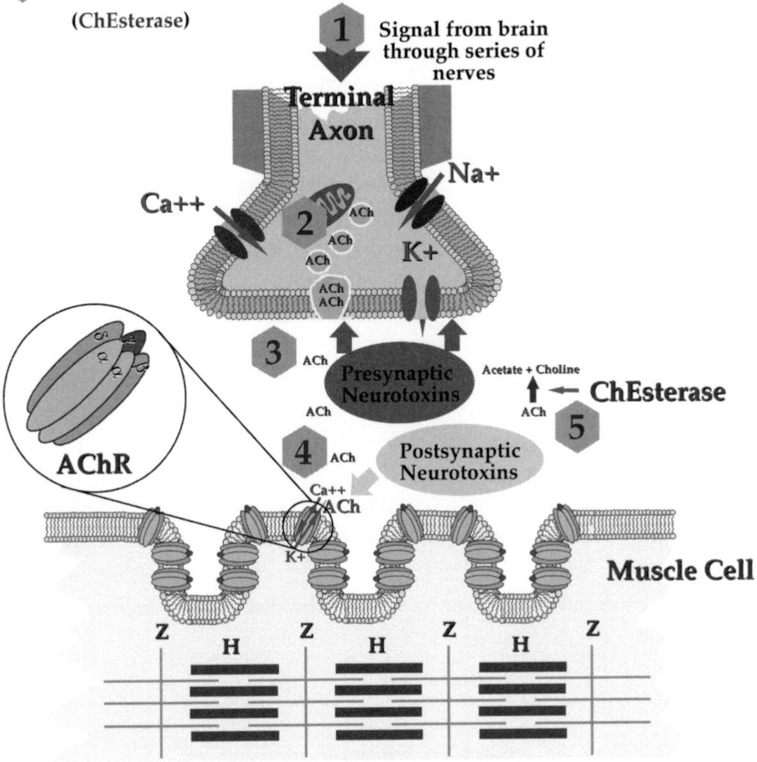

Figure 1. Diagrammatic representation of the site of action of principal neuromuscular junction paralytic neurotoxins (original photo/illustration copyright © Julian White).

failure, hyperkalaemia and cardiotoxicity [21, 28]. In most cases myotoxins are modified phospholipase A_2 (PLA_2) toxins, sometimes closely related to presynaptic neurotoxins [27]. In some cases a single toxin, such as notexin from Australian tiger snake (*Notechis scutatus*) venom, possesses both myotoxic and presynaptic neurotoxic activity, residing in separate portions of the molecule [27, 32]. Most venom myotoxins are found in snake venoms, although only in a minority of species, but myotoxic activity does occasionally occur with envenoming by other animals, including widow spider bites and mass hymenopteran stings [33–39].

Blood toxins

Coagulants and related toxins

Snakes have evolved a wide array of toxins to attack the complex haemostatic system (Fig. 2), and in many cases a variety of distinctly different toxins, with different targets, may coexist within a single venom [40, 41] (Tabs 3 and 4). However, more often a particular toxin will predominate in clinical effects on haemostasis. In the majority of species, this predominant activity will be pro-coagulant, most often causing either clotting through activation of thrombin, or direct attack on fibrinogen. While in the laboratory this may result in rapid plasma clotting, in an *in vivo* setting, like an envenomed human, the effects may be rather different, such as rapid consumption of all fibrinogen, causing hypocoagulability and a tendency to bleed [28, 40–45]. Thus, while these toxins may be characterised as potent clotting agents, their clinical effect may seem quite the opposite, effectively anticoagulating the blood through consumption of fibrinogen. There are exceptions to this, notably the potent clotting toxins in two Caribbean pit-viper venoms, which clinically cause extensive thrombosis, sometimes lethal [46–50]. Snakes are not the only venomous animals to specifically target haemostasis; a South American caterpillar with venom-tipped "hairs" can also cause severe procoagulant coagulopathy and fibrinogen depletion [51, 52]. Coagulopathy is also reported following stings by a few scorpion species, but is less well defined [53–55].

Anticoagulants

In addition to the secondary anticoagulant effects of some procoagulant toxins, some snake venoms contain potent true anticoagulant toxins that work by

Table 3. Summary of common target points for venoms interfering with the human haemostatic system [163]

Class of toxin	Specific activity
Procoagulant	Factor V activating
	Factor X activating
	Factor IX activating
	Prothrombin activating
	Fibrinogen clotting
Anticoagulant	Protein C activating
	Factor IX/X activating
	Thrombin inhibitor
	PLA$_2$
Fibrinolytic	Fibrin(ogen) degradation
	Plasminogen activation
Vessel wall interactive	Haemorrhagins
Platelet activity	Platelet aggregation inducers
	Platelet aggregation inhibitors
Plasma protein activator	SERPIN inhibitors

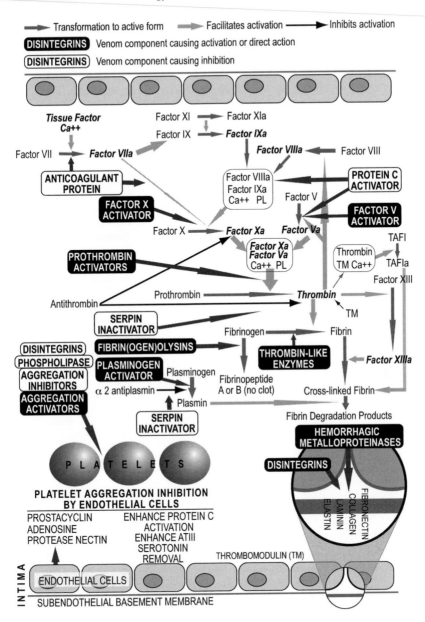

Figure 2. Diagrammatic representation of the human haemostatic pathways within blood vessels and some common targets where venom toxins can interfere with this process (original photo/illustration copyright © Julian White).

inhibiting the haemostatic process (Tabs 3 and 4) [40, 41]. This type of coag-ulopathy is largely restricted to a minority of snake species and, in most cases, causes less severe clinical problems than procoagulants [41, 56, 57].

Table 4. Major venomous animal groups likely to cause primary coagulopathy

Type of animal	Examples	Type of venom action
Colubrid snakes	Boomslang, vine snake	Procoagulant
	Yamakagashi, red necked keelback	Procoagulant
Elapid snakes	Selected Australian snakes; tiger snakes, rough scaled snake, taipans, brown snakes, broad headed snakes	Procoagulant
	Selected Australian snakes; mulga snakes, Collett's snake, black snakes, Papuan black snake	Anticoagulant
Viperid snakes	Saw scaled or carpet vipers	Procoagulant, disintegrins, haemorrhagins
	Gaboon vipers and puff adders	Procoagulant, antiplatelet, disintegrins, haemorrhagins
	Russell's vipers	Procoagulant, haemorrhagins
	Malayan pit viper	Procoagulant, antiplatelet, haemorrhagins
	North American rattlesnakes	Procoagulant, fibrinolytic, antiplatelet, disintegrins, haemorrhagins
	North American copperheads	Procoagulant, anticoagulant, fibrinolytic, disintegrins
	South American pit vipers (selected *Bothrops* spp.)	Procoagulant, Anticoagulant, fibrinolytic, disintegrins, haemorrhagins
	Asian green pit vipers (selected *Trimeresurus* spp.)	Anticoagulant, fibrinolytic, antiplatelet, disintegrins, haemorrhagins
	EuroAsian vipers (selected *Vipera* spp.)	Procoagulant, disintegrins, haemorrhagins,
Insects	Latin American caterpillars, *Lonomia* spp.	Procoagulant

Haemorrhagins

Synergy between diverse toxins can often result in more devastating effects on prey, or humans, and this is clearly the case with haemorrhagins, found in a number of snake venoms, mostly based on a metalloproteinase toxin that directly damages tissue, especially vascular tissue (Tabs 3 and 4) [40, 41, 58–61]. This direct damage promoting bleeding sites when combined with procoagulants that defibrinate, so preventing thrombotic repair of bleeding sites, which can lead to very severe clinical effects, especially locally around the bite site.

Nephrotoxins

Few primary nephrotoxins have been reported from venoms [62, 63], but secondary renal damage is very much a clinical problem with many snakebites, and without renal supportive therapy, such as dialysis, can prove lethal [64–72]. Secondary renal damage can occur through a variety of venom-mediated mechanisms, including coagulopathy, myolysis and hypotension [27, 29]. A particular syndrome, microangiopathic haemolytic anaemia (MAHA), can occur after envenoming by some snake species, and is characterised by intravascular haemolysis, thrombocytopenia and renal failure, but the precise causative mechanisms in envenoming remain to be elucidated [71, 73].

Necrotoxins

Local tissue injury following bites or stings is a common theme across many taxa, including snakes, spiders, scorpions (but only a very few species), centipedes and some marine animals such as the box jellyfish (*Chironex fleckeri*) and some of its relatives, and some stingrays [3, 11, 12, 18, 19, 21, 29, 45, 74–79]. The mechanism of injury is incompletely understood in most cases, although specific necrotoxins, such as sphingomyelinase D (from recluse spiders, *Loxosceles* spp.), are known [80–84], and the role of myotoxic PLA_2 in snake venom indicates a prime role in local tissue injury [81], while hyaluronidases are implicated in other venoms [85]. In many cases it is likely that local tissue necrosis is mediated by a complex interplay between several toxin effects and natural defence mechanisms within the victim.

Other toxins

In addition to the specific toxins and effects listed above, most venoms have a number of other, less well understood components, the clinical significance of which is usually unknown. This group, which may include the bulk of all toxin types, includes many low molecular weight toxins, including peptides. The latter are of increasing interest as potential templates for new pharmaceuticals, but undoubtedly some have significant clinical actions. Also within this group can be included a very diverse and important mix of toxins originating in cone snails (Coniidae; *Conus* spp. and some related hunting marine snails). Broadly classified as "conotoxins", these highly potent toxins are diverse in pharmacological effects and are already proving a rich area for new drug development [86].

Envenoming: A management overview

Envenoming will vary in severity, depending on the relative toxicity of the venom involved, the amount of venom actually delivered, the size of the victim, any pre-existing medical conditions, and environmental/social considerations [21, 28, 29]. It follows that even for a highly dangerous species, such as an Australian taipan snake (*Oxyuranus scutellatus*), the degree of envenoming and risk to life is not constant; while most cases may develop life threatening envenoming, often quite rapidly, there will still be some cases who never develop significant envenoming. Predicting which course each case will take, in the early stages, may be difficult to impossible, so it is a general rule that any case of definite or likely bite/sting by a medically significant venomous animal should be managed initially as a high priority medical emergency. Inevitably, a number of cases, perhaps the majority in some geographic regions, will ultimately prove to be only minor, with minimal or no envenoming. This is not a justification for assigning a low initial priority to bite/sting cases who seem apparently well on presentation. Envenoming can develop quickly, but can also be delayed in onset, yet still potentially lethal. Health professionals, except in a few situations, are unlikely to see or treat large numbers of bite/sting cases, so maintaining knowledge and skill can be problematic. It follows that in most situations, consultation with a doctor who is an expert in clinical toxinology is advisable, if optimal patient outcomes are to be ensured.

First aid

Pre-hospital care can, quite literally, be the difference between life and death in cases of envenoming, particularly for those species causing rapid severe effects such as respiratory paralysis and cardiotoxicity. There are few research-proven first aid methods for envenoming, yet many methods are used or recommended, most of which have either no benefit, or more commonly, cause actual harm [87–106]. Appropriate envenoming first aid should follow three principles; (1) do no harm, (2) immobilise venom to prevent it reaching target sites, and (3) support vital functions (airway, breathing, circulation) [107]. The last of these, supporting vital functions, if adopted universally, would likely save life in many cases of envenoming. It is often overlooked, but the importance of ensuring airway patency, respiration and circulation cannot be overemphasised. Avoiding causing harm is a vital principle, also generally overlooked. Table 5 lists well-known first aid methods that cause actual harm in envenoming and should not be used. Table 6 lists those few first aid methods shown to have value in envenoming.

Approach to management

As outlined earlier, two principles should guide care of the definitely or potentially envenomed patient: (1) all cases should be initially managed as potentially severe, and (2) expert advice should be sought at the earliest opportunity [107]. Locating expert advice will vary between countries, but in most cases, a major poisons information centre may be a reasonable first choice.

Table 5. Harmful or ineffective first aid methods that should not be used; only some prominent methods are listed

Method	Problems
Tourniquet	Direct pressure injury under narrow band tourniquet Severe pain Ischaemic limb damage (may include loss of limb) Potential for massive envenoming on release
Patent suction devices	Local tissue injury Increased local necrosis Painful Only minor venom removal No proven benefit in reducing envenoming
Local scarification, wound excision, amputation	Local tissue injury Painful May increase rate of envenoming May introduce local infection Can cause significant bleeding and blood loss No proven benefit in reducing envenoming
Electric shock	Dangerous No proven benefit in reducing envenoming
Chemical application	Potential toxicity No proven benefit in reducing envenoming
Snake stone	No proven benefit in reducing envenoming
Traditional healers	No proven benefit in reducing envenoming Cause potentially lethal delays in seeking definitive care

Consultant clinical toxinologists are currently a rare commodity within health systems, but this may improve over time, as training courses output more graduates.

The first priority when assessing a case of bite/sting with definite or potential envenoming, is to ensure vital systems functioning (airway, breathing, circulation). One must be aware of the possibility that coagulopathy may be present or develop, and physical interventions, such as i.v. line insertion, should be chosen with care to avoid causing uncontrollable bleeding problems. In the presence of coagulopathy, certain i.v. sites (subclavian, jugular, femoral) and actions (e.g., i.m. injections, fasciotomy, tracheostomy) are hazardous and should be avoided if at all possible. The second priority is establishing a working diagnosis, from which more definitive care, including antivenom therapy, will follow where indicated and available.

Diagnosis of envenoming

Diagnosis is a crucial early step in managing envenoming [28, 107]. Two parts of diagnosis can be discerned: (1) determining the cause of envenoming, from which more specific treatment can follow, and (2) determining the extent of

Table 6. First aid methods considered effective or possibly effective and not harmful

Method	Useful for
Immobilisation of bitten limb and whole patient	All snakebites and other causes of systemic envenoming
Australian pressure immobilisation bandage technique	All non-necrotic or haemorrhagic snakebites, including all Australian snakes, kraits, coral snakes, king cobra, sea snakes, mambas, selected cobras, South American rattlesnakes; Australian funnel-web spiders; Possibly (not proven experimentally or by clinical trial): Buthid scorpions, cone shells, blue ringed octopus
Cardio-pulmonary resuscitation	Any bite/sting causing impaired cardiac or respiratory function
Removal of attached organism	Any bite/sting, to prevent ongoing envenoming; specifically important to remove bee sting/venom gland, paralysis tick, Helodermatid lizard
Hot water (to 45 °C; care to avoid hotter water and thermal injury)	All venomous fish stings, stingray injuries, jellyfish stings (not yet proven for box jellyfish stings)
Direct wound care/staunching bleeding	Injuries affecting major blood vessels, such as some stingray injuries
Copious fluid irrigation of the eye	All cases with venom in the eye, particularly spitting cobras
Removal of rings, other constricting objects from limbs, especially digits	May reduce the chance of local swelling causing ischaemic damage
Reassurance	Calming the patient and keeping them still may reduce the rate of onset of envenoming and development of anxiety-related symptoms
Retrieval of the envenoming animal	If the culprit has been killed or captured and can be safely transported with the patient, do so, as this will assist in accurate diagnosis; CAVEAT: Do not waste time or risk further bites/stings to kill/capture the culprit

envenoming, including severity, progression, systems affected, and evident complications, which will guide the degree and nature of any therapeutic response. All three elements of the diagnostic process, history, examination, and laboratory tests, play a role, but the extent to which each may contribute varies with the venomous animal concerned. For many species, laboratory tests may add little to diagnosis and history will be crucial. However, the history may give no early clue to diagnosis, particularly when the presentation is symptom-driven, perhaps without any suggestion of a bite/sting occurring or being causative. Thus, in unexplained cases of coagulopathy, paralysis, neuroexcitation, myolysis, renal failure, collapse, convulsions, or local tissue injury, envenoming may sometimes be an important differential diagnosis needing consideration and exclusion.

History

Ideally, a toxinological history will answer some or all of the following questions: (1) is a bite/sting a likely diagnosis, (2) do the circumstances (including a description of the assailant, if available) and geographic location of the bite/sting indicate likely assailants, (3) does the patient have any symptomatology suggestive of envenoming, local or systemic, and does the pattern of symptoms indicate likely assailants, (4) are there any patient-related factors that might influence diagnosis, severity of envenoming, or outcome, and (5) is the patient in need of treatment urgently, or likely to need treatment later?

The key areas for questioning are shown in Table 7, but these are designed to fit all common situations, while in the real world, the list of possible assailants will likely be narrower and so the range of questions required will be less. Often the key diagnostic features emerge early and allow a more directed approach to confirm the likely assailant and therapeutic response required. However, some caution is required, because any venomous animal can, on occasion, cause an atypical presentation.

Examination

Examination is directed towards finding evidence that a bite/sting has occurred, and if any local or systemic envenoming effects are present. Where the history has not clearly identified a likely assailant, examination findings may help to narrow diagnostic possibilities. Key areas for examination are shown in Table 8. As for history, this list is designed to cover many common possibilities and in the real world, a more directed examination is often possible. Again, caution is required, to ensure no key signs are missed because early assumptions are made about the likely culprit.

Laboratory tests

Specific testing for evidence of envenoming is only applicable for some animals, mostly snakes, while no lab tests are routinely indicated for bites/stings by many non-snake venomous animals. Key lab tests are shown in Table 9, and as with history and examination, selection of which tests to request, if any, will be determined by the circumstances in each case, particularly the possible assailants to be considered.

Urgent care

The acutely and significantly envenomed patient presents an urgent case requiring prompt, accurate assessment and directed treatment. The patient presenting in extremis will require immediate life supportive care, then best-guess diagnosis of the likely culprit(s) and urgent specific treatment to cover these animals, followed by more considered assessment and treatment, once the acute emergency is controlled. In such a situation, it may still be possible to rapidly ascertain key diagnostic features, such as presence of coagulopathy, paralysis, myo-

Table 7. Important points in a toxinological history

Area of questioning	Relevance
Circumstances of bite/sting	May indicate likely degree of envenoming (brief glancing attack *versus* chewing bite/prolonged sting), but even glancing bite can sometimes cause severe envenoming; May indicate likely culprit
Geographic location	Can narrow range of possible culprits
Description of animal	Can help determine likely culprit, but beware colour variability, especially in snakes
Number of bites/stings	Multiple bites/stings may cause increased envenoming
Immediate symptoms	May indicate possible culprit; May indicate likely severity
First aid, including timing	May influence onset of envenoming symptoms and signs
Onset and nature of any symptoms Specifically enquire about symptoms of: • Paralysis (drooping/heavy eyelids, slurred speech, drooling, difficulty walking, moving limbs, holding head up, breathing, swallowing) • Myolysis (muscle weakness, pain, tenderness, red to black urine) • Coagulopathy (bleeding gums, haematemesis, haematuria, melaena, sudden bruising) • Renal damage (altered urine output, thirst) • Cardiotoxicity (palpitations, collapse) • Necrotoxicity (bite/sting site pain, blistering, bleeding, darkened or blue-black skin, eschar formation) • Neuroexcitatory envenoming (increased sweating, salivation, lacrimation, piloerection, respiratory distress with frothing (pulmonary oedema), fasciculation of muscles, including tongue, nystagmus) • Non-specific (headache, nausea, vomiting, abdominal pain, diarrhoea, dizziness, collapse, convulsions, metallic taste in mouth)	Can determine pattern and severity of envenoming, which can indicate likely identity of culprit and requirement for treatment
Medications	May identify medications that might interact with envenoming or skew interpretation of lab tests (e.g., warfarin and coagulopathy)
Past history	May identify pre-existing conditions of relevance to envenoming
Allergies	Particularly important to determine if there is a potential allergy to any treatment, such as antivenom, OR if the symptoms could be more related to allergy than envenoming

Table 8. Key points in the toxinological examination

Area of examination	Relevance
Bite/sting site	Is there evidence of multiple bites/stings, ongoing bleeding (coagulopathy), bruising (coagulopathy), blistering/bleb formation (necrosis), increased sweating (neuroexcitatory envenoming), major swelling (fluid shifts, impending shock), significant mechanical trauma (stingray), attached tentacle (jellyfish) or stinger (honey bee)?
Bitten/stung region/limb	Is there evidence of venom spread (lymphadenopathy or tenderness, lymphangitic tracking) or regional envenoming (spreading blistering/blebs, ecchymosis, increased sweating)?
Critical systems (cardiac, respiratory)	Is there hyper/hypotension, brady/tachycardia, cardiac arrhythmia, cyanosis/respiratory distress, use of accessory muscles? What is Glascow coma score (GCS)?
Neurological systems	Is there evidence of paralytic neurotoxicity (cranial nerve signs like ptosis, ophthalmoplegia, fixed dilated pupils, drooling, dysarthria, dysphagia, altered taste/smell, limb muscle weakness, reduced or absent deep tendon reflexes)?
	Is there evidence of neuroexcitatory envenoming (increased local, regional, or generalised sweating, piloerection, increased salivation, lacrimation, muscle fasciculation, including tongue, pulmonary oedema)?
Haemostasis systems	Is there evidence of increased bleeding (oozing from bite site, i.v. sites, gums, elsewhere, bruising, CNS signs of intracranial bleeding) OR of thrombotic problems (deep vein thrombosis, pulmonary embolus, stroke)?

lysis, or neuroexcitation, which will guide the therapeutic response. The same rapid assessment techniques can be utilised to effectively triage cases with less life threatening features. Observation of the patient's face can often show if they are in significant pain (grimace), if they have any early developing paralytic features (ptosis, loss of facial tone, partial ophthalmoplegia; Fig. 3), or neuroexcitatory features (increased sweating, lacrimation), or coagulopathy (bleeding bite site, gums; Fig. 4), while a simple check of any i.v. insertion or sampling sites will reveal evidence of coagulopathy (continued ooze, bleeding, extending bruising), and a check of the bite/sting site will reveal if there is rapidly advancing swelling, or early tissue injury features (ecchymotic blistering, marked dark skin colouration, especially if clear demarcating edges; Fig. 5), or early neuroexcitation (increased local sweating, piloerection). If major neuroexcitatory envenoming is a likely diagnosis, chest auscultation (for signs of pulmonary oedema) is required. Except where pulmonary oedema is a significant risk, most envenomed patients will benefit from early i.v. fluid load.

Table 9. Key laboratory investigations to consider in a case of definite or suspected envenoming. The actual choice of tests will be determined partly by the type of organism and the clinical setting

Test	Relevance	Relevant fauna
Whole blood clotting time (WBCT)	If substantially prolonged and/or with weak clot, can indicate coagulopathy (NOTE: always use glass vessel, do control)	Most snakebites, Brazilian *Lonomia* caterpillars, Iranian *Hemiscorpius* and *Nebo* scorpions, recluse spiders
20-minute WBCT (is blood clotted at 20 minutes?)	Simple derivative of WBCT, validated for some snakebites	As above
Coagulation studies • INR/prothrombin time • aPPT/PTTK • d-dimer/XDP/FDP • fibrinogen	Definitive assessment of coagulopathy; d-dimer may be most sensitive early measure of developing coagulopathy	As above
Complete blood examination • platelets • haemoglobin (Hb) • blood film for evidence of haemolysis • white cell and absolute lymphocyte count • reticulocytes (if haemolysis)	Important in assessing if there is haemolysis, MAHA, or isolated thrombocytopenia. Early absolute lymphopenia can be another marker for envenoming	As above, plus other fauna that may cause haemolysis, including severe jellyfish stings, massive hymeno-pteran multiple stings
Blood chemistry, especially • renal function • creatine kinase (CK, for myolysis) • electrolytes (particularly K^+) • bilirubin (if haemolysis) • glucose (if scorpion sting) • liver function tests (LFTs; if haemolysis, myo-lysis, or if pancreatitis is suspected after scorpion sting)	Each parameter specific for particular envenoming/complica-tion, such as renal damage, myolysis, haemolysis, hyperkalaemia	Most snakebites, any major systemic envenoming/ collapse, envenoming where haemolysis suspected, such as mass hymenopteran stings
Arterial blood gases	Principally assessing oxygen-ation, if respiratory compromise, such as in neurotoxic paralysis	Any bite/sting where respiratory failure/paralysis possible, including selected snakebites, Australian funnel-web spider, scorpion, para-lysis tick, cone shell, blue ringed octopus, Irukandji jellyfish envenoming
Bite site wound swabs • venom detection (Australia) • culture and sensitivity	In Australian snakebites, for venom detection; everywhere, if wound is infected	Australian snakes; any infected wound

Specific treatment: Antivenom

In general, the only specific treatment for envenoming is antivenom and this is only available for some venomous animals.

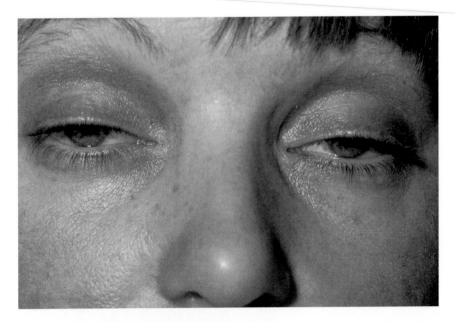

Figure 3. Ptosis, often the first sign of developing neurotoxic envenoming (*Notechis scutatus* bite) (original photo/illustration copyright © Julian White).

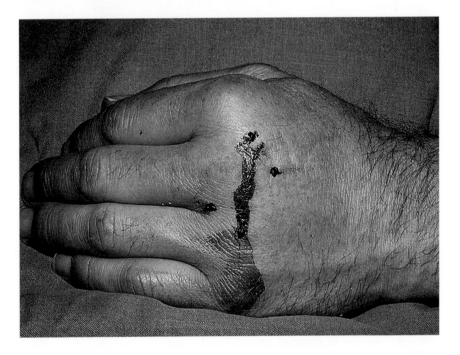

Figure 4. Persistent blood oozing from bite area, often indicative of coagulopathy (*Pseudechis* spp. bite) (original photo/illustration copyright © Julian White).

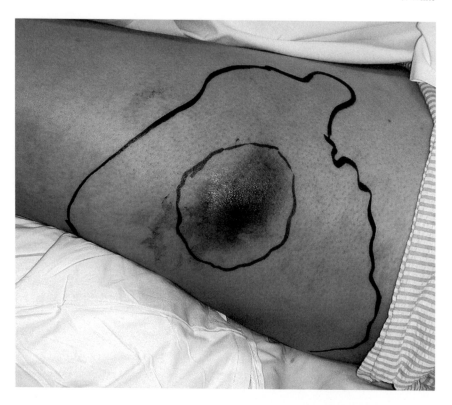

Figure 5. Demarcating area of tissue injury, indicative of an area likely of developing necrosis (*Pseudechis australis* bite) (original photo/illustration copyright © Julian White).

The era of antivenom therapy for envenoming dates back to the work of Calmette and others, in the final years of the 19th century [108]. Antivenom is essentially antibody raised against whole venom(s) or venom fractions in a domesticated animal (horse, sheep, goat, rabbit) and works by binding to toxins, either at the active site (so rendering them inactive), or elsewhere (allowing clearance) [109, 110]. It follows that a given antivenom contains neutralising antibody against only those venoms used in the immunising mix, so utility in treating envenoming by other species is dependent on sufficient antigenic similarities between venoms [111, 112]. For some venoms, there is considerable similarity with venoms from other, usually related, species. This provides cross-specific protection, therefore a particular antivenom may be effective in treating envenoming by a number of different species. However, such cross-specific protection is not a universal, or even particularly common, finding. As a rule, then, antivenom used in treatment should be proven as specific for a particular species, or group of species [110].

There are a variety of ways of producing antivenom, although all currently in use start by hyperimmunising an animal [109, 110, 112]. Nearly all antivenoms are based on mammalian IgG antibody, most commonly equine (horse). The IgG can be refined in a number of ways to eliminate contaminants from plasma that can stimulate adverse reactions. IgG can be further fractionated to yield fractions of IgG, each with distinct properties, advantages and disadvantages. Whole IgG and Fab_2 antivenoms have a prolonged half life, compared to Fab antivenoms, so they maintain clinically useful blood levels over several days, important in neutralising late-released venom from a depot at the bite site, but their larger size limits extravascular spread. Fab antivenoms have better extravascular penetration, but at the cost of short half life, measured in hours, usually necessitating repeat doses or continuous infusion [113–115]. Few Fab antivenoms are available, the principle ones being for North American pit viper bite (CroFab®) and European adder bite (Viperatab®), but early experience with these affinity-column-refined ovine (sheep) antivenoms shows they are relatively safe and effective, but commonly require repeat dosing to counter short half life [113–118]. In North America, an issue of recurrence of coagulopathy has raised questions about effectiveness, since this recurrence is sometimes resistant to further antivenom doses. However, examination of case experience with the previous equine whole IgG antivenom shows recurrence was also an issue and other factors may be at play [114]. Arguments have been mounted that whole IgG antivenoms are the most effective, but traditional manufacture has been associated with high levels of adverse effects [119–122]. As a consequence, many producers have moved to Fab_2 antivenoms, which are as effective, but generally have been considered to have a better adverse effect profile, a view now questioned [119–122]. However, development of caprylic acid treatment of whole IgG antivenoms is claimed to produce a product with high efficacy and a good adverse effect profile, with a further advantage of lower production cost [123–126]. This may swing antivenom production back towards predominantly whole IgG product.

Horses are by far the predominant host animal for antivenom production [109–112, 127–129]. They are relatively easy to manage, provide large plasma volumes with regular venesection or plasma pheresis, are comparatively safe as vectors of disease transmission, and production techniques are well established [130, 131]. However, equine antivenoms, especially whole IgG, have been associated with sometimes very high levels of adverse effects [132]. Because of this, a few producers have explored other animals, notably sheep [113, 115–117, 133]. Ovine antivenoms are now produced by two major producers and have proved safe but, because of an increased risk of disease transmission, particularly viral and prion disease, sheep are only practical in the few countries with certified safe flocks [131]. If new processing steps that can guarantee removal of infectious agents are developed, this may make ovine antivenoms more widespread, but the use of caprylic acid purification of whole IgG equine antivenoms may render such ovine antivenom developments unnecessary. Goats have also been used in the past and one producer currently uses rabbits for a low output specialised antivenom [134]. Current research is investigating camels, as these may be easier than horses in some regions, such as Africa, and camelid IgG can be more readily fractionated into really small molecular size antivenoms that may open up possibilities for combined systemic and local use [135, 136]. This work is purely experimental and it is at present not known if it will translate to commercial production. Another different approach using hens to produce egg-based IgY antivenoms has also been explored, but a number of problems, including widespread major immunity to such a product, with the potential for severe adverse reactions, appears at this time to make commercial IgY antivenoms unlikely [137–140]. The development of genetically engineered antivenom production, using recombinant methods, is at an early stage of development, with no commercial products available as yet, although research is progressing, both into recombinant production of immunising toxins, and complete recombinant production of specific antivenom [141–144].

Antivenom theory
Antivenom works by binding specifically to venom toxins and rendering them inert and/or speeding clearance from the circulation [109, 112, 145]. To be effective, antivenom must rapidly bind and inactivate/remove all circulating venom from the circulation, and as far as possible, the rest of the body. This requires primary intravascular distribution, which is why antivenom should, in most cases, be given only i.v., not used locally or as an i.m. injection. There are a few antivenoms for which i.m. injection is advocated or has shown favourable results [134, 145–158] with some evidence that it is effective, although this is controversial in light of recent studies [158–162]. However, these are for organisms with more slowly developing and, in general, non-lethal envenomings.

The prime requirement for antivenom is therefore i.v. administration of an initial dose expected to fully neutralise all circulating venom. Except for Fab antivenoms, most or all of the antivenom will remain in the circulation, yet for many venoms, key components will exit the circulation to reach their extravascular targets, such as the neuromuscular junction or skeletal muscle. Toxins acting on the haemostatic system and haemorrhagins act within the intravascular system, so are readily accessible to antivenom. Concentration gradients between extravascular and intravascular venom levels are likely to draw extravascular venom back into the circulation, for neutralisation, as intravascular venom levels fall with neutralisation by antivenom. This mechanism requires high levels of antivenom, compared to venom, explaining the clinical requirement for adequate antivenom doses initially. Antivenom administered i.m. will be slow to reach high intravascular concentrations [160, 162], so will be far less efficacious, particularly for rapid, acute, severe envenoming, as caused by many snake species. Similarly, locally injected antivenom is unlikely to reach significant blood levels, so will be ineffective against circulating and distributed venom. Therefore, even if low molecular weight antivenoms are developed for local injection, there will still be a critical need for simultaneous i.v. administration.

What is antivenom effective for?

Antivenom is an effective antidote against venom components that are specifically covered as antigens for a given antivenom [163]. This implies that antivenom must be specific for the type of venomous animal involved, or have proven cross protection for that animal. It also implies antivenom must be able to access the venom. This may be difficult for locally sequestered venom, such as in the bitten limb. It follows that in general, antivenom is far more effective at neutralising systemic effects than local effects, except for low molecular weight antivenoms (Fab), which more readily reach extravascular sites. However, antivenom cannot repair injured tissue, it can only bind to venom with appropriate antigenic matching. Therefore, some venom effects that involve damage to target tissue, such as presynaptic neurotoxicity (terminal axonal damage), myotoxicity (damage to muscle cells), renal toxicity (direct or indirect renal damage) and secondary damage from coagulopathy, are not reversible with antivenom therapy. For this reason it is important to detect systemic envenoming at the earliest opportunity and commence appropriate antivenom therapy, before such tissue damage is extensive. Equally, this explains why late antivenom therapy to remedy such tissue injury is ineffective and generally not warranted. A caveat is that continuing venom absorption from the bite site, causing ongoing envenoming, requires maintenance of adequate antivenom levels, which may warrant repeat dosing, even for whole IgG or Fab_2 antivenoms. Clinically, this seems applicable for continuing myolysis. A list of clinical effects and their responsiveness to antivenom is given in Table 10.

The indications for administering antivenom in a case of envenoming are, to some extent, specific for each type of venomous animal, and discussing requirements for each species or antivenom is beyond the scope of this chapter. There are, however, some broad principles that apply in many circumstances. Firstly, antivenom should only be given if there is evidence of significant envenoming, either systemic, or in some settings, local. It is rarely justified giving antivenom to a patient who exhibits no evidence of envenoming. Bites/stings by nearly all venomous animals have a significant and variable rate of "dry bites", where bite/sting marks may be present, but insufficient venom is injected to cause medically significant envenoming effects. Just because a bite/sting is from a highly dangerous species does not mean significant envenoming will develop. Secondly, in most settings, antivenom should be given as soon as there is evidence of systemic envenoming developing. There are exceptions, particularly for those venomous animals that cause predominantly local effects, but not necrosis, and/or non-specific systemic effects with a low likelihood of threat to life (e.g., headache, nausea, vomiting, diarrhoea, abdominal pain, dizziness). Systemic effects that are virtually always worrying will usually indicate the need for antivenom (Tab. 11).

Choosing an antivenom

The ideal antivenom will be safe and efficacious at neutralising target venoms. In regions where polyvalent antivenoms predominate, covering all major med-

Table 10. Key clinical envenoming effects and their responsiveness to antivenom

Toxin activity type	Clinical effects and responsiveness to antivenom
Paralytic neurotoxin • Presynaptic • Postsynaptic • Anticholinesterase	Flaccid paralysis • Resistant to late antivenom therapy • Often reversal with antivenom therapy • Muscle fasciculation
Excitatory neurotoxin	Often causes "catecholamine storm", massive stimulation of autonomic nervous system; can be very responsive to antivenom, but in some cases (some scorpions) must be given early to be effective
Myotoxin	Systemic skeletal muscle damage; may respond to antivenom, but damage pre-antivenom will remain, causing symptoms and lab test changes (mainly elevated creatine kinase, CK)
Haemostatic system toxins	Interfere with normal haemostasis, causing either bleeding or thrombosis; often respond to antivenom, as only effective treatment, but not effective for all venoms
Haemorrhagins	Damage vascular wall, causing bleeding; role of antivenom uncertain, may be helpful
Nephrotoxins	Direct renal damage; value of late antivenom uncertain
Cardiotoxins	Direct cardiotoxicity; role of antivenom uncertain, controversial
Necrotoxins	Direct tissue injury at the bite site/bitten limb; antivenom, given early, may be of some value, but overall results are not encouraging
Non-specific systemic effects (headache, vomiting etc.)	Often indirectly mediated; antivenom often very effective at controlling symptoms

Table 11. Indicators for antivenom. Note only some indicators will be theoretically applicable for any particular species of venomous animal [191]

Indicators
Any degree of developing or progressing neurotoxic paralysis
Any significant disturbance of haemostasis (except pure secondary disseminated intravascular coagulation, DIC)
Any degree of significant myolysis
Acute renal damage
Acute haemolysis
Prolonged collapse or convulsions in confirmed envenoming
Major and progressive local swelling
Developing necrosis (except if presenting days later)

ically important species of snakes, there is no absolute need to determine the type of snake in choosing an antivenom. However, in this setting, knowledge of the type of snake may allow better prediction of likely progress, complications and prognosis, all valuable for the patient and the therapeutic process.

In regions where there is a choice of several different antivenoms, without one that covers all possible snakes in the region, there is an absolute need to determine the type of snake with a sufficient level of confidence to allow choice of an appropriate antivenom. There are several possible methods for determining the type of snake. All have advantages and risks and wherever possible, combination of several methods is preferred, to assure better accuracy of the result. Venom detection has been used as an experimental technique for many years [164–175]. In Australia and New Guinea there is a unique commercial snake venom detection kit (SVDK), designed specifically to determine the most appropriate antivenom to use [176–185]. While certainly useful, it is not useful in every case and suffers from both false-positive and false-negative results, the likelihood of which are increased with certain test sample choices. This SVDK was not designed to act as a diagnostic screen for snakebite and should not be used as such. It is possible that similar snake venom detection systems may be developed for other regions for which no single universal polyvalent snake antivenom is available.

Given the problems of identifying the snake, if a polyvalent antivenom is not available, why would producers choose to make monovalent or limited polyvalent antivenoms instead of full polyvalent antivenoms? One reason is the practical mechanics of antivenom production. If the range of snakes to be covered is large, and cross protection between species limited, there may be more different venoms required than is practical, both from an immunising and vial size perspective. Inevitably a polyvalent antivenom, covering a number of species, will generally be of higher volume than specific or monovalent antivenoms for each species. That higher volume may translate into higher costs or lower costs (reduced range of products required), but will inevitably result in a higher risk for the patient, because a higher volume of antivenom must be injected, only some of which is actually therapeutically useful (the antibody fraction against the particular snake involved in envenoming that patient). Delayed (type III) hypersensitivity reactions (serum sickness) can occur with any antivenom, but are more common with high volume antivenoms such as polyvalents [109, 117, 121, 136, 139, 148, 152, 160, 163, 186–190]. Therefore, for the patient, to reduce adverse effects and, in some cases, cost, a specific or monovalent antivenom is a better choice, providing the identity of the snake can be reliably determined. Australia and New Guinea have both specific/monovalent and a polyvalent antivenom against regional snakes. The SVDK allows preferential use of specific/monovalent antivenoms, rather than polyvalent antivenom, in most cases, which reduces rates of adverse effects and cost to the health system. Another option in parts of Australia, where the range of important venomous snakes is limited, is to use a mixture of two specific/monovalent antivenoms to cover possible species, where identity of the snake is not assured [134]. A similar approach is possible in some other regions.

For each region, clear delineation of the envenoming profile for each important species can provide the basis for diagnostic algorithms, as used in Australia

(Fig. 6), which can assist in determining the species involved and is a useful confirmatory procedure, even if venom detection is available [134, 191].

While the discussion above has been directed to antivenoms against venomous snakes, the principles apply to all antivenoms. However, for most other venomous animals, if an antivenom exists, it is a specific/monovalent product, because the range of species required to be covered in any region often does not warrant a polyvalent antivenom. There are exceptions to this, such as polyvalent anti-scorpion and/or anti-spider antivenoms, particularly in parts of South America, North Africa and the Middle East [127–130]. Advising on specific choice methods for antivenoms in each region is beyond the scope of this chapter.

Administering antivenom

As discussed earlier, in most settings, acute and rapidly severe envenoming mandates i.v. administration of antivenom to ensure rapid, therapeutically adequate blood levels. For those few antivenoms where the producer recommends an i.m. route, the clinician treating the patient should determine if this is advisable in the individual circumstances, if necessary in consultation with an expert (e.g., through a poisons centre or a clinical toxinology service).

The method of i.v. administration will be dictated by several factors: (1) the volume of the antivenom at the selected dose, (2) the size of the patient, (3) pre-existing health problems for the patient, (4) the availability of i.v. administration equipment, such as sterile i.v. giving sets, i.v. fluids, i.v. pumps etc. High-volume antivenoms in small children may pose fluid overload issues, exacerbated by the common practice of diluting antivenom in an i.v. carrier solution, up to 1:10, such as normal saline or Hartman's solution. In general, where practical, such dilution and administration through a giving set is advantageous, because it allows precise control of rate of infusion and may make adjustments for adverse reactions easier. There are other methods which are also validated, particularly direct slow i.v. injection of antivenom at the bedside, easiest if the total volume is not high [191]. This approach has several advantages; it requires less equipment, so is generally easier and cheaper, particularly in less well resourced health systems, and it forces the doctor, who must give the injection, to be present at the bedside throughout administration. This makes it far more likely that any adverse reaction will be detected early and the injection stopped and the reaction promptly treated. With diluted i.v. infusions there is a risk that staff will start the infusion and then be occupied with other duties or patients, potentially missing early signs of reactions and so missing the opportunity to treat early, when treatment will likely be more effective. In a well-managed hospital setting such risks can be avoided and it is the author's practice, in most cases, to give antivenom by diluted i.v. infusion.

Selection of the dose of antivenom is beyond the scope of this chapter, because it will vary between antivenoms, organisms causing envenoming, and degree of envenoming. There is one important principle that is universal; dose is not determined by patient size, therefore children receive the same dose as

DETERMINING THE MOST LIKELY SNAKE BASED ON CLINICAL FINDINGS

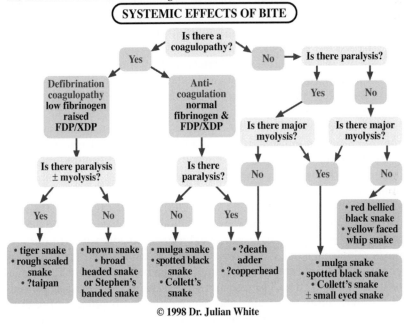

START HERE ➡ **LOCAL EFFECTS OF BITE**

Examine the bite site

Minimal local effects, no significant redness, swelling, bruising

Obvious redness, swelling, ± bruising

Moderate to severe local pain

Minimal or no local pain

Marked swelling after 3+ hours

Only mild swelling after 3+ hours

• ?death adder

• brown snake
• ?taipan

• mulga snake
• red bellied black snake
• yellow faced whip snake

• tiger snake
• rough scaled snake
• ?taipan

PLEASE NOTE:
This chart cannot cover all possible situations and assumes an understanding of the symptoms and signs of local, general and specific envenoming by Australian snakes. If in doubt, seek advice from the **Poisons Information Centre (131126)** and from your local **Critical Care Referral Network**

Combine this information with the result of the systemic effects key (below) to give a best guess for the type of snake most likely to have caused the bite. Accuracy can be improved by matching this with known snake fauna for the region where the bite occured.

SYSTEMIC EFFECTS OF BITE

Is there a coagulopathy?

Yes — No — Is there paralysis?

Defibrination coagulopathy low fibrinogen raised FDP/XDP

Anti-coagulation normal fibrinogen & FDP/XDP

Yes — No

Is there major myolysis?

Is there major myolysis?

Is there paralysis ± myolysis?

Is there paralysis?

No

Yes

No

Yes — No

Yes — No

No — Yes

• red bellied black snake
• yellow faced whip snake

• tiger snake
• rough scaled snake
• ?taipan

• brown snake
• broad headed snake or Stephen's banded snake

• mulga snake
• spotted black snake
• Collett's snake

• ?death adder
• ?copperhead

• mulga snake
• spotted black snake
• Collett's snake
± small eyed snake

© 1998 Dr. Julian White

Figure 6. Diagnostic algorithms for Australian snakebite; an example of what may be possible if detailed profiling of envenoming by snake species is undertaken in a given geographic region (original photo/illustration copyright © Julian White).

adults. There is no paediatric dose for antivenom. Doses should never be reduced because the patient is a child.

Adverse reactions

All antivenoms are, by definition, foreign antigens when they are administered and all have the potential for adverse reactions, both early and late [134, 163, 191, 192]. The more highly purified the antivenom, in general, the lower the rate of reactions, but as noted earlier, whole IgG antivenoms purified with caprylic acid, may enjoy comparatively low reaction rates, especially compared with simple whole IgG antivenoms.

The causes of adverse reactions to antivenom are multiple, but contaminating components in the antivenom are of great importance and may include pyrogens from bacterial or other contamination, other plasma components as contaminants, such as albumin, Fc components of fractionated IgG, and elements of equine plasma that cause allergic responses [109, 119, 121, 136, 191, 192]. In addition, prior exposure to the antivenom or the host animal used in immunising may stimulate an allergic response, even IgE production in rare cases. Modern production methods should exclude contamination with live bacteria or viruses, but prions are harder to exclude, hence the requirement, particularly applicable to ovine antivenoms, that the host animal is from a flock/herd certified free of prion disease [131, 132].

The principle early reactions, in order of frequency and severity, are an erythematous rash, by itself of little consequence, rigors indicative of a pyrogenic reaction, and least common, a significant systemic allergic reaction, often characterised as "anaphylaxis", although true IgE involvement occurs only in the minority of cases, with complement activation by the antivenom being a more common aetiology. The principle delayed reaction is serum sickness and this is partly dependent on the volume of antivenom administered; the higher the volume, the greater the risk.

For early reactions, other than simple rash, the first response should be to stop the antivenom infusion. If there is a major systemic allergic reaction, classic treatment for anaphylaxis is warranted, including adrenaline (epinephrine), i.v. fluids, resuscitation, as indicated. Detailed discussion of the management of anaphylaxis is beyond the scope of this chapter and readers are referred to current published reviews on this topic [193]. Once the reaction is controlled, antivenom infusion can be cautiously restarted, sometimes requiring titration of rate against blood pressure response and i.v. diluted adrenaline infusion [134]. The development of an anaphylactic reaction to antivenom is not a justification for abandoning antivenom therapy in that patient. If antivenom has been commenced on sound clinical grounds, because of major or life threatening envenoming, those grounds remain valid. Nevertheless, it is prudent to re-evaluate the extent/severity of envenoming before committing to restarting antivenom.

For late reactions, notably serum sickness, the patient will often have been discharged prior to onset, so it is essential that all patients receiving antivenom, whatever the type, amount, or route, be informed of the possibility of serum sickness and presenting symptoms, to maximise the probability they will promptly return for treatment. A detailed discussion of management for serum sickness is beyond the scope of this chapter, but oral corticosteroids such as prednisolone, and oral antihistamines are generally the mainstays of treatment. Some doctors advise a short (about 5–7 days) course of oral corticosteroids after administration of antivenom, to reduce the likelihood of serum sickness. This is not a clinical trial-proven therapy, but logically may be of some benefit.

There is a considerable amount of literature on use of prophylaxis prior to antivenom, in an attempt to reduce the rate of adverse reactions. Several key points have emerged. Firstly, sensitivity testing prior to antivenom is a non-predictive and dangerous procedure, which should never be undertaken, even though some antivenom producers still recommend it [163, 191]. Secondly, there is no convincing evidence that antihistamines or steroids such as hydro-cortisone prevent adverse reactions [163, 194]. There is highly conflicting evidence that subcutaneous adrenaline may be useful, but most recent studies and advice from leading authorities is that adrenaline as premedication for antivenom is inappropriate [163, 195].

Other antidotes

Antivenoms are only available to cover some of the more dangerous venomous animals. Even where antivenom is available, there may be other treatments that can be effective as ancillary care, although not as a replacement for antivenom.

For neurotoxic paralysis caused by purely post-synaptic neurotoxins, anti-cholinesterases are theoretically attractive and have shown efficacy for envenoming by some species. By reducing the rate of acetylcholine destruction within the neuromuscular junction (Fig. 1), it is sometimes possible to overwhelm the effect of the toxin in blocking the muscle end-plate acetylcholine receptor, thus reducing the extent of paralytic features. In selected cases this may be enough to wean the patient off the need for ventilatory respiratory support, but frequent re-dosing is usually required. This ancillary treatment has been successful in treating paralysis following bites by Philippines cobras (*Naja philippinensis*), death adders (*Acanthophis* spp.) and sea snakes (New Caledonia; species not certain) and is likely applicable to a wider range of snakes [196–199]. However, recent research indicates at least some death adders also have pre-synaptic neurotoxins in their venom, which may explain cases refractory to both antivenom and anticholinesterase treatment.

For scorpion stings causing neuroexcitatory envenoming, some clinicians report that prazosin is highly effective [200–206]. Experimental studies also indicate prazosin may be effective in countering Irukandji jellyfish (*Carukia barnesi*) envenoming, in cases with significant cardiac involvement [207, 208]. In both these settings there is a form of "catecholamine storm". However, the cardiovascular collapse caused by severe box jellyfish (*Chironex fleckeri*) envenoming is not responsive to prazosin [209, 210].

General treatment

For most cases with significant envenoming it is a reasonable and common practice to give an initial i.v. fluid load (crystalloids), the degree of loading being tempered by patient factors such as presumed degree of dehydration (if any), patient age, size and pre-existing infirmity (such as cardiac disease) [134]. Particularly in children it is important not to overload with fluid.

Analgesia will depend on both the type of envenoming and patient factors [107]. Many envenomings will not result in significant pain, so routine analgesia is not required and where indicated, oral analgesia should be used before considering parenteral analgesia. In all cases, it is best to avoid narcotic analgesia that may cause respiratory depression [107, 163, 211]. However, some forms of envenoming are routinely associated with severe pain, requiring prompt and vigorous analgesia, such as use of i.v. fentanyl for Irukandji stings [212], or regional nerve blocks for intransigent pain from stingray or venomous spined fish wounds [20, 213]. In some cases, antivenom will be the most effective "analgesic", such as in widow spider bites and stonefish stings [9, 20, 134, 152, 214].

Most envenoming cases do not develop significant secondary infection, so routine antibiotic use is generally not warranted [9, 191]. As the organisms involved in those cases that do become infected are highly variable, wherever possible culture and sensitivity should be performed prior to commencing initial antibiotic therapy, often with broad spectrum cover. Some envenomings, notably some snakebites in South America by *Bothrops jararaca, B. jararacusu* and related species can develop significant local sepsis and abscess formation, so routine antibiotic therapy may be appropriate in such bites, although is not always effective [215–219].

All bites and stings are potential sources for tetanus [191, 220, 221] and it is important to ensure current tetanus immunisation status, but care should be taken when giving i.m. tetanus immunisation updates in the presence of active coagulopathy, as caused by many snake species [191, 222–224]; the coagulopathy must first be under control.

Major local limb swelling is a common sequelae of envenoming by many snake species [163, 191, 225, 226]. In the past it has been assumed by some doctors that compartment syndrome would commonly occur, so fasciotomies were frequently performed. This invariably resulted in damaging scarring, which often progressed to long-term functional disability. It is now clear that true compartment syndrome is an infrequent complication of such local snake envenoming and fasciotomy should only be performed in cases where two criteria are met: (1) there is confirmation of compartment syndrome by direct measurement of intracompartmental pressure, and (2) any coagulopathy associated with envenoming has been reversed [163, 191, 225, 226].

Debriding necrotic wounds, should in most cases be done in the first few days, except for loxoscelism (recluse spider bites), where early debridement may spread venom and extend the area of necrosis [9, 227–229]. In these cases it is advisable to wait until the area of necrosis has stabilised. For deep penetrating wounds, such as with some stingray injuries, after debriding damaged and necrotic tissue, it is important to allow wounds to heal by secondary intention [230].

Specific groups of venomous animals

In the following accounts, only selected groups or representatives are discussed, as the vast array of venomous animals is too great to cover in a chapter such as this. Similarly, the range of possible data sources is immense, so readers are referred to a few key texts [15, 22, 27–29, 127–130, 134, 163, 191, 211] and a website (www.toxinology.com), rather than listing many hundreds of further references for individual species or species groups in the remaining portion of this chapter.

Venomous snakes

As discussed earlier, venomous snakes represent the single most important venomous animal group from a medical perspective, accounting for more mortality and serious morbidity than all other groups combined. Amongst the snakes, the majority of species fall into the four broad families containing venomous species [1–3, 163], but true venomous species represent only a minority of the snake fauna, and species dangerous to humans an even smaller proportion.

Colubrid snakes (Colubridae)

Family Colubridae comprises a diverse assemblage of over 1850 snake species, with some recent taxonomic work indicating that the family could be split into an array of further families [231, 232]. The majority of colubrid snakes are considered technically "non-venomous" and lack distinct venom apparatus or fangs [233]. However, it is clear that many other colubrid snakes can produce toxic oral secretions that some authors argue constitutes venom, a view possibly supported by apparent DNA coding for toxins [234]. This issue of what constitutes "venomousness" in colubrid snakes is an ongoing and unresolved issue that will not be further canvassed here. Among those few colubrid snakes with definite venom-producing glands and distinct enlarged teeth (some considered as fangs) for venom delivery, in all cases situated towards the middle to back of the upper mouth (so-called "back-fanged" or opisthoglyphous), several species are capable of causing severe, even lethal systemic envenoming, usually associated with deranged blood coagulation and a bleeding tendency. Colubrid snakes are global in distribution.

Boomslang (*Dispholidus*) and vine snakes (*Thelotornis*): These southern African arboreal snakes have caused a number of fatalities associated with coagulopathy. A specific antivenom is available in South Africa for the boomslang.

Keelbacks (*Rhabdophis*): The keelbacks and yamakagashi were originally thought to be harmless, but several severe, even fatal bites confirmed their potential to cause major envenoming and coagulopathy. A specific antivenom is available in Japan.

Other venomous and toxic colubrids: A number of other colubrid snakes have caused bites with varying degrees of envenoming, although generally not lethal. As more cases are accumulated it is probable that further colubrid species will be added to this list and it is no longer valid to assume a colubrid snake, not previously associated with significant bites, will be always harmless. However, those species that are small in size are less likely to inflict significant bites, although some large species of colubrids are not known to cause medically significant bites. No antivenoms are available for these snakes.

Elapid snakes (Elapidae)

Elapid snakes are, without exception, venomous, possessing well-developed venom glands and paired anterior placed proteroglyphous fangs. Many elapid snakes are small and may not be capable of significantly envenoming humans, but there are also many large species very capable of inflicting lethal bites. The range of elapid snakes is global, reaching a peak of diversity in Australia.

Cobras (*Naja, Hemachatus, Walterinnesia*): Cobras represent the single largest, most widely distributed group of elapid snakes of major medical importance, causing mortality and morbidity in thousands to tens of thousands of humans every year. They cover several genera, but most fall within the single genus *Naja*, with recent taxonomic changes moving several related genera into *Naja*. Clinically cobras divide into two broad types of envenoming: (1) predominantly local envenoming with necrosis, mild to moderate neurotoxicity, and (2) predominantly neurotoxic envenoming, without major local effects. The former group contains many species in Africa and Asia capable of spitting venom and causing severe venom ophthalmia. A variety of antivenoms are available for cobra envenoming, i.e., for covering more common species only, specific for particular species, species groups, or regions. Not all important species are covered and it is important to use the most specific antivenom available, particularly noting differences between African, West Asian and East Asian species, each covered by different products.

King cobra (*Ophiophagus*): The king cobra, although certainly cobra-like in origin and appearance, is separated because of its sheer size, at over 4 m, the longest of all venomous snakes. Found in much of eastern Asia, this snake causes both local effects and severe paralysis. Several specific king cobra antivenoms are available.

Kraits (*Bungarus*): As we understand more about snakebite epidemiology it becomes clear just how important kraits are in Asia as a cause of lethal envenoming. The numerous species are widely distributed and are generally nocturnal hunters, common in rural, even urban areas, where they mostly bite at night, with a painless bite and later development of progressive severe paralysis, often associated with abdominal pain and, at least for some species, myotoxicity as well. Most, but not all, species show some degree of body banding. Antivenom is available for some krait species.

Coral snakes (*Micrurus*, etc.): Coral snakes are of most medical significance in the Americas, especially in South and Central America, where they can cause severe paralysis and/or myolysis, with minimal local effects. There are a few species found in the southern USA, but throughout their range they are an infrequent, although sometimes fatal cause of bites. Several specific coral snake antivenoms are available in South and Central America.

Mambas (*Dendroaspis*): The African mambas (Fig. 7) have a ferocious reputation, but available data indicates they likely cause relatively few bites, although some species have a high lethality potential. The venom causes complex neurotoxicity, leading to both muscle fasciculation and paralysis, but generally few local effects. At least one African polyvalent antivenom covers mambas.

Australian and New Guinea elapids (*Pseudonaja*, *Pseudechis*, *Notechis*, *Tropidechis*, *Austrelaps*, *Hoplocephalus*, *Acanthophis*, *Oxyuranus*, *Micropechis*): Australian and New Guinea elapid snakes have developed rather separately from elapids elsewhere and present a distinct set of clinical problems. Local effects of bites vary, depending on species, from trivial to moderate swelling, but it is systemic effects that dominate, again varying between species, but including pre- and post-synaptic paralysis, severe myotoxicity, coagu-

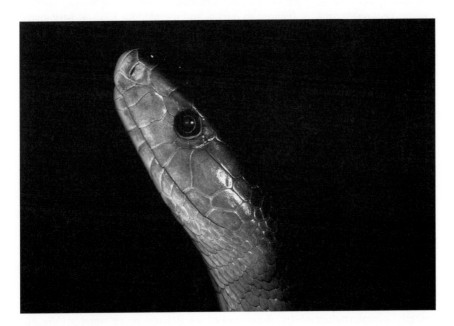

Figure 7. Black mamba, *Dendroaspis polylepis* (original photo/illustration copyright © Julian White).

lopathy and haemorrhage, renal failure and cardiotoxicity. Several "monovalent" and a polyvalent antivenom are available for Australian snakes.

Sea snakes: Long considered a separate family, sea snakes are now included within Elapidae and are thought to have evolved from early Australasian elapids. They are subdivided into two broad groups; the purely marine Hydrophiinae, encompassing the bulk of species, and the Laticaudinae that come onto land during their breeding cycle. Both groups have potent venoms, principally neurotoxins and/or myolysins, this being reflected in clinical envenoming, with both flaccid paralysis (post-synaptic) and systemic myotoxicity possible, either separately, or both together. The myolysis can cause secondary renal failure and cardiac toxicity and be severe enough to cause weakness that can mimic true neurotoxicity. Only one sea snake antivenom is currently available, but while it is made against venom from just one species, it appears to be effective for bites by most other sea snake species.

Other elapids (*Paranaja*, *Pseudohaje*, *Boulengerina*, *Aspidelaps*, *Elapsoidea*, *Homoroselaps*): This mixed group of elapids do not collectively cause significant numbers of bites, but some species can cause moderate to severe envenoming and have lethal potential. The taxonomic status of some genera is in flux; some are proposed to be subsumed within *Naja* (the cobras). There are no antivenoms available for these snakes.

Atractaspid snakes (Atractaspididae)

Burrowing or mole "vipers" have been the subject of considerable taxonomic instability, but currently are considered a distinct family of habitually subterranean venomous snakes, limited to Africa and the Middle East, mostly small and generally not involved in envenomings in humans. There are several larger species within genus *Atractaspis* that have potent venoms and do cause human envenoming and are potentially lethal. Within this group the unique sarafatoxins, similar to human endothelins, can cause severe or lethal cardiac effects. However, local tissue injury and sometimes necrosis is a far more common consequence in envenomed humans. They are adapted for a subterranean existence, burrowing in search of prey and have evolved a unique fang structure allowing side-swiping envenoming.

Viperid snakes (Viperidae)

Vipers comprise a diverse assemblage of venomous snakes, with a wide global distribution. They have front-placed fangs on rotating modified maxillae, allowing the fang to be folded against the roof of the mouth, then erected when biting, an arrangement that permits development of long fangs, and referred to as solenoglyphous dentition (Fig. 8). In some viperids, fangs can exceed 2.5 cm in length and these large fangs are often combined with large venom glands, able to effectively deliver a substantial venom load. While many viper venoms may not be as toxic as selected elapid venoms, this is frequently counterbalanced by their ability to deliver more venom. Viperid snakes are the single most important cause of snakebite to humans globally,

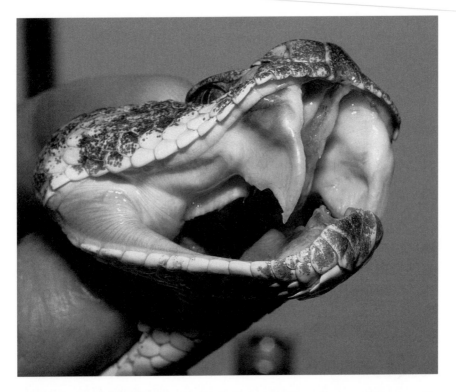

Figure 8. An eastern diamondback rattlesnake, *Crotalus atrox*, with mouth open and fangs moved to erect position, but with fang sheath not yet retracted (original photo/illustration copyright © Julian White).

ahead of elapids. There are two subfamilies of viperid snakes, Viperinae and Crotalinae.

Viperinae
This subfamily contains classic vipers, found throughout much of the "old world" and responsible for a substantial portion of the human snakebite toll, particularly groups like the carpet vipers (genus *Echis*), Russell's vipers (genus *Daboia*) and African adders (genus *Bitis*).

   Classic vipers and adders (*Vipera, Macrovipera*, etc.): These small vipers (or "adders") have a wide distribution from Europe right across northern Asia and south into North Africa and the Middle East. While they can cause severe, even fatal envenoming, in most cases envenoming is less severe and mostly local, with swelling, pain, bruising, and uncommonly necrosis. Systemic effects can include shock, coagulopathy and renal damage, with occasional mild neurotoxic features, such as ptosis, although at least one species (*Vipera ammodytes*) can cause more severe paralysis. Several antivenoms are available.

Puff adders (*Bitis*): These African vipers range from small species to large snakes such as the Gaboon viper, *Bitis gabonica* and the notorious puff adder, *Bitis arietans*, an important cause of sub-Saharan snakebite. These snakes cause severe local envenoming, including swelling, pain, bruising, blistering and necrosis, plus systemic effects including shock, coagulopathy and haemorrhage. Several antivenoms covering the puff adder are available, but not specifically for other species, although cross-reactivity is likely among some of these.

Russell's vipers (*Daboia*): Russell's vipers, *Daboia russelii* and *D. siamensis*, are the most important members of this genus and are found from Sri Lanka, through the Indian subcontinent, to Southeast Asia, Indonesia and Taiwan. Throughout their range they cause a significant number of often severe or fatal bites, characterised by both severe local effect, including blistering and necrosis, and severe systemic effects, including coagulopathy, haemorrhage, shock and renal failure. Some populations, particularly in Myanmar and parts of India, can also cause anterior pituitary infarction, resulting in Sheehan's syndrome. Other populations, notably those in Sri Lanka, can cause myolysis and paralysis. This diversity of venom actions and clinical effects, even intra-species, means that antivenom choice is crucial; the antivenom, to be effective, must be against the particular population of snakes causing the bite. Using specific anti-*Daboia* antivenom from one region, to treat bites by the same species from a different region, can result in treatment failure and death.

Carpet vipers (*Echis*): Carpet or saw-scaled vipers, genus *Echis*, are common, relatively small vipers, with a range extending from west Africa to India, covering a number of species that collectively likely cause more snakebite fatalities than any other genus of snakes. Their bites cause severe local effects, including blistering, haemorrhage and necrosis, plus severe systemic coagulopathy and haemorrhage. Venom variability between species means that antivenom must be sourced from the correct region and species; Indian anti-*Echis* antivenom will not be effective in Africa and *vice versa*.

Other vipers (*Eristocophis, Cerastes, Causus, Pseudocerastes, Atheris, Montatheris, Proatheris, Adenorhinos, Azemiops*): A variety of lesser viperids exist, some of which are not known to cause significant envenoming in humans, while others, such as the horned vipers, *Cerastes* spp., can cause severe, even life-threatening envenoming characterised by coagulopathy and haemorrhage. Antivenoms covering these species are mostly unavailable, although a few antivenoms cover some taxa.

Crotalinae

The other viper subfamily, Crotalinae, contains all the "pit vipers", those vipers with two heat sensing pits on the anterior head, allowing detection of prey by infra-red. Pit vipers occur in both the Old World and New World, although they predominate in the latter, throughout the Americas, where they are the dominant cause of snakebites to humans.

Rattlesnakes (*Crotalus*, *Sistrurus*): The rattlesnakes, genus *Crotalus* (Fig. 9), and the related genus of "pigmy" rattlesnakes, genus *Sistrurus*, are the leading cause of North American snakebite, but are also important in Central and South America. The North American species cause often severe local envenoming, with swelling, bruising, pain, sometimes blistering/bleb formation and occasionally necrosis, particularly for bites to digits. There may be associated shock, and with some species, major coagulopathy. A few species can cause at least minor neurotoxic paralytic features, such as ptosis, but some populations of the Mojave rattlesnake, *Crotalus scutulatus*, can cause severe paralysis, as their venom contains a potent presynaptic neurotoxin. Some rattlesnakes, such as canebrakes, *Crotalus horridus atricaudatus*, can cause major myolysis and secondary renal failure and cardiotoxicity. A single antivenom covering all North American pit vipers is available. In Central and South America, rattlesnake bites have a quite different clinical pattern; major local effects are not common, but severe systemic envenoming is common, including neurotoxic paralysis, myolysis, coagulopathy and renal failure. A variety of South and Central American antivenoms cover one or more of these rattlesnake species.

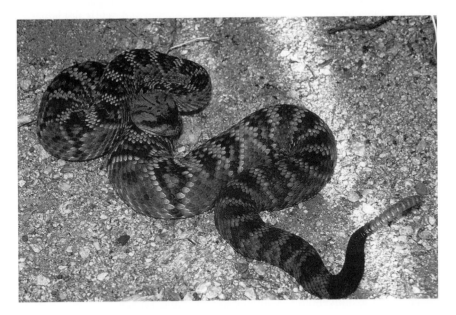

Figure 9. Blacktail rattlesnake, *Crotalus molossus* (original photo/illustration copyright © Julian White).

Lance head pit vipers (*Bothrops*, *Bothriechis*): Snakes of the genus *Bothrops* are the single most important cause of snakebite in South and Central America. Most of the major species cause severe local and systemic effects,

including local tissue injury/necrosis in the bitten limb and systemic coagulopathy and shock. Some species commonly cause local infection with abscess
formation. Renal failure, including permanent injury (bilateral renal cortical
necrosis) is described. Two species in the Caribbean, *Bothrops lanceolatus* and
B. caribbeus, cause thrombotic problems, as discussed earlier in this chapter.
A variety of antivenoms are available in South and Central America to cover
some of the major species of *Bothrops*, but it is important to select an antivenom with coverage for the species involved in a bite. Many of the lesser
Bothrops species, although capable of causing envenoming, seem rarely to do
so and are not specifically covered by any antivenom. The same applies to the
variety of smaller pit vipers, such as the eyelash viper, *Bothriechis schlegeli*.
Some polyvalent antivenoms, particularly from Central America, may provide
some cross neutralisation for some of these species.

Bushmasters (*Lachesis*): The bushmasters are formidable snakes, of large
size, but throughout most of their range, bites are infrequent. Moderate to
severe local effects occur, including bruising, but necrosis is uncommon, while
systemic effects include shock, coagulopathy and haemorrhage. Several
antivenoms covering these snakes are available.

Copperheads, mokasins and cantils (*Agkistrodon*): In parts of North
America, bites by some *Agkistrodon* spp. are common and, while not generally as severe as rattlesnake envenoming, can still cause potentially lethal
effects, particularly in children. Moderate to severe local effects are common,
including tissue injury, but major systemic effects are less common. They are
covered by the North American polyvalent antivenom.

Mamushi, etc. (*Gloydius, Deinagkistrodon*): The snakes currently assigned
to genus *Gloydius*, restricted to Asia, were formerly in genus *Agkistrodon*, and
some species are important as a cause of snakebite, particularly the mamushis
of Japan (*Gloydius blomhoffii blomhoffii*) and China (*G.b. brevicaudus*). The
Japanese subspecies can cause both severe local effects, including blistering,
and systemic effects, including shock, coagulopathy, haemorrhage, renal damage and mild neurotoxicity. The Chinese subspecies causes similarly severe
systemic effects and possibly myolysis as well, but less severe local effects.
Bites by other members of this genus are less well understood. Antivenoms
against the mamushis are available in China and Japan. The hundred pace
snake, *Deinagkistrodon acutus*, also found in parts of Asia, can cause severe or
lethal envenoming, characterised by severe local effects, including blistering
and necrosis, and systemic effects such as shock, coagulopathy and haemorrhage. Specific antivenom is available in China and Taiwan.

Malayan pit viper (*Calloselasma*): In Southeast Asia the Malayan pit viper
is a most important cause of severe and lethal bites. It causes major local
effects, including blistering and necrosis, and systemic effects including
shock, coagulopathy and haemorrhage. Several antivenoms covering this species are available.

Green pit viper (*Trimeresurus, Protobothrops, Crypteletrops, Viridovipera,
Popeia, Garthius, Parias, Peltopelor*): These Asian pit vipers, mostly previ-

ously contained within the single genus *Trimeresurus*, have recently been split into eight distinct genera [235–237]. They encompass a diverse range of mostly arboreal snakes, some of which are important causes of snakebite within their specific distribution. Clinical effects vary between species, from trivial local and no systemic effects, to extensive local swelling and bruising, with systemic coagulopathy and haemorrhage, to severe local effects including necrosis, plus shock, with or without coagulopathy. This latter group includes the habu, *Protobothrops flavoviridis* and *Protobothrops mucrosquamatus*. Antivenoms are available for some of the more medically significant species.

Hump nose vipers (*Hypnale*): Hump nosed vipers from India and Sri Lanka are now recognised as a cause of significant bites, causing both local effects, including blistering, but not necrosis, and systemic effects including shock, coagulopathy, haemorrhage, renal damage and MAHA, although most bites may be less severe. No antivenom is available at present.

Other crotalines (*Atropoides, Cerrophidion, Ermia, Ophryacus, Ovophis, Porthidium, Tropidolaemus*): A number of other New World and Asian pit vipers in several genera can cause bites but are mostly considered of comparatively minor medical importance. None are covered by specific antivenoms.

Venomous lizards

Until recently, only two species of lizards, *Heloderma suspectum* and *H. horridum*, family Helodermatidae, were considered venomous. These large lizards, from arid areas of Mexico and southwestern USA, have venom glands in the lower jaw, which connect to the base of sharp grooved teeth. The venom is likely used in prey acquisition, but bites to humans can result in excruciating local pain and mechanical injury, and in some cases, major systemic effects, including hypotension and shock, but not paralysis, myolysis, or coagulopathy. Treatment is symptomatic and supportive, as no antivenom is available.

Recent controversial research has indicated that several other groups of lizards, notably the varanids/goannas (family Varanidae) and the dragons (family Agamidae) have genes for venom production and may produce oral secretions containing toxins [234]. Some researchers consider that for at least large varanids, such as the massive Komodo dragon (*Varanus komodoensis*), these toxic oral secretions are effectively venom and are used in prey acquisition. Further research is needed to confirm the validity of this work.

Scorpions

Most of the nearly 2000 described species of scorpions are of no medical significance, their stings causing either no effects in humans, or minor or short-lived local pain, rarely with any systemic effects, and the latter are of a minor and self-limiting nature. However, several hundred species, nearly all within family Buthidae, can cause envenoming, varying from mild to severe, even lethal, depending on species and the size of the victim.

Buthid scorpions of medical importance

Buthid scorpions (Fig. 10) capable of causing medically important envenoming occur in the Americas, Africa, the Middle East and Asia. All cause a form of neuroexcitatory envenoming, in many cases characterised as a catecholamine storm effect. A wide variety of scorpion toxins have now been fully elucidated and these include potent potassium and sodium channel neurotoxins. In some regions, such as North Africa, scorpion sting is both more common, and of greater medical importance, than snakebite. In Mexico around 280 000 scorpion sting cases are admitted to hospital every year. With adequate antivenom therapy, mortality is now low, even in those at most risk, younger children, in regions where it is widely used. In contrast, some regions not using antivenom still have significant mortality from scorpion stings. Antivenoms are available for only some major scorpion species, sourced in their native regions. However, the management of scorpion envenoming is controversial, with several different approaches extant. Some clinicians consider antivenom ineffective, instead emphasising both supportive intensive care and use of cardiovascular drugs such as prazosin. Confusing studies suggesting antivenom is ineffective have created more uncertainty about treatment. Nevertheless, evidence from countries including Mexico and Brazil,

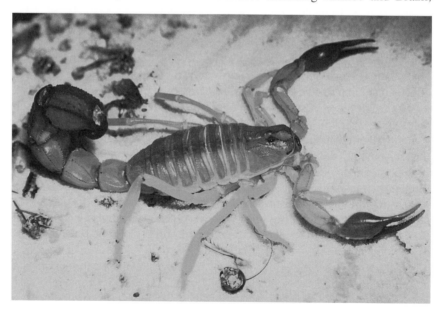

Figure 10. *Androctonus australis* (original photo/illustration copyright © Julian White).

where severe scorpion stings are very common, indicates that the widespread use of antivenom has been associated with a dramatic fall in mortality.

Non-Buthid scorpions of medical importance

The most important non-Buthid scorpion is undoubtedly *Hemiscorpius lepturus*, found in Southwest Iran [238–240]. This scorpion, uniquely within all scorpions, causes local sting-site necrosis and often a systemic syndrome of haemolysis, coagulopathy, renal failure and shock, which can be lethal. It does not cause neuroexcitatory envenoming, unlike other medically important scorpions. A polyvalent scorpion antivenom, which is claimed effective against *Hemiscorpius*, is available in Iran.

Spiders

Spiders undoubtedly cause large numbers of bites to humans, most of which are trivial, requiring no medical treatment, but a few species can cause major effects, and one group is potentially lethal. Spiders are generally grouped into two suborders, Mygalomorphae and Araneomorphae. These two groups can be distinguished by anatomical features and both contain species of medical importance.

Mygalomorphs

These spiders, often described as "primitive", are generally large spiders of robust build, with comparatively long fangs. Most cause minor local effects only on biting humans, but one group, the Australian funnel-web spiders and related mouse spiders are lethal to humans. Some others cause dermal and ophthalmic irritation through shedding abdominal hairs.

Australian funnel-web spiders: These spiders, of genera *Atrax* (Fig. 11) and *Hadronyche*, found only in Australia, are the World's most dangerous spiders. While "dry" or trivial bites are common, they can cause rapidly lethal envenoming, even in healthy adults, with death in less than 30 minutes in some cases in the pre-antivenom era. Envenoming is a rapid, fulminant neuroexcitatory type, with catecholamine storm effects, similar to major scorpion envenoming. It responds rapidly to antivenom, even given late, and since antivenom was introduced, fatalities are now essentially unknown. This specific antivenom actually is effective for all funnel-web species. The related mouse spiders, genus *Missulena*, have a similar venom, also responsive to funnel-web spider antivenom, but clinically significant envenoming is very rare, so antivenom is generally not required for bites by these spiders.

Other mygalomorphs: A number of other large mygalomorph spiders can cause at least local effects such as intense pain, sometimes with non-specific systemic effects, usually mild and of limited duration, but for the majority of species there is no evidence, despite their large size and long fangs, that they are of any medical significance.

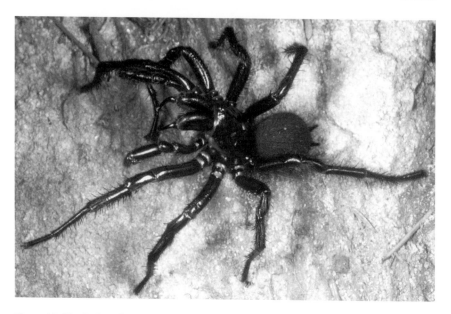

Figure 11. The Sydney funnel-web spider, *Atrax robustus* (original photo/illustration copyright ©
Julian White).

Aranaeomorphs

The bulk of all described spider species are araneomorphs. These diverse spiders span a wide array of families, body size and shape and prey capture methods, the latter ranging from classic web capture, to hunting and stalking. Most
are of no medical significance, but a few groups can cause problem bites.

Widow spiders (*Latrodectus*): Widow spider bite is probably the most common medically important form of spider bite globally. Widow spiders, mostly
of the genus *Latrodectus*, are distributed across most continents, are often
common and adapt well to human habitation, so opportunities for bites can be
many. In Australia more patients are treated with antivenom for widow spider
(red back spider) bite than all other types of envenoming combined (including
snakebite). Although widow spiders are reported to have caused fatalities,
available evidence suggests this is most likely a result of secondary problems,
not direct primary venom toxicity, but there is no doubt that significant widow
spider envenoming, latrodectism, is an unpleasant problem for affected
patients. The venom causes neuroexcitatory envenoming, but usually without
the severe and life threatening systemic effects seen with scorpion and funnel-
web spider envenoming. Instead, envenoming is characterised by local, then
regional or generalised pain, often with associated sweating, sometimes nausea and hypertension, lasting up to several days. A number of antivenoms are
available and evidence suggests any anti-latrodectus antivenom will be effective against bites by all widow spider species. Recent research has questioned
the effectiveness of antivenom for latrodectism, but further research will be

required to resolve this issue, as there is a large body of published case experience (but not randomised control trials) suggesting antivenom is the only effective treatment.

Banana spiders (*Phoneutria*): Banana spiders are restricted to South and Central America, but cause most problems in Brazil, where they are, by far, the most common cause of major spider bite. Effects are similar to widow spiders and most distressing for patients, but with low lethality potential. An antivenom is available in Brazil, but most patients are managed conservatively, including analgesia, without antivenom.

Recluse spiders (*Loxosceles*): Recluse spiders (Fig. 12) are global in distribution, but a more restricted group cause medical problems, which are quite distinctive. An effective bite, although rarely felt at the time, will cause either just local effects, principally necrosis of skin (cutaneous loxoscelism), plus some self limiting systemic effects, or these local effects plus a potentially lethal systemic illness (viscerocutaneous loxoscelism), characterised by haemolysis, coagulopathy, renal failure and shock. An antivenom is available in Brazil, although its effectiveness, given the usual very late presentation, is doubtful. Most cases elsewhere, such as in the USA, are managed conservatively. Early debridement of necrotic areas is generally inadvisable as it can extend the necrotic area. Loxoscelism is sometimes characterised as "necrotic

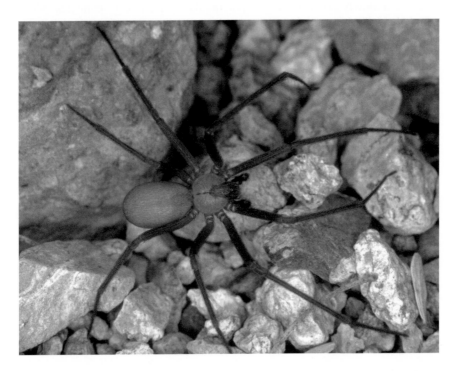

Figure 12. North American recluse spider, *Loxosceles reclusa* (original photo/illustration copyright © Julian White).

arachnidism" (spider bite causing skin necrosis), but is an over-diagnosed condition in some countries, notably the USA, and also in Australia (where *Loxosceles* is not a native species and is likely present, if at all, in very restricted areas and numbers).

Other aranaeomorphs: A number of other larger araneomorph spiders can cause mild local envenoming, usually just local pain and/or swelling, occasionally with mild self-limiting general symptoms. None require antivenom.

Ticks and mites

There are many tick and mite species, all parasites of various hosts, sometimes mammals, but also birds, reptiles, even spiders and insects. Very few produce saliva with toxin (venom) effects in humans. Indeed, medically, ticks are far more important as vectors of disease transmission.

Australian paralysis ticks
Hard bodied ticks of the genus *Ixodes*, limited to eastern Australia, produce a potent paralysing neurotoxin in their saliva, so that when an adult female tick attaches to a human, enough toxic saliva may be inoculated, over several days, to cause a slowly progressive, but potentially lethal, flaccid paralysis. More people have died from tick paralysis in Australia than from funnel-web or red back spider bite. Once the tick is removed, paralysis can still progress for up to 48 hours, before slowly resolving. Severe paralysis can cause respiratory failure, requiring mechanical ventilation. This is the current treatment, as the previously available antivenom was of doubtful effectiveness and has been discontinued.

North American paralysis ticks
North American paralysis ticks are hard bodied species, principally *Dermacentor andersoni* (western North America) and *D. variabilis* (eastern and central North America), causing progressive flaccid paralysis, which regresses immediately on tick removal. No antivenom is available and respiratory support is the mainstay treatment in those rare cases with full respiratory paralysis, often required for only a brief period.

Other paralysis ticks
Tick paralysis is less well described outside North America and Australia, although it is reported to occur, probably rarely, in Africa, possibly elsewhere.

Centipedes

Centipedes have paired fangs and venom glands adjacent to the head, in the maxillipedes; the apparent "venomous" spines at the tail region are not venomous. Bites from large species can cause local mechanical trauma and intense pain from the venom, but systemic effects are not generally seen and local effects usually settle quickly. However, secondary infection is a risk. No antivenom is available or required.

Insects

Insects comprise a large proportion of animal species diversity, so it is hardly surprising some utilise venom for defence or offence. However, comparatively few cause medically significant effects from venom and in most of these, it is allergy, not primary venom toxicity, that is the risk.

Hymenopterans (bees, wasps, ants)
With a few notable exceptions, all the important venomous insects are hymenopterans, either bees, wasps, or stinging ants. In all of these, a single sting in the tail, with an intra-abdominal venom gland, can deliver a small quantity of venom, containing potent and often highly allergenic peptides. Most stinging hymenopterans can sting multiple times, but the honey bee, *Apis mellifera*, is only able to sting once, resulting in the death of the bee, with the sting and pumping venom gland left behind in the skin of the victim. While mass attacks, involving many hundreds, more usually thousands of stings, can result in primary, even lethal venom toxicity, often with fulminant haemolysis, shock and renal failure, these events are generally rare. In a few areas, such as Vietnam and Brazil, such mass attacks by hymenopterans are more common and cause occasional deaths. For most people and regions, it is allergy from a single sting that causes most concern, and most fatalities. In many western countries, bee sting anaphylaxis is considered to kill more people than any form of envenoming. Not all bees sting, nor do all wasps, but some wasps, particularly the large communal species, such as European wasps and North American and Asian hornets, regularly sting humans, either singly, or multiply. Most ants lack effective stinging capacity, although bites can cause local pain and some species can spray venom under pressure from abdominal venom glands. Some species do sting and can cause intense local pain, irritation, redness, and allergic responses in some humans. The pain can last many hours, with "sores" developing around each sting site, which can take days to resolve. A few of these stinging ants, such as the jumping and inch ants (*Myrmecia* spp.) of Australia, can cause major anaphylaxis, more potent than even honey bees. Similarly, the fire ants (*Solenopsis* spp.), originally from South America, but now well established in North America, Australia and elsewhere, can cause intense local pain, sore formation, and major allergic reactions.

Lepidopterans (caterpillars)
Most caterpillars, moths and butterflies are of no medical significance, but the caterpillars of some species have locally irritant hairs and in some cases, notably

Lonomia spp. in Brazil, can cause major, even lethal envenoming, on skin contact with these hairs. *Lonomia* caterpillars cause potentially fatal coagulopathy, with potent procoagulants in their venom; there is a specific antivenom in Brazil. Contact with the hairs of some other caterpillars, across several continents and many species, either through touching the caterpillar, or through shed hairs in the air, can cause not just local skin irritation, but in the eyes, corneal irritation, and if inhaled, bronchial irritation, and potentially severe allergic reactions are also possible. The term lepidopterism is used to cover these diverse clinical effects. In some species, the hairs may be present on the outside of pupae and adverse effects from contact with these is known as erucism.

Coleopterans (beetles)

A variety of beetles can produce toxic secretions, which can cause injury to humans, most commonly skin irritation, staining, blistering or necrosis. Of particular note are beetles of the family Meloidae, the "blister beetles", sometimes known as "Spanish fly". These beetles produce the potent toxin cantharadin, exuded from limb joints (they have no specific venom gland), and direct contact with human skin can cause classic blistering and skin necrosis. Similarly Staphylinidae beetles can cause local effects by squirting toxins, notably pederin, under high pressure from anal glands. These are defensive actions by the beetles, not primary prey acquisition. Management of such local lesions is symptomatic and supportive. No antivenom is available.

Other insects

While a variety of other insect species, across diverse families, possess sucking mouthparts and can attack humans, often as a food source, they are not primarily venomous, though their saliva may contain substances that might be considered toxic. They will not be further discussed here.

Venomous mammals

Several species of mammals, across two suborders, produce toxic secretions. In the case of monotremes, the Australian platypus, *Ornithorhynchus anatinus*, a hind leg spur attached to a venom gland is used in male:male combat and in defence, with accidental stings to humans causing intense local pain lasting many hours. Treatment is symptomatic and no antivenom is available. Toxic oral secretions from shrews can cause local effects in bitten humans, but these are generally minor and managed symptomatically.

Venomous birds

Until 1990, birds were not considered as toxin producers, but the discovery of toxin-producing birds in Papua New Guinea, the pitohuis and infritas, which principally contain batrachotoxins in their feathers and skin, has changed this view. However, in these birds, the toxin is used only in defence, when in contact with the bird. There is also uncertainty about the origin of the toxin (is it made by the bird or concentrated after uptake from the environment). For the present, then, these birds should be considered poisonous rather than venomous.

Venomous amphibians

As with the birds, mentioned above, those frogs possessing toxic secretions are generally considered poisonous, not venomous. Interestingly, some venomous frogs, such as larger *Bufo* toads, can squirt toxic secretions from posterior parotid glands in the head-neck region, as a defensive measure. This can almost be considered venomous, not just poisonous. Toxic secretions in amphibians, including species of frogs (and toads) and newts, can be highly potent, such as the batrachotoxins, pumiliotoxins, samandarines and bufotoxins, many being low molecular weight alkaloids affecting nerve transmission or cardiac function. Many are lethal to humans, even at a low dose, but humans rarely come in contact with these toxins. Most recent reported human deaths from amphibian toxins follow ingestion of herbal medicines or extracts used for recreational drugs containing toad toxins such as bufotoxin and bufogenin. Some of the highly toxic poison arrow frogs from the New World are very colourful and popular in captivity, but generally loose their toxicity after a period of captive care, supporting the environmental origin of the toxins.

Venomous fish

There are numerous fish with venomous spines, in a diverse array of families, in all cases using the venom and spines predominantly for defence, not prey acquisition. Venom glands envelop spines, which are often grooved, and when contact is made with a potential target, as the spine enters the tissue, the gland may be compressed and venom forced subcutaneously into the target. This is particularly effective in fish such as the stonefish (*Synaceia trachynis*), the most venomous of all fish, when a human steps on the dorsal spines. Here, as with other venomous spined fish, the venom causes local pain, which may be excruciating and crippling. Similar, but lesser pain can occur with other species, when stepped on or picked up in the hand. The location of spines varies with species and includes dorsal, ventral, lateral, tail fins and behind the head. Some species, such as lionfish (*Pterois* spp.) can have many spines providing a defensive screen around the fish. Only a few of these fish venoms have been studied, notably the most toxic to humans, the stonefish, which has a potent neurotoxin, although this does not cause paralytic features in envenomed humans.

There are no substantial data on rates of venomous fish stings, but it is likely that minor stings are very common, while severe stings are uncommon to rare. For most of these fish stings, symptomatic care is the only treatment, with hot water immersion widely recommended as both first aid and hospital treatment to abate pain. A specific antivenom is available for stonefish stings and may be useful for severe effects by some closely related species, although this is unproven.

Cnidarians: jellyfish

Jellyfish occur in vast numbers, often in swarms, that can be encountered by swimming humans, often off popular beaches and in bays in summer. The total number of stings to humans is almost certainly measured in the many millions per year, but apart from local pain and wheal formation, generally of short duration and not requiring medical treatment, the vast majority of these stings are of no consequence. However, medically, a few species commonly cause significant effects, even potentially lethal envenoming in the case of the Australian box jellyfish, *Chironex fleckeri*, and Irukandji jellyfish (covers several species, including *Carukia barnesi*).

The box jellyfish (Fig. 13), clearly the most deadly jellyfish globally, can inject large amounts of venom rapidly, some thought to directly enter capillar-

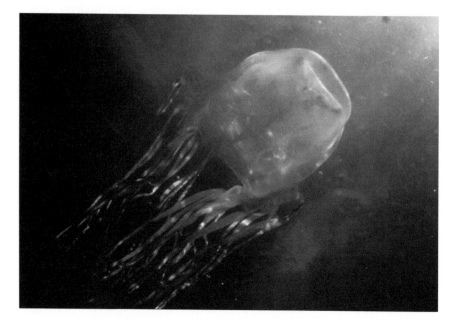

Figure 13. The Australian box jellyfish, *Chironex fleckeri* (original photo courtesy of Jamie Seymour).

ies, because of its large size and great tentacle length. As with other jellyfish, venom is produced in and injected by individual stinging cells, nematocysts (cnidocils), found in vast numbers on the surface of tentacles (Fig. 14). A major box jellyfish sting can inoculate venom from millions of nematocysts instantly. As the tentacle contacts the skin, a trigger on the surface of each nematocyst initiates extrusion at high speed of the everted stinging tube, through the skin, ejecting venom along the extrusion track. A sting is invariably painful, often with distinctive ladder track marks and the pain can be excruciating. Sometimes local necrosis and scarring can occur along tentacle contact tracks. Box jellyfish venom includes toxins that are cardiotoxic and in a major sting, within a few minutes even an adult human can suffer cardiac arrhythmia and arrest, so death can occur within 5 minutes of being stung, probably the most rapid and dramatic lethal envenoming of any venomous animal. This has resulted in great fear of box jellyfish stings, but in reality, such a dire outcome is only likely if the area of tentacle contact is large, usually from a large specimen. Nets around swimming beaches exclude such large specimens and the majority of human box jellyfish stings are comparatively minor. Close relatives of the box jellyfish exist in waters north of Australia and there are reports of fatal jellyfish stings around Southeast Asia, Indonesia and the Philippines. An antivenom is available for Australian box jellyfish stings, but there is recent evidence that while it neutralises the venom effectively, it cannot be given soon enough

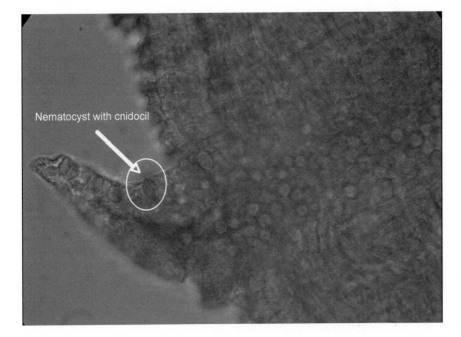

Nematocyst with cnidocil

Figure 14. Photomicrograph of a jellyfish tentacle showing embedded unfired nematocysts (original photo courtesy of Jamie Seymour).

to be effective in a clinical setting, although until further research is performed, this is not a reason to cease using it in severe cases.

The Irukandji syndrome, caused by stings from a variety of jellyfish species, not just *Carukia barnesi*, causes a very different pattern of envenoming. The sting itself may be trivial or not even felt, and involve a tiny area of only a few cm^2. Many, but not all of these Irukandji jellyfish are tiny, so are not excluded by protective nets around beaches. A variable time after the sting, but usually within an hour, systemic effects develop, notably severe muscle pain in the back, limbs, or elsewhere, often accompanied by severe hypotension, sweating, and in severe cases, pulmonary oedema. The whole syndrome is similar to a catecholamine storm and is potentially, but very rarely, lethal. Treatment is supportive and symptomatic, including strong analgesia. There is no antivenom available.

The Portuguese Man-of-War or bluebottle (*Physalia* spp.), is a very common colony organism "jellyfish" that invades swimming areas in mass swarms in summer months mainly, sometimes causing large numbers of humans to be stung. In most cases, local pain, sometimes intense, but usually short lived, often with wheal formation, is the only effect. In a small number of cases, allergy may be stimulated and rarely, anaphylaxis can occur. Recent research indicates that hot water, most commonly a hot shower, can dramatically reduce symptoms, more so than other first aid or treatments. No antivenom is available.

Venomous molluscs

Snails are slow moving, so it is perhaps surprising that more predatory species are not venomous, at least as far as currently known.

Cone snails (Conus)

Of the known venomous predatory marine snails, the vast array of species of cone snails, *Conus* spp., is the most important medically, and the best studied. These snails divide into three broad groups, based on major prey type; fish eaters, snail eaters and worm eaters. All use a system of venom-coated fired "harpoon" like radula "teeth" to acquire prey, but some have such potent venom that they can extrude it into the surrounding water to immobilise or disorient prey such as fish, to facilitate capture. In some cases this may involve stunning multiple small fish simultaneously. To achieve capture of fast moving fish, venom must act almost instantly, which may explain why cone snails have evolved such a diverse and rich array of small peptide-based specialist toxins. These conotoxins are proving of interest as models for new pharmaceutical agents, and have an almost bewildering range of activities and targets, mostly within the nervous system, but often very highly specific, hence their immense value as neuropharmacological tools in research.

Most cone snails appear unable to effectively or significantly envenom humans, but a few species can cause severe or lethal envenoming, although reported cases are few. So from a human epidemiological perspective, their importance is trivial. Most cases occur in the Indo-Pacific, particularly around the Philippines. Envenoming occurs when the snail is interfered with or picked up, with rapid venom inoculation from the fired radula tooth, which may cause either local pain, or minimal local symptoms. Systemic envenoming can develop rapidly, with flaccid paralysis a particular risk. In severe cases, without respiratory support, death may ensue. Treatment is supportive and symptomatic. No antivenom is available.

Blue ringed octopus (Hapalochlaena)

The blue ringed octopuses, genus *Hapalochlaena*, are common in waters around Australia and to the north. They are small and derive their name from dramatic blue rings that form in the skin when the octopus is alarmed. Their saliva contains tetrodotoxin, a potent and rapidly acting neurotoxin that targets sodium channels on nerves, causing flaccid paralysis. It is now considered likely the octopus does not produce the toxin itself, but accumulates it, or a precursor, from the environment. Bites are often apparently trivial, with little or no pain, but in a minority of cases, systemic neurotoxic paralytic envenoming occurs within 10–30 minutes. Without respiratory support, death can rapidly follow. Treatment is supportive. Antivenom is not available.

Other marine venomous animals

A wide variety of marine animals use toxins in defence, to establish territory (such as sedentary corals to maintain or expand living space against competition), or in prey acquisition. However, they are generally of minor or no medical importance and are not discussed further here.

References

1 Chippaux JP (1998) Snake-bites: Appraisal of the global situation. *Bull WHO* 76: 515–524
2 Kasturiratne A, Wickremasinghe AR, de Silva N, Gunawardena NK, Pathmeswaran A, Premaratna R, Savioli L, Lalloo DG, de Silva HJ (2008) The global burden of snakebite: A literature analysis and modelling based on regional estimates of envenoming and deaths. *PLoS Med* 5: e218
3 Mion G, Olive F (1997) Les envenimations par vipéridés en Afrique Noire. In: JM Saissy (ed.): *Réanimation Tropicale*, Arnette, Paris, 349–366
4 Chippaux JP (2005) Ophidian envenomations and emergencies in sub-Saharan Africa. *Bull Soc Pathol Exot* 98: 263–268
5 Siddique AK, Baquo AH, Eusof A, Zaman K (1991) 1988 Floods in Bangladesh: Pattern of illness and causes of death. *J Diarrhoeal Dis Res* 9: 310–314
6 Chippaux JP, Goyffon M (2008) Epidemiology of scorpionism: A global appraisal. *Acta Trop* 107: 71–79
7 Celis A, Gaxiola-Robles R, Sevilla-Godínez E, Orozco Valerio Mde J, Armas J (2007) Trends in mortality from scorpion stings in Mexico, 1979–2003. *Rev Panam Salud Publica* 21: 373–380
8 Goyffon M, Billiald P (2007) Envenomations VI. Scorpionism in Africa. *Med Trop* 67: 439–446
9 White J (1995) Clinical toxicology of spiderbite. In: J Meier, J White (eds): *Handbook of Clinical Toxicology of Animal Venoms and Poisons*, CRC Press, Boca Raton, FL, 259–329

10 Bristoe WS (1958) *The World of Spiders*. Collins, London, UK

11 Vetter RS, Isbister GK (2008) Medical aspects of spider bites. *Annu Rev Entomol* 53: 409–429

12 Isbister GK, White J (2004) Clinical consequences of spider bites: Recent advances in our understanding. *Toxicon* 43: 477–492

13 Isbister GK, Gray MR (2002) A prospective study of 750 definite spider bites, with expert spider identification. *QJM* 95: 723–731

14 Williamson J, Burnett J (1995) Clinical toxicology of marine coelenterate injuries. In: J Meier, J White (eds): *Handbook of Clinical Toxicology of Animal Venoms and Poisons*, CRC Press, Boca Raton, FL, 89–115

15 Williamson JA, Fenner PJ, Burnett JW, Rifkin JF (1996) *Venomous and Poisonous Marine Animals*. Uni NSW Press, Sydney, Australia

16 Fenner PJ, Williamson JA (1996) Worldwide deaths and severe envenomation from jellyfish stings. *Med J Aust* 165: 658–661

17 O'Reilly GM, Isbister GK, Lawrie PM, Treston GT, Currie BJ (2001) Prospective study of jellyfish stings from tropical Australia, including the major box jellyfish *Chironex fleckeri*. *Med J Aust* 175: 652–655

18 Currie BJ, Jacups SP (2005) Prospective study of *Chironex fleckeri* and other box jellyfish stings in the "top end" of Australia's Northern Territory. *Med J Aust* 183: 631–636

19 Williamson JA, Callanan VI, Hartwick RF (1980) Serious envenomation by the Northern Australian box-jellyfish (*Chironex fleckeri*). *Med J Aust* 1: 13–16

20 Williamson J (1995) Clinical toxicology of venomous Scorpaenidae and other selected fish stings. In: J Meier, J White (eds): *Handbook of Clinical Toxicology of Animal Venoms and Poisons*, CRC Press, Boca Raton, FL, 141–158

21 White J (2005) Venom. In: R Byard, T Corey, C Henderson, J Payne-James (eds): *Encyclopedia of Forensic and Legal Medicine*, Academic Press, Burlington, MA

22 Mebs D (2002) *Venomous and Poisonous Animals*. Medpharm, Stuttgart, Germany

23 Chippaux JP, Williams V, White J (1991) Snake venom variability: Methods of study, results and interpretation. *Toxicon* 29: 1279–1303

24 Williams V, White J (1987) Variation in venom constituents within a single isolated population of peninsula tiger snake (*Notechis ater niger*). *Toxicon* 25: 1240–1243

25 Williams V, White J, Schwaner TD, Sparrow A (1988) Variation in venom proteins from isolated populations of tiger snakes (*Notechis ater niger*, *N. scutatus*) in South Australia. *Toxicon* 26: 1067–1075

26 Williams V, White J (1990) Variation in venom composition and reactivity in two specimens of yellow-faced whip snake (*Demansia psammophis*) from the same geographical area. *Toxicon* 28: 1351–1354

27 White J (1987) Elapid snakes: Venom toxicity and actions. In: J Covacevich, P Davie, J Pearn (eds): *Toxic Plants and Animals: A Guide For Australia*, Qld Museum, Brisbane, Australia, 369–389

28 White J (1987) Elapid snakes: Aspects of envenomation. In: J Covacevich, P Davie, J Pearn (eds): *Toxic Plants and Animals: A Guide For Australia*, Qld Museum, Brisbane, Australia, 391–429

29 White J (2004) Overview of venomous snakes of the world. In: R Dart (ed.): *Medical Toxicology*, Lippincott, Williams & Wilkins, Philadelphia, PA, 1543–1559

30 Ramasamy S, Isbister GK, Seymour JE, Hodgson WC (2005) The *in vivo* cardiovascular effects of the Irukandji jellyfish (*Carukia barnesi*) nematocyst venom and a tentacle extract in rats. *Toxicol Lett* 155: 135–141

31 Isbister GK, Gray MR, Balit CR, Raven RJ, Stokes BJ, Porges K, Tankel AS, Turner E, White J, Fisher MM (2005) Funnel-web spider bite: A systematic review of recorded clinical cases. *Med J Aust* 182: 407–411

32 Karlsson E (1979) Chemistry of protein toxins in snake venoms. In: CY Lee (ed.): *Handbook of Experimental Pharmacology: Snake Venoms*, Volume 52, Springer Verlag, Berlin, Germany

33 Gala S, Katelaris CH (1992) Rhabdomyolysis due to redback spider envenomation. *Med J Aust* 157: 66

34 Fouché R, Lucas P, Bernardin G, Roger PM, Corcelle P, Mattéi M (1997) Latrodectism: A rare cause of rhabdomyolysis. *Presse Med* 26: 954

35 Cohen J, Bush S (2005) Case report: Compartment syndrome after a suspected black widow spider bite. *Ann Emerg Med* 45: 414–416

36 Vetter RS, Visscher PK, Camazine S (1999) Mass envenomations by honey bees and wasps. *West*

J Med 170: 223–227

37 Vikrant S, Pandey D, Machhan P, Gupta D, Kaushal SS, Grover N (2005) Wasp envenomation-induced acute renal failure: A report of three cases. *Nephrology* 10: 548–552

38 Grisotto LS, Mendes GE, Castro I, Baptista MA, Alves VA, Yu L, Burdmann EA (2006) Mechanisms of bee venom-induced acute renal failure. *Toxicon* 48: 44–54

39 Das RN, Mukherjee K (2008) Asian wasp envenomation and acute renal failure: A report of two cases. *McGill J Med* 11: 25–28

40 Hutton RA, Warrell DA (1993) Action of snake venom components on the haemostatic system. *Blood Rev* 7: 176–189

41 White J (2005) Snake venoms and coagulopathy. *Toxicon* 45: 951–967

42 White J, Duncan B, Wilson C, Williams V, Lloyd J (1992) Coagulopathy following Australian elapid snakebite; A review of 20 cases. In: P Gopalakrishnakone, CK Tan (eds): *Recent Advances In Toxinology Research*. National University of Singapore, Singapore, 337–344

43 White J, Gilligan JE, Griggs W, Wilson C, Lloyd J (1992) Envenomation by the inland taipan, *Oxyuranus microlepidotus*; A case report. In: P Gopalakrishnakone, CK Tan (eds): *Recent Advances In Toxinology Research*. National University of Singapore, Singapore, 716–721

44 Boyer LV, Seifert SA, Clark RF, McNally JT, Williams SR, Nordt SP, Walter FG, Dart RC (1999) Recurrent and persistent coagulopathy following pit viper envenomation. *Arch Intern Med* 159: 706–710

45 Warrell DA, Davidson NM, Greenwood BM, Ormerod LD, Pope HM, Watkins BJ, Prentice CR (1977) Poisoning by bites of the saw-scaled or carpet viper (*Echis carinatus*) in Nigeria. *QJM* 46: 33–62

46 Estrade G, Garnier D, Bernasconi F, Donatien Y (1989) Pulmonary embolism and disseminated intravascular coagulation after being bitten by a *Bothrops lanceolatus* snake. Apropos of a case. *Arch Mal Coeur Vaiss* 82: 1903–1905

47 Thomas L, Tyburn B, Bucher B, Pecout F, Ketterle J, Rieux D, Smadja D, Garnier D, Plumelle Y (1995) Prevention of thromboses in human patients with *Bothrops lanceolatus* envenoming in Martinique: Failure of anticoagulants and efficacy of a monospecific antivenom. Research Group on Snake Bites in Martinique. *Am J Trop Med Hyg* 52: 419–426

48 Lôbo de Araújo A, Kamiguti A, Bon C (2001) Coagulant and anticoagulant activities of *Bothrops lanceolatus* (Fer de lance) venom. *Toxicon* 39: 371–375

49 Thomas L, Chausson N, Uzan J, Kaidomar S, Vignes R, Plumelle Y, Bucher B, Smadja D (2006) Thrombotic stroke following snake bites by the "Fer-de-Lance" *Bothrops lanceolatus* in Martinique despite antivenom treatment: A report of three recent cases. *Toxicon* 48: 23–28

50 Malbranque S, Piercecchi-Marti MD, Thomas L, Barbey C, Courcier D, Bucher B, Ridarch A, Smadja D, Warrell DA (2008) Fatal diffuse thrombotic microangiopathy after a bite by the "Fer-de-Lance" pit viper (*Bothrops lanceolatus*) of Martinique *Am J Trop Med Hyg* 78: 856–861

51 Arocha-Piñango CL, de Bosch NB, Torres A, Goldstein C, Nouel A, Argüello A, Carvajal Z, Guerrero B, Ojeda A, Rodriguez A (1992) Six new cases of a caterpillar-induced bleeding syndrome. *Thromb Haemost* 67: 402–407

52 Carrijo-Carvalho LC, Chudzinski-Tavassi AM (2007) The venom of the *Lonomia* caterpillar: An overview. *Toxicon* 49: 741–757

53 Devi CS, Reddy CN, Devi SL, Subrahmanyam YR, Bhatt HV, Suvarnakumari G, Murthy DP, Reddy CR (1970) Defibrination syndrome due to scorpion venom poisoning. *BMJ* 1: 345–347

54 Murthy KR, Zolfagharian H, Medh JD, Kudalkar JA, Yeolekar ME, Pandit SP, Khopkar M, Dave KN, Billimoria FR (1988) Disseminated intravascular coagulation and disturbances in carbohydrate and fat metabolism in acute myocarditis produced by scorpion (*Buthus tamulus*) venom. *Indian J Med Res* 87: 318–325

55 Longenecker GL, Longenecker HE Jr (1981) *Centruroides sculpturatus* venom and platelet reactivity: Possible role in scorpion venom-induced defibrination syndrome. *Toxicon* 19: 153–157

56 Isbister GK, Hooper MR, Dowsett R, Maw G, Murray L, White J (2006) Collett's snake (*Pseudechis colletti*) envenoming in snake handlers. *QJM* 99: 109–115

57 Kamiguti AS, Laing GD, Lowe GM, Zuzel M, Warrell DA, Theakston RD (1994) Biological properties of the venom of the Papuan black snake (*Pseudechis papuanus*): Presence of a phospholipase A$_2$ platelet inhibitor. *Toxicon* 32: 915–925

58 Marsh NA (1994) Snake venoms affecting the haemostatic mechanism – A consideration of their mechanisms, practical applications and biological significance. *Blood Coagul Fibrinolysis* 5: 399–410

59 Andrews RK, Berndt MC (2000) Snake venom modulators of platelet adhesion receptors and their ligands. *Toxicon* 38: 775–791

60 Kamiguti AS (2005) Platelets as targets of snake venom metalloproteinases. *Toxicon* 45: 1041–1049

61 Calvete JJ, Marcinkiewicz C, Monleón D, Esteve V, Celda B, Juárez P, Sanz L (2005) Snake venom disintegrins: Evolution of structure and function. *Toxicon* 45: 1063–1074

62 Mandal S, Bhattacharyya D (2007) Ability of a small, basic protein isolated from Russell's viper venom (*Daboia russelli russelli*) to induce renal tubular necrosis in mice. *Toxicon* 50: 236–250

63 De Castro I, Burdmann EA, Seguro AC, Yu L (2004) *Bothrops* venom induces direct renal tubular injury: Role for lipid peroxidation and prevention by antivenom. *Toxicon* 43: 833–839

64 Chugh KS, Aikat BK, Sharma BK, Dash SC, Mathew MT, Das KC (1975) Acute renal failure following snakebite. *Am J Trop Med Hyg* 24: 692–697

65 Sitprija V, Boonpucknavig V (1977) The kidney in tropical snakebite. *Clin Nephrol* 8: 377–383

66 Date A, Shastry JC (1982) Renal ultrastructure in acute tubular necrosis following Russell's viper envenomation. *J Pathol* 137: 225–241

67 White J, Fassett R (1983) Acute renal failure and coagulopathy after snakebite. *Med J Aust* 2: 142–143

68 Tin-Nu-Swe, Tin-Tun, Myint-Lwin, Thein-Than, Tun-Pe, Robertson JI, Leckie BJ, Phillips RE, Warrell DA (1993) Renal ischaemia, transient glomerular leak and acute renal tubular damage in patients envenomed by Russell's vipers (*Daboia russelii siamensis*) in Myanmar. *Trans R Soc Trop Med Hyg* 87: 678–681

69 Pinho FM, Zanetta DM, Burdmann EA (2005) Acute renal failure after *Crotalus durissus* snakebite: A prospective survey on 100 patients. *Kidney Int* 67: 659–667

70 Sitprija V (2006) Snakebite nephropathy. *Nephrology* 11: 442–448

71 Isbister GK, Little M, Cull G, McCoubrie D, Lawton P, Szabo F, Kennedy J, Trethewy C, Luxton G, Brown SG, Currie BJ (2007) Thrombotic microangiopathy from Australian brown snake (*Pseudonaja*) envenoming. *Intern Med J* 37: 523–528

72 Athappan G, Balaji MV, Navaneethan U, Thirumalikolundusubramanian P (2008) Acute renal failure in snake envenomation: A large prospective study. *Saudi J Kidney Dis Transpl* 19: 404–410

73 Schneemann M, Cathomas R, Laidlaw ST, El Nahas AM, Theakston RD, Warrell DA (2004) Life-threatening envenoming by the Saharan horned viper (*Cerastes cerastes*) causing micro-angiopathic haemolysis, coagulopathy and acute renal failure: Clinical cases and review. *QJM* 97: 717–727

74 Giordano AR, Vito L, Sardella PJ (2005) Complication of a Portuguese man-of-war envenomation to the foot: A case report. *J Foot Ankle Surg* 44: 297–300

75 Dall GF, Barclay KL, Knight D (2006) Severe sequelae after stonefish envenomation. *Surgeon* 4: 384–385

76 Barss P (1984) Wound necrosis caused by the venom of stingrays. Pathological findings and surgical management. *Med J Aust* 141: 854–855

77 Rocca AF, Moran EA, Lippert FG 3rd (2001) Hyperbaric oxygen therapy in the treatment of soft tissue necrosis resulting from a stingray puncture. *Foot Ankle Int* 22: 318–323

78 Magalhães KW, Lima C, Piran-Soares AA, Marques EE, Hiruma-Lima CA, Lopes-Ferreira M (2006) Biological and biochemical properties of the Brazilian Potamotrygon stingrays: *Potamotrygon cf. scobina* and *Potamotrygon gr. orbignyi*. *Toxicon* 47: 575–583

79 Pipelzadeh MH, Jalali A, Taraz M, Pourabbas R, Zaremirakabadi A (2007) An epidemiological and a clinical study on scorpionism by the Iranian scorpion *Hemiscorpius lepturus*. *Toxicon* 50: 984–992

80 Hogan CJ, Barbaro KC, Winkel K (2004) Loxoscelism: Old obstacles, new directions. *Ann Emerg Med* 44: 608–624

81 Tambourgi DV, Paixão-Cavalcante D, Gonçalves de Andrade RM, Fernandes-Pedrosa Mde F, Magnoli FC, Paul Morgan B, van den Berg CW (2005) *Loxosceles* sphingomyelinase induces complement-dependent dermonecrosis, neutrophil infiltration, and endogenous gelatinase expression. *J Invest Dermatol* 124: 725–731

82 De Oliveira KC, Gonçalves de Andrade RM, Piazza RM, Ferreira JM Jr, van den Berg CW, Tambourgi DV (2005) Variations in *Loxosceles* spider venom composition and toxicity contribute to the severity of envenomation. *Toxicon* 45: 421–429

83 Paixão-Cavalcante D, van den Berg CW, Gonçalves-de-Andrade RM, Fernandes-Pedrosa Mde F, Okamoto CK, Tambourgi DV (2007) Tetracycline protects against dermonecrosis induced by

Loxosceles spider venom. *J Invest Dermatol* 127: 1410–1418

84 McGlasson DL, Harroff HH, Sutton J, Dick E, Elston DM (2007) Cutaneous and systemic effects of varying doses of brown recluse spider venom in a rabbit model. *Clin Lab Sci* 20: 99–105

85 Malta MB, Lira MS, Soares SL, Rocha GC, Knysak I, Martins R, Guizze SP, Santoro ML, Barbaro KC (2008) Toxic activities of Brazilian centipede venoms. *Toxicon* 52: 255–263

86 Han TS, Teichert RW, Olivera BM, Bulaj G (2008) *Conus* venoms – A rich source of peptide-based therapeutics. *Curr Pharm Des* 14: 2462–2479

87 Sutherland SK, Coulter AR, Harris RD (1979) Rationalisation of first-aid measures for elapid snakebite. *Lancet* 8109: 183–185

88 Sutherland SK, Coulter AR (1981) Early management of bites by the eastern diamondback rattlesnake (*Crotalus adamanteus*): Studies in monkeys (*Macaca fascicularis*). *Am J Trop Med Hyg* 30: 497–500

89 Stewart ME, Greenland S, Hoffman JR (1981) First-aid treatment of poisonous snakebite: Are currently recommended procedures justified? *Ann Emerg Med* 10: 331–335

90 Pearn J, Morrison J, Charles N, Muir V (1981) First-aid for snake-bite: Efficacy of a constrictive bandage with limb immobilization in the management of human envenomation. *Med J Aust* 2: 293–295

91 Anker RL, Straffon WG, Loiselle DS, Anker KM (1983) Snakebite. Comparison of three methods designed to delay uptake of 'mock venom'. *Aust Fam Physician* 12: 365–368

92 Reitz CJ, Willemse GT, Odendaal MW, Visser JJ (1986) Evaluation of the venom ex apparatus in the initial treatment of puff adder envenomation. A study in rabbits. *S Afr Med J* 69: 684–686

93 Moorman CT 3rd, Moorman LS, Goldner RD (1992) Snakebite in the tarheel state. Guidelines for first aid, stabilization, and evacuation. *NC Med J* 53: 141–146

94 Blackman JR, Dillon S (1992) Venomous snakebite: Past, present, and future treatment options. *J Am Board Fam Pract* 5: 399–405

95 Howarth DM, Southee AE, Whyte IM (1994) Lymphatic flow rates and first-aid in simulated peripheral snake or spider envenomation. *Med J Aust* 161: 695–700

96 Tun-Pe, Aye-Aye-Myint, Khin-Ei-Han, Thi-Ha, Tin-Nu-Swe (1995) Local compression pads as a first-aid measure for victims of bites by Russell's viper (*Daboia russelii siamensis*) in Myanmar. *Trans R Soc Trop Med Hyg* 89: 293–295

97 Theakston RD (1997) An objective approach to antivenom therapy and assessment of first-aid measures in snake bite. *Ann Trop Med Parasitol* 91: 857–865

98 Zamudio KR, Hardy DL Sr, Martins M, Greene HW (2000) Fang tip spread, puncture distance, and suction for snake bite. *Toxicon* 38: 723–728

99 Habib AG, Gebi UI, Onyemelukwe GC (2001) Snake bite in Nigeria. *Afr J Med Med Sci* 30: 171–178

100 Juckett G, Hancox JG (2002) Venomous snakebites in the United States: Management review and update. *Am Fam Physician* 65: 1367–1374

101 Bush SP, Green SM, Laack TA, Hayes WK, Cardwell MD, Tanen DA (2004) Pressure immobilization delays mortality and increases intracompartmental pressure after artificial intramuscular rattlesnake envenomation in a porcine model. *Ann Emerg Med* 44: 599–604

102 Alberts MB, Shalit M, LoGalbo F (2004) Suction for venomous snakebite: A study of "mock venom" extraction in a human model. *Ann Emerg Med* 43: 181–186

103 Sharma SK, Koirala S, Dahal G, Sah C (2004) Clinico-epidemiological features of snakebite: A study from Eastern Nepal. *Trop Doct* 34: 20–22

104 Little M (2008) First aid for jellyfish stings: Do we really know what we are doing? *Emerg Med Australas* 20: 78–80

105 Currie BJ, Canale E, Isbister GK (2008) Effectiveness of pressure-immobilization first aid for snakebite requires further study. *Emerg Med Australas* 20: 267–270

106 Simpson ID, Tanwar PD, Andrade C, Kochar DK, Norris RL (2008) The Ebbinghaus retention curve: Training does not increase the ability to apply pressure immobilisation in simulated snake bite – Implications for snake bite first aid in the developing world. *Trans R Soc Trop Med Hyg* 102: 451–459

107 White J (1995) Poisonous and venomous animals – The physician's view. In: J Meier, J White (eds): *Handbook of Clinical Toxicology of Animal Venoms and Poisons*, CRC Press, Boca Raton, FL, 9–26

108 Hawgood BJ (1999) Doctor Albert Calmette 1863–1933: Founder of antivenomous serotherapy and of antituberculous BCG vaccination. *Toxicon* 37: 1241–1258

109 Chippaux JP, Goyffon M (1998) Venoms, antivenoms and immunotherapy. *Toxicon* 36: 823–846

110 Theakston RD, Warrell DA, Griffiths E (2003) Report of a WHO workshop on the standardization and control of antivenoms. *Toxicon* 41: 541–557

111 Nkinin SW, Chippaux JP, Piétin D, Doljansky Y, Trémeau O, Ménez A (1997) Genetic origin of venom variability: Impact on the preparation of antivenin serums. *Bull Soc Pathol Exot* 90: 277–281

112 Chippaux JP, Goyffon M (1991) Antivenom serotherapy: Its applications, its limitations, its future. *Bull Soc Pathol Exot* 84: 286–297

113 Ruha AM, Curry SC, Beuhler M, Katz K, Brooks DE, Graeme KA, Wallace K, Gerkin R, Lovecchio F, Wax P, Selden B (2002) Initial postmarketing experience with crotalidae polyvalent immune Fab for treatment of rattlesnake envenomation. *Ann Emerg Med* 39: 609–615

114 Seifert SA, Boyer LV (2001) Recurrence phenomena after immunoglobulin therapy for snake envenomations: Part 1. Pharmacokinetics and pharmacodynamics of immunoglobulin antivenoms and related antibodies. *Ann Emerg Med* 37: 189–195

115 Consroe P, Egen NB, Russell FE, Gerrish K, Smith DC, Sidki A, Landon JT (1995) Comparison of a new ovine antigen binding fragment (Fab) antivenin for United States Crotalidae with the commercial antivenin for protection against venom-induced lethality in mice. *Am J Trop Med Hyg* 53: 507–510

116 Sjostrom L, al-Abdulla IH, Rawat S, Smith DC, Landon J (1994) A comparison of ovine and equine antivenoms. *Toxicon.* 32: 427–433

117 Cannon R, Ruha AM, Kashani J (2008) Acute hypersensitivity reactions associated with administration of crotalidae polyvalent immune Fab antivenom. *Ann Emerg Med* 51: 407–411

118 Lavonas EJ, Gerardo CJ, O'Malley G, Arnold TC, Bush SP, Banner W Jr, Steffens M, Kerns WP 2nd (2004) Initial experience with Crotalidae polyvalent immune Fab (ovine) antivenom in the treatment of copperhead snakebite. *Ann Emerg Med* 43: 200–206

119 Morais JF, de Freitas MC, Yamaguchi IK, dos Santos MC, da Silva WD (1994) Snake antivenoms from hyperimmunized horses: Comparison of the antivenom activity and biological properties of their whole IgG and F(ab')₂ fragments. *Toxicon* 32: 725–734

120 Otero-Patiño R, Cardoso JL, Higashi HG, Nunez V, Diaz A, Toro MF, Garcia ME, Sierra A, Garcia LF, Moreno AM, Medina MC, Castañeda N, Silva-Diaz JF, Murcia M, Cardenas SY, Dias da Silva WD (1998) A randomized, blinded, comparative trial of one pepsin-digested and two whole IgG antivenoms for *Bothrops* snake bites in Uraba, Colombia. The Regional Group on Antivenom Therapy Research (REGATHER). *Am J Trop Med Hyg* 58: 183–189

121 Otero R, León G, Gutiérrez JM, Rojas G, Toro MF, Barona J, Rodríguez V, Díaz A, Núñez V, Quintana JC, Ayala S, Mosquera D, Conrado LL, Fernández D, Arroyo Y, Paniagua CA, López M, Ospina CE, Alzate C, Fernández J, Meza JJ, Silva JF, Ramírez P, Fabra PE, Ramírez E, Córdoba E, Arrieta AB, Warrell DA, Theakston RD (2006) Efficacy and safety of two whole IgG polyvalent antivenoms, refined by caprylic acid fractionation with or without β-propiolactone, in the treatment of *Bothrops asper* bites in Colombia. *Trans R Soc Trop Med Hyg* 100: 1173–1182

122 León G, Rojas G, Lomonte B, Gutiérrez JM (1997) Immunoglobulin G and F(ab')₂ polyvalent antivenoms do not differ in their ability to neutralize hemorrhage, edema and myonecrosis induced by *Bothrops asper* (terciopelo) snake venom. *Toxicon* 351627–351637

123 Dos Santos MC, D'Império Lima MR, Furtado GC, Colletto GM, Kipnis TL, Dias da Silva W (1989) Purification of F(ab')₂ anti-snake venom by caprylic acid: A fast method for obtaining IgG fragments with high neutralization activity, purity and yield. *Toxicon* 27: 297–303

124 Rojas G, Jiménez JM, Gutiérrez JM (1994) Caprylic acid fractionation of hyperimmune horse plasma: Description of a simple procedure for antivenom production. *Toxicon* 32: 351–363

125 Seddik SS, Malak GA, Helmy MH (2002) Improved purification and yield of the Egyptian snake *Cerastes cerastes* antitoxin by the use of caprylic acid. *J Nat Toxins* 11: 323–328

126 Raweerith R, Ratanabanangkoon K (2003) Fractionation of equine antivenom using caprylic acid precipitation in combination with cationic ion-exchange chromatography. *J Immunol Methods* 282: 63–72

127 Chippaux JP, Goyffon M (1983) Producers of antivenom sera. *Toxicon* 21: 739–752

128 Theakston RD, Warrell DA (1991) Antivenoms: A list of hyperimmune sera currently available for the treatment of envenoming by bites and stings. *Toxicon* 29: 1419–1470

129 Meier J (1995) Commercially available antivenoms (hyperimmune sera, antivenins, antisera) for antivenom therapy. In: J Meier, J White (eds): *Handbook of Clinical Toxicology of Animal Venoms and Poisons*, CRC Press, Boca Raton, FL, 689–721

130 Padilla-Marroquin A (2008) *WHO Guidelines for the Production, Control and Regulation of Snake Antivenom Immunoglobulins.* (http://www.snakebiteinitiative.org/node/24)

131 Burnouf T, Terpstra F, Habib G, Seddik S (2007) Assessment of viral inactivation during pH 3.3 pepsin digestion and caprylic acid treatment of antivenoms. *Biologicals* 35: 329–334

132 Wilde H, Thipkong P, Sitprija V, Chaiyabutr N (1996) Heterologous antisera and antivenins are essential biologicals: Perspectives on a worldwide crisis. *Ann Intern Med* 125: 233–236

133 al-Asmari AK, al-Abdulla IH, Crouch RG, Smith DC, Sjostrom L (1997) Assessment of an ovine antivenom raised against venom from the desert black cobra (*Walterinnesia aegyptia*). *Toxicon* 35: 141–145

134 White J (2002) *CSL Antivenom Handbook.* CSL Ltd, Melbourne, Australia

135 Harrison RA, Hasson SS, Harmsen M, Laing GD, Conrath K, Theakston RD (2006) Neutralisation of venom-induced haemorrhage by IgG from camels and llamas immunised with viper venom and also by endogenous, non-IgG components in camelid sera. *Toxicon* 47: 364–368

136 Herrera M, León G, Segura A, Meneses F, Lomonte B, Chippaux JP, Gutiérrez JM (2005) Factors associated with adverse reactions induced by caprylic acid-fractionated whole IgG preparations: Comparison between horse, sheep and camel IgGs. *Toxicon* 46: 775–781

137 Almeida CM, Kanashiro MM, Rangel Filho FB, Mata MF, Kipnis TL, da Silva WD (1998) Development of snake antivenom antibodies in chickens and their purification from yolk. *Vet Rec* 143: 579–584

138 Maya Devi C, Vasantha Bai M, Krishnan LK (2002) Development of viper-venom antibodies in chicken egg yolk and assay of their antigen binding capacity. *Toxicon* 40: 857–861

139 Sevcik C, Díaz P, D'Suze G (2007) On the presence of antibodies against bovine, equine and poultry immunoglobulins in human IgG preparations, and its implications on antivenom production. *Toxicon* 51: 10–16

140 Meenatchisundaram S, Parameswari G, Michael A, Ramalingam S (2008) Neutralization of the pharmacological effects of Cobra and Krait venoms by chicken egg yolk antibodies. *Toxicon* 52: 221–227

141 Riaño-Umbarila L, Juárez-González VR, Olamendi-Portugal T, Ortíz-León M, Possani LD, Becerril B (2005) A strategy for the generation of specific human antibodies by directed evolution and phage display. An example of a single-chain antibody fragment that neutralizes a major component of scorpion venom. *FEBS J* 272: 2591–2601

142 Alvarenga LM, Diniz CR, Granier C, Chávez-Olórtegui C (2002) Induction of neutralizing antibodies against *Tityus serrulatus* scorpion toxins by immunization with a mixture of defined synthetic epitopes. *Toxicon* 40: 89–95

143 Calderón-Aranda ES, Rivière G, Choumet V, Possani LD, Bon C (1999) Pharmacokinetics of the toxic fraction of *Centruroides limpidus limpidus* venom in experimentally envenomed rabbits and effects of immunotherapy with specific F(ab')₂. *Toxicon* 37: 771–782

144 de Almeida DM, Fernandes-Pedrosa Mde F, de Andrade RM, Marcelino JR, Gondo-Higashi H, de Azevedo Ide L, Ho PL, van den Berg C, Tambourgi DV (2008) A new anti-loxoscelic serum produced against recombinant sphingomyelinase D: Results of preclinical trials. *Am J Trop Med Hyg* 79: 463–470

145 White J (1998) Envenoming and antivenom use in Australia. *Toxicon* 36: 1483–1492

146 Chaves F, Loría GD, Salazar A, Gutiérrez JM (2003) Intramuscular administration of antivenoms in experimental envenomation by *Bothrops asper*: Comparison between Fab and IgG. *Toxicon* 41: 237–244

147 Wiener S (1961) Red back spider bite in Australia: An analysis of 167 cases. *Med J Aust* 48: 44–49

148 Sutherland SK, Trinca JC (1978) Survey of 2144 cases of red-back spider bites: Australia and New Zealand, 1963–1976. *Med J Aust* 2: 620–623

149 Byrne GC, Pemberton PJ (1983) Red-back spider (*Latrodectus mactans hasselti*) envenomation in a neonate. *Med J Aust* 2: 665–666

150 White J, Harbord M (1985) Latrodectism as mimic. *Med J Aust* 142: 75

151 Jelinek GA, Banham ND, Dunjey SJ (1989) Red-back spider-bites at Fremantle Hospital, 1982–1987. *Med J Aust* 150: 693–695

152 Sutherland SK (1992) Antivenom use in Australia. Premedication, adverse reactions and the use of venom detection kits. *Med J Aust* 157: 734–739

153 Mead HJ, Jelinek GA (1993) Red-back spider bites to Perth children, 1979–1988. *J Paediatr Child Health* 29: 305–308

154 Pincus DR (1994) Response to antivenom 14 days after red-back spider bite. *Med J Aust* 161: 226
155 Banham ND, Jelinek GA, Finch PM (1994) Late treatment with antivenom in prolonged red-back spider envenomation. *Med J Aust* 161: 379–381
156 Wells CL, Spring WJ (1996) Delayed but effective treatment of red-back spider envenomation. *Med J Aust* 164: 447
157 Couser GA, Wilkes GJ (1997) A red-back spider bite in a lymphoedematous arm. *Med J Aust* 166: 587–588
158 Ellis RM, Sprivulis PC, Jelinek GA, Banham ND, Wood SV, Wilkes GJ, Siegmund A, Roberts BL (2005) A double-blind, randomized trial of intravenous *versus* intramuscular antivenom for red-back spider envenoming. *Emerg Med Australas* 17: 152–156
159 Isbister GK, Gray MR (2003) Latrodectism: A prospective cohort study of bites by formally identified redback spiders. *Med J Aust* 179: 88–91
160 Isbister GK (2007) Safety of i.v. administration of redback spider antivenom. *Intern Med J* 37: 820–822
161 Brown SG, Isbister GK, Stokes B (2007) Route of administration of redback spider bite antivenom: Determining clinician beliefs to facilitate Bayesian analysis of a clinical trial. *Emerg Med Australas* 19: 458–463
162 Isbister GK, Brown SG, Miller M, Tankel A, Macdonald E, Stokes B, Ellis R, Nagree Y, Wilkes GJ, James R, Short A, Holdgate A (2008) A randomised controlled trial of intramuscular *versus* intravenous antivenom for latrodectism – The RAVE study. *QJM* 101: 557–565
163 White J, Dart RC (2007) *Snakebite: A Brief Medical Guide.* Stirling
164 Theakston RD, Lloyd-Jones MJ, Reid HA (1977) Micro-ELISA for detecting and assaying snake venom and venom-antibody. *Lancet* 8039: 639–641
165 Theakston RD, Reid HA (1979) Enzyme-linked immunosorbent assay (ELISA) in assessing antivenom potency. *Toxicon* 17: 511–515
166 Theakston RD, Pugh RN, Reid HA (1981) Enzyme-linked immunosorbent assay of venom-antibodies in human victims of snake bite. *J Trop Med Hyg* 84: 109–112
167 Theakston RD, Reid HA, Larrick JW, Kaplan J, Yost JA (1981) Snake venom antibodies in Ecuadorian Indians. *J Trop Med Hyg* 84: 199–202
168 Theakston RD (1983) The application of immunoassay techniques, including enzyme-linked immunosorbent assay (ELISA), to snake venom research. *Toxicon* 21: 341–352
169 Dhaliwal JS, Lim TW, Sukumaran KD (1983) A double antibody sandwich micro-ELISA kit for the rapid diagnosis of snake bite. *Southeast Asian J Trop Med Public Health* 14: 367–373
170 Rodriguez-Acosta A, Uzcategui W, Azuaje R, Giron ME, Aguilar I (1998) ELISA assays for the detection of Bothrops lanceolatus venom in envenomed patient plasmas. *Roum Arch Microbiol Immunol* 57: 271–278
171 Selvanayagam ZE, Gnanavendhan SG, Ganesh KA, Rajagopal D, Rao PV (1999) ELISA for the detection of venoms from four medically important snakes of India. *Toxicon* 37: 757–770
172 Khow O, Wongtongkam N, Pakmanee N, Omori-Satoh T, Sitprija V (1999) Development of reversed passive latex agglutination for detection of Thai cobra (*Naja kaouthia*) venom. *J Nat Toxins* 8: 213–220
173 Dong le V, Quyen le K, Eng KH, Gopalakrishnakone P (2003) Immunogenicity of venoms from four common snakes in the South of Vietnam and development of ELISA kit for venom detection. *J Immunol Methods* 282: 13–31
174 Dong le V, Eng KH, Quyen le K, Gopalakrishnakone P (2004) Optical immunoassay for snake venom detection. *Biosens Bioelectron* 19: 1285–1294
175 Chase P, Boyer-Hassen L, McNally J, Vazquez HL, Theodorou AA, Walter FG, Alagon A (2009) Serum levels and urine detection of *Centruroides sculpturatus* venom in significantly envenomated patients. *Clin Tox* 47: 24–28
176 Chandler HM, Hurrell JG (1982) A new enzyme immunoassay system suitable for field use and its application in a snake venom detection kit. *Clin Chim Acta* 121: 225–230
177 Hurrell JG, Chandler HW (1982) Capillary enzyme immunoassay field kits for the detection of snake venom in clinical specimens: A review of two years' use. *Med J Aust* 2: 236–237
178 Marshall LR, Herrmann RP (1984) Cross-reactivity of bardick snake venom with death adder antivenom. *Med J Aust* 140: 541–542
179 White J, Williams V, Passehl JH (1987) The five-ringed brown snake, *Pseudonaja modesta* (Gunther): Report of a bite and comments on its venom. *Med J Aust* 147: 603–605
180 Williams V, White J (1990) Variation in venom composition and reactivity in two specimens of

yellow-faced whip snake (*Demansia psammophis*) from the same geographical area. *Toxicon* 28: 1351–1354

181 Pearn J, McGuire B, McGuire L, Richardson P (2000) The envenomation syndrome caused by the Australian red-bellied black snake *Pseudechis porphyriacus*. *Toxicon* 38: 1715–1729

182 Currie BJ (2004) Snakebite in Australia: The role of the venom detection kit. *Emerg Med Australas* 16: 384–386

183 Jelinek GA, Tweed C, Lynch D, Celenza T, Bush B, Michalopoulos N (2004) Cross reactivity between venomous, mildly venomous, and non-venomous snake venoms with the Commonwealth Serum Laboratories venom detection kit. *Emerg Med Australas* 16: 459–464

184 O'Leary MA, Isbister GK, Schneider JJ, Brown SG, Currie BJ (2006) Enzyme immunoassays in brown snake (*Pseudonaja* spp.) envenoming: Detecting venom, antivenom and venom-antivenom complexes. *Toxicon* 48: 4–11

185 Steuten J, Winkel K, Carroll T, Williamson NA, Ignjatovic V, Fung K, Purcell AW, Fry BG (2007) The molecular basis of cross-reactivity in the Australian snake venom detection kit (SVDK). *Toxicon* 50: 1041–1052

186 Cupo P, Azevedo-Marques MM, de Menezes JB, Hering SE (1991) Immediate hypersensitivity reactions after intravenous use of antivenin sera: Prognostic value of intradermal sensitivity tests. *Rev Inst Med Trop Sao Paulo* 33: 115–122

187 León G, Segura A, Herrera M, Otero R, França FO, Barbaro KC, Cardoso JL, Wen FH, de Medeiros CR, Prado JC, Malaque CM, Lomonte B, Gutiérrez JM (2008) Human heterophilic antibodies against equine immunoglobulins: Assessment of their role in the early adverse reactions to antivenom administration *Trans R Soc Trop Med Hyg* 102: 1115–1119

188 Stewart CS, MacKenzie CR, Hall JC (2007) Isolation, characterization and pentamerization of α-cobrotoxin specific single-domain antibodies from a naïve phage display library: Preliminary findings for antivenom development. *Toxicon* 49: 699–709

189 García M, Monge M, León G, Lizano S, Segura E, Solano G, Rojas G, Gutiérrez JM (2002) Effect of preservatives on IgG aggregation, complement-activating effect and hypotensive activity of horse polyvalent antivenom used in snakebite envenomation. *Biologicals* 30: 143–151

190 Isbister GK, Brown SG, MacDonald E, White J, Currie BJ (2008) Current use of Australian snake antivenoms and frequency of immediate-type hypersensitivity reactions and anaphylaxis. *Med J Aust* 188: 473–476

191 Warrell DA (1999) WHO/SEARO Guidelines for the Clinical Management of snake bites in the Southeast Asian region. *South East Asian J Trop Med Public Health* 30 Suppl 1: 1–84

192 Malasit P, Warrell DA, Chanthavanich P, Viravan C, Mongkolsapaya J, Singhthong B, Supich C (1986) Prediction, prevention, and mechanism of early (anaphylactic) antivenom reactions in victims of snake bites. *Br Med J Clin Res Ed* 29217–29220

193 Sheikh A, Shehata YA, Brown SG, Simons FE (2009) Adrenaline for the treatment of anaphylaxis: Cochrane systematic review. *Allergy* 64: 204–212

194 Fan HW, Marcopito LF, Cardoso JL, França FO, Malaque CM, Ferrari RA, Theakston RD, Warrell DA (1999) Sequential randomised and double blind trial of promethazine prophylaxis against early anaphylactic reactions to antivenom for bothrops snake bites. *BMJ* 318: 1451–1452

195 Isbister GK, Brown SG, MacDonald E, White J, Currie BJ (2008) Current use of Australian snake antivenoms and frequency of immediate-type hypersensitivity reactions and anaphylaxis. *Med J Aust* 188: 473–476

196 Watt G, Theakston RD, Hayes CG, Yambao ML, Sangalang R, Ranoa CP, Alquizalas E, Warrell DA (1986) Positive response to edrophonium in patients with neurotoxic envenoming by cobras (*Naja naja philippinensis*). A placebo-controlled study. *N Engl J Med* 315: 1444–1448

197 Currie B, Fitzmaurice M, Oakley J (1988) Resolution of neurotoxicity with anticholinesterase therapy in death-adder envenomation. *Med J Aust* 148: 522–525

198 Lalloo DG, Trevett AJ, Black J, Mapao J, Saweri A, Naraqi S, Owens D, Kamiguti AS, Hutton RA, Theakston RD, Warrell DA (1996) Neurotoxicity, anticoagulant activity and evidence of rhabdomyolysis in patients bitten by death adders (*Acanthophis* sp.) in southern Papua New Guinea. *QJM* 89: 25–35

199 Trevett AJ, Lalloo DG, Nwokolo NC, Naraqi S, Kevau IH, Theakston RD, Warrell DA (1995) Failure of 3,4-diaminopyridine and edrophonium to produce significant clinical benefit in neurotoxicity following the bite of Papuan taipan (*Oxyuranus scutellatus canni*). *Trans R Soc Trop Med Hyg* 89: 444–446

200 Bawaskar HS, Bawaskar PH (1986) Prazosin in management of cardiovascular manifestations of

scorpion sting. *Lancet* 8479: 510–511

201 Bawaskar HS, Bawaskar PH (2000) Prazosin therapy and scorpion envenomation. *J Assoc Physicians India* 48: 1175–1180

202 Biswal N, Bashir RA, Murmu UC, Mathai B, Balachander J, Srinivasan S (2006) Outcome of scorpion sting envenomation after a protocol guided therapy. *Indian J Pediatr* 73: 577–582

203 Gupta V (2006) Prazosin: A pharmacological antidote for scorpion envenomation. *J Trop Pediatr* 52: 150–151

204 Bawaskar HS, Bawaskar PH (2007) Utility of scorpion antivenin *vs* prazosin in the management of severe *Mesobuthus tamulus* (Indian red scorpion) envenoming at rural setting. *J Assoc Physicians India* 55: 14–21

205 Yildizdas D, Yilmaz HL, Erdem S (2008) Treatment of cardiogenic pulmonary oedema by helmet-delivered non-invasive pressure support ventilation in children with scorpion sting envenomation. *Ann Acad Med Singapore* 37: 230–234

206 al-Asmari AK, al-Seif AA, Hassen MA, Abdulmaksood NA (2008) Role of prazosin on cardiovascular manifestations and pulmonary edema following severe scorpion stings in Saudi Arabia. *Saudi Med J* 29: 299–302

207 Ramasamy S, Isbister GK, Seymour JE, Hodgson WC (2005) The *in vivo* cardiovascular effects of the Irukandji jellyfish (*Carukia barnesi*) nematocyst venom and a tentacle extract in rats. *Toxicol Lett* 155: 135–141

208 Winter KL, Isbister GK, Schneider JJ, Konstantakopoulos N, Seymour JE, Hodgson WC (2008) An examination of the cardiovascular effects of an 'Irukandji' jellyfish, *Alatina nr mordens*. *Toxicol Lett* 179: 118–123

209 Ramasamy S, Isbister GK, Seymour JE, Hodgson WC (2005) Pharmacologically distinct cardiovascular effects of box jellyfish (*Chironex fleckeri*) venom and a tentacle-only extract in rats. *Toxicol Lett* 155: 219–226

210 Ramasamy S, Isbister GK, Seymour JE, Hodgson WC (2005) The *in vivo* cardiovascular effects of an Australasian box jellyfish (*Chiropsalmus* sp.) venom in rats. *Toxicon* 45: 321–327

211 White J (1987) Elapid snakes: Management of bites. In: J Covacevich, P Davie, J Pearn (eds): *Toxic Plants and Animals: A Guide For Australia*, Qld Museum, Brisbane, Australia, 431–457

212 Little M, Mulcahy RF (1998) A year's experience of Irukandji envenomation in far north Queensland. *Med J Aust* 169: 638–641

213 Prentice O, Fernandez WG, Luyber TJ, McMonicle TL, Simmons MD (2008) Stonefish envenomation. *Am J Emerg Med* 26: 972

214 Grandcolas N, Galéa J, Ananda R, Rakotoson R, D'Andréa C, Harms JD, Staikowsky F (2008) Stonefish stings: Difficult analgesia and notable risk of complications. *Presse Med* 37: 395–400

215 de Andrade JG, Pinto RN, de Andrade AL, Martelli CM, Zicker F (1989) Bacteriologic study of abscesses caused by bites of snakes of the genus *Bothrops*. *Rev Inst Med Trop Sao Paulo* 31: 363–367

216 Nishioka Sde A, Silveira PV (1992) A clinical and epidemiologic study of 292 cases of lance-headed viper bite in a Brazilian teaching hospital. *Am J Trop Med Hyg* 47: 805–810

217 Jorge MT, Ribeiro LA, da Silva ML, Kusano EJ, de Mendonça JS (1994) Microbiological studies of abscesses complicating *Bothrops* snakebite in humans: A prospective study. *Toxicon* 32: 743–748

218 Jorge MT, Malaque C, Ribeiro LA, Fan HW, Cardoso JL, Nishioka SA, Sano-Martins IS, França FO, Kamiguti AS, Theakston RD, Warrell DA (2004) Failure of chloramphenicol prophylaxis to reduce the frequency of abscess formation as a complication of envenoming by *Bothrops* snakes in Brazil: A double-blind randomized controlled trial. *Trans R Soc Trop Med Hyg* 98: 529–534

219 Rodríguez Acosta A, Uzcategui W, Azuaje R, Aguilar I, Girón ME (2000) Análisis clínico y epidemiológico de los accidentes por mordeduras de serpientes del género *Bothrops* en Venezuela [A clinical and epidemiological analysis of accidental bites by snakes of the genus *Bothrops* in Venezuela.] *Rev Cubana Med Trop* 52: 90–94

220 Habib AG (2003) Tetanus complicating snakebite in northern Nigeria: Clinical presentation and public health implications. *Acta Trop* 85: 87–91

221 Ehui E, Kra O, Ouattara I, Tanon A, Kassi A, Eholié S, Bissagnéné E, Kadio A (2007) Generalized tetanus complicating a traditional medicine applied for snakebite. *Bull Soc Pathol Exot* 100: 184–185

222 Nazim MH, Gupta S, Hashmi S, Zuberi J, Wilson A, Roberts L, Karimi K (2008) Retrospective review of snake bite victims. *WV Med J* 104: 30–34

223 Brown TP (2005) Diagnosis and management of injuries from dangerous marine life. *MedGenMed* 7: 5

224 Murphey DK, Septimus EJ, Waagner DC (1992) Catfish-related injury and infection: Report of two cases and review of the literature. *Clin Infect Dis* 14: 689–693

225 Warrell DA (1995) Clinical toxicology of snakebite in Africa and the Middle East/Arabian Peninsula. In: J Meier, J White (eds): *Handbook of Clinical Toxicology of Animal Venoms and Poisons*, CRC Press, Boca Raton, FL, 433–492

226 Warrell DA (1995) Clinical toxicology of snakebite in Asia. In: J Meier, J White (eds): *Handbook of Clinical Toxicology of Animal Venoms and Poisons*, CRC Press, Boca Raton, FL, 493–594

227 Wilson DC, King LE Jr (1990) Spiders and spider bites. *Dermatol Clin* 8: 277–286

228 Futrell JM (1992) Loxoscelism. *Am J Med Sci* 304: 261–267

229 Leach J, Bassichis B, Itani K (2004) Brown recluse spider bites to the head: Three cases and a review. *Ear Nose Throat J* 83: 465–470

230 Acott C, Meier J (1995) Clinical toxicology of venomous stingray injuries. In: J Meier, J White (eds): *Handbook of Clinical Toxicology of Animal Venoms and Poisons*, CRC Press, Boca Raton, FL, 135–140

231 Fry BG, Wüster W (2004) Assembling an arsenal: Origin and evolution of the snake venom proteome inferred from phylogenetic analysis of toxin sequences. *Mol Biol Evol* 21: 870–883

232 Jackson K (2007) The evolution of venom-conducting fangs: Insights from developmental biology. *Toxicon* 49: 975–981

233 Weinstein SA, Kardong KV (1994) Properties of Duvernoy's secretions from opisthoglyphous and aglyphous colubrid snakes. *Toxicon* 32: 1161–1185

234 Fry BG, Vidal N, Norman JA, Vonk FJ, Scheib H, Ramjan SF, Kuruppu S, Fung K, Hedges SB, Richardson MK, Hodgson WC, Ignjatovic V, Summerhayes R, Kochva E (2006) Early evolution of the venom system in lizards and snakes. *Nature* 439: 584–588

235 Tu MC, Wang HY, Tsai MP, Toda M, Lee WJ, Zhang FJ, Ota H (2000) Phylogeny, taxonomy, and biogeography of the oriental pitvipers of the genus *trimeresurus* (reptilia: viperidae: crotalinae): A molecular perspective. *Zool Sci* 17: 1147–1157

236 Malhotra A, Thorpe RS (2004) A phylogeny of four mitochondrial gene regions suggests a revised taxonomy for Asian pitvipers (*Trimeresurus* and *Ovophis*). *Mol Phylogenet Evol* 32: 83–100

237 Sanders KL, Malhotra A, Thorpe RS (2004) Ecological diversification in a group of Indomalayan pitvipers (*Trimeresurus*): Convergence in taxonomically important traits has implications for species identification. *J Evol Biol* 17: 721–731

238 Radmanesh M (1990) Clinical study of *Hemiscorpion lepturus* in Iran. *J Trop Med Hyg* 93: 327–332

239 Radmanesh M (1998) Cutaneous manifestations of the *Hemiscorpius lepturus* sting: A clinical study. *Int J Dermatol* 37: 500–507

240 Pipelzadeh MH, Jalali A, Taraz M, Pourabbas R, Zaremirakabadi A (2007) An epidemiological and a clinical study on scorpionism by the Iranian scorpion *Hemiscorpius lepturus*. *Toxicon* 50: 984–992

Molecular, Clinical and Environmental Toxicology. Volume 2: Clinical Toxicology
Edited by A. Luch
© 2010 Birkhäuser Verlag/Switzerland

Mechanistic insights on spider neurotoxins

Andreas Luch

German Federal Institute for Risk Assessment, Berlin, Germany

Abstract. In physiology research, animal neurotoxins historically have served as valuable tools for identification, purification, and functional characterization of voltage-dependent ion channels. In particular, toxins from scorpions, sea anemones and cone snails were at the forefront of work aimed at illuminating the three-dimensional architecture of sodium channels. To date, at least six different receptor binding sites have been identified and – most of them – structurally assigned in terms of protein sequence and spatial disposition. Recent work on Australian funnel-web spiders identified certain peptidic ingredients as being responsible for the neurotoxicity of the crude venom. These peptides, termed δ-atracotoxins (δ-ACTX), consist of 42 amino acids and bind to voltage-gated sodium channels in the same way as classical scorpion α-toxins. According to the 'voltage-sensor trapping model' proposed in the literature, δ-ACTX isoforms interact with the voltage sensor S4 transmembrane segment of α-subunit domain IV, thereby preventing its normal outward movement and concurrent conformational changes required for inactivation of the channel. As consequence prolonged action potentials at autonomic or somatic synapses induce massive transmitter release, resulting in clinical correlates of neuroexcitation (e.g., muscle fasciculation, spasms, paresthesia, tachycardia, diaphoresis, etc.). On the other hand, the major neurotoxin isolated from black widow spiders, α-latrotoxin (α-LTX), represents a 132 kDa protein consisting of a unique N-terminal sequence and a C-terminal part harboring multiple ankyrin-like repeats. Upon binding to one of its specific presynaptic receptors, α-LTX has been shown to tetramerize under physiological conditions to form Ca^{2+}-permeable pores in presynaptic membranes. The molecular model worked out during recent years separates two distinguishable receptor-mediated effects. According to current knowledge, binding of the N terminus of α-LTX at one of its specific receptors either triggers intracellular signaling cascades, resulting in phospholipase C-mediated mobilization of presynaptic Ca^{2+} stores, or leads to the formation of tetrameric pore complexes, allowing extracellular Ca^{2+} to enter the presynaptic terminal. α-LTX-triggered exocytosis and fulminant transmitter release at autonomic synapses may then provoke a clinical syndrome referred to as 'latrodectism', characterized by local and incapacitating pain, diaphoresis, muscle fasciculation, tremor, anxiety, and so forth. The present review aims at providing a short introduction into some of the exciting molecular effects induced by neurotoxins isolated from black widow and funnel-web spiders.

Introduction

Spiders are ubiquitous and abundant worldwide, typically killing their prey by injection of venom. Thus, it should not come as surprise that some spiders are dangerous to humans as well. Although almost all spiders are venomous, fortunately most are incapable of penetrating human skin and injecting sufficient amounts of venom, thus deaths from spider bites are extremely rare, but have been occasionally reported, especially in the pre-antivenom era [1–3]. The venom glands of spiders are associated with specialized fangs, so-called chelicers, that are perfectly adapted to perforate the outer body barriers of insects, other arthropods, or worms. Some of them are even specialized to feed on fish or small terrestrial vertebrates. From the roughly 40 000 described species of spiders worldwide [4, 5], there are 5 genera with some medical significance: *Latrodectus* (Theridiidae, widow spiders), *Loxosceles* (Loxoscelidae, recluse spiders), *Atrax* and *Hadronyche* (Hexathelidae, funnel-web spiders), and *Phoneutria* (Ctenidae, banana spiders).

In North America, bites of widow and brown spiders are most dangerous and painful. The venom of the notorious and abundant black widow spider, e.g., *Latrodectus mactans* (Fig. 1), constitutes a variable mix of neurotoxic proteins, enzymes, and bioactive small molecules such as polyamines that potentiate neurotoxicity, leading to the envenomation syndrome referred to as 'latrodectism'. On the other hand, bites of brown recluse spiders, *Loxosceles* spp., a genus present in most parts of the world, can cause inflammation and hemorrhagic ulceration. Here, in particular the dermonecrotic enzyme sphingomyelinase D, a major component of the venom, hydrolyzes membrane-bound sphingomyelin, induces platelet aggregation, complement-mediated hemolysis, release of tumor necrosis factor α, and triggers inflammation and pain *via* production of prostaglandins [6]. Inflammation and tissue necrosis is the predominating effect of *Loxosceles* bites (so-called 'loxoscelism' or necrotic arachnidism).

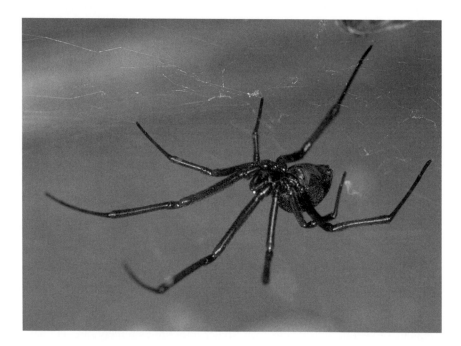

Figure 1. North American black widow spider, female, *Latrodectus mactans* (courtesy of Julian White; original photo/illustration copyright © Julian White).

The endemic funnel-web spiders, e.g., *Atrax robustus*, represent a serious threat and may cause envenoming of humans in Australia. These large and aggressive spiders apply highly toxic venoms that may lead to death if no antivenom can be administered timely. Here, neurotoxic peptides are predominant and responsible for extremely painful bites that eventually may progress toward respiratory and cardiac failure of the human victim. In South America, the Brazilian banana spider *Phoneutria nigriventer* can be compared to *Atrax* in terms of most aspects important from a toxinologist's point of view, such as behavior (extremely aggressive species mostly responsible for serious spider incidents in south Brazil), type and symptoms of human envenoming (neurotoxic, e.g., cramps, tremor, paralysis, arrhythmias, etc.; death is possible if untreated), and toxic ingredients of the venom (i.e., at least 17 different neurotoxic peptides predominantly targeting voltage-dependent sodium or calcium channels) [7].

In general, toxins isolated from animal venoms have been widely used as chemical tools/molecular probes in biomedical research to examine and dissect important physiological pathways. This knowledge can then be beneficially exploited to identify new lead compounds and to develop novel pharmaceutical and agricultural agents, i.e., drugs and biopesticides (anti-arthropod toxins applicable in pest control) [8]. This holds especially true for investigations on the structure, function and manipulation of the nervous system. Due to their toxic effects on neuronal cells, spider venoms are currently in the focus of basic molecular and fundamental mechanistic studies. The present review aims at providing an introduction and a glimpse into the most exciting aspects of the different modes of action of neurotoxins produced by deadly venomous black widow and funnel-web spiders.

Widow spiders

Envenomation

Widow spiders comprising the genus *Latrodectus* (Fig. 1) with about 30 different species are distributed worldwide [9]. In addition to *Latrodectus*, the Theridiidae family includes more than 50 genera with *Steatoda* being closely related to widow spiders, featuring a similar morphology and clinical envenoming syndrome indistinguishable from latrodectism [10]. The venom of widow spiders has been extensively studied and the major neurotoxin, α-latrotoxin (α-LTX), among other toxins, has been isolated and well characterized [8, 11, 12]. α-LTX specifically targets neuronal cell receptors of the presynaptic plasma membrane as part of the synaptic cleft. Once bound to latrophilin 1 or neurexin Iα, α-LTX inserts into the membrane to form Ca^{2+}-permeable pores and to trigger the release of neurotransmitters through vesicle exocytosis, thereby causing massive neurotransmitter excess in the particular synaptic cleft addressed. On the other hand, some of the effects of α-LTX on vesicle exocytosis are mediated independently from toxin pores through receptor binding, subsequent induction of intracellular signaling and release of Ca^{2+} from presynaptic stores (Fig. 2). The overall envenomation syndrome (latrodectism) and clinical effects provoked in humans can persist for hours up to weeks, consisting of incapacitating, local and radiating pain in the extremities affected, local and regional diaphoresis, piloerection, sweating and muscle fasciculation accompanied by nonspecific systemic effects such as anxiety, tremor, dizziness, etc. [2, 13, 14]. In the case of systemic latrodectism pain is the predominating feature. Depending on the site of the bite, the pain initially induced and imposed in a rather circumscribed manner at certain body parts can progress toward generalized abdominal pain that is difficult to distinguish from acute abdominal conditions resulting from a more common etiology. Other systemic

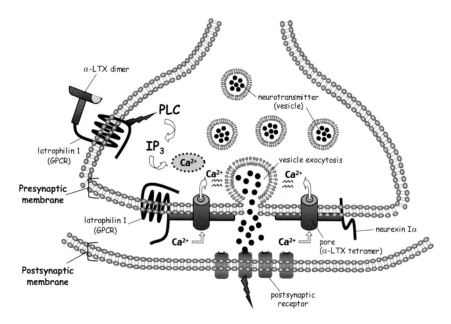

Figure 2. Schematic representation of the effects of α-latrotoxin (α-LTX) at the presynaptic membrane of autonomic or somatic synapses. α-LTX specifically binds to specific neuronal cell receptors, i.e., latrophilin 1 or neurexin Iα. In the presence of divalent cations and upon binding to latrophilin 1 or neurexin Iα, α-LTX tetramerizes and inserts into the presynaptic membrane to form Ca^{2+}-permeable pores. Pore-mediated Ca^{2+} influx into the presynaptic cytosol then triggers massive release of neurotransmitters into the synaptic cleft *via* vesicle exocytosis. On the other hand, binding of α-LTX dimer or tetramer complexes to latrophilin 1 (a G protein-coupled receptor, GPCR) can also trigger vesicle exocytosis *via* GPCR-mediated signaling (flash sign). Receptor-mediated activation of membrane-associated phosphatidylinositide-specific phospholipase C (PLC) leads to increases in presynaptic inositol triphosphate (IP_3) and diacyl glycerol (not shown) levels, subsequent release of Ca^{2+} from intracellular stores and neurotransmitter vesicle exocytosis. Neurotransmitter binding at postsynaptic receptors then induces specific effects depending on the particular neuronal system(s) addressed (flash sign). The overall clinical syndrome entitled 'latrodectism' features a wide range of symptoms, such as pain, sweating, diaphoresis, hypertension, muscle fasciculation, tremor, and dizziness, due to receptor overstimulation at vegetative (automomic) and somatic synapses. Figure adapted according to [23]. See text for further details.

effects such as nausea, vomiting, hypertension, tachycardia, dyspnoea, and insomnia may occur. Apparently the majority of confirmed widow spider bites cause significant clinical effects with severe and persistent pain, hypertension, agitation, irritability, and so forth [15]. This is especially true for children [16]. However, usually, symptoms gradually diminish over time. Only in rare conditions is worsening, long-term persistence, or a fatal outcome possible (e.g., acute renal failure, rhabdomyolysis, paralysis, shock). Despite this potential aggravation, there are no assured reports on deaths resulting from *Latrodectus* envenomation of humans during the past decades [2, 12].

Widow spider neurotoxins

The most important neurotoxin of widow spider venom, α-LTX, isolated from *Latrodectus mactans tredecimguttatus* (Mediterranean species) in the 1970s, was characterized as 130 kDa protein responsible for inducing neurotoxicity in vertebrates with an LD_{50} in mice of about 20–40 μg/kg [17–19]. In 1990, five additional insect-selective, so-called latroinsectotoxins (α-, β-, γ-, δ-, ε-LIT), and the crustacean-selective α-latrocrustotoxin (α-LCT) were purified by Grishin and co-workers [20, 21]. Upon post-translational cleavage of larger precursor proteins the mature proteins range between 110 and 130 kDa. During the 1990s, besides α-LTX [22], three additional latrotoxins were cloned and characterized (α-LIT, δ-LIT, α-LCT) (reviewed in [23]). Latrotoxins such as α-LTX are synthesized as precursor molecules containing an N-terminal recognition site of the eukaryotic endoprotease furin (member of the subtilisin family) that is cleaved-off during post-translational maturation, in a similar manner to that seen in furin-dependent processing and activation of influenza virus hemagglutinin or bacterial toxins such as clostridial or diphtheria toxins [24, 25]. Removal of a 47-residue N-terminal leader and an additional furin-dependent cleavage at another consensus sequence present in the C-terminal part of the precursor (removal of about 200 residues) then produces the mature α-LTX protein consisting of 1179 amino acids and an overall molecular mass of 131.5 kDa [25]. Since α-LTX is produced at cytosolic ribosomes without association to endoplasmic membranes [26], the protein lacks signal peptides or transmembrane domains. According to the current model, upon disintegration of secretory cells, cytoplasmic toxin molecules are released into the lumen of the venom gland as precursors that subsequently undergo truncation at both ends (N and C termini) catalyzed by appropriate (furin-like) proteases. Such proteases have been found in high concentrations in the extracellular compartment of the venom gland [27].

Mature latrotoxins consist of a unique N-terminal region with no substantial homology to any other proteins and a C-terminal region harboring multiple (e.g., 22 in α-LTX) ankyrin-like repeats of about 30–34 amino acids in length. These ankyrin-like repeats are similar to those typical for the eponym (cytoskeletal protein ankyrin) but are also highly common as sequence motif in other proteins with various functions, and are thought to be required as stabilizing 'glue' in intermolecular protein-protein interactions such as those necessary for oligomerization [28, 29]. Studies on the three-dimensional structure revealed that the entire protein is composed of three different domains [30], linked to each other *via* modified (diverged) ankyrin-like repeats, of which the N-terminal 'wing' domain displays a unique, largely α-helical sequence, while the middle 'body' and C-terminal 'head' domains consist mostly of conventional ankyrin repeats producing a rather globular shape at the C terminus. Under physiological conditions, α-LTX forms a complex with two low-molecular mass proteins of 8 and 9.5 kDa, collectively entitled latrodectin [31, 32], neither of which confer toxicity but may augment α-LTX-mediated effects [33–35]. Moreover, the toxin occurs as dimers or (in the presence of divalent cations) as tetramers. Since divalent cations such as Ca^{2+} or Mg^{2+} are required for α-LTX activity, tetrameric complexes most likely represent the fully functional form of the toxin [30, 36]. Cryo-electron microscopy studies on membrane-integrated α-LTX tetramers revealed that the four monomers are symmetrically arranged in a four-bladed (protein monomer) propeller configuration displaying C4 symmetry, leaving a central pore of about 10–35 Å in diameter (depending on section level) collectively lined by the four C-terminal 'head' domains [30]. The entire complex has a diameter of 250 Å and a height of 100 Å, and can fully penetrate lipid bilayers with its hydrophobic base (45 Å deep). The wings protruding from the central mass perpendicular to the axis are attached to the outer membrane surface, slightly dipping into it. A model of the quaternary structure of the toxin and its insertion into lipid bilayers has been comprehensively described by Ushkaryov and co-workers [23, 30].

Studies using recombinant α-LTX forms indicated that three highly conserved cysteine residues within the N-terminal 'wing' domain are crucial for the biological activity of the protein [33]. Replacement of cysteines at positions 14, 71 and 393 completely abolished receptor binding (cf. below) and the ability of α-LTX to release neurotransmitters at synaptosomes [33]. In addition, the sequence and structure of the ankyrin repeat-containing 'body' domain proved crucial for toxin's inherent ability to tetramerize. Introduction of four additional amino acids within a certain tightly packed 'body' domain sequence resulted in a recombinant protein (α-LTX^{N4C}) that initially was thought to be unable to trigger exocytosis [33]. Interestingly, binding to its synaptic receptors and activation of phospholipase C (PLC) signaling was comparable to the wild-type form [33]. Later work revealed, however, that this mutant protein failed to assemble into cylindrical tetramers, but was still capable of strongly inducing transmitter release [37, 38]. This result, therefore, demonstrates that receptor binding and PLC signaling alone, without incorporation of functional tetramers into the membranes as pore complexes, may still be sufficient to trigger neurotransmitter release *via* exocytosis under certain circumstances [37, 38].

About 30 years ago, α-LTX was shown to form Ca^{2+}-permeable pores in membrane bilayers of sensitive cells [39, 40]. Subsequently, continuous efforts have clarified the picture of an amphipathic α-LTX tetramer with a self-organ-izing capacity for the insertion into lipid bilayers in the presence of Ca^{2+} or Mg^{2+} ions [30]. According to the model suggested, purified α-LTX or the entire widow spider venom was expected to trigger massive neurotransmitter release from presynaptic membranes through a sequence of Ca^{2+}-dependent processes, starting with the binding to either one of its various structurally and functionally unrelated specific neuronal receptors, e.g., neurexin Iα and lat-rophilin 1 [35, 41, 42]. Upon binding of its N-terminal 'wing' domain to one of its presynaptic membrane receptors and, most likely facilitated through divalent cation-mediated complexation of appropriate amino acid residues, the above-mentioned tetramers are formed and subsequently integrated into the membrane lipid bilayer [30, 36, 43]. According to the data published, the N-terminal 'wing' would interact with the specific membrane receptor but then rather stay outside the membrane being oriented toward the synaptic cleft. Considering all current literature, Ushkaryov and co-workers nicely summa-rized the most probable mechanism of α-LTX membrane binding and tetrameric complex formation (Fig. 2) [23, 44].

As already indicated, the α-LTX-specific neuronal receptors identified today belong to structurally and functionally unrelated classes of cell surface proteins. The first receptor, neurexin Iα, discovered in 1992 [45] represents a member of a highly variable group of neuronal cell surface receptors compris-ing an extremely wide range of isoforms. This is due to extensive post-tran-scriptional splicing and post-translational modification (O-glycosylation) of the products of three genes at multiple sites [46]. All members of the poly-morphic neurexin family are characterized as Ca^{2+}-dependent neuron-specific cell adhesion molecules containing one transmembrane domain [45]. According to current knowledge, however, from this large group of isoforms only neurexin Iα binds to α-LTX via the so-called LNS-B3 domain as part of its large extracellular sequence [47]. The second neuronal α-LTX-specific receptor characterized, latrophilin 1 [48], represents a member of the group of large heptahelical receptors (containing seven hydrophobic transmembrane domains) that correspond to the peptide hormone-binding secretin family of G protein-coupled receptors (GPCR) [49–51]. In the literature, latrophilin 1 has also been described as Ca^{2+}-independent receptor for latrotoxin (CIRL). Due to an unusual processing while being transported through endoplasmic membranes prior to delivery of the protein to the cell surface, i.e., the consti-tutive post-translational cleavage into a separate cell adhesion-like (extracellu-lar) N-terminal domain and a C-terminal signaling domain [52], latrophilin actually represents a novel and never-before described group of GPCR pro-teins. Upon arrival at the surface membrane, both fragments then can act inde-pendently in close proximity, unless α-LTX binding at the N-terminal frag-ment facilitates reassociation and subsequent G protein activation, PLC sig-naling and Ca^{2+} release from intracellular stores [52]. From the three lat-rophilin isoforms described in the literature, only latrophilin 1 has been found to bind to α-LTX with high affinity and to be enriched in mammalian brain tissue [33, 53, 54]. The protein tyrosine phosphatase σ (PTPσ) represents another, most recently described neuronal cell surface receptor that displays considerable affinity to α-LTX. PTPσ contains a single transmembrane domain, acts independently from Ca^{2+} and binds to the toxin *via* extracellular fibronectin type III repeats [55]; however, it seems to play only a minor role in mediating α-LTX toxicity in mouse brain *in vivo* [56].

The picture of the black widow spider venom that initially emerged suggested that vertebrate-specific multimer α-LTX complexes function as nonselective cation channels allowing Ca^{2+} to enter the presynaptic terminal, to trigger intracellular signaling cascades, and to evoke exocytosis of vesicles and release of transmitters into the synaptic cleft (reviewed in [57]). It further became clear that α-LTX can induce both Ca^{2+}-dependent and -independent neurotransmitter release. The group of Südhof determined the difference between the Ca^{2+}-dependent and the -independent way of α-LTX-triggered exocytosis, the latter being restricted to small presynaptic vesicles that contain glutamate, γ-aminobutyric acid, or acetylcholine [58]. Conversely, emptying of dense core or catecholaminergic vesicles (carrying peptides, noradrenaline, or dopamine) in general required calcium. These data added support to the early observation at frog neuromuscular junctions that – under Ca^{2+}-limited conditions – high doses of α-LTX preferentially induced fulminant release of acetylcholine-containing small synaptic vesicles, thus causing the depletion of cholinergic vesicles and its cargo [59]. The more sophisticated model that has emerged recently separates α-LTX-mediated effects triggered by protein insertion into presynaptic membranes and concomitant (or preceding) formation of tetrameric pore complexes (cf. above) from those effects induced *via* membrane surface receptor binding and initiation of intracellular signaling (reviewed in [23]; Fig. 2). Whereas receptor binding of α-LTX apparently facilitates pore formation, intracellular signaling triggered by α-LTX at its latrophilin 1 receptor most likely occurs independently from tetrameric pore formation. According to recent data, to a great extent made available by the employment of a recombinant protein incapable of forming functional tetramers (i.e., α-LTX^{N4C}, cf. above), it seems plausible that one mode of α-LTX can be narrowed down to its binding of GPCR latrophilin 1 and subsequent receptor-mediated initiation of the following consecutive molecular events: activation of PLC, hydrolysis of phosphatidylinositol phosphates, increases in cytosolic inositol triphosphate (IP_3) and diacyl glycerol concentrations, mobilization of intracellular Ca^{2+} stores, and release of neurotransmitters through bursts (elevated rates and amplitudes) of evoked exocytosis [33, 37, 38, 60]. PLC signaling-mediated intracellular Ca^{2+} waves, however, result in rather small increases of transmitter concentrations emerging in synaptic clefts when compared to huge effects initiated by wild-type protein pore formation and subsequent influx of extracellular Ca^{2+} (reviewed in [23, 44]).

In the absence of extracellular Ca^{2+}, α-LTX can induce massive neurotransmitter release in neuronal cells only when Mg^{2+} functions as substitute so that tetrameric complexes can be formed [30, 36]. However, it is still not clear whether secretion in the absence of extracellular Ca^{2+} can be induced by pore-mediated facilitation of cation conductance and its direct or indirect effects on vesicle exocytosis, or whether this effect results from ion current-driven alterations of membrane depolarization. In addition, intracellular ankyrin-like repeats of the tetrameric pore complex inserted into the neuronal plasma membrane may also directly interfere with the transmitter vesicle exocytosis machinery [43, 61]. Whether or not α-LTX-mediated neurotransmitter release also requires components of the classical synaptic exocytosis machinery, such as the SNARE proteins synaptobrevin/VAMP and SNAP25 [62], as well as the exact contribution of Ca^{2+} to each of the individual modes exerted by α-LTX at synaptic and neuromuscular junctions, both issues require further experimental efforts to be fully and unequivocally established.

Funnel-web spiders

Envenomation

Endemic funnel-web spiders of East Australia represent the most dangerous spider group known to date, responsible for rare, but occasionally severe and life-threatening, sometimes even deadly envenoming of humans [2, 3, 14]. The group encompasses at least 40 species of the genera *Atrax* and *Hadronyche* [63]. Fortunately, adverse health effects induced are mostly mild, mainly consisting of local neurotoxicity (numbness, paresthesia, etc.). However, serious clinical effects have been described, dominated by both autonomic excitation (tachycardia, hypertension, lacrimation, diaphoresis, etc.) and neuromuscular excitation (muscle fasciculation and spasms), and accompanied by systemic symptoms, such as abdominal pain, nausea, headache, and agitation, eventually culminating in elevated intracranial pressure, generalized muscle fasciculations, pulmonary and cranial edema, coma and death [64–66]. Systemic envenomation after bite of these kinds of spiders may develop rapidly within minutes [67]. Prior to the introduction of a specific and effective antivenom in the 1980s, 14 fatal bites of Sydney funnel-web spiders, *Atrax robustus*, had been reported in the medical literature since the 1920s [68]. Although observed deaths were traced back exclusively to male individuals of *A. robustus*, other Australian funnel-web spider species of this or the related *Hadronyche* genus contain similarly effective venom mixtures in their chelicers [69] and induce similar envenomation syndromes [70, 71]. However, these other species have apparently never been reported as the cause of fatalities in Australia, arguably due to their occurrence in remote regions and habitats far away from crowded human settlements [72]. Funnel-web spider venom has long been known for its specific toxicity in primates, only causing comparably mild symptoms in non-primates when administered in high doses [73, 74]. Early studies on the characterization of the venom afforded a component called "atraxin" that gave similar effects in monkeys when compared to the crude mixture [75]. Today, specific peptides, termed as atracotoxins (ACTX), have been shown to be predominantly responsible for the induced neurotoxic envenoming syndrome [12, 72]. Whereas δ-ACTX forms have been identified to predominantly work in primates including humans, the more recently discovered ω- and J-ACTX forms exhibit selectivity toward insects (see next section).

Funnel-web spider neurotoxins

Funnel-web spider venom contains peptide toxins, of which the first to be described were isolated from *Atrax robustus* (δ-ACTX-Ar1, originally termed "robustoxin") and *Hadronyche versuta* (δ-ACTX-Hv1a, originally termed "versutoxin") [76, 77]. Since envenomation symptoms produced in monkeys resembled the neurotoxic syndrome seen in humans after spider bites, these peptides were already suspected at the end of the 1980s of being predominantly responsible for the effects induced by the crude venom *in vivo* [78]. Back at that time, the advent of novel molecular biology tools allowed structural characterization of the peptides and the proposal of a unique sequence of 42 amino acids including 8 cysteine residues [79]. Subsequent analysis of other ACTX homologues gave similar results and demonstrated that 3 of the 8 conserved cysteine residues can be found directly connected to each other in a tricysteinyl triplet [80]. All δ-ACTX isoforms known today represent highly homologous peptides of 42 amino acids in length that are tightly folded due to four conserved intramolecular disulfide bonds. So, all cysteine residues present in those peptides contribute to cystine cross-links. The three-dimensional structures resolved by NMR [81] display a triple-stranded antiparallel β-sheet as core sequence containing disulfide bridges that form a so-called 'pseudo-knot'. Thus, δ-ACTX isoforms share structural features with other neurotoxic and inhibitory polypeptides originating from a variety of phylogenetically related and unrelated sources, such as American funnel-web spiders (e.g., ω-agatoxins from *Agelenopsis aperta*), other arthropods, and cone snails (e.g., ω-conotoxins from *Conus* spp.), which all frequently contain an 'inhibitor cystine knot' (ICK) motif [82, 83]. The biological targets of these ICK motif-containing toxins, however, differ, with membrane ion channels being an important but not the only group of physiological molecules addressed (i.e., inhibited). The relationship between structure and function of individual δ-ACTX forms known and characterized today has been comprehensively reviewed by Nicholson and co-workers [72, 84].

δ-ACTX homologues induce clinical features of envenomation *via* massive transmitter release at both autonomic and somatic synapses (neuroexcitation). This transmitter release is caused by prolonged prejunctional and terminal action potentials triggered through spontaneous repetitive neuronal firing [85, 86]. As most obvious clinical correlates, patients typically display muscle fasciculations, spasms and dysfunction of the autonomic nervous system (cf.

above). Electrophysiological patch-clamp *in vitro* studies revealed that the toxins inhibit conversion of voltage-gated Na^+ channels from an open to an inactivated state, thereby maintaining Na^+ conductance at membrane potentials where inactivation of those channels would normally have been completed (regularly about 2 ms after the start of the action potential). In the presence of δ-ACTX, synaptic Na^+ channels also recover faster from their inactivated state, and voltage-gated Na^+ current inactivation by tetrodotoxin (TTX) can be slowed down [87]. δ-ACTX has been shown to cause an up to 30% increase of Na^+ conductance at the membrane, an additional ion flux that could be inhibited by TTX [88]. Work by Nicholson and co-workers [89, 90] demonstrated that δ-ACTX is capable of inhibiting the binding of mammalian-selective scorpion α-toxins, isolated from *Androctonus australis hector* (AaH-II) or *Leiurus quinquestriatus hebraeus* (LqH-II), to its well-characterized neurotoxin receptor site-3 on voltage-gated Na^+ channels [91] of rat brain synaptosomes at nanomolar concentrations (cf. below). Since they also found that binding of δ-ACTX could be competitively inhibited by scorpion α-toxins, but only allosterically inhibited by brevetoxin PbTx-1 isolated from the dinoflagellate *Ptychodiscus brevis* [92], it was concluded that the binding site of δ-ACTX most likely lies in the proximity of neurotoxin receptor site-3 at the Na^+ channel (Fig. 3) [87]. Thus, from the at least six distinct neurotoxin receptor binding sites at the mammalian voltage-gated sodium channel characterized today [93–95] (cf. next section), classical scorpion α-toxins (e.g., AaH-II and LqH-II), sea anemone toxins (e.g., ApB and anthopleurin-B from *Anthopleura xanthogrammica*) and the funnel-web spider toxins (δ-ACTX) all interact with site-3 on the S3–S4 extracellular loop in domain IV (Fig. 3).

Another δ-ACTX form subsequently isolated from *Hadronyche versuta* venom and with 67% sequence identity to robustoxin, δ-ACTX-Hv1b, showed decreased activity but similar effects at mammalian voltage-gated Na^+ channels when compared to the classical δ-ACTX forms robustoxin and versutoxin [80]. However, in contrast to these classical forms, δ-ACTX-Hv1b proved to be vertebrate-selective and without any activity against sodium channels from insects. Due to varying binding affinities at neuronal sodium channel receptor site-3, toxicity of classical δ-ACTX in insects depends on the source of neuron preparation, e.g., locust *versus* cockroach, thus suggesting subtle alterations between sodium channels from different species [92]. When compared to anti-insect scorpion α-toxin LqHαIT, however, the binding affinity and mode of action of δ-ACTXs characterized in cockroach neuronal preparations are similar and resemble the situation found in rat brain synaptosomes [90, 92, 96].

Based on the presence of certain charged amino acids on the bioactive surface of the toxins and the consideration of possible electrostatic interactions with binding site-3 located at the S3–S4 extracellular loop of domain IV in mammalian voltage-gated sodium channels [97], it was proposed in the 1990s that in particular residues at positions 3–5 (Lys, Lys, Arg) and 13 (Asp) would

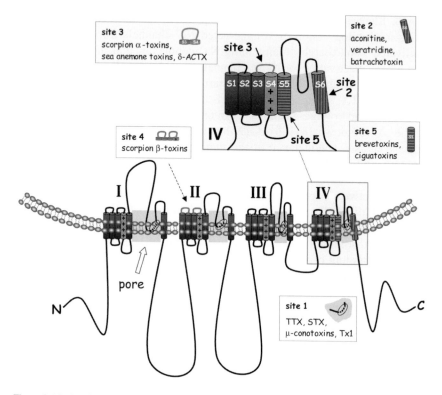

Figure 3. Model of the voltage-gated sodium channel α-subunit and location of the mammalian neurotoxin receptor sites according to the literature (figure adapted from [93]). The α-subunit of the channel is represented by a single pore-forming glycosylated protein consisting of a tandem arrangement of four homologous domains (I–IV), each of which contains six membrane spanning α-helical segments (S1–S6; see cylinders of domain IV enlarged in box). The central channel pore is made from the tetrameric arrangement of the pore-lining S5–S6 segments of all four domains and their reentrant loops in between. The positively charged S4 segments serve as a gating sensor that triggers voltage-dependent activation of the central pore. Neurotoxin receptor binding site 1 is actually part of the inner pore and made of specific sequences of all protein loops interconnecting the four S5 and S6 pairs (encircled in the figure; central pore cavity is indicated by gray shading). Site 1 is targeted, e.g., by tetrodotoxin (TTX), saxitoxin (STX), μ-conotoxins, and Tx1 (toxin of the banana spider *Phoneutria nigriventer*). Neurotoxin binding sites 2 and 5 are represented by certain sequences of transmembrane segments S6 and S5, respectively, within domain IV (see enlarged domain IV in box). These sites are targets of rather lipophilic toxins such as aconitine, veratridine, and batrachotoxin (site 2), or brevetoxins and ciguatoxins (site 5). Toxin binding at sites 2 or 5 triggers an allosterically induced blockage of the sodium channel. Neurotoxin receptor site 3 mainly consists of the S3–S4 extracellular loop within domain IV (see enlarged domain IV in box). At this site, the sodium channel is affected by peptide toxins such as scorpion α-toxin, sea anemone toxins, or δ-atracotoxins (δ-ACTX; isolated from Australian funnel-web spiders, e.g., *Atrax robustus*). Conversely, scorpion β-toxins bind to neurotoxin receptor site 4, consisting of S1–S2 and S3–S4 extracellular loops of domain II. Since neurotoxin receptor site 6 (targeted, e.g., by δ-conotoxins) has as yet not been unambiguously assigned, it is omitted in the cartoon. See text for further details.

represent the toxin's pharmacophore and thus provide the complementary surface (consensus sequence) to crucial residues identified in the S3–S4 loop

[98]. More recent structure-dependent functional research of the two classical δ-ACTX forms in comparison to the scorpion α-toxins AaH-II and LqHαIT emphasizes the importance of residues 3–5 (Lys, Lys, Arg), 6 (Asn), 7 (Trp), 10 (Lys), 12 (Glu), and 22/25 (Tyr), which are all located on the surface of the respective δ-ACTX toxin, thereby being matched by identical amino acids that shape the bioactive surface of scorpion α-toxins [92, 99]. On the other hand, and in view of its ineffectiveness toward insect sodium channels, replacement of cationic amino acid residues at positions 4 and 5 by serine and aspartic acid, respectively, and changes at positions 6 (Gly) and 22 (Lys) in the sequence of δ-ACTX-Hv1b may be regarded as required structural determinants for vertebrate-specific toxicity [80, 84].

Recently, many atracotoxin isoforms of two novel, structurally unrelated, protein families have been isolated from *Hadronyche versuta* venom and termed ω-ACTX [100, 101] or Janus-faced atracotoxins (J-ACTX, also termed κ-ACTX) [102, 103], respectively. In contrast to the well-characterized δ-ACTX-mediated inhibition of Na^+ channels, however, these groups of proteins represent insecticidal neurotoxins that rather target voltage-gated calcium and Ca^{2+}-activated potassium (K_{Ca}) channels, thereby inducing either neurodepression (ω-ACTX-mediated blockage of Ca^{2+} channels) or neuroexcitation (J-ACTX-mediated blockage of K_{Ca} channels). Recent work on insecticidal atracotoxins and the possible implications for future development of novel and highly selective biopesticides have been extensively reviewed elsewhere [104, 105].

Voltage-gated sodium channels: Targets of δ-atracotoxins and beyond?

Voltage-sensitive sodium channels, like similar channels for potassium and calcium, are transmembrane proteins in charge of generating, amplifying and transmitting electric pulses leading to neuronal transmission and muscle contraction. The structures of eukaryotic sodium channels comprise single pore-forming glycosylated proteins of about 220–260 kDa and roughly 2000 amino acid residues in length [95, 106, 107]. These proteins actually represent the pore-forming α subunit that may be associated with one or two smaller auxiliary subunits (β1–β4) of about 33–36 kDa. An α subunit is made of a tandem arrangement of four homologous domains (I–IV), each of which contains six membrane-spanning segments (S1–S6) connected by external and internal peptide loops (Fig. 3). The central channel pore is made from the tetrameric arrangement of the S5–S6 segments, and all four reentrant loops between these four segment pairs together represent the structural correlate of the ion selectivity filter. On the other hand, the four positively charged and highly conserved S4 segments serve as gating voltage sensor that trigger voltage-dependent activation of the central channel pore by moving outward under the influence of changes in the electric field (depolarization phase) [108].

Sodium channels are the target of a wide range of neurotoxins, of both synthetic and biogenic origin. Due to their high affinity and great specificity, however, especially neurotoxins from plant or animal origin have proved to be invaluable as powerful tools to study the structure and function of voltage-gated sodium channels [93–95]. Several groups of natural neurotoxins bind to certain receptor sites thereby altering channel conformation and ultimately ion conductivity (Fig. 3). To date, based on competition binding assays and compound-mediated alterations in voltage-dependent gating (activation) and ion permeation (conductance), or channel inactivation (pore block), at least six different neurotoxin receptor sites have been identified, of which four are involved in peptide toxin binding (Fig. 3) [95, 109]. Moreover, the interaction of a certain neurotoxin at one particular site may induce conformational changes that, in turn, cause altering of voltage-dependent gating of the channel and – at the same time – might also affect the binding affinity of other proximal receptor sites.

Neurotoxin receptor site 1 (Fig. 1) of sodium channels represents the target of the small water-soluble guanidinium alkaloids TTX and saxitoxin (STX) isolated from a range of different so-called puffer fish (and other animals) and the dinoflagellates *Gonyaulax* spp., respectively [93–95]. These toxins have long been known as for their ability to physically occlude the ion channel. In addition, the peptidic µ-conotoxins, produced from piscivore cone snails (*Conus geographus* and others), and Tx1 from the banana spider *Phoneutria nigriventer* (cf. above) can block sodium conductance, thereby competing with each other for the same binding site [110–112]. However, although µ-conotoxins were also shown to competitively inhibit TTX binding, the two groups of toxins (small molecules *versus* peptides) are unlikely to address identical receptor sites, but rather share overlapping channel sequences for interaction [93–95].

Soluble lipophilic toxins that were found to bind to intramembrane receptor sites 2 or 5 alter voltage-dependent gating *via* allosterically induced blockage of sodium channel inactivation and shifting of the channel activation toward more negative potentials (hyperpolarizing shift in voltage dependence of activation). In this group of allosteric modulators, among others, alkaloid toxins such as aconitine (from *Aconitum napellus*, Monkshood plant), veratridine (from *Veratrum* spp. and other plants of the Liliaceae family) and batrachatoxin (from *Phyllobates* spp., poison dart frogs) for site 2, and the ladder-shaped cyclic polyether compounds produced from dinoflagellates, e.g., brevetoxins (from *Ptychodiscus brevis*) and ciguatoxins (from *Gamierdiscus toxicus*) for site 5 have been identified (Fig. 3) [93–95, 113]. All of these toxins bind with high affinity at sites distant from the inner pore or the voltage sensors, and can cause persistent activation (open state) of the sodium channel at normal resting potential as well as allosterically triggered interactions with receptor binding site 3 (see below) [109].

Various peptide toxins isolated from venoms of sea anemones and terrestrial invertebrates, such as scorpions and spiders, are capable of inducing prolongation of the action potential *via* binding to receptor site 3 that mainly consists of the S3–S4 extracellular loop within domain IV (cf. above) [87, 88, 97]. These toxins slow down or block sodium channel inactivation; thus, patch clamp studies are suitable for demonstrating residual currents beyond 2 ms after depolarization. Such toxins include the classical scorpion α-toxins (e.g., AaH-II, LqH-II), sea anemone toxins (e.g., Ae1, Af1, ApA, ApB, ApC) and funnel-web spider toxins (e.g., δ-ACTX-Ar1, δ-ACTX-Hv1a) (Fig. 3) [84, 93–95, 109, 114]. Scorpion toxins comprise a class of structurally and functionally related polypeptides consisting of about 60–76 amino acids and four disulfide cross-links [115, 116]. Based on functional differences two different types, α- and β-toxins, have been distinguished. Whereas β-toxins bind to receptor site 4 (cf. below), α-toxins are capable of interacting with site 3 to decrease the rate of channel conversion to an inactive state. Scorpion toxins have been highly instrumental in characterizing sodium channel structures and functions [93–95]. Receptor site 3 was the first binding site on mammalian sodium channels identified by the use of photoreactive derivatives of neurotoxic α-toxins and sequence-specific antibodies. It was demonstrated that their binding affinity depends on the membrane potential, as does the channel activation itself. Since membrane potential affects binding affinities of scorpion α-toxins *via* alteration of receptor site 3 conformation and, at the same time, voltage gating and channel activation–inactivation loops rely on conformational changes of site 3, it was concluded already 30 years ago that, inversely, binding of α-toxins prevents conformational changes required for fast channel inactivation [93, 117].

By employing allosteric modulators of receptor site 3, such as veratridine (site 2 toxin) or brevetoxin PbTx-1 (site 5 toxin), the binding (consensus) sequences of all of the above-mentioned scorpion α-toxins, sea anemone toxins, and funnel-web spider toxins have been shown to overlap with neurotoxin receptor site 3 [93, 118]. Site-directed mutagenesis studies subsequently shed further light on the exact amino acid residues involved in shaping the toxin binding surface of site 3 in rat brain sodium channels. Glutamic acid at position 1613 (E1613) located in the extracellular loop between transmembrane segments S3 and S4 of domain IV represents a major determinant for scorpion α-toxins and sea anemone toxins [97]. However, further deciphering of the S3–S4 loop by replacing each amino acid residue individually revealed overlapping binding sites of both kinds of toxins rather than identical sites (reviewed in [93, 95]). The overall picture that has emerged suggests that scorpion α-toxins and sea anemone toxins electrostatically interact with E1613 in rat brain sodium channels and with aspartic acids D1612 and D1428 in cardiac and skeletal sodium channels, respectively, all of which are located within the S3–S4 loop of domain IV. In addition, some minor contacts occur with loops S5–S6 in domains I and IV (Fig. 3). By interacting with the positively charged and highly conserved voltage sensors (S4 segments) of the Na^+ channel, the toxins most likely hinder the normal outward movement of the segment and thus conformational changes required for fast inactivation of the channel (voltage-sensor trapping model) [95, 97, 119].

Another group of peptide toxins, i.e., δ-conotoxins (e.g., TxVIA), were again isolated from the venom of cone snails (e.g., *Conus textile*) and also shown to specifically bind to rat brain sodium channels and inhibit sodium current inactivation [120, 121]. Since binding of TxVIA to the channel proved to be rather voltage independent, and allosteric modulation by site 2 or site 5 toxins did not fully resemble the situation described above, another binding site, receptor site 6, was proposed. Recent data, however, provide some hint that δ-conotoxins bind in close proximity to receptor site 3 and may thus trap the S4 segment of domain IV in a similar way (conformation) as shown for scorpion α-toxins, sea anemone toxins or funnel-web spider toxins (cf. above) [122]. Further experimental efforts are required to establish the exact differences between δ-conotoxins and classical site 3 toxins with regard to target sites and molecular effects.

The main receptor site 4 binding neurotoxins are represented by scorpion β-toxin peptides [95, 123, 124]. Their targets are the S1–S2 and S3–S4 extracellular loops of domain II (Fig. 3). According to the most currently proposed mechanism, β-toxins predominantly interact with the S4 segment of domain II in activated sodium channels at residues that become accessible during depolarization, thereby facilitating and retaining channel activation *via* trapping and stabilizing S4 in its outward position (activated state). Concurrently, the voltage dependence of activation becomes negatively shifted toward more hyperpolarized potentials. Along with other site 3 or site 4 binding neurotoxins, such as the funnel-web spider δ-ACTX toxins (cf. above), both classes of scorpion toxins, i.e., α and β, therefore belong to the group of gating modifiers that confer toxicity *via* execution of a voltage-sensor trapping mechanism. Through binding to the extracellular ends of the S4 segments of sodium channels they either block channel inactivation by holding this transmembrane segment in its inward position (α-toxins, S4 of domain IV), or they enhance channel activation by trapping it in its outward position (β-toxins, S4 of domain II). Based on these insights and similar findings with other voltage-gated cation channels, it has been proposed that polypeptide toxins altering the voltage dependence of ion channels in general may act *via* voltage-sensor trapping mechanisms at accessible extracellular S3–S4 loops [95].

Conclusion

Evolution has shaped the development of a great variety of versatile and extremely potent venoms in a wide range of different groups of invertebrates, such as scorpions, jellyfish, sea anemones, cone snails, scorpions, hymenopteran insects, and spiders. These venoms, in general, comprise complex mixtures of bioactive ingredients administered *via* claws, stingers, fangs, chelicers, or other injection devices such as harpoons, nematocysts, etc. As exemplified for spider venoms, which are actually applied by the creature to immobilize and predigest small prey, the present chapter has addressed two different groups of neurotoxins that have become infamous over the last few decades due to their importance and role in rare but significant, and potentially deadly, incidents of human envenoming.

The most important and well-studied neurotoxins produced by black widow spiders of the genus *Latrodectus*, or by funnel-web spiders of the genus *Atrax* and *Hadronyche*, are represented by the protein α-LTX (1179 amino acid residues) and the peptides δ-ACTX (42 amino acid residues), respectively. These toxins proved effective in mammals either by targeting presynaptic vesicle exocytosis *via* neuronal cell receptors at the presynaptic membrane, or through increasing ion conductance at voltage-gated sodium channels *via* trapping the channel's voltage sensor domain IV S4 segment in an inward conformation, thereby evoking fulminant neurotransmitter release at autonomic and/or somatic synapses. While protein toxins such as α-LTX and the set of recently characterized insect- or crustacean-selective latrotoxins hold great potential as versatile tools to further elucidate and characterize the molecular basics of receptor-mediated presynaptic signaling and neuroexocytosis in vertebrates and invertebrates alike [125], peptide toxins such as those isolated from scorpion venoms have historically been applied in the purification and characterization of voltage-gated ion channels. Invertebrate venoms often consist of vast arrays of tightly folded and stabilized polypeptides, such as those found in scorpions, cone snails, sea anemones, and funnel-web or banana spiders. Besides contributing as valuable molecular probes in illuminating the three-dimensional architecture of ion channels, structurally and functionally diverse peptide mixtures present in animal venoms are now also starting to serve as new drug discovery platforms that hold great promise for identifying new lead structures in the development of highly effective and potent neuropharmacological drugs or biopesticides [109, 126–129].

References

1 Currie BJ (2008) Snakes, jellyfish and spiders. *Adv Exp Med Biol* 609: 43–53
2 Isbister GK, White J (2004) Clinical consequences of spider bites: Recent advances in our understanding. *Toxicon* 43: 477–492
3 Isbister GK, Gray MR, Balit CR, Raven RJ, Stokes BJ, Porges K, Tankel AS, Turner E, White J, Fisher MM (2005) Funnel-web spider bite: A systematic review of recorded clinical cases. *Med J Aust* 182: 407–412
4 Coddington JA, Levi HW (1991) Systematics and evolution of spiders (Araneae). *Annu Rev Ecol Syst* 22: 565–592
5 Platnick NI (2006) *The World Spider Catalog,* Version 10.0 (online available at: http://research. amnh.org/entomology/spiders/catalog/COUNTS.html, accessed at July 29, 2009)
6 Fernandes Pedrosa Mde F, Junqueira de Azevedo Ide L, Conçalves de Andrade RM, van den Berg CW, Ramos CR, Ho PL, Tambourgi DV (2002) Molecular cloning and expression of a functional dermonecrotic and haemolytic factor from *Loxosceles laeta* venom. *Biochem Biophys Res Commun* 298: 638–645
7 Gomez MV, Kalapothakis E, Guatimosim C, Prado MA (2002) *Phoneutria nigriventer* venom: A cocktail of toxins that affect ion channels. *Cell Mol Neurobiol* 22: 579–588
8 Rash LD, Hodgson WC (2002) Pharmacology and biochemistry of spider venoms. *Toxicon* 40: 225–254
9 Garb JE, Gonzalez A, Gillespie RG (2004) The black widow spider genus *Latrodectus* (Araneae:

Theridiidae): Phylogeny, biography, and invasion history. *Mol Phylogenet Evol* 31: 1127–1142

10 Warrell DA, Shaheen J, Hillyard PD, Jones D (1991) Neurotoxic envenoming by an immigrant spider (*Steatoda nobilis*) in southern England. *Toxicon* 29: 1263–1265

11 Grishin EV (1998) Black widow spider toxins: The present and the future. *Toxicon* 36: 1693–1701

12 Nicholson GM, Graudins A (2002) Spiders of medical importance in the Asia-Pacific: Atracotoxin, latrotoxin and related spider neurotoxins. *Clin Exp Pharmacol Physiol* 29: 785–794

13 Maretic Z (1983) Latrodectism. Variations in clinical manifestations provoked by *Latrodectus* species of spiders. *Toxicon* 21: 457–466

14 Vetter RS, Isbister GK (2008) Medical aspects of spider bites. *Annu Rev Entomol* 53: 409–429

15 Isbister GK, Gray MR (2003) Latrodectism: A prospective cohort study of bites by formally identified redback spiders. *Med J Aust* 179: 88–91

16 Trethewy CE, Bolisetty S, Wheaton G (2003) Red-back spider envenomation in children in Central Australia. *Emerg Med* 15: 170–175

17 Grasso A (1976) Preparation and properties of a neurotoxin purified from the venom of black widow spider (*Latrodectus mactans tredecimguttatus*). *Biochim Biophys Acta* 439: 406–412

18 Frontali N, Ceccarelli B, Gorio A, Mauro A, Siekevitz P, Tzeng MC, Hurlbut WP (1976) Purification from black widow spider venom of a protein factor causing the depletion of synaptic vesicles at neuromuscular junctions. *J Cell Biol* 68: 462–479

19 Ushkarev IA, Grishin EV (1986) Neurotoxin of the black widow spider and its interaction with receptors from the rat brain. *Bioorg Khim* 12: 71–80

20 Krasnoperov VG, Shamotienko OG, Grishin EV (1990) Isolation and properties of insect-specific neurotoxins from venoms of the spider *Latrodectus mactans tredecimguttatus*. *Bioorg Khim* 16: 1138–1140

21 Krasnoperov VG, Shamotienko OG, Grishin EV (1990) A crustacean-specific neurotoxin from the venom of the black widow spider *Latrodectus mactans tredecimguttatus*. *Bioorg Khim* 16: 1567–1569

22 Kiyatkin NI, Dulubova IE, Chekhovskaya IA, Grishin EV (1990) Cloning and structure of cDNA encoding α-latrotoxin from black widow spider venom. *FEBS Lett* 270: 127–131

23 Ushkaryov YA, Volynski KE, Ashton AC (2004) The multiple actions of black widow spider toxins and their selective use in neurosecretion studies. *Toxicon* 43: 527–542

24 Stieneke-Gröber A, Vey M, Angliker H, Shaw E, Thomas G, Roberts C, Klenk HD, Garten W (1992) Influenza virus hemagglutinin with multibasic cleavage site is activated by furin, a subtilisin-like endoprotease. *EMBO J* 11: 2407–2414

25 Volynski KE, Nosyreva ED, Ushkaryov YA, Grishin EV (1999) Functional expression of α-latrotoxin in baculovirus system. *FEBS Lett* 442: 25–28

26 Cavalieri M, Corvaja N, Grasso A (1990) Immunocytological localization by monoclonal antibodies of α-latrotoxin in the venom gland of the spider *Latrodectus tredecimguttatus*. *Toxicon* 28: 341–346

27 Duan ZG, Yan XJ, He XZ, Zhou H, Chen P, Cao R, Xiong JX, Hu WJ, Wang XC, Liang SP (2006) Extraction and protein component analysis of venom from the dissected venom glands of *Latrodectus tredecimguttatus*. *Comp Biochem Physiol B Biochem Mol Biol* 145: 350–357

28 Sedgwick SG, Smerdon SJ (1999) The ankyrin repeat: A diversity of interactions on a common structural framework. *Trends Biochem Sci* 24: 311–316

29 Li J, Mahajan A, Tsai MD (2006) Ankyrin repeat: A unique motif mediating protein-protein interactions. *Biochemistry* 45: 15168–15178

30 Orlova EV, Rahman MA, Gowen B, Volynski KE, Ashton AC, Manser C, van Heel M, Ushkaryov YA (2000) Structure of α-latrotoxin oligomers reveals that divalent cation-dependent tetramers form membrane pores. *Nat Struct Biol* 7: 48–53

31 Volkova TM, Pluzhnikov KA, Woll PG, Grishin EV (1995) Low molecular weight components from black widow spider venom. *Toxicon* 33: 483–489

32 Pescatori M, Bradbury A, Bouet F, Gargano N, Mastrogiacomo A, Grasso A (1995) The cloning of cDNA encoding a protein (latrodectin) which co-purifies with the α-latrotoxin from the black widow spider *Latrodectus tredecimguttatus* (Theridiidae). *Eur J Biochem* 230: 322–328

33 Ichtchenko K, Khvotechev M, Kiyatkin N, Simpson L, Sugita S, Südhof TC (1998) α-Latrotoxin action probed with recombinant toxin: Receptors recruit α-latrotoxin but do not transduce an exocytotic signal. *EMBO J* 17: 6188–6199

34 Kiyatkin NI, Kulikovskaya IM, Grishin EV, Beadle DJ, King LA (1995) Functional characterization of black widow spider neurotoxins synthesised in insect cells. *Eur J Biochem* 230: 854–859

35 Volynski KE, Meunier FA, Lelianova VG, Dudina EE, Volkova TM, Rahman MA, Manser C, Grishin EV, Dolly JO, Ashley RH, Ushkaryov YA (2000) Latrophilin, neurexin, and their signaling-deficient mutants facilitate α-latrotoxin insertion into membranes but are not involved in pore formation. *J Biol Chem* 275: 41175–41183

36 Ashton AC, Rahman MA, Volynski KE, Manser C, Orlova EV, Matsushita H, Davletov BA, van Heel M, Grishin EV, Ushkaryov YA (2000) Tetramerisation of α-latrotoxin by divalent cations is responsible for toxin-induced non-vesicular release and contributes to the Ca^{2+}-dependent vesicular exocytosis from synaptosomes. *Biochimie* 82: 453–468

37 Volynski KE, Capogna M, Ashton AC, Thomson D, Orlova EV, Manser CF, Ribchester RR, Ushkaryov YA (2003) Mutant α-latrotoxin (LTX^{N4C}) does not form pores and causes secretion by receptor stimulation: This action does not require neurexins. *J Biol Chem* 278: 31058–31066

38 Capogna M, Volynski KE, Emptage NJ, Ushkaryov YA (2003) The α-latrotoxin mutant LTX^{N4C} enhances spontaneous and evoked transmitter release in CA3 pyramidal neurons. *J Neurosci* 23: 4044–4053

39 Finkelstein A, Rubin LL, Tzeng MC (1976) Black widow spider venom: Effect of purified toxin on lipid bilayer membranes. *Science* 193: 1009–1011

40 Grasso A, Alemà S, Rufini S, Senni MI (1980) Black widow spider toxin-induced calcium fluxes and transmitter release in a neurosecretory cell line. *Nature* 283: 774–776

41 Petrenko AG, Kovalenko VA, Shamotienko OG, Surkova IN, Tarasyuk TA, Ushkaryov YA, Grishin EV (1990) Isolation and properties of the α-latrotoxin receptor. *EMBO J* 9: 2023–2027

42 Van Renterghem C, Iborra C, Martin-Moutot N, Lelianova V, Ushkaryov Y, Seagar M (2000) α-Latrotoxin forms calcium-permeable membrane pores *via* interactions with latrophilin or neurexin. *Eur J Neurosci* 12: 3953–3962

43 Khvotchev M, Südhof TC (2000) α-Latrotoxin triggers transmitter release *via* direct insertion into the presynaptic plasma membrane. *EMBO J* 19: 3250–3262

44 Rohou A, Nield J, Ushkaryov YA (2007) Insecticidal toxins from black widow spider venom. *Toxicon* 49: 531–549

45 Ushkaroyov YA, Petrenko AG, Geppert M, Südhof TC (1992) Neurexins. Synaptic cell surface proteins related to the α-latrotoxin receptor and laminin. *Science* 257: 50–56

46 Missler M, Südhof TC (1998) Neurexins: Three genes and 1001 products. *Trends Genet* 14: 20–26

47 Davletov BA, Krasnoperov V, Hata Y, Petrenko AG, Südhof TC (1995) High affinity binding of α-latrotoxin to recombinant neurexin Iα. *J Biol Chem* 270: 23903–23905

48 Davletov BA, Shamotienko OG, Lelianova VG, Grishin EV, Ushkaryov YA (1996) Isolation and biochemical characterization of a Ca^{2+}-independent α-latrotoxin-binding protein. *J Biol Chem* 271: 23239–23245

49 Lelianova VG, Davletov BA, Sterling A, Rahman MA, Grishin EV, Totty NF, Usaharyov YA (1997) α-Latrotoxin receptor, latrophilin, is a novel member of the secretin family of G protein-coupled receptors. *J Biol Chem* 272: 21504–21508

50 Sugita S, Ichtechenko K, Khvotchev M, Südhof TC (1998) α-Latrotoxin receptor CIRL/latrophilin 1 (CL1) defines an unusual family of ubiquitous G-protein-linked receptors. G-protein coupling not required for triggering exocytosis. *J Biol Chem* 273: 32715–32724

51 Krasnoperov VG, Bittner MA, Beavis R, Kuang Y, Salnikow KV, Chepurny OG, Little AR, Plotnikov AN, Wu D, Holz RW, Petrenko AG (1997) α-Latrotoxin stimulates exocytosis by the interaction with a neuronal G-protein-coupled receptor. *Neuron* 18: 925–937

52 Volynski KE, Silva JP, Lelianova VG, Rahman MA, Hopkins C, Ushkaryov YA (2004) Latrophilin fragments behave as independent proteins that associate and signal on binding of LTX^{N4C}. *EMBO J* 23: 4423–4433

53 Ichtchenko K, Bittner MA, Krasnoperov V, Little AR, Chepurny O, Holz RW, Petrenko AG (1999) A novel ubiquitously expressed α-latrotoxin receptor is a member of the CIRL family of G-protein-coupled receptors. *J Biol Chem* 274: 5491–5498

54 Matsushita H, Lelianova VG, Ushkaryov YA (1999) The latrophilin family: Multiply spliced G protein-coupled receptors with differential tissue distribution. *FEBS Lett* 443: 348–352

55 Krasnoperov VG, Bittner MA, Mo W, Buryanovsky L, Neubert TA, Holz RW, Ichtchenko K, Petrenko AG (2002) Protein-tyrosine phosphatase-σ is a novel member of the functional family of α-latrotoxin receptors. *J Biol Chem* 277: 35887–35895

56 Tobaben S, Südhof TC, Stahl B (2002) Genetic analysis of α-latrotoxin receptors reveals functional interdependence of CIRL/latrophilin 1 and neurexin Iα. *J Biol Chem* 277: 6359–6365

57 Rosenthal L, Meldolesi J (1989) α-Latrotoxin and related toxins. *Pharmacol Ther* 42: 115–134

58 Khvotchev M, Lonart G, Südhof TC (2000) Role of calcium in neurotransmitter release evoked by
α-latrotoxin or hypertonic sucrose. *Neuroscience* 101: 793–802.

59 Matteoli M, Haimann C, Torri-Tarelli F, Polak JM, Ceccarelli B, de Camilli P (1988) Differential
effect of α-latrotoxin on exocytosis from small synaptic vesicles and from large dense-core vesicles containing calcitonin gene-related peptide at the frog neuromuscular junction. *Proc Natl Acad
Sci USA* 85: 7366–7370

60 Ashton AC, Volynski KE, Lelianova VG, Orlova EV, van Renterghem C, Canepari M, Seagar M,
Ushkaryov YA (2001) α-Latrotoxin, acting *via* two Ca²⁺-dependent pathways, triggers exocytosis
of two pools of synaptic vesicles. *J Biol Chem* 276: 44695–44703

61 Li G, Lee D, Wang L, Khvotchev M, Chiew SK, Arunachalam L, Collins T, Feng ZP, Sugita S
(2005) N-terminal insertion and C-terminal ankyrin-like repeats of α-latrotoxin are critical for
Ca²⁺-dependent exocytosis. *J Neurosci* 25: 10188–10197

62 Deák F, Liu X, Khvotchev M, Li G, Kavalali ET, Sugita S, Südhof TC (2009) α-Latrotoxin stimulates a novel pathway of Ca²⁺-dependent synaptic exocytosis independent of the classical synaptic fusion machinery. *J Neurosci* 29: 8639–8648

63 Gray MR (1998) Aspects of the systematics of the Australian funnel-web spiders (Araneae:
Hexathelidae: Atracinae) based upon morphological and electrophoretic data. In: AD Austin, NW
Heather (eds): *Australian Arachnology*. The Australian Entomological Society, Brisbane,
Australia, 113–125

64 Torda TA, Loong E, Greaves I (1980) Severe lung oedema and fatal consumption coagulopathy
after funnel-web spider bite. *Med J Aust* 2: 442–444

65 Sutherland SK (1983) Genus Atrax Cambridge, the funnel-web spiders. In: SK Sutherland (ed.):
Australian Animal Toxins. Oxford University Press, Melbourne, Australia, 255–298

66 White J, Carduso JL, Fan HW (1995) Clinical toxicology of spider bites. In: J Meier, J White
(eds): *Handbook of Clinical Toxicology of Animal Venoms and Poisons*. CRC Press, New York,
259–329

67 Sutherland SK, Tibballs J (2001) The genera *Atrax* and *Hadronyche*, funnel-web spiders. In: SK
Sutherland, J Tibballs (eds): *Australian Animal Toxins: The Creatures, Their Toxins and Care of
the Poisoned Patient*. Oxford University Press, Melbourne, Australia, 402–464

68 Sutherland SK (1980) Antivenom to the venom of the male Sydney funnel-web spider *Atrax
robustus*. Preliminary report. *Med J Aust* 2: 437–441

69 Graudins A, Wilson D, Alewood PF, Broady KW, Nicholson GM (2002) Cross-reactivity of
Sydney funnel-web spider antivenom: Neutralization of the *in vitro* toxicity of other Australian
funnel-web (*Atrax* and *Hadronyche*) spider venoms. *Toxicon* 40: 259–266

70 Miller MK, Whyte IM, White J, Keir PM (2000) Clinical features and management of *Hadronyche*
envenomation in man. *Toxicon* 38: 409–427.

71 Isbister GK, Gray MR (2004) Bites by Australian mygalomorph spiders (Araneae, Mygalomorphae), including funnel-web spiders (Atracinae) and mouse spiders (Actinopodidae:
Missulena spp). *Toxicon* 43: 133–140

72 Nicholson GM, Graudins A, Wilson HI, Little M, Broady KW (2006) Arachnid toxinology in
Australia: From clinical toxicology to potential applications. *Toxicon* 48: 872–898

73 Wiener S (1957) The Syndney funnel-web spider (*Atrax robustus*). I. Collection of venom and its
toxicity in animals. *Med J Aust* 44: 377–382

74 Duncan AW, Tibballs J, Sutherland SK (1980) Effects of funnel-web spider envenomation in monkeys, and their clinical implications. *Med J Aust* 2: 429–435

75 Mylecharane EJ, Spence I, Gregson RP (1984) *In vivo* actions of atraxin, a protein neurotoxin
from the venom glands of the funnel-web spider (*Atrax robustus*). *Comp Biochem Physiol C* 79:
395–399

76 Sheumack DD, Baldo BA, Carroll PR, Hampson F, Howden ME, Skorulis A (1984) A comparative study of properties and toxic constituents of funnel-web spider (*Atrax*) venoms. *Comp
Biochem Physiol C* 78: 55–68

77 Brown MR, Sheumack DD, Tyler MI, Howden MEH (1988) Amino acid sequence of versutoxin,
a lethal neurotoxin from the venom of the funnel-web spider *Atrax versutus*. *Biochem J* 250:
401–405

78 Mylecharane EJ, Spence I, Sheumack DD, Claassens R, Howden MEH (1989) Actions of robustoxin, a neurotoxic polypeptide from the venom of the male funnel-web spider (*Atrax robustus*),
in anaesthetized monkeys. *Toxicon* 27: 481–492

79 Sheumack DD, Claassens R, Whiteley NM, Howden MEH (1985) Complete amino acid sequence

of a new type of lethal neurotoxin from the venom of the funnel-web spider *Atrax robustus*. *FEBS Lett* 181: 154–156

80 Szeto TH, Birinyi-Strachan LC, Smith R, Connor M, Christie MJ, King GF, Nicholson GM (2000) Isolation and pharmacological characterisation of δ-atracotoxin-Hv1b, a vertebrate-selective sodium channel toxin. *FEBS Lett* 470: 293–299

81 Pallaghy PK, Alewood D, Alewood PF, Norton RS (1997) Solution structure of robustoxin, the lethal neurotoxin from the funnelweb spider *Atrax robustus*. *FEBS Lett* 419: 191–196

82 Pallaghy PK, Neilsen KJ, Craik DJ, Norton RS (1994) A common structural motif incorporating a cystine knot and a triple-stranded β-sheet in toxic and inhibitory polypeptides. *Protein Sci* 3: 1833–1839

83 Norton RS, Pallaghy PK (1998) The cystine knot structure of ion channel toxins and related polypeptides. *Toxicon* 36: 1573–1583

84 Nicholson GM, Little MJ, Birinyi-Strachan LC (2004) Structure and function of δ-atracotoxins: Lethal neurotoxins targeting the voltage-gated sodium channel. *Toxicon* 43: 587–599

85 Grolleau F, Stankiewicz M, Birinyi-Strachan L, Wang XH, Nicholson GM, Pelhate M, Lapied B (2001) Electrophysiological analysis of the neurotoxic action of a funnel-web spider toxin, δ-atracotoxin-Hv1a, on insect voltage-gated Na⁺ channels. *J Exp Biol* 204: 711–721

86 Alewood D, Birinyi-Strachan LC, Pallaghy PK, Norton RS, Nicholson GM, Alewood PF (2003) Synthesis and characterization of δ-atracotoxin-Ar1a, the lethal neurotoxin from venom of the Sydney funnel-web spider (*Atrax robustus*). *Biochemistry* 42: 12933–12940

87 Nicholson GM, Walsh R, Little MJ, Tyler MI (1998) Characterisation of the effects of robustoxin, the lethal neurotoxin from the Sydney funnel-web spider *Atrax robustus*, on sodium channel activation and inactivation. *Pflügers Arch* 436: 117–126

88 Nicholson GM, Little MJ, Tyler M, Narahashi T (1996) Selective alteration of sodium channel gating by Australian funnel-web spider toxins. *Toxicon* 34: 1443–1453

89 Little MJ, Wilson H, Zappia C, Cestèle S, Tyler MI, Martin-Eauclaire MF, Gordon D, Nicholson GM (1998) δ-Atracotoxins from Australian funnel-web spiders compete with scorpion α-toxin binding on both rat brain and insect sodium channels. *FEBS Lett* 439: 246–252

90 Little MJ, Zappia C, Gilles N, Connor M, Tyler MI, Martin-Eauclaire MF, Gordon D, Nicholson GM (1998) δ-Atracotoxins from Australian funnel-web spiders compete with scorpion α-toxin binding but differentially modulate alkaloid toxin activation of voltage-gated sodium channels. *J Biol Chem* 273: 27076–27083

91 Gordon D (1997) Sodium channels as targets for neurotoxins: Mode of action and interaction of neurotoxins with receptor sites on sodium channels. In: P Lazarowici, Y Gutman (eds): *Toxins and Signal Transduction*. Harwood Press, Amsterdam, The Netherlands, 119–149

92 Gilles N, Harrison G, Karbat I, Gurevitz M, Nicholson GM, Gordon D (2002) Variations in receptor site-3 on rat brain and insect sodium channels highlighted by binding of a funnel-web spider δ-atracotoxin. *Eur J Biochem* 269: 1500–1510

93 Cestèle S, Catterall WA (2000) Molecular mechanisms of neurotoxin action on voltage-gated sodium channels. *Biochimie* 82: 883–892

94 Blumenthal KM, Seibert AL (2003) Voltage-gated sodium channel toxins. *Cell Biochem Biophys* 38: 215–237

95 Catterall WA, Cestèle S, Yarov-Yarovoy V, Yu FH, Konoki K, Scheuer T (2007) Voltage-gated ion channels and gating modifier toxins. *Toxicon* 49: 124–141

96 Eitan M, Fowler E, Herrmann R, Duval A, Pelhate M, Zlotkin E (1990) A scorpion venom neurotoxin paralytic to insects that affects sodium current inactivation: Purification, primary structure, and mode of action. *Biochemistry* 29: 5941–5947

97 Rogers JC, Qu Y, Tanada TN, Scheuer T, Catterall WA (1996) Molecular determinants of high affinity binding of α-scorpion toxin and sea anemone toxin in the S3–S4 extracellular loop in domain IV of the Na⁺ channel α subunit. *J Biol Chem* 271: 15950–15962

98 Fletcher JI, Chapman BE, Mackay JP, Howden MEH, King GF (1997) The structure of versutoxin (δ-atracotoxin-Hv1): Implications for binding of site-3 toxins to the voltage-gated sodium channel. *Structure* 5: 1525–1535

99 Gilles N, Leipold E, Chen H, Heinemann SH, Gordon D (2001) Effect of depolarization on binding kinetics of scorpion α-toxin highlights conformational changes of rat brain sodium channels. *Biochemistry* 40: 14576–14584

100 Fletcher JI, Smith R, O'Donoghue SI, Nilges M, Connor M, Howden ME, Christie MJ, King GF (1997) The structure of a novel insecticidal neurotoxin, ω-atracotoxin-Hv1, from the venom of

an Australian funnel-web spider. *Nat Struct Biol* 4: 559–566

101 Wang XH, Connor M, Wilson D, Wilson HI, Nicholson GM, Smith R, Shaw D, Mackay JP, Alewood PF, Christie MJ, King GF (2001) Discovery and structure of a potent and highly specific blocker of insect calcium channels. *J Biol Chem* 276: 40306–40312

102 Wang X, Connor M, Smith R, Maciejewski MW, Howden ME, Nicholson GM, Christie MJ, King GF (2000) Discovery and characterization of a family of insecticidal neurotoxins with a rare vicinal disulfide bridge. *Nat Struct Biol* 7: 505–513

103 Gunning SJ, Maggio F, Windley MJ, Valenzuela SM, King GF, Nicholson GM (2008) The Janus-faced atracotoxins are specific blockers of invertebrate K_{ca} channels. *FEBS J* 275: 4045–4059

104 King GF, Tedford HW, Maggio F (2002) Structure and function of insecticidal neurotoxins from Australian funnel-web spiders. *J Toxicol Toxin Rev* 21: 359–389

105 Tedford HW, Sollod BL, Maggio F, King GF (2004) Australian funnel-web spiders: Master insecticide chemists. *Toxicon* 43: 601–618

106 Catterall WA (1992) Cellular and molecular biology of voltage-dependent sodium channels. *Physiol Rev* 72: S15–48

107 Catterall WA (2000) From ionic currents to molecular mechanisms: The structure and function of voltage-gated sodium channels. *Neuron* 26: 13–25

108 Yang N, George AL Jr, Horn R (1996) Molecular basis of charge movement in voltage-gated sodium channels. *Neuron* 16: 113–122

109 Nicholson GM (2007) Insect-selective spider toxins targeting voltage-gated soidum channels. *Toxicon* 49: 490–512

110 Dudley SC Jr, Todt H, Lipkind G, Fozzard HA (1995) A μ-conotoxin-insensitive Na^+ channel mutant: Possible localization of a binding site at the outer vestibule. *Biophys J* 69: 1657–1665

111 Martin-Moutot N, Mansuelle P, Alcaraz G, Dos Santos RG, Cordeiro MN, De Lima ME, Seagar M, van Renterghem C (2006) *Phoneutria nigriventer* toxin 1: A novel, state-dependent inhibitor of neuronal sodium channels that interacts with μ conotoxin binding sites. *Mol Pharmacol* 69: 1931–1937

112 Chahine M, Chen LQ, Fotouhi N, Walsky R, Fry D, Santarelli V, Horn R, Kallen RG (1995) Characterizing the μ-conotoxin binding site on voltage-sensitive sodium channels with toxin analogs and channel mutations. *Receptors Channels* 3: 161–174

113 Nicholson GM, Lewis RJ (2006) Ciguatoxins: Cyclic polyether modulators of voltage-gated ion channel function. *Mar Drugs* 4: 82–118

114 Smith JJ, Blumenthal KM (2007) Site-3 anemone toxins: Molecular probes of gating mechanisms in voltage-dependent sodium channels. *Toxicon* 49: 159–170

115 Srinivasan KN, Gopalakrishnakone P, Tan PT, Chew KC, Cheng B, Kini RM, Koh JL, Seah SH, Brusic V (2002) SCORPION, a molecular database of scorpion toxins. *Toxicon* 40: 23–31

116 Tan PT, Veeramani A, Srinivasan KN, Ranganathan S, Brusic V (2006) SCORPION2: A database for structure-function analysis of scorpion toxins. *Toxicon* 47: 356–363

117 Catterall WA (1979) Binding of scorpion toxin to receptor sites associated with sodium channels in frog muscle. Correlation of voltage-dependent binding with activation. *J Gen Physiol* 74: 375–391

118 Cestèle S, Khalifa RB, Pelhate M, Rochat H, Gordon D (1995) α-Scorpion toxins binding on rat brain and insect sodium channels reveal divergent allosteric modulations by brevetoxin and veratridine. *J Biol Chem* 270: 15153–15161

119 Sheets MF, Kyle JW, Kallen RG, Hanck DA (1999) The Na channel voltage sensor associated with inactivation is localized to the external charged residues of domain IV, S4. *Biophys J* 77: 747–757

120 Hasson A, Fainzilber M, Gordon D, Zlotkin E, Spira ME (1993) Alteration of sodium currents by new peptide toxins from the venom of a molluscivorous *Conus* snail. *Eur J Neurosci* 5: 56–64

121 Fainzilber M, Kofman O, Zlotkin E, Gordon D (1996) A new neurotoxin receptor site on sodium channels is identified by a conotoxin that affects sodium channel inactivation in molluscs and acts as an antagonist in rat brain. *J Biol Chem* 269: 2574–2580

122 Leipold E, Hansel A, Olivera BM, Terlau H, Heinemann SH (2005) Molecular interaction of δ-conotoxins with voltage-gated sodium channels. *FEBS Lett* 579: 3881–3884

123 Cestèle S, Qu Y, Rogers JC, Rochat H, Scheuer T, Catterall WA (1998) Voltage-sensor-trapping: Enhanced activation of sodium channels by β-scorpion toxin bound to the S3–S4 loop in domain II. *Neuron* 21: 919–931

124 Cestèle S, Yarov-Yarovoy V, Qu Y, Sampieri F, Scheuer T, Catterall WA (2006) Structure and

function of the voltage sensor of sodium channels probed by a β-scorpion toxin. *J Biol Chem* 281: 21332–21344

125 Ushkaryov YA, Rohou A, Sugita S (2008) α-Latrotoxin and its receptors. *Handb Exp Pharmacol* 184: 171–206

126 Lewis RJ, Garcia ML (2003) Therapeutic potential of venom peptides. *Nat Rev Drug Discov* 2: 790–802

127 Han TS, Teichert RW, Olivera BM, Bulaj G (2008) *Conus* venoms – A rich source of peptide-based therapeutics. *Curr Pharm Des* 14: 2462–2479

128 Lewis RJ (2009) Conotoxins: Molecular and therapeutic targets. *Prog Mol Subcell Biol* 46: 45–65

129 Escoubas P, King GF (2009) Venomics as a drug discovery platform. *Expert Rev Proteomics* 6: 221–224

Molecular, Clinical and Environmental Toxicology. Volume 2: Clinical Toxicology
Edited by A. Luch

Analytical toxicology

Hans H. Maurer

*Department of Experimental and Clinical Toxicology, Institute of Experimental and Clinical
Pharmacology and Toxicology, Saarland University, Homburg, Germany*

Abstract. This paper reviews procedures for screening, identification and quantification of
drugs, poisons and their metabolites in biosamples, and the corresponding work-up procedures. Gas chromatography–mass spectrometry and liquid chromatography–mass spectrometry are mostly used today in analytical toxicology. Selection of the most appropriate
biosample, e.g., ante/postmortem blood, urine, or tissues or alternative matrices like hair,
sweat and oral fluid, nails or meconium, is discussed. The importance of quality control and
possibilities and limitations of interpretation of the analytical result are also discussed.

Introduction

Analytical toxicology deals with screening, confirmation, identification and
quantification of foreign compounds (xenobiotics), such as drugs, poisons,
pesticides, pollutants and their metabolites in biological and related samples,
followed by the pharmacological and toxicological interpretation of the analytical result [1–4]. The particular task of analytical toxicology is to analyze
complex biological matrices such as ante- or postmortem blood, urine, or tissues or alternative matrices such as hair, sweat and oral fluid, nails or meconium [5–17]. Appropriate sample preparation prior to instrumental analysis is
therefore a key step in such analytical methods [11, 14]. In modern clinical and
forensic toxicology, and in the field of doping control, analytical procedures
must not only be sensitive but also highly specific, because in most cases the
analytes are not known in advance and many other xenobiotics or endogenous
biomolecules may interfere with their detection. The result of toxicological
analysis can have serious clinical and/or legal consequences, so the quality
must be strictly controlled [2, 18, 19].

The demand of detecting and thereby protecting from poisons is as old as
mankind [20]. In former times, animals or even humans were used to sample
food, drinks or medications in advance, and sometimes even amulets were
believed to indicate poisonings. With the development of sciences such as
chemistry and botany in the modern era, chemical or botanic procedures for
detection of poisons were called for. The pioneer of inorganic analytics was the
British chemist James Marsh and of organic analytics, the Belgian chemist
Jean Servais Stas [20]. With the development of chromatographic procedures
in the 20th century, analytical toxicology developed into a modern science.

Hyphenation of chromatographic procedures with various detection systems, particularly with spectrometric detectors, was another milestone in detection of poisons. Thin-layer chromatography [21] and gas chromatography (GC) alone using common detectors [22] are now rarely used in routine of analytical toxicology, but liquid chromatography (LC) with diode-array detection (DAD) is still in use for screening and quantification, particularly in laboratories with no or limited access to liquid chromatography with mass spectrometry (LC-MS). Pragst et al. developed a screening procedure using a DAD reference library [23, 24]. A significant breakthrough in achieving these tasks was hyphenation of GC with MS in the 1960s. GC-MS is still the most frequently used technique in analytical toxicology [8, 17, 20, 25, 26]. It took more than 30 years to combine LC-MS for routine application. Today, liquid chromatography combined with single-stage or tandem mass spectrometry (LC-MS, LC-MS/MS) have left the development stage and are becoming increasingly important in routine toxicological analysis, especially for quantification of the identified analytes [9, 13, 17, 20, 25, 27]. Electrokinetic techniques (e.g., capillary electrophoresis-mass spectrometry, CE-MS) are, due to the limited sensitivity, used only for particular applications [28].

In clinical toxicology, rational diagnosis or definite exclusion of an acute or chronic intoxication must be supported by efficient toxicological analysis. The analytical strategy includes screening, confirmation/identification, followed by quantification of relevant compounds and interpretation of the results [29]. Several papers have been published on strategies of clinical toxicological analysis services [25, 29–37], showing that, depending on the country and/or the tasks to be covered, different statements have been made. The tasks may cover, besides support for diagnosis and prognosis of poisonings, help for indication for (invasive) treatment, monitoring of the efficiency of detoxication and support in differential diagnostic for exclusion of certain poisons. Furthermore, patients addicted to alcohol, medicaments or illegal drugs have to be monitored [25]. For determination of clinical brain death, as a prerequisite for explantation of organs, the presence of drugs that may depress the central nervous system (CNS) must be excluded [38]. The compliance of patients can be monitored by determination of the prescribed drugs. Finally, monitoring of drugs with a narrow therapeutic range, so-called therapeutic drug monitoring (TDM) [27], can be performed by the clinical toxicologist. Reliable analytical and reference data are thus a prerequisite for correct interpretation of toxicological findings not only in the daily routine work, but also in the evaluation of scientific studies.

Similar problems arise in forensic toxicology, where proof of abuse of illegal drugs or of murder by poisoning are important tasks [3]. Furthermore, drugs, which may reduce the penal responsibility of a defendant, or which may reduce the fitness to drive a car, must be monitored in body fluids or tissues [8, 17]. In doping controls, the use or abuse of drugs that may stimulate the build-up of muscles, enhance the endurance during competition, lead to reduction of body weight, or reduce pain caused by overexertion must be monitored [13,

39]. In the following, important aspects of analytical toxicology are reviewed and critically discussed.

Biosamples used in analytical toxicology

Various types of specimens have to be analyzed, depending of the task to be fulfilled. It is obvious that any mistake made during specimen selection, collection, preservation, storage, transport and work-up cannot be compensated by the best analytical procedure. Therefore, the analytical toxicologist must be familiar with all these pre-analytical steps, the analyte stability, the risk of infection, and also with the pharmaco/toxicokinetic properties of the analyte [3, 33, 34, 40]. Proper documentation of the history of the sample including chain of custody is essential.

Blood is the sample of choice, at least for living humans and animals, because the analyte concentration in blood correlates best with its biological effect. Besides whole blood, plasma (the fluid obtained by centrifugation of anticoagulated whole blood), or serum (the fluid remaining when blood has clotted) are widely used. Special regard is needed when analyzing and interpreting postmortem specimens, because they may be substantially decomposed or contaminated with analytes from gastric contents or adjacent tissues. Nevertheless, it is expected that analysts produce results that can be of use in the case investigation since many of these cases are of forensic interest and may involve criminal prosecutions. Subsequently, it is expected that any bioanalytical procedures and results that come from these investigations can meet the rigor of court cross-examination and medicolegal scrutiny [5].

Blood (plasma, serum), being the sample of choice for quantification, can also be used for drug screening if the concentration is high enough. This is especially advantageous if only blood samples are available and/or if the procedures allow simultaneous screening and quantification [9, 17, 20, 25, 31, 41]. In cases of 'driving under the influence of drugs' (DUID), blood analysis is even mandatory in some countries [17].

Excretions (e.g., urine, exhaled air, feces, meconium), secretions (e.g., saliva, sweat, breast milk, bile), or vitreous humor, nails, hairs, etc. are less important for quantitative interpretation, but very useful for screening for and identification of xenobiotics. Drug screening in alternative matrices like hair, sweat and saliva, meconium or nails has also been described [6, 7, 9, 10, 12], but a comprehensive screening for series of various drugs has not yet been described in alternative matrices, probably because of the too-low concentrations.

Urine is, therefore, still the sample of choice for target drug screening, e.g., by immunoassay, GC-MS or LC-MS and particularly for non-target comprehensive screening for and identification of unknown drugs or poisons, mainly because concentrations of drugs are relatively high in urine and the samples can be taken non-invasively [9, 17, 20, 25, 41, 42]. However, in postmortem forensic toxicology or in cases of an acute overdose leading to rapid death, urinalysis may not be appropriate. In human and horse doping controls, urine is also the common sample for drug screening [13, 43–45].

A comprehensive overview of recommendations for sample collection, transport, and storage, of advantages and disadvantages of different sample types, and of information requested for general toxicological analysis have recently been published by Flanagan et al. [3].

Sample work-up

Immunoassays used for drug screening or quantification mostly need no sample work-up. In contrast, suitable sample preparation is an important prerequisite for all chromatographic approaches in biosamples. For GC-MS, work-up may include cleavage of conjugates, extraction and derivatization preceded or followed by clean-up steps [3, 26, 41, 46]. LC-MS was claimed to be less demanding with respect to sample preparation. However, a more or less selective extraction is also important for LC-MS [8, 9, 13, 14, 17, 27, 47], especially to avoid ion suppression effects [9, 17, 20, 48–53].

Cleavage of conjugates can be performed by fast acid hydrolysis or by gentle but time-consuming enzymatic hydrolysis [26]. It was amazing to read that nearly all LC-MS (/MS) urine screening procedures also needed time-consuming enzymatic cleavage of conjugates [9, 45, 54–56]. Enzymatic hydrolysis of acyl glucuronides [ester glucuronides of carboxy derivatives like nonsteroidal anti-inflammatory drugs (NSAIDs)] may be hindered due to acyl migration [57], an intramolecular transesterification at the hydroxy groups of the glucuronic acid that leads to β-glucuronidase-resistant derivatives. If the analysis must be done within a rather short time, like in emergency toxicology, it is preferable to cleave the conjugates by rapid acid hydrolysis [26, 41, 58]. Alkaline hydrolysis is only suitable for cleavage of ester conjugates. However, the formation of artifacts during chemical hydrolysis must be considered [26]. Acyl glucuronides, e.g., of acidic drugs, were readily cleaved under the conditions of extractive alkylation (alkaline pH, elevated temperature) and needed no extra cleavage step [59].

Isolation can be performed by liquid-liquid extraction (LLE) at a pH at which the analyte is non-ionized or by solid-phase extraction (SPE) preceded or followed by clean-up steps. Sample pretreatment for SPE depends on the sample type: whole blood and tissue (homogenates) need deproteinization and filtration/centrifugation steps before application to SPE columns, whereas for urine usually a simple dilution step and/or centrifugation are satisfactory. Details on the pros and cons of various extraction procedures have recently been discussed elsewhere [3, 14].

Solid-phase microextraction (SPME) is becoming a modern alternative to SPE and LLE. SPME is a solvent-free and concentrating extraction technique especially for rather volatile analytes. It is based on the adsorption of the analyte on a stationary phase coating a fine rod of fused silica. The analytes can be desorbed directly in the GC injector. Fast GC-MS procedures for screening, e.g., for drugs of abuse, have been published recently [11, 60]; however, this technique has not been tested for comprehensive screening procedures. SPME as a method for sample preparation for LC-MS/MS determination has been described for phenothiazines in body fluids [61]. Details on the pros and cons of various SPME procedures have recently been discussed [11, 60].

Extractive alkylation has proved to be a powerful procedure for simultaneous extraction and derivatization of acidic compounds [59, 62–65]. The acidic compounds are extracted at alkaline pH as ion pairs with a phase-transfer catalyst into the organic phase. In the organic phase, the phase-transfer catalyst is easily solvated due to its lipophilic groups, whereas the poor solvation of the anionic analytes leads to a high reactivity with the alkylation reagent. Part of the phase-transfer catalyst can also reach the organic phase as an ion pair with the iodide anion formed during the alkylation reaction or with anions of the urine matrix. Therefore, the remaining part had to be removed using suitable SPE to prevent a loss of the separation power of the GC column and to exclude interactions with analytes in the GC injection port.

Derivatization steps are necessary if relatively polar compounds containing, for example, carboxylic, hydroxy, primary or secondary amino groups are to be determined by GC-MS, and/or if electronegative moieties (e.g., halogen atoms) have to be introduced into the molecule for sensitive negative ion chemical ionization (NICI) detection [66–71]. The following procedures are typically used for basic compounds: acetylation (AC), trifluoroacetylation (TFA), pentafluoropropionylation (PFP), heptafluorobutyration (HFB), trimethylsilylation (TMS), or for acidic compounds: methylation (ME), extractive methylation, PFP, TMS or *tert*-butyldimethylsilylation. Further details on derivatization methods can be found in [26, 72].

Screening and identification procedures

In clinical and forensic toxicology and in doping control, the compounds to be analyzed are often unknown. Therefore, the first step before quantification is identifying the compounds of interest. High-throughput procedures in analytical toxicology mean that thousands of relevant toxicants can be simultaneously screened using one single procedure (so-called systematic toxicological analysis, STA) [20, 25, 26, 41]. The choice of a method in analytical toxicology depends on the problems to be solved. The analytical strategy often includes a screening test and a confirmatory test before quantification. If only a single drug or category has to be monitored, immunoassays can be used for preliminary screening to differentiate between negative and presumptively positive samples. Positive results must be confirmed by a second independent method that is at least as sensitive as the screening test and that provides the highest level of confidence in the result. Use of a second immunoassay system to confirm another immunoassay is not regarded as acceptable, even though the assays differ somewhat in principle. Use of only immunoassays for toxicological screening is not sufficient, because not all relevant drugs are detectable by immunoassays [42]; in addition, the samples can easily be adulterated, many interferences are described with other drugs or food additives [73], and differentiation of common metabolites (e.g., of opiates) can be difficult [74].

Up to now, GC-MS, especially in the electron ionization (EI) mode, has been the method most often used for confirmation of positive screening tests [8, 17, 25]. Immunoassay prescreening followed by mass spectral confirmation is employed if only those drugs or poisons have to be determined that are scheduled, e.g., by law or by international sport organizations, and for which immunoassays are commercially available. If these demands are not met, the screening strategy must be more extensive, because several thousands of drugs or pesticides are on the market worldwide. For these reasons, STA procedures are necessary that allow the simultaneous detection of as many toxicants as possible in biosamples.

The most comprehensive GC-MS screening procedure allows detection of over 2000 different drugs, poisons and/or their metabolites [25, 30, 75–89]. One prerequisite for this procedure is the mass spectral elucidation of the metabolism of the covered drugs and poisons. Another prerequisite for full-scan screening procedures is the availability of a suitable reference mass spectra collection as discussed below. Use of extensive mass spectral reference libraries from the fields of toxicology [90] and general chemistry [91] often allow detecting even unexpected compounds amenable to GC and EI. This comprehensive GC-MS screening method was developed and has been improved and extended over the last few years. For cleavage of conjugates, rapid acid hydrolysis is used to save time, which is relevant, for example, in emergency toxicology. The extraction mixture has proved to be very efficient in extracting compounds with very different chemical properties from biomatrices [25, 30, 75–89]. Acetylation has proved to be very suitable for robust derivatization to improve the GC properties, and thereby the detection limits, of thousands of drugs and their metabolites [26]. The use of microwave irradiation reduced the incubation time from 30 to 5 min [26], so that derivatization should no longer be renounced due to expense of time.

This comprehensive full-scan GC-MS screening procedure allows, within one run, the simultaneous screening and library-assisted identification of the following categories of drugs: tricyclic antidepressants, selective serotonin reuptake inhibitors (SSRIs), butyrophenone neuroleptics, phenothiazine neuroleptics, benzodiazepines, barbiturates and other sedative-hypnotics, anticonvulsants, antiparkinsonian drugs, phenothiazine antihistamines, alkanolamine antihistamines, ethylenediamine antihistamines, alkylamine antihistamines, opiates and opioids, non-opioid analgesics, stimulants and hallucinogens, designer drugs of the amphetamine type, the piperazine type, the phenethylamine type, the phencyclidine type, *Eschscholtzia californica* ingredients, nutmeg ingredients, β-blockers, antiarrhythmics, and diphenol laxatives [26, 41].

In addition, a further series compounds can be detected if they are present in the extract and their mass spectra are contained in the used reference libraries [90–92].

It is evident that most compounds with acidic or zwitterionic properties cannot be analyzed with this general screening procedure. Extractive alkylation has proved to be a powerful procedure for simultaneous extraction and derivatization of acidic compounds such as angiotensin-converting enzyme (ACE) inhibitors and AT_1 blockers, coumarin anticoagulants of the first generation, dihydropyridine calcium channel blockers, NSAIDs, barbiturates, diuretics, antidiabetics of the sulfonylurea type (sulfonamide part), and finally after enzymatic cleavage of the acetalic glucuronides, anthraquinone and diphenol laxatives or buprenorphine [26, 41]. In addition, various other acidic compounds could also be detected [26, 90]. Further GC-MS screening procedures are described or reviewed elsewhere [17, 25, 41].

In the early 1990s, several working groups started using LC-MS in analytical toxicology [93, 94]. Some of them started with a transfer of existing LC-UV or GC-MS procedures so that the scientific and/or practical progress was rather limited, particularly when considering the limitations of this new technique such as the rather poor spectral information (in single-stage apparatus), the poor reproducibility of the ionization, and the susceptibility to matrix effects (ion suppression or enhancements). Details have already been discussed elsewhere [20]. Nowadays, the apparatus have been improved and analysts have learned to more or less overcome the disadvantages and challenges with LC-MS analysis [20]. For example, relevant matrix effects can often be avoided by suitable specimen clean-up, chromatographic changes, reagent modifications, and effective internal standardization [95]. After 15 years, single-stage or tandem LC-MS with electrospray ionization (ESI) or atmospheric pressure chemical ionization (APCI) have now definitively left the development stage and are becoming increasingly important in routine toxicological analysis, especially for quantification of the identified analytes [20, 25, 31, 32, 96]. They have even opened the door to new fields of toxicological interpretation and expertise such as sensitive detection of chemical agents in hair in the case of drug-facilitated crimes [7] or determination of a chronic alcohol consumption by determination of ethanol conjugates in plasma, urine, or hair [97]. The question of whether ESI or APCI is more suitable for developing a new procedure cannot be answered in general. APCI is more appropriate for unionized analytes. The sensitivity depends on the analyte structure and the apparatus type used and should always be tested for. Dams et al. [50] found that ESI and APCI showed matrix effects, with ESI being much more susceptible than APCI. Finally, Beyer et al. [98] showed that the accuracy and precision data of a plasma quantification method for toxic alkaloids were very similar when using LC-APCI-MS or LC-ESI-MS/MS.

Most LC-MS(/MS) screening procedures focus on multi-target screening procedures rather than on STA. This means that they allow screening for a certain number of analytes in the selected-ion monitoring (SIM) or multiple-reaction monitoring (MRM) mode, whereas analytes not included *a priori* cannot be detected. Nevertheless, such methods have helped to extend the spectrum of sensitive and specific MS-based methods to analytes, which are not amenable to GC-MS analysis because of hydrophilic or thermolabile properties. For STA, the best strategies are based on tandem MS with MRM as survey scan and an enhanced product ion (EPI) scan in an information-dependent acquisition (IDA) and identification of the product ion spectra by library search using the authors' EPI spectra libraries [99, 100]. Possibilities and limitations of such methods have been extensively discussed elsewhere [9, 17, 20, 25, 96].

Few years ago, the working group of Ojanpera started the development of urine screening procedures based on enzymatic cleavage of conjugates and mixed-mode SPE using a time-of-flight (TOF) mass analyzer based on measurement of the accurate mass and the retention times and their comparison with reference data [54, 101]. In two recent papers, advances in these procedures were presented [102, 103]. They relied on a large target database of exact masses of reference drugs and their metabolites. Using LC-Fourier transform MS (LC-FTMS), they were able to confirm the findings with a higher mass accuracy than provided by the LC-TOF [102]. Mass spectral identification was based on matching measured accurate mass and isotopic pattern of a sample component with those in the database using a newly developed software for automated reporting of findings in an easily interpretable form [103]. However, it must be considered that there are several potential drugs with the same empirical formula and molecular mass (e.g., morphine and hydromorphone) [104] and that their metabolites (e.g., hydroxy or demethyl metabolites) may also have the same masses, so that in many cases other procedures are needed for confirmation.

A strategy for rapid and selective testing for drugs of abuse in urine as an alternative to immunoassay prescreening has been developed [105–111]. Multi-analyte screening methods for directly injected diluted urine samples have been reported that were based on classic triple-quadrupole LC-MS/MS in the MRM mode. Meanwhile, corresponding studies have been performed and showed no serious matrix effect if the analytes were separated from the solvent front [108–111]. Therefore, it can be concluded that this strategy may in future replace the common immunoassay prescreening for drugs of abuse in urine, at least in specialized laboratories with a high sample throughput for which screening by LC-MS may be profitable.

Quantification procedures

Use of only immunoassays for quantification is also limited, because the given drug levels, e.g., of tricyclic antidepressants, cannot be interpreted, as different drugs of the corresponding group may have quite different cross-reactivity and/or pharmacological potency. In the case of combinations of drugs of the same group (e.g., benzodiazepines, one was taken by the patient, one was administered by the emergency doctor), the given drug levels cannot be differentiated. In summary, conclusions based on immunoassay results are not state-of-the-art in clinical and forensic toxicology.

As discussed in detail by Peters et al. [19], quantitative procedures must be validated and at least the following parameters should be evaluated: selectivity, calibration model (linearity), stability, accuracy (bias), precision (repeatability, intermediate precision) and the lower limit of quantification (LLOQ). Additional parameters that may be relevant include limit of detection (LOD), recovery, reproducibility, and ruggedness (robustness). As already mentioned above, experiments for assessment of matrix effects are mandatory for LC-MS methods. In addition, the applicability to real samples should also be documented for all bioanalytical procedures.

In most chromatographic assays, internal standards (IS) are mandatory for reliable quantification compensating all variability (work-up and measurement). They should have similar physicochemical properties, their signal should not interfere with that of the analyte, their mass spectra should not contain fragment ions corresponding to those of the analyte and finally they should not cause relevant ion suppression/enhancement in LC-MS approaches [32]. Non-labeled therapeutic drugs should not be used as IS because even if a drug is not marketed in a certain country, its presence in the specimen to be analyzed can never be fully excluded in times of increasing international travel and globalization. In this case, the signal of the IS will be overestimated, inevitably leading to underestimation of the analyte concentration in the sample. In methods employing MS, the IS should always be chosen from the pool of available isotopically labeled compounds. Nowadays these are available in a large variety of structures with different physicochemical properties so it should not be a problem to find an appropriate IS in this pool of compounds. They can ideally compensate for variability during sample preparation and measurement, but still be differentiated from the target analyte by MS detection. However, isotopically labeled compounds may contain the non-labeled compound as an impurity or their mass spectra may sometimes contain fragment ions with the same mass-to-charge ratios (m/z) as the monitored ions of the target analyte. In both cases, the peak area of the analyte peak would be overestimated, thus compromising quantification. The absence of such interference caused by the IS should be checked by analyzing so-called zero samples, i.e., blank samples spiked with the IS [19]. In a way similar to that described above, the analyte might interfere with a stable-isotope-labeled IS. This even becomes a principle problem with deuterated analogues when the number of deuterium atoms of the analogue or one of its monitored fragments is three or less [112]. Blank samples spiked with the analyte at the upper limit of the calibration range, but without IS, can be used to check for absence of such interferences [19].

Another problem that may arise is when a metabolite is the active component or contributes to the pharmacological and/or toxic effect (e.g.,

O-desmethyltramadol [113, 114]). For reliable assessment, such metabolites must also be determined, but reference standards are needed. However, such metabolite standards are often not commercially available, particularly in the case of new therapeutic drugs or drugs of abuse. The classic chemical synthesis of drug metabolites can be cumbersome and stereochemically demanding, and hence go beyond the possibilities of most biochemistry- or pharmacology/toxicology-oriented laboratories. Custom made metabolite standards are a possible, but usually time-consuming and very expensive, solution. Biotechnological synthesis of drug metabolites using cytochrome P450 (CYP) enzymes could be a versatile alternative to classic chemical synthesis and possibly have important advantages over the latter. Firstly, they would yield the metabolites of interest as products, at least if the CYP isozymes responsible for the *in vivo* formation of the respective metabolites were used. Secondly, one would expect only one (major) product when using specific isozymes, because they usually catalyze one metabolic step with high preference or even exclusively. Moreover, the metabolic reactions are generally highly stereoselective. Finally, they can be carried out under mild conditions in comparison to classic chemical reactions that often require high temperatures, high pressure or aggressive and/or toxic chemicals. Peters et al. [115–117] developed an interesting alternative by evaluating the feasibility of biotechnological synthesis of drug metabolites using human CYP2D6, CYP2B6, CYP2C9, CYP2C19, or CYP3A4 heterologously expressed in the fission yeast *Schizosaccharomyces pombe* as model enzymes because they are involved in the metabolism of many therapeutic and illicit drugs in humans.

Quantification in urine is of lesser importance than in blood, because the concentrations may vary considerably depending on the hydration status of the body and the urinary pH. Moreover, compounds in urine have already been eliminated from the body, so that their concentrations are of little relevance with respect to toxic effects. Nevertheless, detection procedures are developed as quantitative assays, particularly for confirmation of immunoassay results and/or for determinations that must meet certain cut-off values. Such procedures have recently been critically reviewed and basic information is given there [9, 13].

Reliable quantification of drugs, poisons and/or their pharmacologically active metabolites in blood, plasma or serum is mandatory for correct interpretation of toxicological findings because the analyte concentration in blood correlates best with the biological effect. Series of mono-analyte and several multi-analyte procedures have been published for a wide range of drugs or poisons, and they are critically reviewed elsewhere [5, 8, 9, 17, 27, 28, 97, 118]. Therefore, only some typical state-of-the-art procedures are given here as examples.

As an example for multi-analyte GC-MS procedures, a screening and simultaneous quantification procedure was selected for various central stimulants and designer drugs [119]. This assay was fully validated according to international criteria and its applicability was proven by analyzing authentic blood plasma samples as well as a certified reference sample. Corresponding chiral procedures have been developed by the same working group and also fully validated [67–69].

As examples for multi-analyte LC-MS procedures, the following assays were selected. Sauvage et al. [120] developed a fully automated turbulent flow LC-MS/MS procedure for monitoring 13 antidepressants and 4 of their pharmacologically active metabolites in serum for therapeutic drug monitoring (TDM), but also useful in clinical and forensic toxicology. The analytes were divided in two groups depending on their lipophilicity, so that two injections would be necessary to monitor all compounds. Turbulent flow chromatography is based on direct injection of biological samples without previous extraction onto a column packed with large particles of a stationary-phase material and a high mobile-phase flow rate. This allows retention of the small analytes and exclusion of large matrix compounds, thus helping to avoid matrix effects. The procedure was validated including testing for matrix effects. Finally, the authors compared drug concentrations in external quality control samples measured with this new procedure and the consensus mean of all laboratories participating in this proficiency test. Certainly, the method performance in such external quality control schemes is one of the most convincing ways to demonstrate its reliability [38].

Beyer et al. [121] developed a multi-analyte LC-MS/MS procedure for the detection and validated quantification of ephedrine-derived phenalkylamines in plasma. The method was exemplarily validated according to international guidelines recently reviewed by Peters et al. [19]. The same authors developed similar procedures for the detection and quantification of toxic alkaloids including the hallucinogenic and mydriatic alkaloids atropine and scopolamine in plasma [98]. They fully validated the procedure for two different apparatus types, on LC-ESI-MS/MS and LC-APCI-MS with conditions similar to their routine multi-analyte procedures [122–125]. Except for its greater sensitivity and higher identification power, LC-ESI-MS/MS had no major advantages over the much cheaper LC-APCI-MS. Figure 1 shows chromatograms of a plasma extract after SPE indicating a toxic concentration of colchicine, a therapeutic concentration of atropine, a toxic concentration of scopolamine, and a common smoker's concentration of cotinine determined using single-stage or tandem MS.

Laloup et al. [126] developed an LC-MS/MS assay for determination of 26 benzodiazepines and zolpidem and zopiclone in blood, urine and hair samples. The procedure was fully validated for all the biosamples and showed acceptable results for most analytes and/or biosamples. Musshoff et al. [127] described an LC-MS/MS method for quantitative determination of opioids and some of their metabolites including the pharmacologically active morphine-6-glucuronide in plasma. They used automatically performed SPE and validated their assay also according to the recommendations of Peters et al. [19]. Kristoffersen et al. [128] recently described a single-stage LC-MS assay for cardiovascular drugs in postmortem whole blood after precipitation and

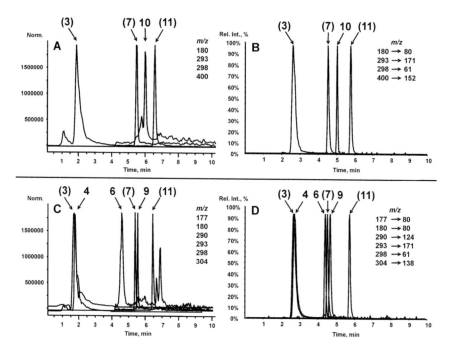

Figure 1. (A) Smoothed, normalized and merged chromatograms with the given ions of a plasma extract after solid-phase extraction (SPE) indicating a toxic concentration of 24 ng/ml colchicine (peak 10) determined using single-stage mass spectrometry (MS). (B) Smoothed, normalized and merged chromatograms of the given transitions of the same extract indicating a toxic concentration of 25 ng/ml colchicine (peak 10) determined using tandem MS. (C) Smoothed, normalized and merged chromatograms with the given ions of a plasma extract after SPE indicating a therapeutic concentration of 6.4 ng/ml atropine (peak 9), a toxic concentration of 5.6 ng/ml of scopolamine (peak 6), and a common smoker's concentration of 321 ng/ml cotinine (peak 4) determined using single-stage MS. (D) Smoothed, normalized and merged chromatograms of the given transitions of the same extract indicating a therapeutic concentration of 6.1 ng/ml atropine (peak 9), a toxic concentration of 5.9 ng/ml scopolamine (peak 6), and a common smoker's concentration of 319 ng/ml cotinine (peak 4) determined using tandem MS. The peaks are numbered as follows: cotinine-d_3 (3), cotinine (4), scopolamine (6), benzoylecgonine-d_3 (7), atropine (9), colchicine (10), and trimipramine-d_3 (11) (reproduced from [98] with permission of the copyright owner John Wiley & Sons Limited).

mixed-mode SPE. They validated the procedure and tested for robustness by systematically searching for satisfactory conditions using experimental designs including factorial and response surface designs. They found that the assay showed satisfactory robustness to small changes in the procedure only for some analytes, but that the LC separation was robust with regard to consistency of retention order and no co-elution under the used pH and buffer ionic strength. As they used SIM with only two ions per analyte, selectivity was tested intensively using drug-free postmortem whole blood samples of eight different sources directly or after spiking with a series of drugs. No interferences with endogenous or exogenous compounds were detected.

Quality control

Analytical methods to be used in clinical and/or forensic toxicology require careful method development and thorough validation of the final method as recommended by Peters et al. [18, 19, 95]. This is especially true in the context of quality management and accreditation, which have become matters of increasing relevance in analytical toxicology in recent years. As already mentioned, validation should include, when appropriate, recovery, selectivity, calibration model, the assessment of accuracy and precision, limits of detection and quantitation, stability, and, additionally for LC-MS procedures, matrix effect. Authentic samples must be analyzed and their sources described, and relevant data should be presented. Methods for routine analysis need to be submitted to internal and external quality control, e.g., by regular participation in proficiency test programs [2].

Interpretation of the analytical result

Interpretation of analytical results in the context of clinical case data as well as of pharmacological and toxicological data of the involved drug or toxicant is a sophisticated task and needs good cooperation of the toxicologists with the clinicians. The main questions are which substances are present, whether the quantity of the identified drug and/or poison explains the patient's condition, what are the consequences for a rational therapy, and what is the prognosis? Several aspects must be considered here and are summarized elsewhere [2]. One important issue is to consider what was already done therapeutically and which medication was administered. Another is to discuss whether the mode of action of the drug and/or poison fit with the shown symptoms, which diseases may also lead to the shown symptoms, and whether the patient may suffer from a further disease in addition to the poisoning. Influences of shock, insufficiency of liver or kidney, variations of drug metabolism due to interactions and/or genetic polymorphisms must be considered in toxicokinetic calculations using reference data from population kinetics. Reference blood levels of drugs or poisons used for interpretation should carefully be checked for plausibility and validity and discussed critically. In case of organ-toxic compounds, risks should be considered for long-term toxicity.

Unreliable clinical and analytical data and/or their interpretation could lead to wrong treatment of the patient or might be contested in court and, finally, they could lead to unjustified legal consequences for the defendant [2]. Reference data for toxicological interpretation of poisonings in humans come mainly from case reports. In contrast to other clinical or experimental sciences, controlled clinical studies [129–131] or prospective cohort studies [132] are rare in clinical toxicology on ethical grounds. This is a general problem in toxicological risk assessment, because human data cannot be generated in controlled studies for correlation of toxic concentrations of drugs, poisons or chemicals in body samples and the corresponding clinical effect. Correlation studies, e.g., between the dose of drugs of abuse, alcohol or medicaments and the clinical effect and behavior (e.g., drugs and driving studies) are only possible after strict evaluation of the study protocols. Therefore, toxicological data are generally collected from animal or *ex vivo* studies and correlated with human data of poisoning cases. To improve the toxicological risk assessment of chemicals, some national chemical acts demand that poisonings with chemicals must be reported to the responsible governmental institution. Such reports as well as case reports, and retrospective or prospective studies published in scientific journals must yield sufficient information on the clinical, the toxicological and analytical part, otherwise they provide only unreliable data for assessing the clinical outcome in the sense of evidence-based medicine. In addition, such data are mandatory for any forensic conclusion made by extrapolating published case data (e.g., blood levels correlated to observed clinical signs) with a current case to be evaluated, e.g., for court. Possible individual variations in the pharmacological or toxicological responses caused by body mass, age, gender, kidney and liver function, drug-drug (food-drug) interactions, and genetic variability should be discussed [74, 133].

Conclusions and perspectives

Analytical sciences are an important part of clinical and forensic toxicology as well as in doping control, and food and environmental toxicology. Selection of the most appropriate technique with careful method development and thorough validation followed by internal and external quality control is the basis for successful application of toxicological analysis in these fields. The analytical results can only help in diagnosis of acute or chronic poisonings, and drug abuse, as well as drug monitoring if they are reliable. GC-MS and increasingly LC-MS are the gold standards, providing best selectivity, sensitivity and universality. Appropriate selection and work-up of the biosample to be assayed are important prerequisites. Careful interpretation of the analytical results completes the tasks of analytical toxicology.

Recent and future developments in analytical technologies such as high-resolution MS, chip technologies for separation, automation, miniaturization, etc., will also improve the power of analytical toxicology if appropriately applied.

Acknowledgments
The author would like to thank Dr. Markus Meyer for his suggestions.

References

1 Maurer HH (2007) Analytical toxicology. *Anal Bioanal Chem* 388: 1311
2 Maurer HH (2007) Demands on scientific studies in clinical toxicology. *Forensic Sci Int* 165: 194–198

3 Flanagan RJ, Taylor AA, Watson ID, Whelpton R (2009) *Fundamentals of Analytical Toxicology.* John Wiley & Sons, Chichester, UK

4 Kuelpmann, WR (2009) *Clinical Toxicological Analysis – Procedures, Results, Interpretation.* Wiley-VCH, Weinheim, Germany

5 Drummer OH (2007) Requirements for bioanalytical procedures in postmortem toxicology. *Anal Bioanal Chem* 388: 1495–1503

6 Gray T, Huestis M (2007) Bioanalytical procedures for monitoring *in utero* drug exposure. *Anal Bioanal Chem* 388: 1455–1465

7 Kintz P (2007) Bioanalytical procedures for detection of chemical agents in hair in the case of drug-facilitated crimes. *Anal Bioanal Chem* 388: 1467–1474

8 Kraemer T, Paul LD (2007) Bioanalytical procedures for determination of drugs of abuse in blood. *Anal Bioanal Chem* 388: 1415–1435

9 Maurer HH (2007) Current role of liquid chromatography–mass spectrometry in clinical and forensic toxicology. *Anal Bioanal Chem* 388: 1315–1325

10 Musshoff F, Madea B (2007) Analytical pitfalls in hair testing. *Anal Bioanal Chem* 388: 1475–1494

11 Pragst F (2007) Application of solid-phase microextraction in analytical toxicology. *Anal Bioanal Chem* 388: 1393–1414

12 Samyn N, Laloup M, de Boeck G (2007) Bioanalytical procedures for determination of drugs of abuse in oral fluid. *Anal Bioanal Chem* 388: 1437–1453

13 Thevis M, Schanzer W (2007) Current role of LC-MS in doping control. *Anal Bioanal Chem* 388: 1351–1358

14 Wille SM, Lambert WE (2007) Recent developments in extraction procedures relevant to analytical toxicology. *Anal Bioanal Chem* 388: 1381–1391

15 Drummer OH (2008) Introduction and review of collection techniques and applications of drug testing of oral fluid. *Ther Drug Monit* 30: 203–206

16 Moeller KE, Lee KC, Kissack JC (2008) Urine drug screening: Practical guide for clinicians. *Mayo Clin Proc* 83: 66–76

17 Maurer HH (2009) Mass spectrometric approaches in impaired driving toxicology. *Anal Bioanal Chem* 393: 97–107

18 Peters FT, Maurer HH (2002) Bioanalytical method validation and its implications for forensic and clinical toxicology – A review. *Accred Qual Assur* 7: 441–449

19 Peters FT, Drummer OH, Musshoff F (2007) Validation of new methods. *Forensic Sci Int* 165: 216–224

20 Maurer HH (2006) Hyphenated mass spectrometric techniques – Indispensable tools in clinical and forensic toxicology and in doping control. *J Mass Spectrom* 41: 1399–1413

21 Pelander A, Ojanpera I, Sistonen J, Rasanen I, Vuori E (2003) Screening for basic drugs in 2-mL urine samples by dual-plate overpressured layer chromatography and comparison with gas chromatography–mass spectrometry. *J Anal Toxicol* 27: 226–232

22 Rasanen I, Kontinen I, Nokua J, Ojanpera I, Vuori E (2003) Precise gas chromatography with retention time locking in comprehensive toxicological screening for drugs in blood. *J Chromatogr B Analyt Technol Biomed Life Sci* 788: 243–250

23 Pragst F, Herzler M, Erxleben BT (2004) Systematic toxicological analysis by high-performance liquid chromatography with diode array detection (HPLC-DAD). *Clin Chem Lab Med* 42: 1325–1340

24 Pragst F, Herzler M, Herre S, Erxleben BT, Rothe M (2007) *UV Spectra of Toxic Compounds: Database of Photodiode Array UV Spectra of Illegal and Therapeutic Drugs, Pesticides, Ecotoxic Substances and Other Poisons.* Verlag Toxicological Chemistry, Berlin, Germany

25 Maurer HH (2004) Position of chromatographic techniques in screening for detection of drugs or poisons in clinical and forensic toxicology and/or doping control. *Clin Chem Lab Med* 42: 1310–1324

26 Maurer, HH, Pfleger, K, Weber, AA (2007) *Mass Spectral and GC Data of Drugs, Poisons, Pesticides, Pollutants and Their Metabolites.* 3rd edn., Wiley-VCH, Weinheim, Germany

27 Saint-Marcoux F, Sauvage FL, Marquet P (2007) Current role of LC-MS in therapeutic drug monitoring. *Anal Bioanal Chem* 388: 1327–1349

28 Tagliaro F, Bortolotti F, Pascali JP (2007) Current role of capillary electrophoretic/electrokinetic techniques in forensic toxicology. *Anal Bioanal Chem* 388: 1359–1364

29 Maurer HH, Kraemer T, Kratzsch C, Paul LD, Peters FT, Springer D, Staack RF, Weber AA (2002)

What is the appropriate analytical strategy for effective management of intoxicated patients? In: *Proceedings of the 39th International TIAFT Meeting in Prague (2001)*, 61–75

30 Maurer HH, Peters FT (2005) Towards high-throughput drug screening using mass spectrometry. *Ther Drug Monit* 27: 686–688

31 Maurer HH (2005) Multi-analyte procedures for screening for and quantification of drugs in blood, plasma, or serum by liquid chromatography–single stage or tandem mass spectrometry (LC-MS or LC-MS/MS) relevant to clinical and forensic toxicology. *Clin Biochem* 38: 310–318

32 Maurer HH (2005) Advances in analytical toxicology: Current role of liquid chromatography–mass spectrometry for drug quantification in blood and oral fluid. *Anal Bioanal Chem* 381: 110–118

33 Flanagan RJ (2004) Developing an analytical toxicology service: Principles and guidance. *Toxicol Rev* 23: 251–263

34 Flanagan RJ, Connally G, Evans JM (2005) Analytical toxicology: Guidelines for sample collection postmortem. *Toxicol Rev* 24: 63–71

35 Wu AH, McKay C, Broussard LA, Hoffman RS, Kwong TC, Moyer TP, Otten EM, Welch SL, Wax P (2003) National Academy of clinical biochemistry laboratory medicine practice guidelines: Recommendations for the use of laboratory tests to support poisoned patients who present to the emergency department. *Clin Chem* 49: 357–379

36 Boyer EW, Shannon MW (2003) Which drug tests in medical emergencies? *Clin Chem* 49: 353–354

37 Bailey B, Amre DK (2005) A toxicologist's guide to studying diagnostic tests. *Clin Toxicol* 43: 171–179

38 Peters FT, Jung J, Kraemer T, Maurer HH (2005) Fast, simple, and validated gas chromatographic-mass spectrometric assay for quantification of drugs relevant to diagnosis of brain death in human blood plasma samples. *Ther Drug Monit* 27: 334–344

39 Segura J, Pascual JA, Gutierrez-Gallego R (2007) Procedures for monitoring recombinant erythropoietin and analogues in doping control. *Anal Bioanal Chem* 388: 1521–1529

40 Peters FT (2007) Stability of analytes in biosamples: An important issue in clinical and forensic toxicology? *Anal Bioanal Chem* 388: 1505–1519

41 Maurer HH (2007) Forensic screening with GC-MS. In: M Bogusz (ed.): *Handbook of Analytical Separation Sciences: Forensic Sciences*, 2nd edn., Elsevier Science, Amsterdam, 429–449

42 von Mach MA, Weber C, Meyer MR, Weilemann LS, Maurer HH, Peters FT (2007) Comparison of urinary on-site immunoassay screening and gas chromatography–mass spectrometry results of 111 patients with suspected poisoning presenting at an emergency department. *Ther Drug Monit* 29: 27–39

43 Stanley SD, McKemie D, Skinner W (2003) Large-volume injection gas chromatography–mass spectrometry for automated broad-spectrum drug screening in horse urine. *J Anal Toxicol* 27: 325–331

44 Thevis M, Schanzer W (2007) Mass spectrometry in sports drug testing: Structure characterization and analytical assays. *Mass Spectrom Rev* 26: 79–107

45 Thevis M, Opfermann G, Schanzer W (2003) Liquid chromatography/electrospray ionization tandem mass spectrometric screening and confirmation methods for β2-agonists in human or equine urine. *J Mass Spectrom* 38: 1197–1206

46 Peters FT, Drvarov O, Lottner S, Spellmeier A, Rieger K, Haefeli WE, Maurer HH (2009) A systematic comparison of four different workup procedures for systematic toxicological analysis of urine samples using gas chromatography–mass spectrometry. *Anal Bioanal Chem* 393: 735–745

47 Decaestecker TN, Coopman EM, van Peteghem CH, van Bocxlaer JF (2003) Suitability testing of commercial solid-phase extraction sorbents for sample clean-up in systematic toxicological analysis using liquid chromatography–(tandem) mass spectrometry. *J Chromatogr B Analyt Technol Biomed Life Sci* 789: 19–25

48 Annesley TM (2003) Ion suppression in mass spectrometry. *Clin Chem* 49: 1041–1044

49 Liang HR, Foltz RL, Meng M, Bennett P (2003) Ionization enhancement in atmospheric pressure chemical ionization and suppression in electrospray ionization between target drugs and stable-isotope-labeled internal standards in quantitative liquid chromatography/tandem mass spectrometry. *Rapid Commun Mass Spectrom* 17: 2815–2821

50 Dams R, Huestis MA, Lambert WE, Murphy CM (2003) Matrix effect in bio-analysis of illicit drugs with LC-MS/MS: Influence of ionization type, sample preparation, and biofluid. *J Am Soc Mass Spectrom* 14: 1290–1294

51 Müller C, Schäfer P, Störtzel M, Vogt S, Weinmann W (2002) Ion suppression effects in liquid chromatography–electrospray-ionisation transport-region collision induced dissociation mass spectrometry with different serum extraction methods for systematic toxicological analysis with mass spectra libraries. *J Chromatogr B Analyt Technol Biomed Life Sci* 773: 47–52

52 Mortier KA, Clauwaert KM, Lambert WE, van Bocxlaer JF, van den Eeckhout EG, van Peteghem CH, de Leenheer AP (2001) Pitfalls associated with liquid chromatography/electrospray tandem mass spectrometry in quantitative bioanalysis of drugs of abuse in saliva. *Rapid Commun Mass Spectrom* 15: 1773–1775

53 King R, Bonfiglio R, Fernandez-Metzler C, Miller-Stein C, Olah T (2000) Mechanistic investigation of ionization suppression in electrospray ionization. *J Am Soc Mass Spectrom* 11: 942–950

54 Pelander A, Ojanpera I, I, Laks S, Rasanen I, Vuori E (2003) Toxicological screening with formula-based metabolite identification by liquid chromatography/time-of-flight mass spectrometry. *Anal Chem* 75: 5710–5718

55 Josefsson M, Kronstrand R, Andersson J, Roman M (2003) Evaluation of electrospray ionisation liquid chromatography–tandem mass spectrometry for rational determination of a number of neuroleptics and their major metabolites in human body fluids and tissues. *J Chromatogr B Analyt Technol Biomed Life Sci* 789: 151–167

56 Thevis M, Opfermann G, Schanzer W (2001) High speed determination of β-receptor blocking agents in human urine by liquid chromatography/tandem mass spectrometry. *Biomed Chromatogr* 15: 393–402

57 Spahn LH, Benet LZ (1992) Acyl glucuronides revisited: Is the glucuronidation process a toxification as well as a detoxification mechanism? *Drug Metab Rev* 24: 5–47

58 Maurer HH, Bickeboeller-Friedrich J (2000) Screening procedure for detection of antidepressants of the selective serotonin reuptake inhibitor type and their metabolites in urine as part of a modified systematic toxicological analysis procedure using gas chromatography–mass spectrometry. *J Anal Toxicol* 24: 340–347

59 Maurer HH, Tauvel FX, Kraemer T (2001) Screening procedure for detection of non-steroidal antiinflammatory drugs (NSAIDs) and their metabolites in urine as part of a systematic toxicological analysis (STA) procedure for acidic drugs and poisons by gas chromatography–mass spectrometry (GC-MS) after extractive methylation. *J Anal Toxicol* 25: 237–244

60 Risticevic S, Niri VH, Vuckovic D, Pawliszyn J (2009) Recent developments in solid-phase microextraction. *Anal Bioanal Chem* 393: 781–795

61 Kumazawa T, Seno H, Watanabe-Suzuki K, Hattori H, Ishii A, Sato K, Suzuki O (2000) Determination of phenothiazines in human body fluids by solid-phase microextraction and liquid chromatography/tandem mass spectrometry. *J Mass Spectrom* 35: 1091–1099

62 Maurer HH, Arlt JW (1998) Detection of 4-hydroxycoumarin anticoagulants and their metabolites in urine as part of a systematic toxicological analysis procedure for acidic drugs and poisons by gas chromatography–mass spectrometry after extractive methylation. *J Chromatogr B Biomed Sci Appl* 714: 181–195

63 Maurer HH, Arlt JW (1999) Screening procedure for detection of dihydropyridine calcium channel blocker metabolites in urine as part of a systematic toxicological analysis procedure for acidics by gas chromatography–mass spectrometry (GC-MS) after extractive methylation. *J Anal Toxicol* 23: 73–80

64 Beyer J, Peters FT, Maurer HH (2005) Screening procedure for detection of stimulant laxatives and/or their metabolites in human urine using gas chromatography–mass spectrometry after enzymatic cleavage of conjugates and extractive methylation. *Ther Drug Monit* 27: 151–157

65 Beyer J, Bierl A, Peters FT, Maurer HH (2005) Screening procedure for detection of diuretics and uricosurics and/or their metabolites in human urine using gas chromatography–mass spectrometry after extractive methylation. *Ther Drug Monit* 27: 509–520

66 Peters FT, Samyn N, Kraemer T, Riedel W, Maurer HH (2007) Negative-ion chemical ionization gas chromatographic–mass spectrometric assay for enantioselective determination of amphetamines in oral fluid: Application to a controlled study with MDMA and driving under the influence of drugs cases. *Clin Chem* 53: 702–710

67 Peters FT, Samyn N, Lamers C, Riedel W, Kraemer T, de Boeck G, Maurer HH (2005) Drug testing in blood: Validated negative-ion chemical ionization gas chromatographic–mass spectrometric assay for enantioselective determination of the designer drugs MDA, MDMA (ecstasy) and MDEA and its application to samples from a controlled study with MDMA. *Clin Chem* 51: 1811–1822

68 Peters FT, Samyn N, Wahl M, Kraemer T, de Boeck G, Maurer HH (2003) Concentrations and ratios of amphetamine, methamphetamine, MDA, MDMA, and MDEA enantiomers determined in plasma samples from clinical toxicology and driving under the influence of drugs cases by GC-NICI-MS. *J Anal Toxicol* 27: 552–559

69 Peters FT, Kraemer T, Maurer HH (2002) Drug testing in blood: Validated negative-ion chemical ionization gas chromatographic–mass spectrometric assay for determination of amphetamine and methamphetamine enantiomers and its application to toxicology cases. *Clin Chem* 48: 1472–1485

70 Maurer HH (2002) The role of gas chromatography–mass spectrometry with negative ion chemical ionization (GC-MS-NCI) in clinical and forensic toxicology, doping control and biomonitoring. *Ther Drug Monit* 24: 247–254

71 Maurer HH, Kraemer T, Kratzsch C, Peters FT, Weber AA (2002) Negative ion chemical ionization gas chromatography–mass spectrometry (NICI-GC-MS) and atmospheric pressure chemical ionization liquid chromatography–mass spectrometry (APCI-LC-MS) of low-dosed and/or polar drugs in plasma. *Ther Drug Monit* 24: 117–124

72 Segura J, Ventura R, Jurado C (1998) Derivatization procedures for gas chromatographic–mass spectrometric determination of xenobiotics in biological samples, with special attention to drugs of abuse and doping agents. *J Chromatogr B* 713: 61–90

73 Fuentes-Block L (2000) Drug screening: Interactions, pitfalls, and techniques. *MLO Med Lab Obs* 32: 26–35

74 Maurer HH, Sauer C, Theobald DS (2006) Toxicokinetics of drugs of abuse: Current knowledge of the isoenzymes involved in the human metabolism of tetrahydrocannabinol, cocaine, heroin, morphine, and codeine. *Ther Drug Monit* 28: 447–453

75 Ewald AH, Peters FT, Weise M, Maurer HH (2005) Studies on the metabolism and toxicological detection of the designer drug 4-methylthioamphetamine (4-MTA) in human urine using gas chromatography–mass spectrometry. *J Chromatogr B Analyt Technol Biomed Life Sci* 824: 123–131

76 Theobald DS, Staack RF, Puetz M, Maurer HH (2005) New designer drug 2,5-dimethoxy-4-ethylthio-β-phenethylamine (2C-T-2): Studies on its metabolism and toxicological detection in rat urine using gas chromatography/mass spectrometry. *J Mass Spectrom* 40: 1157–1172

77 Theobald DS, Fehn S, Maurer HH (2005) New designer drug 2,5-dimethoxy-4-propylthio-phenethylamine (2C-T-7): Studies on its metabolism and toxicological detection in rat urine using gas chromatography/mass spectrometry. *J Mass Spectrom* 40: 105–116

78 Ewald AH, Fritschi G, Maurer HH (2006) Designer drug 2,4,5-trimethoxyamphetamine (TMA-2): Studies on its metabolism and toxicological detection in rat urine using gas chromatographic/mass spectrometric techniques. *J Mass Spectrom* 41: 1140–1148

79 Ewald AH, Fritschi G, Bork WR, Maurer HH (2006) Designer drugs 2,5-dimethoxy-4-bromoamphetamine (DOB) and 2,5-dimethoxy-4-bromomethamphetamine (MDOB): Studies on their metabolism and toxicological detection in rat urine using gas chromatographic/mass spectrometric techniques. *J Mass Spectrom* 41: 487–498

80 Sauer C, Peters FT, Staack RF, Fritschi G, Maurer HH (2006) New designer drug (1-(1-phenylcyclohexyl)-3-ethoxypropylamine (PCEPA): Studies on its metabolism and toxicological detection in rat urine using gas chromatography/mass spectrometry. *J Mass Spectrom* 41: 1014–1029

81 Theobald DS, Putz M, Schneider E, Maurer HH (2006) New designer drug 4-iodo-2,5-dimethoxy-β-phenethylamine (2C-I): Studies on its metabolism and toxicological detection in rat urine using gas chromatographic/mass spectrometric and capillary electrophoretic/mass spectrometric techniques. *J Mass Spectrom* 41: 872–886

82 Theobald DS, Maurer HH (2006) Studies on the metabolism and toxicological detection of the designer drug 4-ethyl-2,5-dimethoxy-β-phenethylamine (2C-E) in rat urine using gas chromatographic–mass spectrometric techniques. *J Chromatogr B Analyt Technol Biomed Life Sci* 842: 76–90

83 Ewald AH, Fritschi G, Maurer HH (2007) Metabolism and toxicological detection of the designer drug 4-iodo-2,5-dimethoxy-amphetamine (DOI) in rat urine using gas chromatography–mass spectrometry. *J Chromatogr B Analyt Technol Biomed Life Sci* 857: 170–174

84 Sauer C, Peters FT, Meyer MR, Maurer HH (2007) Studies on the CYP isoform dependent metabolism of the new phencyclidine-derived designer drug PCEPA. *Ther Drug Monit* 29: 463

85 Ewald AH, Ehlers D, Maurer HH (2008) Metabolism and toxicological detection of the designer drug 4-chloro-2,5-dimethoxyamphetamine in rat urine using gas chromatography–mass spectrometry. *Anal Bioanal Chem* 390: 1837–1842

86 Ewald AH, Fritschi G, Maurer HH (2008) Studies on the metabolism and toxicological detection

of the designer drug DOI in rat urine using GC-MS techniques. *Proceedings of the XVth GTFCh Symposium in Mosbach (2007)*, 259–262

87 Sauer C, Peters FT, Staack RF, Fritschi G, Maurer HH (2008) Metabolism and toxicological detection of a new designer drug, *N*-(1-phenylcyclohexyl)propanamine, in rat urine using gas chromatography–mass spectrometry. *J Chromatogr A* 1186: 380–390

88 Sauer C, Peters FT, Staack RF, Fritschi G, Maurer HH (2008) New designer drugs *N*-(1-phenyl-cyclohexyl)-2-ethoxyethanamine (PCEEA) and *N*-(1-phenylcyclohexyl)-2-methoxyethanamine (PCMEA): Studies on their metabolism and toxicological detection in rat urine using gas chro-matographic/mass spectrometric techniques. *J Mass Spectrom* 43: 305–316

89 Sauer C, Peters FT, Staack RF, Fritschi G, Maurer HH (2008) Metabolism and toxicological detection of the designer drug *N*-(1-phenylcyclohexyl)-3-methoxypropanamine (PCMPA) in rat urine using gas chromatography–mass spectrometry. *Forensic Sci Int* 181: 47–51

90 Maurer HH, Pfleger K, Weber AA (2007) *Mass Spectral Library of Drugs, Poisons, Pesticides, Pollutants and Their Metabolites*. 4th edn., Wiley-VCH, Weinheim, Germany

91 McLafferty FW (2001) *Registry of Mass Spectral Data*. 7th edn., John Wiley & Sons, New York, NY

92 U.S. Department of Commerce (2005) *NIST/EPA/NIH Mass Spectral Library 2005*. John Wiley & Sons, New York, NY

93 Hoja H, Marquet P, Verneuil B, Lotfi H, Penicaut B, Lachatre G (1997) Applications of liquid chromatography–mass spectrometry in analytical toxicology: A review. *J Anal Toxicol* 21: 116–126

94 Maurer HH (1998) Liquid chromatography–mass spectrometry in forensic and clinical toxicolo-gy. *J Chromatogr B Biomed Sci Appl* 713: 3–25

95 Peters FT (2006) Method validation using LC-MS. In: A Polettini (ed.): *Applications of Liquid Chromatography–Mass Spectrometry in Toxicology*, Pharmaceutical Press, London, 71–95

96 Wood M, Laloup M, Samyn N, Mar Ramirez FM, De Bruijn EA, Maes RA, de Boeck G (2006) Recent applications of liquid chromatography–mass spectrometry in forensic science. *J Chromatogr A* 1130: 3–15

97 Politi L, Leone F, Morini L, Polettini A (2007) Bioanalytical procedures for determination of con-jugates or fatty acid esters of ethanol as markers of ethanol consumption: A review. *Anal Biochem* 368: 1–16

98 Beyer J, Peters FT, Kraemer T, Maurer HH (2007) Detection and validated quantification of toxic alkaloids in human blood plasma – Comparison of LC-APCI-MS with LC-ESI-MS/MS. *J Mass Spectrom* 42: 621–633

99 Mueller CA, Weinmann W, Dresen S, Schreiber A, Gergov M (2005) Development of a multi-tar-get screening analysis for 301 drugs using a QTrap liquid chromatography/tandem mass spec-trometry system and automated library searching. *Rapid Commun Mass Spectrom* 19: 1332–1338

100 Sauvage FL, Saint-Marcous F, Duretz B, Deporte D, Lachatre G, Marquet P (2006) Screening of drugs and toxic compounds with liquid chromatography–linear ion trap tandem mass spectro-metry. *Clin Chem* 52: 1735–1742

101 Gergov M, Boucher B, Ojanpera I, Vuori E (2001) Toxicological screening of urine for drugs by liquid chromatography/time-of-flight mass spectrometry with automated target library search based on elemental formulas. *Rapid Commun Mass Spectrom* 15: 521–526

102 Ojanpera I, Pelander A, Laks S, Gergov M, Vuori E, Witt M (2005) Application of accurate mass measurement to urine drug screening. *J Anal Toxicol* 29: 34–40

103 Ojanpera S, Pelander A, Pelzing M, Krebs I, Vuori E, Ojanpera I (2006) Isotopic pattern and accurate mass determination in urine drug screening by liquid chromatography/time-of-flight mass spectrometry. *Rapid Commun Mass Spectrom* 20: 1161–1167

104 Pfleger, K, Maurer, HH, Weber, A (1992) *Mass Spectral and GC Data of Drugs, Poisons, Pesticides, Pollutants and their Metabolites*. 2nd edn., Wiley-VCH, Weinheim, Germany

105 Nordgren HK, Beck O (2003) Direct screening of urine for MDMA and MDA by liquid chro-matography–tandem mass spectrometry. *J Anal Toxicol* 27: 15–19

106 Nordgren HK, Beck O (2004) Multicomponent screening for drugs of abuse: Direct analysis of urine by LC-MS-MS. *Ther Drug Monit* 26: 90–97

107 Nordgren HK, Holmgren P, Liljeberg P, Eriksson N, Beck O (2005) Application of direct urine LC-MS-MS analysis for screening of novel substances in drug abusers. *J Anal Toxicol* 29: 234–239

108 Gustavsson E, Andersson M, Stephanson N, Beck O (2007) Validation of direct injection elec-

trospray LC-MS/MS for confirmation of opiates in urine drug testing. *J Mass Spectrom* 42: 881–889

109 Andersson M, Gustavsson E, Stephanson N, Beck O (2008) Direct injection LC-MS/MS method for identification and quantification of amphetamine, methamphetamine, 3,4-methylene-dioxyamphetamine and 3,4-methylenedioxymethamphetamine in urine drug testing. *J Chromatogr B Analyt Technol Biomed Life Sci* 861: 22–28

110 Bjornstad K, Helander A, Beck O (2008) Development and clinical application of an LC-MS-MS method for mescaline in urine. *J Anal Toxicol* 32: 227–231

111 Stephanson N, Josefsson M, Kronstrand R, Beck O (2008) Accurate identification and quantification of 11-nor-Δ^9-tetrahydrocannabinol-9-carboxylic acid in urine drug testing: Evaluation of a direct high efficiency liquid chromatographic–mass spectrometric method. *J Chromatogr B Analyt Technol Biomed Life Sci* 871: 101–108

112 Bogusz MJ (1997) Large amounts of drugs may considerably influence the peak areas of their coinjected deuterated analogues measured with APCI-LC-MS. *J Anal Toxicol* 21: 246–247

113 Musshoff F, Madea B, Stuber F, Stamer UM (2006) Enantiomeric determination of tramadol and *O*-desmethyltramadol by liquid chromatography–mass spectrometry and application to postoperative patients receiving tramadol. *J Anal Toxicol* 30: 463–467

114 Stamer UM, Musshoff F, Kobilay M, Madea B, Hoeft A, Stuber F (2007) Concentrations of tramadol and *O*-desmethyltramadol enantiomers in different CYP2D6 genotypes. *Clin Pharmacol Ther* 82: 41–47

115 Peters FT, Dragan CA, Wilde DR, Meyer MR, Bureik M, Maurer HH (2007) Biotechnological synthesis of drug metabolites using human cytochrome P450 2D6 heterologously expressed in fission yeast exemplified for the designer drug metabolite 4'-hydroxymethyl-α-pyrrolidinobutyrophenone. *Biochem Pharmacol* 74: 511–520

116 Peters FT, Dragan CA, Kauffels A, Schwaninger AE, Zapp J, Bureik M, Maurer HH (2009) Biotechnological synthesis of the designer drug metabolite 4'-hydroxymethyl-α-pyrrolidinohexanophenone in fission yeast heterologously expressing human cytochrome P450 2D6 – A versatile alternative to multi-step chemical synthesis. *J Anal Toxicol* 33: 190–197

117 Peters FT, Dragan CA, Schwaninger AE, Sauer C, Zapp, J., Bureik M, Maurer HH (2009) Use of fission yeast heterologously expressing human cytochrome P450 2B6 in biotechnological synthesis of the designer drug metabolite 2-[(1-phenylcyclohexyl)amino]ethanol. *Forensic Sci Int* 184: 69–73

118 Beyer J, Drummer OH, Maurer HH (2009) Analysis of toxic alkaloids in body samples. *Forensic Sci Int* 185: 1–9

119 Peters FT, Schaefer S, Staack RF, Kraemer T, Maurer HH (2003) Screening for and validated quantification of amphetamines and of amphetamine- and piperazine-derived designer drugs in human blood plasma by gas chromatography/mass spectrometry. *J Mass Spectrom* 38: 659–676

120 Sauvage FL, Gaulier JM, Lachatre G, Marquet P (2006) A fully automated turbulent-flow liquid chromatography–tandem mass spectrometry technique for monitoring antidepressants in human serum. *Ther Drug Monit* 28: 123–130

121 Beyer J, Peters FT, Kraemer T, Maurer HH (2007) Detection and validated quantification of herbal phenalkylamines and methcathinone in human blood plasma by LC/MS/MS. *J Mass Spectrom* 42: 150–160

122 Kratzsch C, Weber AA, Peters FT, Kraemer T, Maurer HH (2003) Screening, library-assisted identification and validated quantification of fifteen neuroleptics and three of their metabolites in plasma by liquid chromatography/mass spectrometry with atmospheric pressure chemical ionization. *J Mass Spectrom* 38: 283–295

123 Kratzsch C, Tenberken O, Peters FT, Weber AA, Kraemer T, Maurer HH (2004) Screening, library-assisted identification and validated quantification of 23 benzodiazepines, flumazenil, zaleplone, zolpidem and zopiclone in plasma by liquid chromatography/mass spectrometry with atmospheric pressure chemical ionization. *J Mass Spectrom* 39: 856–872

124 Maurer HH, Kratzsch C, Kraemer T, Peters FT, Weber AA (2002) Screening, library-assisted identification and validated quantification of oral antidiabetics of the sulfonylurea-type in plasma by atmospheric pressure chemical ionization liquid chromatography–mass spectrometry (APCI-LC-MS). *J Chromatogr B Analyt Technol Biomed Life Sci* 773: 63–73

125 Maurer HH, Tenberken O, Kratzsch C, Weber AA, Peters FT (2004) Screening for, library-assisted identification and fully validated quantification of twenty-two β-blockers in blood plasma by liquid chromatography–mass spectrometry with atmospheric pressure chemical ionization. *J*

Chromatogr A 1058: 169–181

126 Laloup M, Ramirez Fernandez MM, de Boeck G, Wood M, Maes V, Samyn N (2005) Validation of a liquid chromatography–tandem mass spectrometry method for the simultaneous determination of 26 benzodiazepines and metabolites, zolpidem and zopiclone, in blood, urine, and hair. *J Anal Toxicol* 29: 616–626

127 Musshoff F, Trafkowski J, Kuepper U, Madea B (2006) An automated and fully validated LC-MS/MS procedure for the simultaneous determination of 11 opioids used in palliative care, with 5 of their metabolites. *J Mass Spectrom* 41: 633–640

128 Kristoffersen L, Oiestad EL, Opdal MS, Krogh M, Lundanes E, Christophersen AS (2007) Simultaneous determination of 6 β-blockers, 3 calcium-channel antagonists, 4 angiotensin-II antagonists and 1 antiarrhytmic drug in post-mortem whole blood by automated solid phase extraction and liquid chromatography mass spectrometry method development and robustness testing by experimental design. *J Chromatogr B Analyt Technol Biomed Life Sci* 850: 147–160

129 Halcomb SE, Sivilotti ML, Goklaney A, Mullins ME (2005) Pharmacokinetic effects of diphenhydramine or oxycodone in simulated acetaminophen overdose. *Acad Emerg Med* 12: 169–172

130 Ginsburg BY, Leybell I, Hoffman RS (2005) Comment on "Effect of anticholinergic drugs on the efficacy of activated charcoal". *Clin Toxicol* 43: 313

131 Green R, Sitar DS, Tenenbein M (2004) Effect of anticholinergic drugs on the efficacy of activated charcoal. *J Toxicol Clin Toxicol* 42: 267–272

132 Eddleston M, Eyer P, Worek F, Mohamed F, Senarathna L, von Meyer L, Juszczak E, Hittarage A, Azhar S, Dissanayake W, Sheriff MH, Szinicz L, Dawson AH, Buckley NA (2005) Differences between organophosphorus insecticides in human self-poisoning: A prospective cohort study. *Lancet* 366: 1452–1459

133 Evans WE, McLeod HL (2003) Pharmacogenomics-drug disposition, drug targets, and side effects. *N Engl J Med* 348: 538–549

Molecular, Clinical and Environmental Toxicology. Volume 2: Clinical Toxicology
Edited by A. Luch
© 2010 Birkhäuser Verlag/Switzerland

Household chemicals: management of intoxication and antidotes

Christine Rauber-Lüthy and Hugo Kupferschmidt

Swiss Toxicological Information Centre, Zürich, Switzerland

Abstract. Exposure to household products is very common, but in industrialized countries severe or fatal poisoning with household products is rare today, due to the legal restriction of sale of hazardous household products. The big challenge for physicians, pharmacologists and toxicologists is to identify the few exceptional life-threatening situations where immediate intervention is needed. Among thousands of innocuous products available for the household only very few are hazardous. Substances found in these products include detergents, corrosives, alcohols, hydrocarbons, and some of the essential oils. The ingestion of batteries and magnets and the exposure to cyanoacrylates (super glue) can cause complications in exceptional situations. Among the most dangerous substances still present in household products are ethylene glycol and methanol. These substances cause major toxicity only through their metabolites. Therefore, initial symptoms may be only mild or absent. Treatment even in asymptomatic patients has to be initiated as early as possible to inhibit production of toxic metabolites. For all substances not only the compound itself but also the route of exposure is relevant for toxicity. Oral ingestion and inhalation generally lead to most pronounced symptoms, while dermal exposure is often limited to mild irritation. However, certain circumstances need special attention. Exposure to hydrofluoric acid may lead to fatal hypocalcemia, depending on the concentration, duration of exposure, and area of the affected skin. Accidents with hydrocarbon pressure injectors and spray guns are very serious events, which may lead to amputation of affected limbs. Button batteries normally pass the gastrointestinal tract without problems even in toddlers; in rare cases, however, they get lodged in the esophagus with the risk of localized tissue damage and esophageal perforation.

Introduction

Exposure to household products is very common. Of all exposures reported to poisons centers, in Switzerland 25.7% [1] and in the USA 8.7% [2] are related to household chemicals. In industrialized countries severe or fatal poisoning with household products is rare today due to the legal restriction of the sale of hazardous household products, safety packaging and prevention efforts. The big challenge is therefore to identify the few exceptional life-threatening situations where immediate intervention is needed.

Detergents

Detergents are widely used in the household. Three types exist: non-ionic, anionic, and cationic detergents. While anionic and non-ionic detergents enable the cleaning solution to wet the surface and hold soil in suspension so that dirt can be removed and rinsed away, cationic detergents are particularly used for their disinfectant properties.

Anionic and non-ionic detergents

Toxic principle

Detergents have a slightly irritant effect on mucous membranes and the eyes. Furthermore, the foam produced in the stomach can lead to vomiting and tracheobronchial aspiration. The incidence of exposure to detergents is very high, especially in children. The Swiss Toxicological Information Centre (STIC) has recorded 11 225 cases within 10 years (1999–2008) with only one single fatal outcome. The annual report 2007 of the American Association of Poison Control Centers (AAPCC) describes three cases where anionic/non-ionic detergents were undoubtedly or probably responsible for death, among altogether 51 928 cases with anionic/non-ionic detergent exposures [2].

Substances (examples) include: ammonium lauryl sulfate, perfluorooctanesulfonate, octyl glucoside, cetyl alcohol, and alkyl polyethylene oxide.

Sources in the household

Soaps, shower gels, multi purpose cleaners, washing powder, and dishwashing liquids (but not electric dishwasher soaps) represent household examples.

Symptoms

The toxicity of household products containing anionic and non-ionic detergents is very low, and severe or fatal outcomes even after ingestion of bigger amounts are extremely rare. After ingestion, detergents have an irritant effect on mucous membranes, which eventually leads to abdominal pain, nausea, vomiting, and diarrhea. Complications including dehydration and electrolyte abnormalities are rare. After vomiting, aspiration of foam can result in chemical pneumonitis leading to respiratory failure and death in rare cases [3]. In case of ocular exposure, mild irritation is common but self-limiting.

Treatment

To limit foam production in the stomach, drinking of more than one mouthful of liquid should be avoided. Administration of dimethicon reduces foam production. Induced emesis for gastrointestinal decontamination is contraindicated, and activated charcoal of no use. In symptomatic patients treatment is supportive: intravenous fluids to correct dehydration, oxygen and artificial ventilation in case of respiratory failure due to pneumonitis. There is no indication for antibiotics unless signs of bacterial superinfection are present. In case of ocular exposure irrigation with water over 10–15 minutes is generally sufficient. If pain persists the patient should be seen by an ophthalmologist.

Cationic detergents

Toxic principle
Depending on the concentration, cationic detergents have an irritant or corrosive effect on eyes and mucous membranes. In household products their concentration is generally low. As most products containing cationic detergents also contain other toxicologically relevant substances (such as alcohols and other disinfectants), it is often difficult to distinguish between the effect of the former from the latter. Exposures to cationic detergents are considerably less frequent than those with anionic and non-ionic detergents. The AAPCC reports 6371 cases for 2007 [2].

Substances (examples) include: benzalkonium chloride, benzethonium chloride, cetyl trimethylammonium bromide, polyethoxylated tallow amine, diqualinum chloride, cetrimonium bromide, cetylpyridinum bromide, stearalkonium chloride, and alkyl dimethyl benzyl ammonium chloride.

Sources in the household
Sanitizers for bathrooms, toilets and swimming pools, disinfectants, and ingredients of washing powder (based on the bacteriostatic effect) represent household examples.

Symptoms
In low concentrations cationic detergents are mildly irritant. However, at higher concentrations (around >7.5%) or after ingestion of a greater amount in suicidal intention, cationic detergents may be corrosive on skin, eyes and mucous membranes. As little as two teaspoonfuls of a solution containing 10% benzalkonium chloride given to a newborn caused edematous epiglottis leading to respiratory insufficiency [4]. Ingestion can lead to gastrointestinal bleeding, perforation, and stricture formation. Airway compromise may occur due to edema of the epiglottis. Eye contact may cause corneal damage.

Treatment
Similar to that for irritants and caustic substances (see below).

Irritants and caustic substances

Toxic principle

Caustic substances include alkalis, acids, and oxidizing agents. They cause tissue destruction through liquefaction (alkalis), coagulation necrosis (acids), or through redox reactions and generation of free radicals. The extent of damage depends on the type, pH, concentration, duration of contact, titrable acid or alkaline reserve (TAR), the amount of the substance ingested, and the presence or absence of food in the stomach.

Examples of alkalis include: sodium hydroxide, calcium hydroxide, potassium hydroxide, ammonia, sodium metasilicate, sodium carbonate, sodium tripolyphosphate, and cement. Examples of acids include: acetic acid, hydrofluoric acid, hydrochloric acid, hydrobromic acid, sulfuric acid, nitric acid, phosphoric acid, chromic acid, lactic acid, citric acid, formic acid, oxalic acid, amidosulfonic acid, and zinc chloride. Other caustic substances include: sodium hypochlorite, hydrogen peroxide, formaldehyde, methylene chloride, phenol, potassium permanganate, and ethanolamine.

Sources in the household

Disinfectants, drain cleaners, decalcifiers, hair-bleachers, permanent wave neutralizers, oven cleaners, rust removers, toilet bowl cleaners, bleaches, automatic dishwasher soaps, automobile air bags (sodium azide), and battery liquid represent household examples.

Symptoms

Corrosive substances can lead to local effects, depending on the site of exposure (skin, eyes, respiratory or gastrointestinal tract), and systemic effects due to absorption of the agents.

Oral exposure

Ingestion of caustic substances may lead to mild irritation of the mucous membranes of the gastrointestinal tract with nausea, pharyngeal, retrosternal and abdominal pain, dysphagia, vomiting and diarrhea; in severe cases ulceration, bleeding and perforation may result (Tab. 1). The absence of oral cavity symptoms (reddening, pain, ulceration) is no warrant for a benign course. A study at the STIC showed absence of oral findings in 30% of cases with severe gastrointestinal burns [5]; however, completely asymptomatic patients are at very low risk for severe injury and complications. Only two cases were found in the literature of patients developing strictures after an uneventful initial course [6, 7]. In the case of acid ingestion, the oral cavity and the esophagus are the most common sites affected, and with alkaline ingestion the stomach shows the greatest damage. In severe cases, necrosis can extend to the small and large intestine, liver, spleen, and pancreas.

Edema of the epiglottis and perforation of the gastrointestinal wall are early complications after corrosive ingestion. Epiglottal edema necessitating intubation occurs within the first 6 hours. Although perforation can occur at this early stage, it is most frequent between days 7 and 21. Strictures are an intermediate-term complication. They generally develop within 3 weeks after ingestion and can persist for years. An elevated risk for esophageal cancer is a late com-

Table 1. Concentration of caustics and risk of injury after ingestion

Substance	Concentration with no caustic effect after accidental ingestion of a small amount
Acetic acid	<50%
Ammonium hydroxide	<3%
Formic acid	<10%
Hydrochloric acid	<10%
Hydrogen peroxide	<10%
Oxalic acid	<10%
Phosphoric acid	<60%
Potassium hydroxide	<1%
Sodium hypochlorite	<10%
Sodium metasilicate	<10%
Sulfuric acid	<10%
Sulfamic acid	<15%
Zinc chloride	<10%

plication that has been associated with severe caustic injury of the esophagus from lye [8] but also from acid [9] ingestion.

Eye exposure

Eye exposures cause conjunctival irritation, itching, pain and chemosis. In the case of exposure to strong caustics or prolonged contact with any corrosive substance conjunctival edema and corneal clouding may ensue with the risk of irreversible damage.

Dermal exposure

Dermal exposure causes symptoms similar to those seen with thermal burns. Depending on the substances and time of exposure pain, erythema, blistering and necrosis may occur. Systemic toxicity is also possible in cases of extensive dermal exposure to strong acids.

Inhalation

Inhalation of irritants or caustic substances may cause minor symptoms such as cough, stridor, dyspnea and pain. Major clinical manifestations include hypoxia, bronchospasm and acute lung injury (ALI) formerly called pulmonary edema. The most frequent inhalation hazard in the household is mixing a mild acid with sodium hypochlorite. The resulting formation of chlorine vapors may lead to strong irritation of the upper airways, but usually the symptoms resolve quickly as exposure is short. Irritative symptoms occurring within a short time after exposure are a sufficient warning signal to leave the danger zone. In contrast, poorly water soluble substances reach the lower respiratory tract and therefore carry a much higher risk of causing ALI, sometimes with a delayed appearance of symptoms.

Systemic effects

Systemic effects are due to either massive tissue breakdown or other toxic properties of absorbed corrosive substances. Metabolic acidosis and hemolysis with or without renal failure are common complications of ingestion or large cutaneous contamination with strong acids. Specific effects depend on the nature of the agent involved. Oral or large dermal exposures with hydrofluoric acid lead to profound hypocalcemia, hypomagnesemia and hyperkalemia with cardiac dysrhythmias and death. Phosphoric acid ingestion is associated with the risk of hyperphosphatemia and hypocalcemia. Permanganate or nitric acid ingestions may lead to methemoglobinemia. Ingestion of oxalic acid produces oxaluria with oxalate crystal formation and renal failure. Methylene chloride is metabolized to carbon monoxide and may cause central nervous system (CNS) depression and cardiac arrhythmias. Phenol can cause seizures, coma, and renal and liver injury.

Treatment

Oral exposure

The general outline is depicted in Figure 1. Dilution with 100–150 mL (toddler) or 200–300 mL (adult) water shortly after ingestion is recommended. In one study [10], milk and water had the same effect, but as water is more readily available there is no need for milk. In the case of hydrofluoric acid inges-

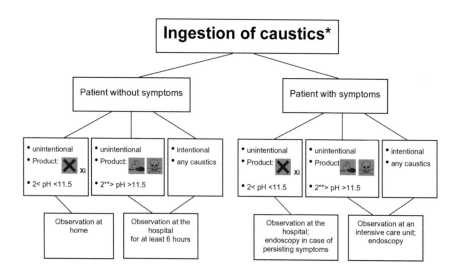

*Shortly after ingestion dilution with 1-1.5 dL (toddler) or 2-3 dL (adult) water
**Not applicable for all acids, e.g. sulfamic acid at concentrations of 15% has pH <2 but is only irritant

Figure 1. Algorithm for the management of caustic ingestion.

tion, first aid consists in fluid aspiration from the stomach with a nasogastric tube and instillation of 200 mL 5% calcium glubionate or calcium gluconate.

Since local tissue destruction is the main problem with ingestion of caustics, activated charcoal does not influence the outcome positively. Vomiting induced by activated charcoal may even worsen injury. Moreover, administration of charcoal complicates endoscopy by deteriorating visibility. If symptoms persist or if a corrosive substance has been ingested in high concentration or amount, early endoscopy is recommended to determine the extent of injury. As the risk of iatrogenic perforation increases with time, endoscopy should be performed within the first 24 hours after ingestion.

While the administration of corticosteroids is generally agreed if epiglottal edema starts to occur, the use of corticosteroids for prevention of stricture formation is controversial. All studies performed so far have limitations, either with respect to distinction of the degree of burns, or with respect to the distinction between acid and alkaline exposures. Nevertheless, most recent meta-analyses [11, 12] and our own data suggest that there is no benefit from using corticosteroids to prevent the development of strictures. Further management consists of early intubation or surgical cricothyroidotomy in the case of upper airway obstruction, emergency surgery in the case of perforation, placement of an esophageal stent depending on the degree of injury, and nutritional support, monitoring of pH, fluid and electrolyte status, methemoglobin level in the case of ingestion of permanganate, plasma phosphate concentration for phosphoric acid exposure, and urgent plasma calcium level in the case of hydrofluoric acid exposure. Note: As ingestion of hydrofluoric acid can be fatal within a few minutes after ingestion, calcium should be administrated upon clinical signs of hypocalemia even if the plasma calcium concentration is not yet available.

Eye exposure

The initial approach after eye exposures with caustics is immediate irrigation with copious amounts of water. Although the duration of irrigation depends on the substance, 10–20 minutes are generally sufficient. In the hospital setting the topical administration of local anesthetics can improve compliance and the effectiveness of irrigation. After exposure to hydrofluoric acid the application of calcium glubionate or gluconate drops (1%) in addition to irrigation with water could theoretically be beneficial, although no studies exist demonstrating a better outcome. Two studies show that amphoteric eyewash solutions could improve pH [13] and stop penetration [14], but comparative studies on the outcome of corneal damage are lacking.

Dermal exposure

Immediate removal of all wet clothing and irrigation of exposed skin with copious amounts of water is critical for external decontamination. The subsequent treatment is identical to the treatment of thermal burns. In the case of extensive cutaneous exposure to strong acids with systemic toxicity refer to oral exposures for treatment guidelines. Calcium gluconate gel 2.5–3.0% should be applied topically in cases of hydrofluoric acid exposure as early as possible. If pain persists, intradermal injection of a calcium gluconate (10%) or calcium glubionate (13%) solution is advised. If the wound is large or an extremity involved, intra-arterial application of calcium gluconate or glubionate (2%) should be considered. Calcium chloride is contraindicated due to its strong irritating effect.

Inhalation

Intubation and the administration of oxygen, bronchodilators, and steroids in case of airway obstruction should be performed based on clinical status. For ALI, corticosteroids were not beneficial compared to supportive care in a systematic Cochrane review [15]. Only in one small study, in which corticosteroids were given for late phase acute respiratory distress syndrome (ARDS) hospital mortality could be reduced, but no cases with inhalation poisoning were included [16]. Reviews such as [16] covered all causes for ALI and ARDS but not predominantly inhalation poisoning. As long as there is no clear evidence for the benefit of corticosteroids in inhalation poisoning, it cannot be recommended since the risk of adverse effects in the case of infection cannot be excluded.

Alcohols and glycols

While the toxicity of ethanol is primarily caused by the parent compound, other more toxic alcohols and glycols induce their toxicity mainly through metabolites.

Ethanol

Toxic principle

The toxicity of ethanol is primarily caused *via* γ-aminobutyric acid A (GABA$_A$) receptors, while *N*-methyl-D-aspartate (NMDA), serotonin (5-HT$_3$) and glycine are involved to a lesser intent. Ethanol is mainly metabolized by alcohol dehydrogenase (ADH), a liver enzyme that is also present in the gastric mucosa. The latter is responsible for oxidation of a small percentage of ethanol prior to systemic absorption. This pathway is responsible for the gender difference in alcohol toxicokinetics [17], leading to higher concentrations in females.

Sources in the household

Drinking alcohol, disinfectant, fuel, solvent in pharmaceuticals, personal care products (perfume, aftershave and mouthwash) and cleaning agents represent examples of such household toxins.

Symptoms

Minor to moderate signs of intoxication include inebriation, flush, confusion, ataxia, somnolence, hypoglycemia (especially in toddlers), nausea and vomiting. Severe signs of intoxication are coma, respiratory failure accompanied by hypothermia, metabolic acidosis, and electrolyte disturbances. Excessive exposures through the dermal (especially in toddlers) or respiratory route may produce similar symptoms, with irritation of the respiratory tract and the skin in the case of inhalation and dermal exposure, respectively.

Laboratory tests include: blood ethanol concentrations of 2–3‰ (g/L) in adults and 1.5–2‰ (g/L) in toddlers may produce severe poisoning; 5–6‰ (g/L) in adults and 3‰ (g/L) in toddlers are potentially fatal. If determination of plasma ethanol concentrations is not available, an approximation can be made using Widmark's equation [18] (Fig. 2). The osmolar gap is elevated but it is not routinely measured because blood ethanol concentrations are more accurate and available in most laboratories. Hypoglycemia may be present, sometimes accompanied by ketonuria.

$$\text{blood ethanol concentration [g/L]} = \frac{\text{amount of ethanol ingested [g]}}{\text{body weight [kg]} \times r}$$

$r = 0.55$ (for females), 0.68 (for males)

Figure 2. Estimation of blood ethanol concentration by Widmark's equation. r = Widmark's factor (0.55 for females, 0.68 for males) [18].

Treatment

In the majority of cases supportive care is sufficient. This includes dextrose, infusion, oxygen, intubation and ventilation if needed. In patients with a history of chronic ethanol abuse thiamine is indicated. Activated charcoal does not adsorb ethanol and therefore cannot be used for gastrointestinal decontamination. As ethanol is rapidly absorbed from the gut, gastric lavage is only indicated immediately after ingestion. Alternatively aspiration of the gastric fluid by a nasogastric tube can be performed, but there is no evidence for its benefit. Although hemodialysis is very efficient for enhanced extracorporeal elimination of ethanol, it is rarely used and indicated only in cases of severe intoxication with coma and respiratory failure.

Ethylene glycol

Toxic principle

Ethylene glycol (syn. 1,2-ethanediol, ethane-1,2-diol, glycol alcohol) is a colorless liquid of sweet taste with no warning or deterrent effect. While ethylene glycol itself produces only slight signs of intoxication similar to those of ethanol, its metabolites are responsible for toxicity. Ethylene glycol is metabolized to glycol aldehyde by ADH in a first step, and then rapidly to glycolic acid and further to different metabolites, but most importantly to glyoxylic acid and oxalic acid. Oxalic acid may convert to calcium oxalate and form oxalate crystals. Glyoxylic acid and oxalic acid are responsible for acidosis, and oxalate crystals for acute renal failure and the neurological manifestations including confusion, hallucinations, seizures, and coma.

There are large differences in the incidence of ethylene glycol poisoning in individual countries depending on its availability. In Switzerland, where ethylene glycol has been replaced with other alcohols in antifreeze, the STIC recorded only 207 cases in the last 10 years (1999–2008) with no fatal and only 6 severe outcomes. In the USA, contrarily, ethylene glycol was responsible for 33 fatalities among 5406 cases with ethylene glycol exposure in 2007 alone [2].

Sources in the household

Household sources include: antifreeze agents, brake fluids, inks and cleaning agents.

Symptoms

Ethylene glycol has low volatility and poorly penetrates the skin, making the oral route the only relevant one. One exceptional case has been described where inhalation of aerosolized ethylene glycol from a leaking automobile heater core resulted in a serum ethylene glycol concentration of 28 mg/100 mL [19]. After ingestion, first signs may be inebriation, euphoria, nausea and vomiting, as for ethanol ingestion, but these symptoms may be absent after ingestion of small amounts until the accumulation of toxic metabolites leads to specific symptoms and pathological laboratory findings. Metabolic acidosis and an elevated anionic gap is the hallmark of toxicity. Acidosis generally develops within a few hours but may be delayed up to 12 hours, especially in case of combined ingestion of ethylene glycol and ethanol. Severe intoxication includes coma, tachycardia, hypo- or hypertension, seizures, and hyperventilation. Hypoxia, ARDS, and multiple organ failure are poor prognostic signs. Oliguria, acute tubular necrosis and renal failure may develop 1–3 days after ingestion.

A pathognomonic sign for ethylene glycol poisoning is metabolic acidosis with an elevated anion gap (Fig. 3). In the early phase when ethylene glycol is not yet metabolized to anions the osmolar gap is elevated. With ongoing metabolism of ethylene glycol, the osmolar gap decreases, while the anion gap increases. Due to considerable individual variability a normal osmolar gap should never be used to exclude ethylene glycol poisoning. The detection of calcium oxalate crystals in the urine may be helpful in such cases. Plasma ethylene glycol concentrations are of great use for prognosis and for the decision to stop antidote treatment, but are nor easily available. A bedside test in use in veterinary medicine has been described to be a reliable qualitative test in cases of suspected human ethylene glycol poisoning [20]. The minimal ingested

$$Anion\ Gap = [Na^+] - ([Cl^-] + [HCO_3^-])$$

$$Osmolar\ Gap = 2\times[Na^+] + [glucose] + [BUN] + 1.25\times[ethanol]$$

Figure 3. Upper panel (anion gap): Calculation of the anion gap. All concentrations are in mmol/L. Because of electroneutrality net positive charges must equal net negative charges in the serum. The sum of all unmeasured charged particles corresponds to the anion gap. Normal values are in the range of 7 ± 4 mEq/L. It might be elevated due to an increased presence of unmeasured anions or a decreased presence of unmeasured cations. Lower panel (osmolar gap): Calculation of the osmolar gap. All concentrations are in mmol/L. The difference between the values for the measured osmolality and the calculated osmolarity is called the osmolar gap. Normal values are in the range of 2 ± 6 mOsm/L. Due to limitations in osmolar gap calculation and a large individual variability, small (or even negative) osmolar gaps never rule out toxic alcohol ingestion. In addition, common conditions such as alcoholic ketoacidosis, lactic acidosis, renal failure, and shock, are all associated with elevated osmolar gaps. The presence of very high osmolar gaps (>50–70 mOsm/L) is usually due to toxic alcohol ingestion. BUN, blood urea nitrogen.

dose or serum ethylene concentration leading to severe intoxication is not known, but there is consensus among experts that 20 mg/100 mL (3.2 mmol/L) should be the threshold for treatment. The minimal concentration that leads to severe intoxication has been estimated to be about twice this dose. Calculating back to ingested dose on the basis of the volume of distribution, a plasma ethylene glycol concentration of 20 mg/100 mL corresponds to an ingested dose of 0.11–0.18 mL/kg body weight. For comparison, the smallest ever reported dose leading to death was 60 mL evenly shared by two adults [21].

Treatment
For a general outline see Figure 4. Activated charcoal does not adsorb ethylene glycol and, therefore, has no role in gastrointestinal decontamination. In large ingestions, liquid gastric content can be removed with a nasogastric tube. The main goal of treatment is to reduce production of toxic metabolites as early as possible. Since ADH has a 67-fold higher affinity for ethanol compared to ethylene glycol, metabolism of ethylene glycol can be inhibited by administration of ethanol. Ethanol should be titrated to a plasma alcohol level of 1‰ (g/L). The recommended loading dose is 750–1000 mg/kg by i.v. drip, using 5–10% ethanol, followed by 66 and 154 mg/kg per hour in non-drinkers and drinkers, respectively. It is necessary to follow plasma ethanol levels closely. During hemodialysis ethanol administration has to be increased to 169 and 257 mg/kg per hour in non-drinkers and drinkers, respectively [22]. Whenever available, fomepizole (4-methylpyrazole) should be used to inhibit ADH. The advantages of using fomepizole over ethanol are that it can be administered twice a day in a fixed dosage regimen, it does not cause inebriation, and it has fewer side effects. The loading dose is 15 mg/kg, followed by

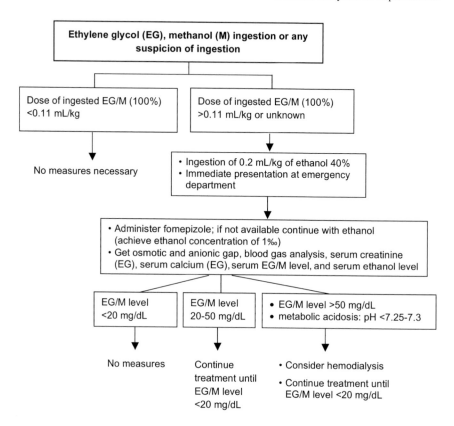

Figure 4. Algorithm for the management of ethylene glycol or methanol ingestion.

a maintenance dose of 10 mg/kg every 12 hours for four doses, then 15 mg/kg every 12 hours thereafter until ethylene glycol concentrations are undetectable or below 20 mg/100 mL, and the patient is asymptomatic with normal arterial pH. All doses should be administered as a slow intravenous infusion over 30 minutes. In individuals on hemodialysis, because fomepizole is dialyzable, its dose has to be increased according to the recommendations of the manufacturer, and the dosing interval must be reduced to every 4 hours.

Although ethylene glycol is dialyzable, hemodialysis is often not necessary if antidote therapy is started early, i.e., before metabolic acidosis appears. If the ethylene glycol concentration is >50 mg/100 mL, hemodialysis may be indicated to shorten the course. Hemodialysis is clearly indicated in cases of severe metabolic acidosis for a faster elimination of metabolites and to clear acidosis. It may also be indicated as a supportive measure in the case of renal failure. Supportive care further includes administration of pyridoxine (100 mg/day i.v.) and thiamine (100 mg/day i.v.) for facilitating metabolism of toxic metabolites.

Methanol

Toxic principle

Methanol (syn. hydroxymethane, methyl alcohol, methyl hydrate, wood alcohol, carbinol) itself may produce only minor signs of intoxication, similar to those occurring with ethanol. Severe toxicity is mainly due to its metabolites. Methanol is initially metabolized by ADH to formaldehyde and then rapidly by aldehyde dehydrogenase to formic acid. Formic acid is then further metabolized to carbon dioxide and water. Formic acid is responsible for metabolic acidosis, coma and, if untreated, for respiratory and circulatory arrest, and for blindness.

The incidence of exposure is very low. The STIC recorded 224 cases in the last 10 years (1999–2008), with only one fatal outcome, while AAPCC in their annual report of 2007 lists 16 deaths among 3638 cases with methanol exposure where methanol was undoubtedly or probably responsible [2].

Sources in the household

Paint solvent, fuel for model aircrafts, and inadequate distillation of drinking alcohol are household sources of methanol. Methanol has been banned in most countries as a denaturing agent for industrial ethanol.

Symptoms

Poisoning is possible by oral, dermal and inhalative exposures, but most intoxications are through the oral route. After inhalation of methanol vapors, plasma methanol concentrations are usually low. Three workers were exposed to methanol vapors while repairing a spillage of 300 L of methanol in an enclosed ill-ventilated room of 600 m^3 for 60 minutes. Blood was drawn about 3 hours after exposure. Despite this prolonged exposure, methanol blood levels were 3.0, 1.4 and 0.3 mg/100 mL and thus far below a dangerous level. All three patients had a normal blood gas analysis. Nevertheless, abuse of methanol vapors and extreme occupational settings may lead to severe intoxications [23, 24]. First signs include inebriation, euphoria, nausea und vomiting, similar to ethanol intoxication, but can be absent after ingestion of only small amounts until the accumulation of toxic metabolites (i.e., formic acid) leads to specific symptoms and pathological laboratory findings. Metabolic acidosis and an elevated anionic gap are the hallmarks of toxicity. Acidosis may be delayed up to 24 hours, especially in the case of combined ingestion of methanol and ethanol. Severe intoxication may include profound metabolic acidosis, coma and, when untreated, bradycardia, cardiovascular shock, respiratory and circulatory arrest, and (delayed) blindness due to the unique susceptibility of retinal pigmented epithelial cells and optic nerve cells.

A pathognomonic sign for methanol poisoning is metabolic acidosis with an elevated anion gap. For detailed information on the calculation refer to the section on ethylene glycol (Fig. 3). Serum methanol levels are of value for prognoses and concerning the decision for stopping specific treatment. The minimal ingested dose or serum methanol concentration leading to severe intoxication is not known, but there is consensus among experts that 20 mg/100 mL (6.3 mmol/L) should be the threshold for treatment. Calculating back to the ingested dose on the basis of the volume of distribution a plasma methanol concentration of 20 mg/100 mL corresponds to an ingested dose of 0.12–0.15 mL/kg body weight. The smallest ever mentioned dose leading to death in an adult is 15 mL of 40% methanol [25].

Treatment

For a general outline see Figure 4. Activated charcoal does not adsorb most alcohols and therefore has no role in gastrointestinal decontamination of methanol poisoning. Aspiration of gastric contents with a nasogastric tube after substantial ingestions can be considered within the first 30 minutes after ingestion, although there is no evidence supporting its benefit. The main goal of treatment is to reduce production of toxic metabolites as early as possible. Since ADH has a 15-fold higher affinity for ethanol compared to methanol, metabolism of methanol can be inhibited by administration of ethanol. If available, fomepizole should be used to inhibit ADH. For detailed information on dosing of ethanol or fomepizole refer to the section on ethylene glycol (see above).

Although methanol is dialyzable, hemodialysis is often not necessary if antidote therapy is started early, i.e., before metabolic acidosis appears. If the methanol concentration is >50 mg/100 mL, hemodialysis may be indicated to shorten the course. Hemodialysis is clearly indicated in cases of severe metabolic acidosis to eliminate metabolites faster and to clear acidosis. Supportive care further includes correction of acid-base disturbances, and the administration of folinic acid (if not available, use folic acid) to enhance formic acid metabolism. However, there is no evidence on the benefit of folinic acid in humans.

1-Propanol, 2-propanol

Toxic principle

The isomers 1-propanol (syn. propyl alcohol) and 2-propanol (syn. isopropyl alcohol, isopropanol) are often used in combination in household disinfectants. Since they are metabolized by ADH to different end products (propionic acid from 1-propanol, and acetone from 2-propanol), their toxic effects are also different: 1-propanol leads to metabolic acidosis, whereas 2-propanol leads to ketosis and ketonuria. The fact that AAPCC reports no fatal outcome among 13 271 isopropanol exposures in their 2007 annual report demonstrates the relative benignity of this substance [2]. The STIC recorded 698 cases in the last 10 years (1999–2008) with no fatalities and only two cases with severe symptoms after exposure to products containing 2-propanol as toxicologically the most important ingredient.

Sources in the household

Household sources include for 1-propanol: disinfectant, and cleaning agents; and for 2-propanol: rubbing alcohol, disinfectant, skin lotion, aftershave, cleaning agents, and antifreeze agents.

Symptoms

The capacity to penetrate skin decreases with chain length in higher alcohols, and they are less likely to be inhaled. Yet systemic intoxications with excessive cutaneous use of rubbing alcohol (2-propanol) have been described [26]. Both propanol isomers may lead to somnolence, ataxia, nausea, vomiting, diarrhea, and hypo- or hyperglycemia, and in severe cases to hemorrhagic gastritis, coma, hypotension and respiratory depression. Laboratory findings are characteristic for an elevated osmolar gap. In addition, 1-propanol leads to an elevated anion gap and metabolic acidosis, while 2-propanol causes ketosis and ketonuria, and, in severe cases, rarely lactic acidosis.

Information on toxic doses is limited. For pure 1-propanol no data on minimal toxic dose exist. The oral LD_{50} for rats is 1870 mg/kg. Case reports on poisoning with 1-propanol are all related to exposures with combined products, mostly with 2-propanol. For 2-propanol, as little as 20 mL may cause symptoms, but as much as 150–240 mL is estimated to be lethal for adults [27].

Treatment

Activated charcoal does not bind most alcohols and therefore has no role in gastrointestinal decontamination of 1- or 2-propanol poisoning. Aspiration of gastric contents with a nasogastric tube after substantial ingestions can be considered in the first 30 minutes after ingestion, although there is no evidence supporting this measure. First symptoms after ingestion of 1- or 2-propanol occur within 20–60 minutes. In most cases the course is favorable with supportive care only. In severely poisoned patients with coma and hypotension hemodialysis should be considered [27]. However, the necessity of this measure is still discussed controversially in the literature and some authors reject the indication for hemodialysis [28].

Since 2-propanol is metabolized to acetone, relevant 2-propanol intoxication can be excluded if ketone bodies are absent in the urine 3 hours after ingestion [29]. This rule cannot be used in case of coingestion with other alcohols, particularly ethanol, because of delayed metabolism due to ADH inhibition. In such cases ketonuria may appear as late as 12 hours after ingestion [30].

Hydrocarbons

Toxic principle

From a toxicological point of view, there are three basic types of hydrocarbons, all of which are also used in the household: aliphatic, aromatic and halogenated hydrocarbons. Both aliphatic and aromatic hydrocarbons are composed of only carbon and hydrogen atoms. Aromatic hydrocarbons consist of at least one aromatic ring (i.e., benzene), while aliphatic compounds do not contain aromatic rings. Many are straight chains, but cyclic (such as cyclohexane) and branched species exist. In addition to their carbon and hydrogen moiety, halogenated hydrocarbons contain halogen atoms (in household products mostly fluorine or chlorine). All types of hydrocarbons are absorbed by the oral, dermal and inhalative route. The ability to be absorbed depends on the structure and on molecular weight. Aliphatic hydrocarbons with 14 carbon atoms have an intestinal absorption rate of about 60%. Shorter hydrocarbons are absorbed better; no absorption was observed for hydrocarbons with more than 30 carbons [31]. Most hydrocarbons lead to irritation of mucous membranes. Short contact to skin may lead to defatting, prolonged contact to irritation and dermal burns. Most hydrocarbons commonly used in households are only partly absorbed from the gastrointestinal tract and thus do not cause systemic toxicity unless large amounts are ingested, as in suicidal attempts.

Systemic toxicity includes euphoria, CNS depression and cardiac arrhythmias. Additionally some of the halogenated hydrocarbons display specific organ toxicities. Chlorinated hydrocarbons are in particular nephro- and hepatotoxic. Carbon tetrachloride causes liver injury *via* radical formation. Trichloroethylene can induce dose-independent hepatitis, possibly immune-mediated, as well as dose-dependent toxic liver injury. Methylene chloride is metabolized to carbon monoxide, which mediates some of its toxicity. Freons (chlorofluorocarbons) as well as butane and propane are rather non-toxic volatile compounds, but may lead to asphyctic effects in case of prolonged exposure in enclosed, ill-ventilated rooms. After inhalation, systemic toxicity can occur because hydrocarbons are easily absorbed through the respiratory tract. Significant exposures occur at the workplace in the case of prolonged use of products containing solvents in insufficiently ventilated areas, and in the case of substance abuse (sniffing, huffing, and bagging).

The most feared complication after ingestion of highly volatile hydrocarbons with low viscosity is aspiration and chemical pneumonitis. Products with a viscosity of $<7 \times 10^{-6}$ m^2/s or <60 Saybolt Seconds Universal (SSU) are associated with a high aspiration potential. The mechanism of lung injury is not completely clear. Based on animal studies with intratracheal instillation of hydrocarbons the mechanism is only partly understood. Pathologically, a generalized hyperemia and focal bronchopneumonia, and physiologically, a significant decrease in thoracic gas volume, total lung capacity and compliance have been described [32, 33].

Examples include: substances with low viscosity, e.g., gasoline, kerosene, naphtha, xylene and toluene; substances with high viscosity, e.g., lubricating oil and mineral oil. Halogenated hydrocarbons include: carbon tetrachloride, trichloroethylene, tetrachloroethylene, methylene chloride, and freon.

Sources in the household

Household sources of aliphatic and aromatic hydrocarbons include: lamp oil, lighter fluid, thinner, brush cleaner, fuel, lubricants, furniture polisher, fuel paste, ignition means, fire eating fluid, degreasers, solvents in paints, pesticides, petrol, glue, shoe shiner and many other household products. Examples of household halogenated hydrocarbons include: solvents (trichloroethylene, methylene chloride), drycleaning (tetrachloroethylene), paint stripper (methylene chloride), degreaser (methylene chloride), and cooling agent in air conditioning and refrigeration (freons).

Symptoms

Oral exposure
Ingestion leads to nausea, vomiting, diarrhea, and abdominal pain. After ingestion of large amounts of short chain hydrocarbons, as in suicidal attempts, systemic toxicity (see inhalation exposure below) is possible. The major hazard after ingestion of hydrocarbons with low viscosity is pneumonitis. Already very small doses bear the risk of aspiration, which occurs while swallowing the liquid, but also in the case of vomiting. Fire eating or aspirating gasoline with a small tube from a tank represents a particular risk. In most instances aspiration only leads to transient coughing, gagging, choking or dyspnea. Clinical findings may furthermore include bronchospasm, rales, rhonchi, tachypnea, cyanosis, leukocytosis and fever. In severe cases, hemoptysis, ALI, ARDS, pneumatoceles [34, 35], lipoid pneumonia, or respiratory arrest may develop. Pulmonary toxicity is not only due to hydrocarbon aspiration but can also be the consequences of intravenous injection of hydrocarbons [36, 37]. Radiographic findings after aspiration can be seen 30 minutes after aspiration and are present in 98% of patients 12 hours after exposure [38, 39]. The most frequent signs visible on chest radiographs are bilateral alveolar opacities of the middle and lower lobes, other finding are pleural effusion, pneumatoceles, pneumothorax, and pneumomediastinum, but these are rare. Computed tomography of hydrocarbon pneumonia shows patchy opacities [35]. At the time when symptoms of aspiration appear, the subsequent course of intoxication is not predictable. Decisions about management have to be based on clinical status. In symptomatic patients symptoms generally progress over 24–48 hours and then resolve within 3–5 days.

Eye exposure
Eye exposure causes mild transient irritation. Damage of the cornea has been described in cases of exposure to combined products with hydrocarbons and other substances [40].

Dermal exposure

Dermal exposure may lead to severe cutaneous burns. The STIC recorded a case of a toddler who splashed a greater quantity of lamp oil over his clothes. The mother changed pants and T-shirt but left the diaper. Several hours later the child began to cry and on arriving at the hospital, severe burns with blistering under the diaper were present.

Special situations are injuries resulting from the use of high pressure injectors and spray guns with products that contain hydrocarbons. These are rare but serious events, which may lead to amputation [41].

Inhalation

Inhalation exposure may lead to mild symptoms like headache, nausea, obtundation, lethargy or euphoria; in severe cases followed by coma. Cardiac arrhythmia can be fatal. Seizures are rare and most probably due to hypoxia. Halogenated hydrocarbons such as trichloroethylene and tetrachloroethylene may lead to renal and hepatic damage, but also to cranial and peripheral neuropathies, and fatal abdominal compartment syndrome as reported in a single case [42].

Treatment

Charcoal does not effectively adsorb hydrocarbons. Gastric lavage for gastrointestinal decontamination is not indicated for accidental ingestion, because toxicity is relatively low and the major goal is to prevent any measures that increase the risk of aspiration. If large amounts of hydrocarbons have been ingested capable of causing systemic toxicity, gastric lavage under airway protection has to be considered. Anas and co-workers proposed gastrointestinal decontamination after ingestion of more than 1 mL/kg [43].

Patients who are asymptomatic or who have only minor gastrointestinal symptoms after accidental ingestion may be managed at home. Patients who have ingested hydrocarbons in a suicidal attempt and all patients with coughing, gagging, choking or dyspnea must have a medical follow-up. Treatment after ingestion and inhalation is mainly symptomatic and includes bronchodilators, oxygenation, intubation, ventilation (with positive end-expiratory pressure, PEEP). Ventricular fibrillation due to hydrocarbon-induced sensitization of the myocardium is of special concern. Catecholamines should be avoided for treatment. Some authors suggest the use of amiodarone, lidocaine or β-adrenergic antagonists [44, 45].

Antibiotics are not indicated in cases of chemical pneumonitis or for prophylaxis. Secondary bacterial infection following kerosene-induced pneumonitis is rare [46]. Artificial surfactant has been successfully used for treatment of hydrocarbon aspiration in a sheep model [47] but studies in humans are not available. For dermal exposure, removal of the involved clothing and washing the skin with soap and water is sufficient. In the case of high pressure injury, immobilization, tetanus and antimicrobial prophylaxis, analgesia, and minimizing the time to definitive surgical treatment is important [48].

Essential oils

Toxic principle

While most of the essential oils have only minor to moderate toxicity with irritant effects on skin and mucous membranes, a small number can cause systemic toxicity. CNS depression and seizures are the most common symptoms. In particular, oil of wintergreen causes salicylate poisoning due to its content of methyl salicylate, with nausea, vomiting, tinnitus, hyperpnoea, alkalosis, later acidosis, coma and seizures. Little is known about the dose of essential oils and the mechanisms that cause systemic toxicity. An exception is thujone, which is quite well studied, most likely related to the debate about the toxicity of absinthe (a liquor made from wormwood *Artemisia absinthum*). The isomer α-thujone seems to act as a $GABA_A$ receptor chloride channel blocker [49].

Examples of these oils include: those with low toxicity, e.g., essential oils from orange, lemon, chamomile, citronella, myrtle, cypress, and dill; and those with high toxicity, e.g., camphor, thujone, eucalyptus, and oil of wintergreen.

Sources in the household

Air fresheners, liniments, rubefacients, cold preparations, vaporizer solutions and insecticides represent household sources.

Symptoms

Oral exposure

Oral exposure may lead to gastrointestinal irritation with epigastric and abdominal pain, nausea, vomiting, and diarrhea. Vertigo, ataxia, drowsiness are quite frequent neurological findings. Seizures, significant CNS depression, and coma are described after eucalyptus, thujone, camphor, lavender and menthol ingestions [50–54]. Complications described in the medical literature include rhabdomyolysis and renal failure due to seizures and, in rare cases, aspiration pneumonitis probably promoted by emesis and gastric lavage [55]. The minimal toxic dose for essential oils is not known. For eucalyptus the lowest reported dose that led to coma is 5 mL [51]. Manoguerra and co-workers recommend that patients who have ingested more than 30 mg/kg of a camphor-containing products or who are exhibiting symptoms of moderate to severe toxicity should be referred to an emergency department for observation and treatment [56]. For essential oils with low toxicity there are no case reports of severe course. Thus, patients with accidental ingestion have to be referred to the hospital only in case of persistent symptoms.

Eye exposure

Eye exposures cause conjunctivitis with erythema and severe pain.

Dermal exposure

Short skin contact may lead to defatting; with longer contact irritation and dermal burns may occur.

Treatment

Emesis and gastric lavage for gastrointestinal decontamination should be avoided to minimize risk of aspiration. Activated charcoal could be considered in case of large ingestions. However, for camphor, which is one of the potentially dangerous essential oils based on an animal studies [57], and in light of missing human evidence in support of, or against, the use of activated charcoal, latest evidence-based practice guidelines suggest that activated charcoal should not be administered unless there are other ingredients in the product that can be effectively adsorbed [56]. For seizure control i.v. benzodiazepines (diazepam, midazolam or lorazepam) are the treatment of choice.

In the case of ocular exposure irrigation with water for 10–15 minutes is generally sufficient. If pain, redness or other discomfort persists, an ophthalmological examination is recommended. After dermal exposure immediate removal of all wet clothing and irrigation of exposed skin with copious amounts of water is sufficient.

Cyanoacrylates

Toxic principle

Cyanoacrylates are widely used as super glue. The acrylate monomer polymerizes within seconds to produce adhesion and heat. Adhesion generally occurs only on skin, hair and eyes, and not on mucous membranes. The non-polymerized form is mildly irritant, and production of heat may contribute to minimal skin irritation.

Examples are ethyl-2-cyanoacrylates and methyl-2-cyanoacrylates.

Sources in the household

Glue is the major household source.

Symptoms

Oral exposure

Oral exposure does not pose a great risk. Due to rapid polymerization in the mouth adhesion to mucosa (wet surface) is limited. However, an exceptional course with tracheal and bronchial obstruction after ingestion and aspiration of cyanoacrylate in a toddler has been described in the literature [58].

Eye exposure

Eye exposure may cause conjunctivitis in some cases. Corneal abrasions resolve within a few days.

Dermal exposure

Dermal exposures usually do not cause symptoms. In rare cases mild irritation is possible. More severe cutaneous lesions may be seen due to mechanical manipulation in order to remove the glue or due to pulling body parts apart (e.g., two fingers stuck together).

Note: Pressure necroses may occur if the polymerized glue is trapped in narrow body cavities. The STIC has recorded a case of a mother who applied cyanoacrylate-containing glue to her child instead of ear drops; within hours the child developed pressure necroses in the ear that necessitated surgical treatment.

Treatment

Dermal, mucosal and ocular exposure is preferably managed without mechanical manipulation. The use of swabs soaked in normal saline helps to remove the glue [59], but it also comes off spontaneously within 1–4 days. In exceptional cases where removal is essential or highly desirable, acetone could be used. However, as acetone itself has an irritating effect, administration must be short and washing with soap and water after removal is essential.

Batteries

Toxic principle

There are a lot of types of batteries. They can be distinguished by their ability to be rechargeable, by their size (button batteries, PP3, AAA, AA, C and D batteries) and by their use (car batteries). The toxic ingredients are always acids (sulfuric acid, ammonium chloride, zinc chloride) or alkalis (potassium or sodium hydroxide) and metals (nickel, cadmium, lithium, manganese, and – in older batteries – mercury and lead). The caustics may cause dermal burns, most often during handling of car batteries that generally contain sulfuric acid.

Dermal or mucosal burns are also seen with leaking batteries. Mucosal burns of the tongue or the oral mucosa develop when toddlers put them into their mouth. Heavy metals are minor in terms of acute effects. The amounts leaking from a battery are usually small and rarely cause significant elevation of blood metal levels. A single case with elevated blood mercury levels and the need of chelating therapy after battery ingestion has been described in the literature [60]. Contrarily, intoxications with heavy metals may occur in industrial workers from chronic exposures in battery manufactories.

Besides chemical-inherent acute toxic effects, there are other mechanisms involved in tissue damage after ingestion of batteries. *In situ* formation of caustic substances due to external electrical current [61] and pressure necrosis may play a role. An allergic enterocolitis caused by manganese leak from a disk battery has been described in a single case [62].

The incidence of exposures to batteries is very high, particularly in children. The STIC recorded 2065 cases in the last 10 years (1999–2008). In 766 cases a button battery was involved. Two cases with severe outcome were registered. One person suffered from dermal ulceration, and one developed a hand lesion after battery explosion, eventually leading to the amputation of an endphalangx. In the AAPCC annual report for 2007, 476 button battery exposures were reported among 6779 battery exposures in total, with no fatal outcome [2].

Symptoms

Cutaneous exposure may lead to dermal burns similar to those described in the section on irritants and caustic substances (see above). Small batteries, especially button batteries, normally pass the gastrointestinal tract without problems. In rare cases they get lodged in the esophagus, giving rise to immediate symptoms. Patients complain of discomfort, retrosternal pain and dysphagia, and may vomit or choke. If this occurs a chest radiograph followed by an emergent endoscopic removal is required. Localized tissue damage with the risk of esophageal perforation, tracheoesophageal fistula and stricture formation are possible complications. In rare cases, death may result [63, 64].

Management

Some authors propose an initial radiograph for localization of the battery in all cases of battery ingestion. Based on experience and consideration of case reports on button batteries lodged in the esophagus (in all cases initial symptoms were present, sometimes only discrete) the STIC proposes stool examination as the only measure if the patient remains completely asymptomatic. In most cases the battery passes the gastrointestinal tract without problems. Radiological location and surgical intervention is only necessary if the battery does not pass the body within a few days after ingestion. There are no case reports in the literature nor does the STIC have any own documented cases of batteries causing relevant mucosal damage in asymptomatic patients when remained in the gut for a few days. Batteries trapped in the nose or the ear are rare events. They must be removed urgently due to the risk of pressure necrosis.

Magnets

Ingested magnets pose no toxicological problem but lead to an increasing number of inquiries at poison centers. Ingestion of single magnet represents a foreign body which rarely causes any symptoms and that will leave the gastrointestinal tract within some days. There are only two occasions when swallowed magnets lead to a medical emergency. When a magnet gets lodged in the esophagus it may produce pressure necrosis if not removed within short time. If more than one magnet is ingested, they can get mutually attracted across loops of the intestine, thus causing necrosis and perforation [65].

Asymptomatic patients who have ingested one magnet can stay at home. Symptomatic patients or patients with more than one magnet ingested, or after ingestion of a magnet and other metallic subjects, should be subjected to medical examination with radiographic localization of foreign bodies. If trapping or lodging is suspected, urgent surgical removal is advocated.

References

1 STIC (2008) Swiss Toxicological Information Centre. Annual Report 2008. Available at: http://www.toxi.ch (accessed August 14, 2009)
2 Bronstein AC, Spyker DA, Cantilena LR, Green JL, Rumack BH, Heard SE (2008) 2007 Annual Report of the American Association of Poison Control Centers' National Poison Data System (NPDS): 25th Annual Report. Clin Toxicol 46: 927–1057
3 Schaper A, Renneberg B, Desel H, Langer C (2006) Intoxication-related fatalities in Northern Germany. Eur J Intern Med 17: 474–8
4 Okan F, Coban A, Ince Z, Can G (2007) A rare and preventable cause of respiratory insufficiency: Ingestion of benzalkonium chloride. Pediatr Emerg Care 23: 404–406
5 Rauber-Lüthy C (1997) Schwere und tödliche Säure- und Laugenverätzungen: Eine retrospektive Fallanalyse aus dem Schweizerischen Toxikologischen Informationszentrum (STIZ). University of Zürich 1997, MD thesis (in German), available at: http://www.toxi.ch (accessed August 14, 2009)
6 Gaudreault P, Parent M, McGuigan, Chicoine L, Lovejoy FH Jr (1983) Predictability of esophageal injury from signs and symptoms: A study of caustic ingestion in 378 children. Pediatrics 71: 767–770
7 Stiff G, Rees BI, Alwafi A, Lari J (1996) Corrosive injuries of the oesophagus and stomach: Experience in management at a regional paediatric centre. Ann R Coll Surg Engl 78: 119–123
8 Appelqvist P, Salmo M (1980) Lye corrosion carcinoma of the esophagus: A review of 63 cases. Cancer 45: 2655–2658
9 Kochhar R, Sethy PK, Kochhar S, Nagi B, Gupta NM (2006) Corrosive induced carcinoma of oesophagus: Report of three patients and review of literature. J Gastroenterol Hepatol 21: 777–780
10 Homan CS, Maitra SR, Lane BP, Thode HC, Sable M (1994) Therapeutic effects of water and milk

for acute alkali injury of the esophagus. *Ann Emerg Med* 24: 14–20

11 Pelclová D, Navrátil T (2005) Do corticosteroids prevent oesophageal stricture after corrosive ingestion? *Toxicol Rev* 24: 125–129

12 Fulton JA, Hoffman RS (2007) Steroids in second degree caustic burns of the esophagus: A systematic pooled analysis of fifty years of human data: 1956–2006. *Clin Toxicol* 45: 402–408

13 Spöler F, Frentz M, Först M, Kurz H, Schrage NF (2008) Analysis of hydrofluoric acid penetration and decontamination of the eye by means of time-resolved optical coherence tomography. *Burns* 34: 549–555

14 Rihawi S, Frentz M, Schrage NF (2006) Emergency treatment of eye burns: Which rinsing solution should we choose? *Graefe's Arch Clin Exp Ophthalmol* 244: 845–854

15 Adhikari N, Burns KE, Meade MO (2004) Pharmacologic therapies for adults with acute lung injury and acute respiratory distress syndrome. *Cochrane Database Syst Rev* 18: CD004477.

16 Meduri GU, Headley AS, Golden E, Carson SJ, Umberger RA, Kelso T, Tolley EA (1998) Effect of prolonged methylprednisolone therapy in unresolving acute respiratory distres syndrome: A randomized controlled trial. *J Am Med Assoc* 280: 159–165

17 Baraona E, Abittan CS, Dohmen K (2001) Gender differences in pharmacokinetics of alcohol. *Alcohol Clin Exp Res* 25: 502–507

18 Andréasson R, Jones AW, Erik MP (1995) Widmark (1889–1945) Swedish pioneer in forensic alcohol toxicology. *Forensic Sci Int* 72: 1–14

19 Hodgman M, Wezorek C, Krenzelok E (1997) Toxic inhalation of ethylene glycol: A pharmacological improbability. *J Toxicol Clin Toxicol* 35: 109–111

20 Long H, Nelson LS, Hoffman RS (2008) A rapid qualitative test for suspected ethylene glycol poisoning. *Acad Emerg Med* 5: 688–690

21 Widman C (1946) A few cases of ethylene glycol intoxication. *Acta Med Scand* 126: 293–306

22 Barceloux DG, Krenzelok EP, Olson K, Watson W (1999) American Academy of Clinical Toxicology practice guidelines on the treatment of ethylene glycol poisoning. *J Toxicol Clin Toxicol* 37: 537–560

23 Aufderheide TP, White SM, Brady WJ, Stueven HA (1993) Inhalational and percutaneous methanol toxicity in two firefighters. *Ann Emerg Med* 22: 1916–1918

24 Frenia ML, Schauben JL (1993) Methanol inhalation toxicity. *Ann Emerg Med* 22: 1919–1923

25 Bennett IL, Cary FH, Mitchell GL, Cooper MN (1953) Acute methyl alcohol poisoning: A review based on experiences in an outbreak of 323 cases. *Medicine* 32: 431–463

26 Dyer S, Mycyk MB, Ahrens WR, Zell-Kanter M (2002) Hemorrhagic gastritis from topical isopropanol exposure. *Ann Pharmacother* 36: 1733–1735

27 Lacouture PG, Wason S, Abrams A, Lovejoy FH (1983) Acute isopropyl alcohol intoxication. Diagnosis and management. *Am J Med* 75: 680–686

28 Trullas JC, Aguilo S, Castro P, Nogue S (2004) Life-threatening isopropyl alcohol intoxication: Is hemodialysis really necessary? *Vet Hum Toxicol* 46: 282–284

29 Jerrard D, Verdile V, Yealy D, Krenzelok E, Menegazzi J (1992) Serum determinations in toxic isopropanol ingestion. *Am J Emerg Med* 10: 200–202

30 Vujasinovic M, Kocar M, Kramer K, Bunc M, Brvar M (2007) Poisoning with 1-propanol and 2-propanol. *Hum Exp Toxicol* 26: 975–978

31 Barrowman JA, Rahman A, Lindstrom MB, Borgstrom B (1989) Intestinal absorption and metabolism of hydrocarbons. *Prog Lipid Res* 28: 189–203

32 Scharf SM, Prinsloo I (1982) Pulmonary mechanics in dogs given different doses of kerosene intratracheally. *Am Rev Respir Dis* 126: 695–700

33 Scharf SM, Heimer D, Goldstein J (1981) Pathologic and physiologic effects of aspiration of hydrocarbons in the rat. *Am Rev Respir Dis* 124: 625–629

34 Kamijo Y, Soma K, Asari Y, Ohwada T (2000) Pulse steroid therapy in adult respiratory distress syndrome following petroleum naphtha ingestion. *J Toxicol Clin Toxicol* 38: 59–62

35 Facon Coumbaras J, Bigot E, Bahlouli F, Boissonnas A, Bellin MF (2005) Acute hydrocarbon pneumonia after white spirit aspiration: Sequential HRCT findings. *Eur Radiol* 15: 31–33

36 Domej W, Mitterhammer H, Stauber R, Kaufmann P, Smolle KH (2007) Successful outcome after intravenous gasoline injection. *J Med Toxicol* 3: 173–177

37 Neeld EM, Limacher MC (1978) Chemical pneumonitis after the intravenous injection of hydrocarbon. *Radiology* 129: 36

38 Victoria MS, Nangia BS (1987) Hydrocarbon poisoning: A review. *Pediatr Emerg Care* 3: 184–186

39 Truemper E, Reyes de la Rocha S, Atkinson SD (1987) Clinical characteristics, pathophysiology, and management of hydrocarbon ingestion: Case report and review of the literature. *Pediatr Emerg Care* 3: 187–193

40 Ansari EA (1997) Ocular injury with xylene – A report of two cases. *Hum Exp Toxicol* 16: 273–275

41 Pinto M, Turkula-Pinto L, Cooney W, Wood MB, Dobyns JH (1993) High-pressure injection injuries of the hand. Review of 25 patients managed by open wound technique. *J Hand Surg* 18: 125–130

42 Liotier J, Barbier M, Plantefeve G, Duale C, Deteix P, Souweine B, Coudoré F (2008) A rare cause of abdominal compartment syndrome: Acute trichloroethylene overdose. *Clin Toxicol* 46: 905–907

43 Anas N, Namasonthi V, Ginsburg CM (1981) Criteria for hospitalizing children who have ingested products containing hydrocarbons. *J Am Med Assoc* 246: 840–843

44 Edwards KE, Wenstone R (2000) Successful resuscitation from recurrent ventricular fibrillation secondary to butane inhalation. *Br J Anaesth* 84: 803–805

45 Mortiz F, de La Chapelle A, Bauer F (2000) Esmolol in the treatment of severe arrhythmia after acute trichloroethylene poisoning. *Intensive Care Med* 26: 256

46 Wolfsdorf J (1976) Experimental kerosene pneumonitis in primates: Relevance to the therapeutic management of childhood poisoning. *Clin Exp Pharmacol Physiol* 3: 539–544

47 Widner LR, Goodwin SR, Berman LS, Banner MJ, Freid EB, KcKee TW (1996) Artificial surfactant for therapy in hydrocarbon-induced lung injury in sheep. *Crit Care Med* 24: 1524–1529

48 Fialkov JA, Freiberg A. (1991) High pressure injection injuries: An overview. *J Emerg Med* 9: 367–371

49 Höld KM, Sirisoma NS, Ikeda T, Narahashi T, Casida JE (2000) α-Thujone (the active component of absinthe): γ-Aminobutyric acid type A receptor modulation and metabolic detoxification. *Proc Natl Acad Sci USA* 97: 3826–3831

50 Landelle C, Francony G, Sam-Laï NF, Gaillard Y, Vincent F, Wrobleski I, Danel V (2008) Poisoning by lavandin extract in a 18-month-old boy. *Clin Toxicol* 46: 279–281

51 Spoerke DG, Vandenberg SA, Smolinske SC, Kulig K, Rumack BH (1989) Eucalyptus oil: 14 cases of exposure. *Vet Hum Toxicol* 31: 166–168

52 Khine H, Weiss D, Graber N, Hoffman RS, Esteban-Cruciani N, Avner JR (2009) A cluster of children with seizures caused by camphor poisoning. *Pediatrics* 123: 1269–1272

53 Weisbord SD, Soule JB, Kimmel PL (1997) Poison on line – Acute renal failure caused by oil of wormwood purchased through the internet. *N Engl J Med* 337: 825–827

54 O'Mullane NM, Joyce P, Kamath SV, Tham MK, Knass D (1982) Adverse CNS effects of menthol-containing olbas oil. *Lancet* 1: 1121

55 Temple WA, Smith NA, Beasley M (1991) Management of oil of citronella poisoning. *J Toxicol Clin Toxicol* 29: 257–262

56 Manoguerra AS, Erdman AR, Wax PM (2006) Camphor poisoning: An evidence-based practice guideline for out-of-hospital management. *Clin Toxicol* 44: 357–370

57 Dean BS, Burdick JD, Geotz CM, Bricker JD, Krenzelok EP (1992) *In vivo* evaluation of the adsorptive capacity of activated charcoal for camphor. *Vet Hum Toxicol* 34: 297–300

58 Vitale C, George M, Sheroff A, Hernon C, Boyer E (2008) Tracheal and bronchial obstruction following cyanoacrylate aspiration in a toddler. *Clin Toxicol* 46: 560–562

59 Cousin GC (1990) Accidental application of cyanoacrylate to the mouth. *Br Dent J* 169: 293–294

60 Mant TG. Lewis JL, Mattoo TK, Rigden SP, Volans GN, House IM, Wakefield AJ, Coel RS (1987) Mercury poisoning after disc-battery ingestion. *Hum Toxicol* 6: 179–181

61 Yamashita M, Saito S, Koyama K (1987) Esophageal electrochemical burn by button-type alkaline batteries in dogs. *Vet Hum Toxicol* 29: 226–230

62 Altaf MA, Goday PS, Telega G (2008) Allergic enterocolitis and protein-losing enteropathy as the presentations of manganese leak from an ingested disk battery: A case report. *J Med Case Reports* 27: 286

63 Anand TS, Kumar S, Wadhwa V, Dhawan R (2002) Rare case of spontaneous closure of tracheoesophageal fistula secondary to disc battery ingestion. *Int J Ped Otorhinolaryngol* 63: 57–59

64 Shabino CL, Feinberg AN (1979) Esophageal perforation secondary to alkaline battery ingestion. *JACEP* 8: 360–362.

65 Dutta S, Barzin A (2008) Multiple magnet ingestion as a source of severe gastrointestinal complications requiring surgical intervention. *Arch Pediatr Adolesc Med* 162: 123–125

Molecular, Clinical and Environmental Toxicology. Volume 2: Clinical Toxicology
Edited by A. Luch

Heavy metal poisoning: management of intoxication and antidotes

Daniel E. Rusyniak[1], Anna Arroyo[1], Jennifer Acciani[1], Blake Froberg[2], Louise Kao[1] and Brent Furbee[1]

[1] *Department of Emergency Medicine, Indiana University School of Medicine, Indianapolis, USA*
[2] *Department of Pediatrics, Indiana University School of Medicine, Indianapolis, USA*

Abstract. Of the known elements, nearly 80% are either metals or metalloids. The highly reactive nature of most metals result in their forming complexes with other compounds such oxygen, sulfide and chloride. Although this reactivity is the primary means by which they are toxic, many metals, in trace amounts, are vital to normal physiological processes; examples include iron in oxygen transport, manganese and selenium in antioxidant defense and zinc in metabolism. With these essential metals toxicity occurs when concentrations are either too low or too high. For some metals there are no physiological concentrations that are beneficial; as such these metals only have the potential to cause toxicity. This chapter focuses on four of these: arsenic, mercury, lead and thallium.

Arsenic poisoning

Arsenic's history is marked by great successes and tremendous tragedies. Used by Greek and Roman physicians as far back as 400 B.C. [1], arsenic is still used in traditional Chinese and Indian folk medicine [2, 3]. In western medicine it has recently been used as a treatment for late-stage African trypanosomiasis (melarsoprol) [4] and for acute promyelocytic leukemia (arsenic trioxide, Trisenox®) [5]. Arsenic also enjoys an illustrious place in history as a frequently employed homicidal agent. The historical use of arsenic as a poison has earned it the title of "Poison of Kings and the King of Poisons" [6].

Toxicology

As the 20th most abundant element in the earth's crust, arsenic can be found in all living organisms as one of several varieties: elemental, organic, inorganic, and gaseous [7, 8]. In nature arsenic is found in rocks, soil, minerals, and metals ores such as lead and copper; environmental arsenic contamination may occur through water runoff and leaching, wind, and volcanic eruptions. Mining and smelting of arsenic-containing ores, combustion of fossil fuels in coal-fired power plants and incinerators, as well as the use of organic arsenic in pesticides and animal feed contribute to environmental contamination [6, 9, 10].

Human exposure to arsenic primarily occurs through food, particularly seafood, rice, mushrooms, and poultry. Air and water represent alternative sources of exposure. In Bangladesh tube-wells were built to provide safe drinking water, but inadvertently exposed the population to elevated arsenic from contaminated ground water [11, 12]. Generally, residents of the United States consume only about 50 µg of arsenic per day with 3.5 µg being inorganic. Occupational contact represents an additional route of arsenic exposure with metal workers, electronic workers, and glass and ceramic manufacturing workers being at highest risk.

Elemental arsenic is nontoxic. Organic arsenicals can be found in fish and shellfish, in the form of arsenobetaine and, like elemental arsenic, these forms pose a low risk for human toxicity [9]. Arsenic toxicity primarily results from exposure to inorganic arsenicals, which are found in trivalent (As^{3+}, arsenite, more toxic) and pentavalent (As^{5+}, arsenate, less toxic) forms. Arsenate compounds have little protein binding and are free to be excreted. Arsenite compounds on the other hand have high protein binding, resulting in both toxicity and a potential storage depot for further exposure [13]. Once arsenic reaches hepatocytes, it undergoes conversion from an inorganic compound to an organic compound through alternating reduction and methylation reactions. This process detoxifies the parent compound but creates carcinogenic metabolites [6, 7, 13]. Arsenate is reduced to the more toxic arsenite form prior to being converted into monomethyl arsenic (MMA) and ultimately dimethyl arsenic (DMA). Both MMA and DMA can be reduced into the more toxic trivalent form [6, 13, 14]. The final effects of this bioactivation and detoxification pathway depends on the rate of each step in the tissue exposed [14].

Arsenic disrupts cellular functioning though two distinct mechanisms of action. Arsenic, particularly trivalent forms, binds sulfhydryl groups, disrupting essential enzyme activity, and leads to impaired gluconeogenesis and oxidative phosphorylation. Pentavalent arsenic can serve as a phosphorous substitute, forming less stable bonds in high energy compounds such as ATP. This 'arsenolysis' causes rapid hydrolysis of these bonds, uncoupling oxidative phosphorylation [15].

Clinical presentation

The clinical presentation of arsenic toxicity differs depending on the species of arsenic, the amount, and the route and duration of exposure. Acute occupational contact to arsenic may occur following inhalational exposure to inorganic arsenic or arsine gas [6, 9, 16]. Symptoms from arsine gas exposure differ from other types of arsenic exposure, and are discussed separately.

Acute arsenic toxicity from ingestion is characterized by gastrointestinal (GI) symptoms, including abdominal pain, nausea, emesis, and profuse watery or bloody diarrhea [6, 17, 18]. Subsequent hypotension, heart failure, pulmonary edema and shock can be seen as a result of capillary dilation with third spacing of fluid, cardiomyopathy, and ventricular arrhythmias [6, 18]. Altered mental status with confusion can be seen [17] and "seizures" or hypoxic convulsions may signal a pre-terminal event [8, 19]. Cardiac abnormalities have been noted following arsenic exposure, particularly following treatment with arsenic trioxide. These abnormalities may include QTc prolongation, pericardial effusion, myocarditis and serositis, T-wave abnormalities, second-degree heart block, QRS widening, non-conducted P-waves, torsade de pointes, and asystole [18, 20–24]. There are multiple theories regarding the etiology of these cardiac abnormalities. Patients receiving arsenic trioxide may have been exposed to other cardiotoxic medication in their previous chemotherapeutic regimen. In addition, arsenic trioxide therapy itself is associated with hypokalemia and hypomagnesemia [14]. The combination of these two factors may account for cardiac effects seen with arsenic trioxide in chemotherapy patients. Arsenic has also been shown to have direct cardiac effects including blockade (I_{Kr} and I_{Ks}) and activation (I_{K-ATP}) of cardiac ion channels – effects that may account for arsenic's variability of QT prolongation [18].

Peripheral neuropathy typically occurs 2–8 weeks after arsenic exposure, although it may occur within hours of a severe exposure [6, 25]. Early symptoms consist of a symmetric sensorimotor neuropathy, which may be initially misdiagnosed as Guillain-Barré syndrome [6, 26]. Patients who develop arsenic-induced neuropathy note pain, numbness, and paresthesias in a stocking glove distribution [6, 17]. Electrophysiological studies are consistent with axonal degeneration, showing a decrease in amplitude, and with severe poisonings velocity [6]. Arsenic-induced cellular toxicity results in cytoskeleton protein changes, which may be the etiology of arsenic-induced neuropathy [6].

Chronic arsenic toxicity is characterized by macrocytosis, pancytopenia, hyperkeratotic lesions noted on the extremities, hyperpigmented melanosis described as "raindrops in the dust", bronze pigmentation, GI symptoms, anemia, and liver disease [6, 27, 28]. In addition, Mees' lines – transverse white striae on the fingernails (Fig. 1), a sensation of a metallic taste [6] and peripheral neuropathy have all been characterized in chronic arsenic exposure [27].

Long-term effects

Arsenic is considered a known human carcinogen by the U.S. Department of Health and Human Services, the International Agency for Research on Cancer (IARC), and the U.S. Environmental Protection Agency (EPA) [9]. Specifically, arsenic has been shown to alter gene expression through induction, down-regulation, and up-regulation of various genes involved in damage response, apoptosis, cell cycle regulation, cell signaling, and growth factor response [13]. Multiple cancers have been linked to arsenic in populations with increased occupational or environmental arsenic exposure, including

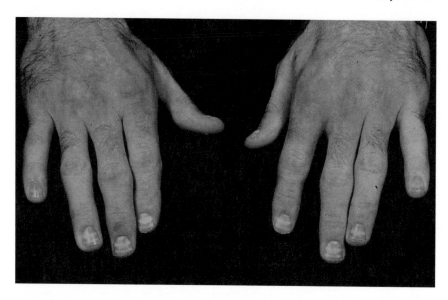

Figure 1. Mees' lines from two separate incidences of arsenic poisoning (courtesy of R. Pascuzzi, MD, Indianapolis, IN).

liver, bladder, lung, digestive tract, lymphatic, hematopoietic, and skin cancer [9, 11, 29–31].

Diagnosis

The diagnosis of arsenic toxicity depends on combining the clinical history with the possibility of exposure. If the exposure is recent, urine and blood testing can confirm or refute suspected arsenic toxicity [6, 9]. Arsenic has been shown to clear from blood in three phases [32]. Due to the rapid clearance seen during phases 1 and 2, blood testing may only be reliable during the early stages (typically <7–10 days after acute arsenic poisoning) [8]. The long half-life of arsenic in phase 3 of elimination (estimated 230 hours), however, may make urinary arsenic concentrations detectable for weeks after an acute exposure [32]. Arsenic speciation may be helpful to separate inorganic and organic arsenic species, since only inorganic arsenic is of toxicological concern. If the sample was collected in a metal-free container and there was no recent seafood ingestion, a urinary arsenic level greater than 50 µg/L in a random sample or greater than 100 µg in a 24-hour sample should be considered elevated [6]. In cases of suspected chronic arsenic toxicity, hair and nails can also be used to confirm the diagnosis [6]. Since hair grows at rate of 0.4 mm a day, hair studies may be used to help determine an approximate time of exposure based on the distance of an arsenic peak from the hair root [33].

Treatment

As with any toxin, it is important to remove the patient from the source of their exposure. While not well studied, gastric lavage and activated charcoal have been used to decrease absorption [6]. Initial treatment of arsenic toxicity is geared towards intensive supportive care. Additionally, hemodialysis has shown some benefit in treating arsenic-poisoned patients who present with significant renal dysfunction. Once renal function recovers, urinary arsenic excretion may exceed the amount removed by dialysis [34].

Since arsenic is a metalloid, chelation therapy may be used [6]. Dimercaprol (2,3-dimercaptopropanol, British Anti-Lewisite, BAL), at a dose of 3–4 mg/kg intramuscularly every 4–12 hours can be used as a chelator following acute arsenic toxicity [8, 19]. In a patient able to take an oral medication, dimercaprol may be discontinued, and *meso*-2,3-dimercaptosuccinic acid (DMSA) given at a dose of 10 mg/kg every 8 hours for 5 days then every 12 hours can be applied [8]. Treatment duration is based on clinical course and may be influenced by urinary arsenic levels [19]. However, increased urinary arsenic clearance has not been consistently demonstrated following DMSA therapy [33, 35]. Neuropathy progression despite chelation therapy has been reported [17, 33]. DMSA is only U.S. Food and Drug Administration (FDA) approved for the treatment of lead toxicity in children but has orphan status for the treatment of mercury poisoning [35]. While historically D-penicillamine was also recommended as an oral chelating agent, animal studies have suggested it to be inferior to dimercaprol and DMSA [36].

Arsine gas

Arsine gas is liberated when an acid contacts arsenic containing compounds or when water contacts metallic arsenide. Industrial processes at risk of generating arsine gas include galvanizing, soldering, etching, and lead plating. Arsine gas is colorless, nonirritating, and possesses a slight garlic odor, which may not be detected following an industrial exposure [37]. Arsine toxicity presents very differently from arsenic toxicity. Within hours of significant arsine exposure, patients develop headache, abdominal pain, nausea, and emesis, followed by hemolysis, gross hematuria, scleral icterus, bronze skin discoloration, and acute renal failure. A classic triad of abdominal/flank pain, hematuria, and jaundice has been described. While recovery is possible, patients may experience chronic renal dysfunction [38] and peripheral neuropathy following arsine exposure [39].

Laboratory evaluation following exposure to arsine gas reveals a Coombs negative hemolytic anemia with mildly elevated serum bilirubin and lactate dehydrogenase levels. Erythrocyte lysis and renal failure may lead to massive elevations of serum potassium requiring treatment. Urinalysis reveals hemoglobinuria, albuminuria, and occasional tubular casts consisting of erythrocytes and hemoglobin [37].

Treatment of exposed individuals begins with removing the patient from the source of their exposure. Exchange transfusion can restore functional red blood cells [39, 40] and remove hemoglobin pigment and the toxic products formed from the effect of arsine on hemoglobin [39]. The successful use of plasmapheresis in addition to red blood cell (RBC) exchange has also been described [37, 38]. Hemodialysis should be considered in any patient experiencing renal failure [40]. Chelation therapy is controversial in the acute management of arsine toxicity, and may not influence outcomes or the development of peripheral neuropathy [39].

Chromated copper arsenate

First used as a wood preservative during the 1930s, chromated copper arsenate (CCA) became the main preservative used in residential settings in the United States by the 1970s [41, 42]. Despite its popularity, concern arose regarding the potential for arsenic toxicity from its use in children's playground equipment. While this potential exposure is smaller than what children receive through food and water [9], a 2001 petition was presented to the Consumer Product Safety Commission requesting a ban on the use of CCA in playground equipment [42]. Although chronic arsenic toxicity has only occurred following the burning of CCA-treated wood in an enclosed environment [43], production of CCA for consumer products was halted in December of 2003 following a voluntary agreement between CCA manufacturers and the Environmental Protection Agency [42]. Today, CCA-treated wood can still be found in industrial settings [9].

Mercury poisoning

Mercury is a naturally occurring metal that exists in three forms: elemental, inorganic salt, and organic. Documented use of mercury dates back to 1500 B.C. and over the ensuing centuries it has been used as decoration, in cosmetics, and even as a medicine. The clinical syndromes associated with mercury exposure vary with the dose, length of exposure, and form of mercury [44–47].

Elemental mercury

Elemental mercury (quicksilver or liquid mercury) is a silver colored liquid at room temperature. The primary means by which elementary mercury is absorbed is through inhalation of its vapor. The vapor pressure of mercury approximately doubles for every 10 °C temperature increase, so that its heating greatly increases exposure and toxicity. Approximately 80% of inhaled vapor is absorbed by the alveoli and passes rapidly into the blood where it is taken up by red blood cells and converted to a less lipid soluble divalent (mercuric) form. A small amount of non-oxidized mercury vapor can penetrate the blood-brain barrier leading to central nervous system (CNS) toxicity in high-dose exposures [48]. Inhaled vapor is largely eliminated in the urine with an elimination half-life of about 60 days [49]. Compared to the respiratory tract, GI absorption is negligible [50] and represents little risk for patients with intact GI mucosa [51]. Toxicity can occur if the GI mucosa is not intact [52]. Two less common sources of exposure are intravenous (i.v.) and subcutaneous injection. Intravenous injection can lead to potentially fatal pulmonary emboli and mercury poisoning [53, 54]. Although small amounts can enter through intact skin [55], subcutaneous injection of elemental mercury tends to be limited to local symptoms; it may, however, cause increases in blood and urine mercury concentrations.

Toxicology
Target organs for elemental mercury vapor include the lungs, brain, and to a lesser degree the kidneys [47, 56, 57]. It appears to cross the blood-brain barrier in its vapor form concentrating in neuronal lysosomal dense bodies. Elemental mercury combines with sulfhydryl groups on cell membranes and interferes with protein and nucleic acid synthesis, calcium homeostasis and protein phosphorylation. Elemental mercury causes cellular damage and oxidant stress [58].

Clinical presentation
The dose and length of exposure are responsible for the wide variability in symptoms from elemental mercury toxicity. Within hours of an acute exposure, chills, GI upset, weakness, cough and dyspnea may develop. Adult respiratory distress syndrome and renal failure may occur in severe cases. Depending on the level of exposure, chronic mercury toxicity may develop over weeks to months. Early symptoms such as GI upset, poor appetite, abdominal pain, headache, dry mouth, and myalgia may mimic a viral illness. Two distinct syndromes, acrodynia and erethism have been associated with chronic exposure (Fig. 2). 'Acrodynia', alternately known as pink disease, Feer syndrome, or Feer-Swift disease, is a complex of symptoms that may be seen in chronic exposure to either elemental or inorganic mercury. It usually occurs in infants and children, but has been reported in adults. The symptom complex includes the following: (1) Autonomic changes – sweating, hypertension, tachycardia; (2) dermatological/dental changes – pruritus, erythematous rash on palms/soles, erythematous gingiva, ulceration of oral mucosa, loose teeth; (3) musculoskeletal – weakness, poor muscle tone.

Many of the adrenergic symptoms are thought to be due to mercury's inactivation of coenzyme *S*-adenosylmethionine, which causes inhibition of catechol *O*-methyltransferase (COMT). A reduction in the breakdown of catecholamines produces the sympathetic symptoms such as hypertension and may result in a clinical picture mimicking pheochromocytoma [59–61].

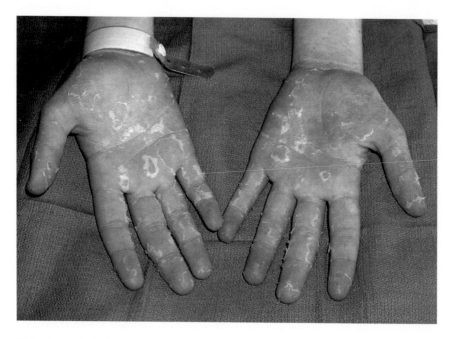

Figure 2. Acrodynia from elemental mercury vapor toxicity (courtesy of D. Rusyniak, MD, Indiana-polis, IN).

'Erethism' refers to personality changes in affected individuals. They may exhibit memory loss, drowsiness, lethargy, depression, withdrawal, and irritability. Other neuropsychiatric findings are also reported: insomnia, shyness, confusion, hallucinations, manic-depressive episodes, emotional lability [56]. Some authors have suggested a link between mercury exposure, erethism, and parkinsonism [56, 62, 63]. Two studies from the 1980s [64, 65] and two case reports [62, 63] suggest this link; however, causation has not been established.

Diagnosis

The diagnosis of elemental mercury poisoning is based upon history, physical findings, and the demonstration of a significantly increased body burden of mercury.

After an acute exposure, whole blood mercury is reliably elevated for 2–3 days (the usual reference range is 0–10 µg/L). Urine 24-hour collection is the most useful indication of exposure to elemental and inorganic mercury. Samples need to be refrigerated to decrease bacterial reduction of mercury to volatile elemental mercury [66]. Excretion in excess of 50 µg/L is considered elevated but reference ranges vary and an exact threshold for toxicity does not exist [47, 56]. Care must be taken in interpretation of urine testing for metals as specimens collected after administration of chelators can increase excretion of various metals even in patients without excessive exposure [67, 68]. The results of such tests should *not* be applied to reference ranges for non-chelated specimens.

Treatment

Removal of the patient from the source is a key intervention [47, 56, 57, 69]. Decontamination is of little use in either respiratory or GI exposure. While chelation is considered a mainstay of therapy, it is still somewhat controversial. DMSA, dimercaprol, and D-penicillamine have all been used; DMSA is considered the current treatment of choice in the United States. Chelation may take several months and studies showing a clear long-term benefit are lacking [57, 70]. Dialysis with or without the inclusion of a chelating agent, may be required in patients with renal failure.

Dental amalgam

Also known as mercury or silver amalgam, dental amalgam consists of up to 50% elemental mercury, copper or silver and also contains lesser concentrations of other metals such as zinc. For over a century, this durable compound has been widely used in dental restorations because it can be tightly inserted and expands in place to fill defects. In the latter part of the 19th century concerns were raised as to the potential mercury toxicity in dental fillings [71]. A German chemist, Alfred Stock, who suffered from erethism as a result of years of exposure to mercury, is credited with first recognizing that dental amalgam could elevate urine mercury concentrations [71]. In more recent years, animal studies have confirmed that mercury is released from amalgam fillings with the amount increasing with the size and number of fillings [72]. Some authors have suggested a causal relationship between a variety of diseases and dental amalgam including autoimmune disorders, renal disease, Alzheimer's disease, and autism [73]. Multiple human studies, however, have failed to establish causation [74–81]. Some studies have reported improvement in a variety of symptoms after the removal of mercury amalgam; however, these studies have not clearly established a link between amalgam removal and improvement of symptoms [82, 83]. It should be noted that removal of mercury amalgam appears to increase plasma mercury by three- to fourfold for a short time after removal [84, 85].

Inorganic mercury

Mercury occurs naturally as mercuric and mercurous salts. Cinnabar [mercury (II) sulfide, HgS] is the most common natural source. This mineral is used as the pigment vermilion. A wide variety of mercurial salts have been used in a variety of industries including medicine as antiseptics (i.e., mercuric chloride); cosmetics, explosives, dyes and pigments, and as antifungals in paints [47, 56, 86, 87].

Clinical presentation

Inorganic mercury may be absorbed *via* the GI or respiratory tracts as well as dermally. Ingestion is the most common route. Unlike the elemental form, mercury salts are very corrosive to the gut [56, 88]. Presenting complaints following ingestion may include nausea, vomiting, abdominal pain, or hematemesis. Colitis with necrosis or mucosal sloughing may occur in severe cases, leading to excessive volume loss [56, 88, 89].

Prolonged cutaneous application can cause hyperpigmentation, swelling, and vesicular or scaly rash. Hyperpigmentation is seen as a gray-brown discoloration of skin folds of the face and neck. Used as a topical analgesic for teething in the 19th century, calomel (mercuric chloride) caused loosening of teeth, bluish discoloration of the gingiva, and systemic toxicity [56, 90].

The half-life of inorganic mercury is 24–40 hours in the blood. It is excreted by the kidneys, which results in concentration and injury of the distal portions of the proximal convoluted tubules [91, 92]. These effects can be seen within 2 weeks of exposure and may reverse over time [93]. Chronic exposure can also cause membranous glomerulonephritis and nephrotic syndrome. Animal studies suggest that this is an autoimmune process. Spontaneous resolution of the nephrotic syndrome has been reported following termination of mercury exposure [47, 94]. Acrodynia and erethism have also been reported with inorganic mercury exposure [47, 56].

Diagnosis

As with elemental mercury exposures, 24-hour urine testing is the preferred method of measuring body burden. However, there is no clear threshold for toxicity (see diagnosis under elemental mercury).

Treatment

The GI tract and kidneys are the target organs of inorganic mercury. Injury to the gut in severe poisoning may require aggressive fluid resuscitation. Renal injury may necessitate hemodialysis. Dimercaprol has been reported to be most effective if started within 4 hours of oral exposure [95]. DMSA may be substituted when patients can tolerate oral medication.

Organic mercury

Recognition of organic mercury toxicity has been relatively recent. Organic mercurial compounds are used as preservatives, antiseptics and seed dressings. Two historical episodes of methylmercury exposure brought to the light the toxicity related to organic mercury. The first event occurred in the community of Minamata Bay, Japan. During the 1950s and 60s a local chemical company disposed waste into the neighboring bay where resident bacteria converted the inorganic mercury into methylmercury, which eventually found its way up the food chain and concentrated in larger fish. Over 2265 people who consumed contaminated fish developed toxicity known as Minamata disease. Symptoms included ataxia, sensory disturbances, dysarthria, visual field constriction, auditory disturbances and tremor. Children born to mothers who were exposed to methylmercury *in utero* developed congenital Minamata disease characterized by spasticity, seizures, deafness and severe mental deficiency [96, 97].

The second event occurred in Iraq in 1971 when bread that was made from seed grain treated with a methylmercury fungicide was consumed by over 6500 people [98]. Studies from the Iraqi victims were used as the first standards for defining safe organic mercury exposure in adults. The FDA used these data to propose an acceptable daily intake of 0.4 µg/kg body weight per day [96].

Toxicology
Studies from the disasters in Japan and Iraq show that methylmercury primarily targets the CNS with fetal brain tissue being more susceptible than the adult CNS. Up to 90% of organic mercury is absorbed from the GI tract [99] after which it readily crosses the blood-brain barrier and placenta reaching levels in the brain three to six times those in the blood [100].

Clinical presentation
The most common presentation of organic mercury poisoning is concentric constriction of the bilateral visual fields, paresthesias of extremities and mouth, incoordination, ataxia, tremor, dysarthria and auditory impairment [97, 98]. Postmortem findings demonstrate neuronal damage in gray matter of the cerebral and cerebellar cortex, with the calcarine region of the occipital lobe and the pre- and postcentral and temporal cortex are the most affected. Granule cells in the cerebellum are lost, while neighboring Purkinje cells are preserved. Sensory fibers of the peripheral nerves may also be damaged [101, 102].

Among children with Minamata disease, all had mental retardation, cerebellar ataxia, primitive reflexes, limb deformities, and dysarthria. Chorea and hypersalivation were seen in 95%, while 60% had microcephaly [97, 103, 104]. Pathological changes were similar in adults and children: cortical atrophy and hypoplasia of the corpus callosum, demyelination of the pyramidal tracts, and hypoplasia of the granular cell layer of the cerebellum [103].

Diagnosis
Ninety percent of methylmercury is bound to hemoglobin in red blood cells [99]. Most elimination occurs through the GI tract rather than the kidneys. For that reason, whole blood mercury rather than urine mercury is a better indication of organic mercury burden. Whole blood mercury concentrations are usually less than 6 ng/mL, but diets rich in fish can increase levels to 200 ng/mL or higher [7].

Treatment
Chelating agents including D-penicillamine, N-acetyl-D,L-penicillamine, 2,3-dimercaptopropane sulfonate, and DMSA have all be utilized in cases of

organic mercury toxicity [98, 105, 106]. While all appear to increase excretion, none have been shown to lead to clinical improvement. Most cases are discovered after symptoms are pronounced, and treatment is likely more effective when begun early [107, 108].

Thimerosal and vaccines

Thimerosal is an organic mercury compound that contains ethylmercury bound to thiosalicylate. Since the 1930s it has been widely used as a preservative in certain vaccines. *In vitro* studies showed thimerosal to be 40–50 times as effective as phenol as an antimicrobial against *Staphylococcus aureus*. Before the introduction of thimerosal, there were several episodes of bacterial contamination of vaccines that resulted in illness and death in recipients [96]. Thimerosal is 50% mercury by weight and found in concentrations of 0.003–0.01% in vaccines. A vaccine containing 0.01% thimerosal contains 25 µg mercury per 0.5 mL dose. Before the marketing of thimerosal, high-dose toxicity studies were performed on animals, but no clinical studies formally evaluated its safety in humans. In 1929, a trial of high-dose thimerosal was given intravenously to 22 patients with meningococcal meningitis. Although not effective as treatment, these patients seemed to tolerate such high doses without observed toxic effects [96].

Toxicity has been observed with large amounts of thimerosal in reports of both accidental and intentional exposure [109–113]. There are limited data on toxicity from low dose exposures similar to that seen with vaccines. A formal review of thimerosal by the FDA in 1976 stated "no dangerous quantity of mercury is likely to be received from biological products in a lifetime" [114]. The low concentration of mercury within the vaccines was considered both safe and effective in practice.

The calculations used by the EPA, Agency for Toxic Substances and Disease Registry (ATSDR), World Health Organization (WHO) and the FDA were based on the assumption that ethylmercury was similar in toxicity to methylmercury; this was based on their related chemical structure and similar clinical effects at high doses [115, 116]. These two compounds, however, are not equivalent and have significant differences in pharmacokinetics. Ethylmercury has a half-life somewhere between 7 and 18 days whereas that of methylmercury can be as long as 1.5 months. In addition, ethylmercury has less movement across the blood-brain barrier in the CNS [116].

A review of the FDA risk assessment found that the only established harm from thimerosal at doses found in vaccines is a delayed-type hypersensitivity reaction. However, because thimerosal vaccines could expose infants to cumulative mercury at levels that exceed the EPA recommendations (but not the ATSDR, WHO, or FDA) it was recommended that thimerosal be withdrawn from US vaccines. In July 1999, the American Academy of Pediatrics along with the Public Health Service called for the removal of thimerosal from further use in vaccines targeted for children [115]. Even though thimerosal was removed from childhood vaccines in the US in 1999, with the rise in neurodevelopmental disorders including autism, thimerosal has been questioned as a potential risk factor for these disorders. Several studies looking at the association between autism and thimerosal have found no causal relationship [117–119]. Several organizations including the WHO and the Institute of Medicine (IOM) have developed statements addressing the safety of thimerosal-containing vaccines. The IOM concludes that the evidence to date indicates no causal relationship between these vaccines and autism [120]. The WHO also supports that "the most recent pharmacokinetic and developmental studies do not support concerns over the safety of thimerosal (ethylmercury) in vaccines" [121].

Fish consumption

Human exposure to methylmercury is almost exclusively from the consumption of fish and other seafood. Pregnant women who eat fish expose the fetus to methylmercury which crosses the placenta as well as the blood-brain barrier [122, 123]. Although Minamata bay clearly showed the dangers of eating fish with exceptionally high levels of methylmercury, the fetal risks of current day maternal fish consumption are unknown. In 1989, the Seychelles Child Development Study (SCDS) was designed to study maternal methylmercury exposure due to fish consumption and its impact on fetal neurodevelopment; inhabitants of the Seychelles rely primarily on fish as a source of protein. Assessments were made at 6, 19, 29, and 66 months that showed no association between prenatal maternal hair mercury levels and neurodevelopmental outcome [124]. The findings reported in the 9-year follow-up of the SCDS found 2 of 21 endpoints were associated with prenatal methylmercury exposure and developmental outcomes at 9 years of age. In one test for speed and coordination, there was diminished performance in children of mothers with higher mercury concentrations; however, these children also did better on ratings of hyperactivity as compared to children of mothers with lower concentrations. The authors contributed both findings to chance, and in their conclusion state that their data do not support a relationship of impaired neurodevelopment from prenatal exposure to methylmercury in fish consumption in the Seychelles islands [122, 123].

The second large longitudinal study conducted in the Faroe Islands produced results that differed from those of the Seychelles study. The Faroe children showed deficits in language, attention and memory at age seven [125]. Some have suggested that the positive findings in the Faroe Island study may be related to differences in diet. The Faroe Island inhabitants eat more shark and whale meat, which contains higher concentrations of methylmercury than the fish consumed in Seychelles. Others have suggested the difference in neurodevelopmental testing may account for these differences [96, 122, 125].

The EPA, ATSDR, FDA and WHO have each developed recommendations for limits of exposure to methylmercury in the diet ranging from 0.1 to 0.47 µg/kg body weight per day [115].

Lead poisoning

Lead is a gray-silver heavy metal with a variety of industrial uses. As it has no known physiological role, any lead present in the human body can be viewed as contamination. Lead has been utilized by humans because of its properties of malleability and resistance to corrosion. From the mining of lead by the ancient Egyptians, Phoenicians, Greeks, and Romans to the use of lead machinery and lead-containing products during the Industrial Revolution and the widespread use of leaded gasoline and lead-based paint in the United States in the 20th century, the human use of lead has led to unfortunate consequences. It is speculated that some of the leaders of ancient Rome suffered neurotoxicity and sterility as a result of lead poisoning [126]. In the 1700s in England an outbreak of lead toxicity occurred due to lead contaminated cider; the victims of this outbreak suffered from severe abdominal pain and were said to have "Devonshire Colic" [127]. In the United States, Benjamin Franklin was aware of the effects of lead poisoning and described both lead-inflicted abdominal colic and peripheral neuropathy in 1763 [128]. Despite recognition of lead toxicity in the United States, lead-based paints were not banned until 1978 and leaded gasoline not until the 1990s [129]. The elimination of lead along with initiatives focused on limiting lead exposure, screening appropriate populations for lead exposure, and intervening when elevated blood lead levels (BLLs) are detected, has resulted in a decrease in the number of U.S. lead toxicity cases [130]. There continues to be at-risk populations in the U.S. including patients age 1–5 years and older than 60 years, minorities, lower socioeconomic populations, and recent immigrants [130]. This, along with continued environmental lead contamination, mandates clinicians to continue to be aware of the presentation, care, and prevention of lead toxicity.

Toxicology

Pediatric exposure to lead is often a result of oral ingestion of lead-containing material, including lead-based paints and contaminated soil [129, 131]. Children, particularly from the ages of 18–36 months, are more susceptible than adults to exposure to lead because of their increased hand-to-mouth activity. Children are also more susceptible to toxicity from lead secondary to their increased GI absorption of lead, active growth of their organ systems, immature blood-brain barrier, and propensity for iron deficiency – which increases GI lead absorption [132]. Children tend to have higher BLLs in the summer months due to increased exposure to lead-contaminated soil and dust [131]. Pediatric lead exposure has been reported with ingestion of larger lead-containing objects such as necklace charms [133], window curtain weights, bullets [134], and fishing weights (Fig. 3). Lead exposure can also occur by tap water contamination in residences that still have lead plumbing.

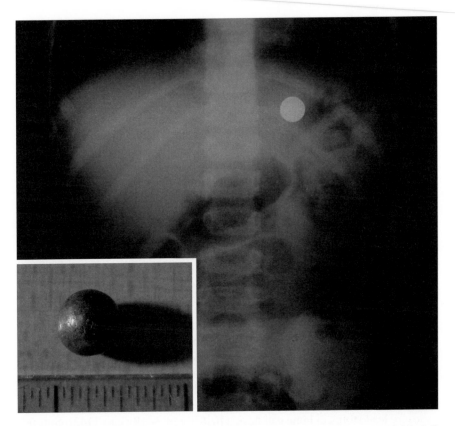

Figure 3. A 3-year-old swallowed a lead musket ball (insert). Two days later an x-ray revealed the ball in the stomach. The lead ball was removed by endoscopy without complication. A venous blood lead level, approximately 48-hour post ingestion, was at 89 μg/dL. The child underwent chelation therapy with succimer and a repeat lead level 1 week after chelation was 5 μg/dL. The child never developed symptoms and no other sources of lead were found in his environment (courtesy of C. Holstege, MD, Charlottesville, VA).

Lead exposure in adults usually occurs *via* the respiratory route through many occupations: battery plant worker, metal welder, painter, construction worker, lead miner, firing range worker, glass blower, and ship builder. Another source of lead poisoning in adults is ingestion of "moonshine" alcohols that have been distilled in lead-containing pipes [135, 136]. Exposure to leaded gasoline can increase organic lead exposure.

After absorption, lead can have detrimental effects to many organ systems including the nervous, hematological, renal, cardiovascular, GI, and endocrine systems. Lead can cause a decrease in the integrity of the blood-brain barrier by disrupting the intracellular junction of capillary endothelium. This results in increased capillary leak into the CNS and a resultant increase in intracranial fluid. Lead can also disrupt several neurotransmitter systems in the CNS by increasing spontaneous release of dopamine, acetylcholine, and γ-aminobutyric acid (GABA), by blocking N-methyl D-aspartate (NMDA) glutamate receptors and increasing levels of protein kinase C. A process termed "pruning" in which necessary neural pathways are protected and unnecessary neural pathways are destroyed, peaks when children are around 2 years of age. By interfering with the neurotransmitters of the CNS, lead causes ineffective "pruning" in which necessary neural pathways are destroyed and unnecessary neural pathways are enhanced [132, 137].

Microcytic anemia is a classic finding in lead toxicity. Lead inhibits several heme synthesis enzymes: aminolevulinic acid (ALA) synthetase, δ-ALA dehydratase, coproporphyrinogen decarboxylase, and ferrochelatase, leading to elevated erythrocyte protoporphyrin levels [138, 139]. In addition to decrease heme synthesis, lead weakens erythrocyte membranes shortening the erythrocyte life span. A clinical finding in, but not unique to, plumbism is basophilic stippling [140]. Basophilic stippling is a result of the inhibition of pyrimidine-5-nucleotidase. In children, the anemia caused by lead is often complicated by iron deficiency and other nutritional deficiencies that decrease effective hemoglobin synthesis [141].

Lead-protein complexes deposit in the proximal tubular cells of the kidney and are accompanied by mitochondrial swelling in this same region. Lead interferes with mitochondrial respiration and phosphorylation in the kidney, leading to glycosuria, aminoaciduria, and phosphaturia. Chronic high-dose lead exposure has been shown in animal models to cause renal failure through tubular atrophy, interstitial fibrosis, and glomerular sclerosis. These findings can also be seen in other forms of kidney failure [142].

The skeletal system serves as the main reservoir for lead. With chronic lead exposure lead stores in bone can have a half-life of 5–19 years [143]. Soft tissues may be subjected to increased lead exposure during times of accelerated bone turnover, such as during childhood growth, after a long bone fracture, or during pregnancy [144]. In children lead causes increased calcification of cartilage in the bone metaphysis resulting in increased metaphysis density [145].

Hypertension has been associated with chronic lead exposure. Lead likely affects vascular smooth muscle cells by causing a decrease in Na^+/K^+-ATPase activity with a subsequent increase in Na^+/Ca^{2+} pump activity, and increased calcium-mediated contractility. Lead may also alter vascular smooth muscle activity by increasing protein kinase C [146].

Clinical presentation

The clinical aspects of lead toxicity are widely described; however, there is no clear "toxidrome" and it is difficult to define expected symptoms at certain BLLs. The reason for this difficulty likely involves the many variables affecting the clinical effects of lead exposure: age at time of exposure, length of exposure time, genetic predisposition to effects, environmental factors, nutritional status, and underlying medical problems of the patient. Lead toxicity can present with symptoms in a variety of different organs. There are both similarities and differences in the way that children and adults are affected by lead toxicity.

In children, the neurological consequences of plumbism are the greatest concern. Serious neurological problems from lead toxicity are most commonly described in children between the ages of 18–36 months. Symptoms at BLLs of 50–100 μg/dL may be obvious or subtle and can include intermittent irritability, hyperactivity, and developmental delay in one particular skill [132, 137]. Higher levels or more chronic exposure can result in ataxia, lethargy, seizures, and coma. There is controversy over the cognitive effects of lower BLLs (BLLs less than 10 μg/dL). Some epidemiological studies have reported an inverse correlation between elevated BLLs in children and IQ [147], but not all published data are in agreement with this association [148]. Epidemiological studies that examine this topic have the difficult task of trying to control for all possible confounding variables [149].

Adults can also experience neurological symptoms with plumbism. Signs of encephalopathy including seizure, coma, and papilledema usually occur at BLLs over 150 μg/dL. At BLLs above 80 μg/dL memory problems, insomnia, and personality changes have been reported [150]. More subtle signs are seen in adults with BLLs of 40–70 μg/dL and can be similar to those symptoms seen with depression [151, 152].

Other clinical manifestations of lead poisoning in children and adults include a normocytic or microcytic anemia, abdominal pain, constipation, hepatotoxicity, and pancreatitis. Peripheral neuropathy, with resultant foot and wrist drop, is well described in adults and is occasionally seen in children – particularly those with underlying sickle cell disease [153]. Nephrotoxicity has been reported in all age groups with lead toxicity; a Fanconi's syndrome with aminoaciduria, glycosuria, and phosphaturia has been more commonly described in the adult population [142]. Saturnine gout is a phenomenon seen in adult patients and is due to impaired uric acid clearance by the kidneys. There is concern that chronic lead exposure can raise blood pressure; however, two recent meta-analyses found a less than robust association [154, 155]. Sperm abnormalities have also been associated with BLL of ≥40 μg/dL in work-exposed men [156]. Lead can cross the placenta and has been associated with spontaneous abortion, prematurity, and developmental delay. Lead is also excreted in breast milk [157].

Lead exposure does not have any clear association with carcinogenicity in humans. Inorganic lead is classified as a probable carcinogen (group 2A) and organic lead is not classifiable in regards to carcinogenicity (group 3) by the IARC [158]. These data coupled with clinical studies suggest that lead is, at worst, a weak carcinogen [159].

Organic lead, such as tetraethyl lead, at high doses can cause predominately neurological symptoms similar to a generalized encephalopathy including delirium, ataxia, and seizures. Neurological symptoms from organic lead are reported at lower levels than what would be typically expected with inorganic lead [160].

Diagnosis

The best initial test for evaluating a patient with suspected lead poisoning is a whole BLL obtained by venipuncture. A BLL should be sent in a lead-free tube and is usually measured by atomic absorption spectrophotometry. It is important to recognize that whole BLLs can be used to guide management but may not reflect lead in other organ systems, such as the CNS or bone. Capillary lead levels can be used for screening purposes, but may be falsely elevated if there is lead on the skin where the sample is drawn from [161]. A disadvantage of BLLs is that most laboratories are not equipped to report same-day results. BLLs that are done during chelation therapy can be elevated from lead that is pulled out of soft tissues and into the bloodstream. Zinc or erythrocyte protoporphyrin may also be elevated with lead toxicity but are not a sensitive test and can be elevated in other conditions that interfere with heme synthesis such as iron deficiency, sickle cell anemia, and vanadium toxicity. The protoporphyrin tests are more likely to be elevated with chronic lead toxicity than with acute lead toxicity [162].

Additional laboratory tests that may be useful in the evaluation of a patient with suspected plumbism should be guided by the history and physical exam, and may include a complete blood count, a comprehensive metabolic panel, and a urinalysis. These tests can also provide a baseline for management of possible side effects if chelation therapy is initiated.

Radiographic imaging may help to support the diagnosis of lead poisoning and can also help to illicit the etiology of exposure in some cases. In a patient with the possible ingestion of a lead-containing object, an abdominal x-ray should be obtained. Any patient with suspected plumbism and a history of bullet wound, should have an x-ray of the area of bullet impact to visualize any retained bullet fragments [134] (Fig. 3). Radiographs of long bones of children with BLLs of 70 µg/dL or greater may show increased densities at the metaphyses, also referred to as "lead lines". Findings indistinguishable from "lead lines" are also seen with bismuth, phosphate, and fluoride toxicity [145]. Chronic lead exposure may be quantified using bone x-ray fluorescence technology. This is a test that has been used in research studies and is not typically utilized in the clinical setting [163]. A head computed tomography scan should be obtained on any patient with suspected plumbism and acute CNS symptoms to evaluate for evidence of cerebral edema.

Treatment

The management of children with elevated BLLs should follow the guidelines set forth by the Centers of Disease Control and Prevention [164]. Some state health departments have slight variations in these guidelines. It is important to recognize that the first step in management of a patient with elevated lead levels is prompt removal from the source. The local health department should be contacted and should assist with identification of the source and containment of the lead source in a pediatric patient with a BLL greater than 20 µg/dL or with two separate BLLs within the 15–19 µg/dL range. A recent Cochrane review of 12 studies concluded that there was no clear benefit of educational initiatives and/or dust control measures, and there was insufficient evidence to comment on soil abatement in regards to lowering pediatric BLLs in a population [165]. Chelation therapy in asymptomatic children is usually not initiated unless a patient has a BLL of 45 µg/dL or greater; chelating patients with levels less than this does not show any benefit on cognitive outcomes [166]. Oral chelation is recommended for those patients who are asymptomatic and have BLLs of 45–69 µg/dL. Patients who have BLLs greater than 69 µg/dL or who are symptomatic should have parenteral chelation [150].

Screening of adults that have workplace lead exposure should be guided by Occupational Safety and Health Administration's recommendations: Asymptomatic adults with BLLs less than 70 µg/dL do not require chelation, oral chelation is recommended for mild symptoms or BLLs of 70–100 µg/dL, and parenteral chelation therapy is advised for symptoms of lead-induced encephalopathy and/or BLLs greater than 100 µg/dL [150].

The oral chelator that is approved by the FDA for lead poisoning in children over 1 year of age is DMSA. The pediatric dose of DMSA is 10 mg/kg per dose every 8 hours for 5 days followed by 10 mg/kg per dose every 12 hours for 14 days. Although DMSA is not officially recommended in adults, the dose that has been most widely used is 10–30 mg/kg per day for 5 days. Adverse reactions are not limited to, but include, neutropenia, hemolytic anemia, and elevation of aspartate and alanine aminotransferase [167]. Edetate calcium disodium (Calcium EDTA) is a parenteral chelator approved by the FDA for adult and pediatric plumbism. Edetate calcium disodium can be administered intravenously or intramuscularly. The recommended intravenous dose in adults for severe lead poisoning is 1–1.5 g/m^2 per day infused over 8–12 hours for a total of 5 days; after 2 days a repeat 5-day course can be administered if indicated. The recommended pediatric intravenous dose for severe lead poisoning is 1–1.5 g/m^2 per day divided into equal doses infused every 8 or 12 hours, an additional 5-day course can be given after 2 days if indicated. The following serious side effects have been reported with edetate calcium disodium: fever, hypersensitivity immune reaction, hypotension, nephrotoxicity, and thrombophlebitis. Care should be taken when using edetate calcium disodium in a patient with renal insufficiency, and the dose may need to be modified or an alternative chelator may need to be used. Edetate calcium disodium may increase intracranial pressure and, in patients with cerebral edema, the manufacturer recommends using the intramuscular route or alternatively using the intravenous route with a slow infusion rate. It has been reported that edetate calcium disodium may exacerbate symptoms when given as the sole chelator to a patient with a high BLL, and that dimercaprol should be given in conjunction with edetate calcium disodium in the patient who has symptomatic lead poisoning or a BLL over 70 µg/dL. If the patient can take oral medications, DMSA can be used instead of dimercaprol [168]. Edetate disodium without calcium should not be used because of the risk of hypocalcemia [169, 170]. Another FDA approved chelator for lead toxicity is dimercaprol. It is administered by deep intramuscular (i.m.) injection. In severe plumbism dimercaprol is administered at a dose of 4 mg/kg i.m. every 4 hours for 2–7 days in both pediatric and adult patients. In mild lead poisoning the recommended dose is 4 mg/kg i.m. for the first dose followed by 3 mg/kg i.m. every 4 hours for 2–7 days. Adverse reactions with dimercaprol include fever, hypertension, tachycardia, and injection site abscesses. Dimercaprol is administered in peanut oil and should usually be avoided in patients with peanut allergies [171]. Secondary to the number of side effects associated with dimercaprol, its use should be limited to symptomatic patients who cannot take oral DMSA. D-Penicillamine is not approved by the FDA for lead poisoning and should only be used in cases of serious lead poisoning in which other chelators have had unacceptable side effects. D-Penicillamine can cause the life-threatening side effect of agranulocytosis and can also cause severe dermatological and renal conditions [172].

Bowel irrigation with a polyethylene glycol-electrolyte solution should be considered if a patient has lead-containing objects in the GI tract that could easily transit through the GI tract. A gastroenterologist or surgeon may need to be contacted for removal of a larger lead-containing object out of the GI tract if it is likely that the object will not move adequately with GI peristalsis [173]. Likewise patients with evidence of lead poisoning may require surgical removal of lead containing bullet fragments lodged in soft tissues and/or joint spaces [134].

Thallium poisoning

In the late 19th century the spectro-chemical analysis of deposits from a sulfuric acid chamber resulted in the discovery of thallium [174]. Although useful in the manufacture of optic lenses, semiconductors and in very low concentrations as a radiocontrast agent, thallium is best known for its toxicity.

Toxicology

Thallium salts are tasteless, odorless, water soluble and rapidly absorbed and distributed throughout the body. By interfering with potassium and sulfhydryl-containing enzymes, thallium impairs energy production resulting, in severe cases, in cell death [175–178]. Although high concentrations of thallium are toxic to all organs, the peripheral nervous system and hair are particularly sensitive. Thallium does not undergo significant renal excretion, rather it undergoes entero-hepatic circulation with the primary means of elimination being fecal [179]. This makes treatment with the standard heavy metal chelators (DMSA, dimercaprol, edetate calcium disodium) less effective.

Clinical presentation

One of the earliest findings in thallium poisoning – typically within 2–3 days of exposure – is the development of a rapidly progressive painful peripheral neuropathy [180–182]. Symptoms begin in the feet and legs and may progress over time to involve the hands. The pain associated with thallium is described as "pins and needles" and may be severe enough to make the weight of a bed sheet intolerable [181–184]. With large exposures, motor nerves can also be affected including those innervating respiratory muscles [172, 185–187]. In these cases, the clinical picture of a rapidly progressive neuropathy can be misdiagnosed as Guillain-Barré [184]. Along with peripheral neuropathies, cranial neuropathies have also been reported [184, 186–191].

Perhaps the best-known complication of thallium poisoning is alopecia (Fig. 4). Beginning 5–14 days after exposure, victims begin painlessly losing

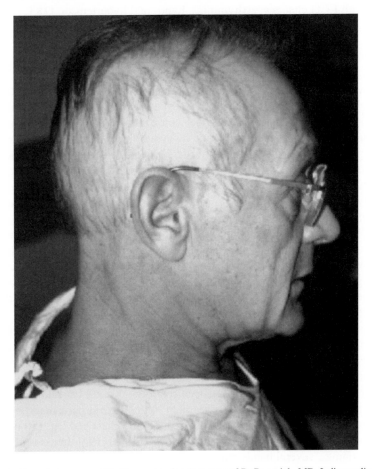

Figure 4. Alopecia in a case of thallium poisoning (courtesy of D. Rusyniak, MD, Indianapolis, IN).

their hair in clumps [182, 185, 187]. By 2–3 weeks patients may have developed total body alopecia – including axillary hair, pubic hair, and the lateral eyebrows [192–194]. The medial part of the eyebrow is typically spared as these hairs are commonly in a resting non-growth phase [194, 195]. While the exact cause of alopecia is not known, thallium's interruption of keratin synthesis and its interruption of hair matrix metabolism are likely responsible [196, 197]. While the most recognizable feature of thallium poisoning is alopecia, in mild cases peripheral neuropathies can occur without the development of hair loss [182].

Along with the peripheral nerves and hair, thallium can affect most major organ systems. Included amongst these are the CNS with hallucinations, altered mental status, insomnia, psychosis, ataxia and coma [181, 185–187, 189, 190, 198]; the GI tract with abdominal pain, vomiting, loose stools, and constipation or obstipation [182, 183, 186, 187, 194]; muscular systems with myalgias and pleuritic chest pain [182, 183, 199]; and the cardiovascular systems with ECG changes, arrhythmias, hypo- and hypertension [183, 200].

Diagnosis

Making the diagnosis of thallium poisoning early enough to institute effective therapy requires the early recognition of symptoms combined with neurological and clinical testing and analytical confirmation. This can be difficult as thallium poisoning is uncommon and its symptoms may be attributed to other etiologies [182]. Further hampering the early diagnosis, alopecia – the most recognizable feature of thallium poisoning [201] (Fig. 4) – may not be evident for up to 5–14 days after the exposure [197]. Despite these difficulties, two readily available tests may aid in making the early diagnosis of thallium poisoning: nerve conduction studies (NCS) and microscopic hair analysis.

NCS are useful in diagnosing and monitoring the recovery of patients with thallium poisonings [182]. They typical reveal a sensorimotor axonopathy with the severity of neuropathy correlating with the severity of other symptoms and findings. In cases of severe poisoning, a nerve biopsy may reveal Wallerian degeneration with axonal destruction and secondary myelin loss, although these findings are not specific to thallium [189, 202, 203].

Once it has been established that patients have a neuropathy suspicious for thallium, simply visually inspecting pulled hair under a low-powered light microscope may help make the diagnosis. When viewed under low power with a light microscope, the hair roots of thallium-poisoned patients appear darkened [182, 194]. This finding has been reported as early as 4 days after poisoning [194]. The darkened roots are seen in the highest percentage in pulled hair from the scalp (95%), followed by hairs of the chest and legs (50 to 60%), and less commonly from eyebrows and eyelids (30%) [194]. In cases of repeated poisonings, several bands may likewise be seen [194]. The blackened roots are not the accumulation of a pigment or the metal itself but rather represent an optical phenomenon. As the interruption of cellular processes disorganizes the hair root matrix, the hair root accumulates gaseous inclusions which diffract light and cause the appearance of a black stain [192, 197]. Treatment with acid or mechanical pressure will cause the accumulated gas to escape the hair and subsequently the hair root darkening disappears [204].

The definitive diagnosis of thallium poisoning requires the identification of elevated concentrations of thallium in urine or hair. Like many other metals, a 24-hour urine is considered the gold standard in thallium poisoning. In most persons, there should be no detectable levels of thallium, but levels up to a level 20 μg/specimen may be considered normal depending on occupational or environmental exposures. Hair analysis is not thought to be as reliable as urine and a negative hair test should not exclude the possibility of thallium poisoning. Hair levels less than 15 ng thallium/gram hair are considered normal [178]. Along with hair and urine, postmortem tissues including paraffin tissue blocks and even cremated ashes can be used to confirm elevations of thallium in suspected criminal poisonings [203, 205].

Treatment

The primary objective in treating thallium-poisoned patients is to increase thallium's elimination preventing further toxicity. The best-studied and most effective antidote is a complex of potassium hexacyanoferrate known as Prussian blue. Recently, the FDA approved Prussian blue for the treatment of cesium or thallium poisoning under the brand name Radiogardase®, the recommended dose is 3 g orally three times a day. Poorly absorbed, Prussian blue exchanges potassium for thallium in the gut increasing the fecal excretion of a thallium-Prussian blue complex. Numerous animal studies have shown that Prussian blue increases fecal elimination, decreases mortality, and decreases brain thallium concentrations [206–213]. Although clinical trials are not possible for thallium poisoning, human case reports support the safety and efficacy of Prussian blue [180, 210, 214]. Based on its affinity for sulfhydryl groups, several sulfur chelators have been studied in animal models of thallium poisoning. None have shown significant improvement [213, 215–217], and some may actually increase toxicity [208]. As Prussian blue may not be stocked in some hospitals, activated charcoal can be used until Prussian blue is available. *In vitro* studies demonstrate that activated charcoal effectively adsorbs thallium [170, 218], although its benefit in animal studies is contradictory [207, 215] and benefits in human cases are anecdotal [182, 185].

Summary

Acute and chronic toxicity from exposure to arsenic, mercury, lead and thallium still occur and pose significant morbidity and mortality if they are not recognized and treated. With each of these, the diagnosis is based on combining clinical suspicion with analytical testing. If a patient is suspected of poisoning, they should be removed from the source and if symptoms are severe, treatment, including chelation, should begin prior to analytical confirmation.

References

1 Hunt E, Hader SL, Files D, Corey GR (1999) Arsenic poisoning seen at Duke Hospital, 1965–1998. *NC Med J* 60: 70–74
2 Lynch E, Braithwaite R (2005) A review of the clinical and toxicological aspects of 'traditional' (herbal) medicines adulterated with heavy metals. *Expert Opin Drug Saf* 4: 769–778
3 Wong ST, Chan HL, Teo SK (1998) The spectrum of cutaneous and internal malignancies in chronic arsenic toxicity. *Singapore Med J* 39: 171–173
4 Klasco RK (2009) DRUGDEX® System. Thomson Reuters, Greenwood Village, CO (online available at: http://csi.micromedex.com/help/DKS/DKRefEntir.htm)
5 FDA (2001) *Trisenox Consumer Information Sheet.* U.S. Food and Drug Administration Center for Drug Evaluation and Research (http://www.fda.gov/)
6 Vahidnia A, van der Voet GB, de Wolff FA (2007) Arsenic neurotoxicity – A review. *Hum Exp Toxicol* 26: 823–832
7 Baselt RC (2002) *Disposition of Toxic Drugs and Chemicals in Man.* 6th edn., Biomedical Publications, Foster City, CA
8 Ford M (2006) Arsenic. In: NE Flomenbaum, LR Goldfrank, RS Hoffman, MA Howland, NA Lewin, LS Nelson (eds): *Goldfrank's Toxicologic Emergencies.* 8th edn., McGraw-Hill, New York, 1251–1264
9 ATSDR (2007) *Toxicological Profile for Arsenic.* U.S. Department of Health and Human Services, Public Health Service, Agency for Toxic Substances and Disease Registry, Atlanta, GA
10 Peters GR, McCurdy RF, Hindmarsh JT (1996) Environmental aspects of arsenic toxicity. *Crit Rev Clin Lab Sci* 33: 457–493
11 Khan MM, Sakauchi F, Sonoda T, Washio M, Mori M (2003) Magnitude of arsenic toxicity in tube-well drinking water in Bangladesh and its adverse effects on human health including cancer: Evidence from a review of the literature. *Asian Pac J Cancer Prev* 4: 7–14
12 Jones H, Visoottiviseth P, Bux MK, Fodenyi R, Kovats N, Borbely G, Galbacs Z (2008) Case reports: Arsenic pollution in Thailand, Bangladesh, and Hungary. *Rev Environ Contam Toxicol* 197: 163–187
13 Ghosh P, Banerjee M, Giri AK, Ray K (2008) Toxicogenomics of arsenic: Classical ideas and recent advances. *Mutat Res* 659: 293–301
14 Vahter M, Concha G (2001) Role of metabolism in arsenic toxicity. *Pharmacol Toxicol* 89: 1–5
15 ter Welle HF, Slater EC (1967) Uncoupling of respiratory-chain phosphorylation by arsenate. *Biochim Biophys Acta* 143: 1–17
16 Pullen-James S, Woods SE (2006) Occupational arsine gas exposure. *J Natl Med Assoc* 98: 1998–2001
17 Vantroyen B, Heilier JF, Meulemans A, Michels A, Buchet JP, Vanderschueren S, Haufroid V, Sabbe M (2004) Survival after a lethal dose of arsenic trioxide. *Clin Toxicol* 42: 889–895
18 ATSDR (1990) *Case Studies in Environmental Medicine. Arsenic Toxicity.* U.S. Department of Health and Human Services, Public Health Service, Agency for Toxic Substances and Disease Registry, Atlanta, GA
19 Klaassen CD (2006) Heavy metals and heavy-metal antagonists. In: LL Brunton, JS Lazo, KL Parker (eds): *Goodman & Gilman's The Pharmacological Basis of Therapeutics.* McGraw-Hill, New York, 1753–1775
20 Hall JC, Harruff R (1989) Fatal cardiac arrhythmia in a patient with interstitial myocarditis related to chronic arsenic poisoning. *South Med J* 82: 1557–1560
21 Beckman KJ, Bauman JL, Pimental PA, Garrard C, Hariman RJ (1991) Arsenic-induced torsade de pointes. *Crit Care Med* 19: 290–292
22 Little RE, Kay GN, Cavender JB, Epstein AE, Plumb VJ (1990) Torsade de pointes and T-U wave alternans associated with arsenic poisoning. *Pacing Clin Electrophysiol* 13: 164–170

23 Goldsmith S, From AH (1980) Arsenic-induced atypical ventricular tachycardia. *N Engl J Med* 303: 1096–1098

24 St Petery J, Gross C, Victorica BE (1970) Ventricular fibrillation caused by arsenic poisoning. *Am J Dis Child* 120: 367–371

25 Kishi Y, Sasaki H, Yamasaki H, Ogawa K, Nishi M, Nanjo K (2001) An epidemic of arsenic neuropathy from a spiked curry. *Neurology* 56: 1417–1418

26 Donofrio PD, Wilbourn AJ, Albers JW, Rogers L, Salanga V, Greenberg HS (1987) Acute arsenic intoxication presenting as Guillain-Barre-like syndrome. *Muscle Nerve* 10: 114–120

27 Heaven R, Duncan M, Vukelja SJ (1994) Arsenic intoxication presenting with macrocytosis and peripheral neuropathy, without anemia. *Acta Haematol* 92: 142–143

28 Alain G, Tousignant J, Rozenfarb E (1993) Chronic arsenic toxicity. *Int J Dermatol* 32: 899–901

29 Ferreccio C, Sancha AM (2006) Arsenic exposure and its impact on health in Chile. *J Health Popul Nutr* 24: 164–175

30 Rahman MM, Ng JC, Naidu R (2009) Chronic exposure of arsenic *via* drinking water and its adverse health impacts on humans. *Environ Geochem Health*

31 Ferreccio C, Gonzalez C, Milosavjlevic V, Marshall G, Sancha AM, Smith AH (2000) Lung cancer and arsenic concentrations in drinking water in Chile. *Epidemiology* 11: 673–679

32 Mealey J Jr, Brownell GL, Sweet WH (1959) Radioarsenic in plasma, urine, normal tissues, and intracranial neoplasms; distribution and turnover after intravenous injection in man. *AMA Arch Neurol Psychiatry* 81: 310–320

33 Stenehjem AE, Vahter M, Nermell B, Aasen J, Lierhagen S, Morland J, Jacobsen D (2007) Slow recovery from severe inorganic arsenic poisoning despite treatment with DMSA (2.3-dimercaptosuccinic acid). *Clin Toxicol* 45: 424–428

34 Vaziri ND, Upham T, Barton CH (1980) Hemodialysis clearance of arsenic. *Clin Toxicol* 17: 451–456

35 FDA (2007) Approved Drug Products. Label for CHEMET. NDA no. 019998 (http://www.fda.gov/)

36 Kreppel H, Reichl FX, Forth W, Fichtl B (1989) Lack of effectiveness of D-penicillamine in experimental arsenic poisoning. *Vet Hum Toxicol* 31: 1–5

37 Klimecki WT, Carter DE (1995) Arsine toxicity: Chemical and mechanistic implications. *J Toxicol Environ Health* 46: 399–409

38 Parish GG, Glass R, Kimbrough R (1979) Acute arsine posioning in two workers cleaning a clogged drain. *Arch Environ Health* 34: 224–227

39 Ibrahim D, Froberg B, Wolf A, Rusyniak DE (2006) Heavy metal poisoning: Clinical presentations and pathophysiology. *Clin Lab Med* 26: 67–97

40 Fowler BA, Weissberg JB (1974) Arsine poisoning. *N Engl J Med* 291: 1171–1174

41 EPA Web Page – Chromated Copper Arsenate (CCA), U.S. Environmental Protection Agency (http://www.epa.gov/)

42 CPSC (U.S. Consumer Product Safety Commission) Fact Sheet, *Chromated Copper Arsenate (CCA) – Treated Wood Used in Playground Equipment*, http://www.cpsc.gov/phth/ccafact.html

43 Hall AH (2002) Chronic arsenic poisoning. *Toxicol Lett* 128: 69–72

44 O'Shea JG (1990) "Two minutes with Venus, two years with mercury" – Mercury as an antisyphilitic chemotherapeutic agent. *J R Soc Med* 83: 392–395

45 Risher J, De Woskin R (1999) *Toxicological Profile for Mercury.* Agency for Toxic Substances and Disease Registry (ATSDR), U.S. Department of Health and Human Services, Public Health Service, Atlanta, GA

46 Goldwater LJ (1955) Hat industry: *Mercury; a History of Quicksilver.* York Press, Baltimore, MD

47 Graeme KA, Pollack CV (1998) Heavy metal toxicity, Part I: Arsenic and mercury. *J Emerg Med* 16: 45–56

48 Caravati EM, Erdman AR, Christianson G, Nelson LS, Woolf AD, Booze LL, Cobaugh DJ, Chyka PA, Scharman EJ, Manoguerra AS, Troutman WG, American Association of Poison Control Centers (2008) Elemental mercury exposure: An evidence-based consensus guideline for out-of-hospital management. *Clin Toxicol* 46: 1–21

49 Bluhm RE, Breyer JA, Bobbitt RG, Welch LW, Wood AJ, Branch RA (1992) Elemental mercury vapour toxicity, treatment, and prognosis after acute, intensive exposure in chloralkali plant workers. Part II: Hyperchloraemia and genitourinary symptoms. *Hum Exp Toxicol* 11: 211–215

50 Song Y, Li A (2007) Massive elemental mercury ingestion. *Clin Toxicol* 45: 193

51 Rusyniak DE, Nanagas KA (2008) Conservative management of elemental mercury retained in

the appendix. *Clin Toxicol* 46: 831–833

52 Bredfeldt JE, Moeller DD (1978) Systemic mercury intoxication following rupture of a Miller-Abbott tube. *Am J Gastroenterol* 69: 478–480

53 dell'Omo M, Muzi G, Bernard A, Lauwerys RR, Abbritti G (1996) Long-term toxicity of intravenous mercury injection. *Lancet* 348: 64

54 Kedziora A, Duflou J (1995) Attempted suicide by intravenous injection of mercury: A rare cause of cardiac granulomas. A case report. *Am J Forensic Med Pathol* 16: 172–176

55 Hursh JB, Clarkson TW, Miles EF, Goldsmith LA (1989) Percutaneous absorption of mercury vapor by man. *Arch Environ Health* 44: 120–127

56 Boyd AS, Seger D, Vannucci S, Langley M, Abraham JL, King LE Jr (2000) Mercury exposure and cutaneous disease. *J Am Acad Dermatol* 43: 81–90

57 Rishler JF, Amler SN (2005) Mercury exposure: Evaluation and intervention in the inappropriate use of chelation agents in the diagnosis and treatment of putative mercury poisoning. *Neurotoxicology* 26: 691–699

58 Chang LW, Verity MA (1995) Mercury neurotoxicity: Effects and mechanisms. In: LW Chang, RS Dyer (eds): *Handbook of Neurotoxicology*. Marcel Dekker, New York, 31–59

59 Henningsson C, Hoffmann S, McGonigle L (1993) Acute mercury poisoning (acrodynia) mimicking pheochromocytoma in an adolescent. *J Pediatr* 122: 252–253

60 Torres AD, Ashok NR, Hardiek ML (2000) Mercury intoxication and arterial hypertension: Report of two patients and review of the literature. *Pediatrics* 105: E34

61 Wossmann W, Kohl M, Gruning G, Bucsky P (1999) Mercury intoxication presenting with hypertension and tachycardia. *Arch Dis Childhood* 80: 556–557

62 Finkelstein Y, Vardi J, Kesten MM, Hod I (1996) The enigma of parkinsonism in chronic borderline mercury intoxication, resolved by challenge with penicillamine. *Neurotoxicology* 17: 291–295

63 Miller K, Ochudlo S, Opala G, Smolicha W, Siuda J (2003) Parkinsonism in chronic occupational metallic mercury intoxication. *Neurol Neurochir Pol* 37 Suppl 5: 31–38

64 Ngim CH, Devathasan G (1989) Epidemiologic study on the association between body burden mercury level and idiopathic Parkinson's disease. *Neuroepidemiology* 8: 128–141

65 Ohlson CG, Hogstedt C (1981) Parkinson's disease and occupational exposure to organic solvents, agricultural chemicals and mercury – A case-referent study. *Scand J Work Environ Health* 7: 252–256

66 Cornelis R, Heinzow B, Herber R, Christensen J, Paulsen O, Sabbioni E, Templeton D, Thomassen Y, Vahter M, Vesterberg O (1995) Sample collection guidelines for trace elements in blood and urine. *Pure Appl Chem* 67: 1575–1608

67 Allain P, Mauras Y, Premel-Cabic A, Islam S, Herve JP, Cledes J (1991) Effects of an EDTA infusion on the urinary elimination of several elements in healthy subjects. *Br J Clin Pharmacol* 31: 347–349

68 Sata F, Araki S, Murata K, Aono H (1998) Behavior of heavy metals in human urine and blood following calcium disodium ethylenediamine tetraacetate injection: Observations in metal workers. *J Toxicol Environ Health A* 54: 167–178

69 Clarkson TW, Magos L, Myers GJ (2003) The toxicology of mercury – Current exposures and clinical manifestations. *N Engl J Med* 349: 1731–1737

70 Kosnett MJ (1992) Unanswered questions in metal chelation. *Clin Toxicol* 30: 529–547

71 Clarkson TW, Magos L (2006) The toxicology of mercury and its chemical compounds. *Crit Rev Toxicol* 36: 609–662

72 Vimy MJ, Takahashi Y, Lorscheider FL (1990) Maternal-fetal distribution of mercury (^{203}Hg) released from dental amalgam fillings. *Am J Physiol* 258: R939–945

73 Mutter J, Naumann J, Guethlin C (2007) Comments on the article "The toxicology of mercury and its chemical compounds" by Clarkson and Magos (2006) *Crit Rev Toxicol* 37: 537–552

74 Bates MN, Fawcett J, Garrett N, Cutress T, Kjellstrom T (2004) Health effects of dental amalgam exposure: A retrospective cohort study. *Int J Epidemiol* 33: 894–902

75 Bjorkman L, Pedersen NL, Lichtenstein P (1996) Physical and mental health related to dental amalgam fillings in Swedish twins. *Commun Dent Oral Epidemiol* 24: 260–267

76 Factor-Litvak P, Hasselgren G, Jacobs D, Begg M, Kline J, Geier J, Mervish N, Schoenholtz S, Graziano J (2003) Mercury derived from dental amalgams and neuropsychologic function. *Environ Health Perspect* 111: 719–723

77 Fung YK, Meade AG, Rack EP, Blotcky AJ (1997) Brain mercury in neurodegenerative disorders. *J Toxicol Clin Toxicol* 35: 49–54

78 Fung YK, Meade AG, Rack EP, Blotcky AJ, Claassen JP, Beatty MW, Durham T (1996) Mercury determination in nursing home patients with Alzheimer's disease. *Gen Dent* 44: 74–78

79 Nitschke I, Müller F, Smith J, Hopfenmüller W (2000) Amalgam fillings and cognitive abilities in a representative sample of the elderly population. *Gerodontology* 17: 39–44

80 Saxe SR, Snowdon DA, Wekstein MW, Henry RG, Grant FT, Donegan SJ, Wekstein DR (1995) Dental amalgam and cognitive function in older women: Findings from the Nun Study. *J Am Dent Assoc* 126: 1495–1501

81 Saxe SR, Wekstein MW, Kryscio RJ, Henry RG, Cornett CR, Snowdon DA, Grant FT, Schmitt FA, Donegan SJ, Wekstein DR, Ehmann WD, Markesbery WR (1999) Alzheimer's disease, dental amalgam and mercury. *J Am Dent Assoc* 130: 191–199

82 Langworth S, Bjorkman L, Elinder CG, Jarup L, Savlin P (2002) Multidisciplinary examination of patients with illness attributed to dental fillings. *J Oral Rehabil* 29: 705–713

83 Lygre GB, Gjerdet NR, Bjorkman L (2005) A follow-up study of patients with subjective symptoms related to dental materials. *Commun Dent Oral Epidemiol* 33: 227–234

84 Berglund A, Molin M (1997) Mercury levels in plasma and urine after removal of all amalgam restorations: The effect of using rubber dams. *Dent Mater* 13: 297–304

85 Molin M, Bergman B, Marklund SL, Schutz A, Skerfving S (1990) Mercury, selenium, and glutathione peroxidase before and after amalgam removal in man. *Acta Odontol Scand* 48: 189–202

86 DeBont B, Lauwerys R, Govaerts H, Moulin D (1986) Yellow mercuric oxide ointment and mercury intoxication. *Eur J Pediatr* 145: 217–218

87 Yip L, Dart R, Sullivan JJ (2001) Mercury. In: JJ Sullivan, G Drieger (eds): *Clinical Environmental Health and Toxic Exposures*. Lippincott Williams & Wilkins, Philadelphia, PA, 867–879

88 Dargan P, Giles L, Wallace C, House I, Thomson A, Beale R, Jones A (2003) Case report: Severe mercuric sulphate poisoning treated with 2,3-dimercaptopropane-1-sulphonate and haemodiafiltration. *Crit Care* 7: R1–R6

89 Endo T, Nakaya S, Kimura R, Murata T (1984) Gastrointestinal absorption of inorganic mercuric compounds *in vivo* and *in situ*. *Toxicol Appl Pharmacol* 74: 223–229

90 Martin-Gil J, Martin-Gil FJ, Delibes-de-Castro G, Zapatero-Magdaleno P, Sarabia-Herrero FJ (1995) The first known use of vermillion. *Experientia* 51: 759–761

91 Sanchez-Sicilia L, Seto D, Nakamoto S, Kolff W (1963) Acute mercurial intoxication treated by hemodialysis. *Ann Intern Med* 59: 692–706

92 Schreiner G, Maher J (1965) Toxic nephropathy. *Am J Med* 38: 409–449

93 Newton JA, House IM, Volans GN, Goodwin FJ (1983) Plasma mercury during prolonged acute renal failure after mercuric chloride ingestion. *Hum Toxicol* 2: 535–537

94 Lund A (1956) The effect various substances on the excretion and the toxicity of thallium in the rat. *Acta Pharmacol Toxicol* 12: 260–268

95 Longcope WT, Luetscher JA Jr (1949) The use of BAL in the treatment of the injurious effects of arsenic, mercury and other metallic poisons. *Ann Intern Med* 31: 545–554

96 Baker JP (2008) Mercury, vaccines, and autism: One controversy, three histories. *Am J Pub Health* 98: 244–253

97 Harada M (1995) Minamata disease: Methylmercury poisoning in Japan caused by environmental pollution. *Crit Rev Toxicol* 25: 1–24

98 Bakir F, Damluji SF, Amin-Zaki L, Murtadha M, Khalidi A, al-Rawi NY, Tikriti S, Dahahir HI, Clarkson TW, Smith JC, Doherty RA (1973) Methylmercury poisoning in Iraq. *Science* 181: 230–241

99 Aberg B, Ekman L, Falk R, Greitz U, Persson G, Snihs JO (1969) Metabolism of methyl mercury (^{203}Hg) compounds in man. *Arch Environ Health* 19: 478–484

100 Berlin M, Carlson J, Norseth T (1975) Dose-dependence of methylmercury metabolism. A study of distribution: Biotransformation and excretion in the squirrel monkey. *Arch Environ Health* 30: 307–313

101 Eto K (2000) Minamata disease. *Neuropathology* 20: S14–19

102 Eto K, Tokunaga H, Nagashima K, Takeuchi T (2002) An autopsy case of minamata disease (methylmercury poisoning) – Pathological viewpoints of peripheral nerves. *Toxicol Pathol* 30: 714–722

103 Harada M (1978) Congenital Minamata disease: Intrauterine methylmercury poisoning. *Teratology* 18: 285–288

104 Kondo K (2000) Congenital Minamata disease: Warnings from Japan's experience. *J Child*

Neurol 15: 458–464

105 Bakir F, Rustam H, Tikriti S, Al-Damluji SF, Shihristani H (1980) Clinical and epidemiological aspects of methylmercury poisoning. *Postgrad Med J* 56: 1–10

106 Nierenberg DW, Nordgren RE, Chang MB, Siegler RW, Blayney MB, Hochberg F, Toribara TY, Cernichiari E, Clarkson T (1998) Delayed cerebellar disease and death after accidental exposure to dimethylmercury. *N Engl J Med* 338: 1672–1676

107 Aaseth J, Frieheim EA (1978) Treatment of methyl mercury poisoning in mice with 2,3-dimercaptosuccinic acid and other complexing thiols. *Acta Pharmacol Toxicol* 42: 248–252

108 Zimmer LJ, Carter DE (1978) The efficacy of 2,3-dimercaptopropanol and D-penicillamine on methyl mercury induced neurological signs and weight loss. *Life Sci* 23: 1025–1034

109 Axton JH (1972) Six cases of poisoning after a parenteral organic mercurial compound (Merthiolate). *Postgrad Med J* 48: 417–421

110 Fagan DG, Pritchard JS, Clarkson TW, Greenwood MR (1977) Organ mercury levels in infants with omphaloceles treated with organic mercurial antiseptic. *Arch Dis Child* 52: 962–964

111 Lowell JA, Burgess S, Shenoy S, Peters M, Howard TK (1996) Mercury poisoning associated with hepatitis-B immunoglobulin. *Lancet* 347: 480

112 Pfab R, Mückter H, Roider G, Zilker T (1996) Clinical course of severe poisoning with thiomersal. *J Toxicol Clin Toxicol* 34: 453–460

113 Rohyans J, Walson PD, Wood GA, MacDonald WA (1984) Mercury toxicity following merthiolate ear irrigations. *J Pediatr* 104: 311–313

114 Gibson S (1976) Memorandum from Assistant Diretor, Bureau of Biologics, FDA to Director, Bureau of Biologics, FDA entitled "Use of thimerosol in biologics production". February 27, 1976

115 Ball LK, Ball R, Pratt RD (2001) An assessment of thimerosal use in childhood vaccines. *Pediatrics* 107: 1147–1154

116 Bigham M, Copes R (2005) Thiomersal in vaccines: Balancing the risk of adverse effects with the risk of vaccine-preventable disease. *Drug Saf* 28: 89–101

117 Hviid A, Stellfeld M, Wohlfahrt J, Melbye M (2003) Association between thimerosal-containing vaccine and autism. *J Am Med Assoc* 290: 1763–1766

118 Thompson WW, Price C, Goodson B, Shay DK, Benson P, Hinrichsen VL, Lewis E, Eriksen E, Ray P, Marcy SM, Dunn J, Jackson LA, Lieu TA, Black S, Stewart G, Weintraub ES, Davis RL, DeStefano F (2007) Early thimerosal exposure and neuropsychological outcomes at 7 to 10 years. *N Engl J Med* 357: 1281–1292

119 Verstraeten T, Davis RL, DeStefano F, Lieu TA, Rhodes PH, Black SB, Shinefield H, Chen RT (2003) Safety of thimerosal-containing vaccines: A two-phased study of computerized health maintenance organization databases. *Pediatrics* 112: 1039–1048

120 Immunization Safety Review Committee (2004) *Vaccines and Autism.* The National Academies Press, Institute of Medicine (online available at: http://www.nap.edu/openbook.php?isbn= 030909237X)

121 Global Advisory Committee on Vaccine Safety (2003) *Statement on Thimerosal.* World Health Organization (online available at: http://www.who.int/vaccine_safety/topics/thiomersal/statment _jul2006/en/index.html)

122 Lyketsos CG (2003) Should pregnant women avoid eating fish? Lessons from the Seychelles. *Lancet* 361: 1667–1668

123 Myers GJ, Davidson PW, Cox C, Shamlaye CF, Palumbo D, Cernichiari E, Sloane-Reeves J, Wilding GE, Kost J, Huang LS, Clarkson TW (2003) Prenatal methylmercury exposure from ocean fish consumption in the Seychelles child development study. *Lancet* 361: 1686–1692

124 Davidson PW, Myers GJ, Cox C, Axtell C, Shamlaye C, Sloane-Reeves J, Cernichiari E, Needham L, Choi A, Wang Y, Berlin M, Clarkson TW (1998) Effects of prenatal and postnatal methylmercury exposure from fish consumption on neurodevelopment: Outcomes at 66 months of age in the Seychelles Child Development Study. *J Am Med Assoc* 280: 701–707

125 Grandjean P, Weihe P, White RF, Debes F, Araki S, Yokoyama K, Murata K, Sorensen N, Dahl R, Jorgensen PJ (1997) Cognitive deficit in 7-year-old children with prenatal exposure to methylmercury. *Neurotoxicol Teratol* 19: 417–428

126 Hernberg S (2000) Lead poisoning in a historical perspective. *Am J Ind Med* 38: 244–254

127 Waldron HA (1969) James Hardy and the Devonshire Colic. *Med Hist* 13: 74–81

128 Felton JS (1967) Man, medicine, and work in America: A historical series. 3. Benjamin Franklin and his awareness of lead poisoning. *J Occup Med* 9: 543–554

129 Jacobs DE, Clickner RP, Zhou JY, Viet SM, Marker DA, Rogers JW, Zeldin DC, Broene P, Friedman W (2002) The prevalence of lead-based paint hazards in U.S. housing. *Environ Health Perspect* 110: A599–606

130 CDC (2005) Blood lead levels – United States, 1999–2002. *MMWR – Morb Mortal Wkly Rep* 54: 513–516

131 Haley VB, Talbot TO (2004) Seasonality and trend in blood lead levels of New York State children. *BMC Pediatr* 4: 8

132 Goldstein GW (1992) Neurologic concepts of lead poisoning in children. *Pediatr Ann* 21: 384–388

133 CDC (2004) Lead poisoning from ingestion of a toy necklace – Oregon, 2003. *MMWR – Morb Mortal Wkly Rep* 53: 509–511

134 Sokolowski MJ, Sisson G Jr (2005) Systemic lead poisoning due to an intra-articular bullet. *Orthopedics* 28: 411–412

135 CDC (1992) Elevated blood lead levels associated with illicitly distilled alcohol – Alabama, 1990–1991. *MMWR – Morb Mortal Wkly Rep* 41: 294–295

136 Holstege CP, Ferguson JD, Wolf CE, Baer AB, Poklis A (2004) Analysis of moonshine for contaminants. *J Toxicol Clin Toxicol* 42: 597–601

137 Lidsky TI, Schneider JS (2003) Lead neurotoxicity in children: Basic mechanisms and clinical correlates. *Brain* 126: 5–19

138 Piomelli S (1981) Chemical toxicity of red cells. *Environ Health Perspect* 39: 65–70

139 Albahary C (1972) Lead and hemopoiesis. The mechanism and consequences of the erythropathy of occupational lead poisoning. *Am J Med* 52: 367–378

140 Cheson BD, Rom WN, Webber RC (1984) Basophilic stippling of red blood cells: A nonspecific finding of multiple etiology. *Am J Ind Med* 5: 327–334

141 Levander OA (1979) Lead toxicity and nutritional deficiencies. *Environ Health Perspect* 29: 115–125

142 Loghman-Adham M (1997) Renal effects of environmental and occupational lead exposure. *Environ Health Perspect* 105: 928–939

143 Rabinowitz MB (1991) Toxicokinetics of bone lead. *Environ Health Perspect* 91: 33–37

144 Rastogi S, Nandlike K, Fenster W (2007) Elevated blood lead levels in pregnant women: Identification of a high-risk population and interventions. *J Perinat Med* 35: 492–496

145 Sachs HK (1981) The evolution of the radiologic lead line. *Radiology* 139: 81–85

146 Prozialeck WC, Edwards JR, Nebert DW, Woods JM, Barchowsky A, Atchison WD (2008) The vascular system as a target of metal toxicity. *Toxicol Sci* 102: 207–218

147 Canfield RL, Henderson CR Jr, Cory-Slechta DA, Cox C, Jusko TA, Lanphear BP (2003) Intellectual impairment in children with blood lead concentrations below 10 microg per deciliter. *N Engl J Med* 348: 1517–1526

148 Pocock SJ, Smith M, Baghurst P (1994) Environmental lead and children's intelligence: A systematic review of the epidemiological evidence. *BMJ* 309: 1189–1197

149 Koller K, Brown T, Spurgeon A, Levy L (2004) Recent developments in low-level lead exposure and intellectual impairment in children. *Environ Health Perspect* 112: 987–994

150 Henretig FM (2006) Lead. In: NE Flomenbaum, LR Goldfrank, RS Hoffman, MA Howland, NA Lewin, LS Nelson (eds): *Goldfrank's Toxicologic Emergencies*. 8th edn., McGraw-Hill, New York, 1308–1334

151 Cullen MR, Robins JM, Eskenazi B (1983) Adult inorganic lead intoxication: Presentation of 31 new cases and a review of recent advances in the literature. *Medicine (Baltimore)* 62: 221–247

152 Baker EL, Feldman RG, White RA, Harley JP, Niles CA, Dinse GE, Berkey CS (1984) Occupational lead neurotoxicity: A behavioural and electrophysiological evaluation. Study design and year one results. *Br J Ind Med* 41: 352–361

153 Erenberg G, Rinsler SS, Fish BG (1974) Lead neuropathy and sickle cell disease. *Pediatrics* 54: 438–441

154 Nawrot TS, Thijs L, Den Hond EM, Roels HA, Staessen JA (2002) An epidemiological re-appraisal of the association between blood pressure and blood lead: A meta-analysis. *J Hum Hypertens* 16: 123–131

155 Navas-Acien A, Schwartz BS, Rothenberg SJ, Hu H, Silbergeld EK, Guallar E (2008) Bone lead levels and blood pressure endpoints: A meta-analysis. *Epidemiology* 19: 496–504

156 Assennato G, Paci C, Baser ME, Molinini R, Candela RG, Altamura BM, Giorgino R (1987) Sperm count suppression without endocrine dysfunction in lead-exposed men. *Arch Environ*

Health 42: 124–127

157 Counter SA, Buchanan LH, Ortega F (2004) Current pediatric and maternal lead levels in blood and breast milk in Andean inhabitants of a lead-glazing enclave. *J Occup Environ Med* 46: 967–973

158 IARC (1987) *Overall Evaluation of Carcinogenicity: An Updating of IARC Monographs*, Vols. 1 to 42. International Agency for Research on Cancer (IARC), Lyon, 230–232

159 Steenland K, Boffetta P (2000) Lead and cancer in humans: Where are we now? *Am J Ind Med* 38: 295–299

160 Boeckx RL, Postl B, Coodin FJ (1977) Gasoline sniffing and tetraethyl lead poisoning in children. *Pediatrics* 60: 140–145

161 Anderson MK, Amrich M, Decker KL, Mervis CA (2007) Using state lead poisoning surveillance system data to assess false positive results of capillary testing. *Matern Child Health J* 11: 603–610

162 Martin CJ, Werntz CL 3rd, Ducatman AM (2004) The interpretation of zinc protoporphyrin changes in lead intoxication: A case report and review of the literature. *Occup Med* 54: 587–591

163 Hu H, Shih R, Rothenberg S, Schwartz BS (2007) The epidemiology of lead toxicity in adults: Measuring dose and consideration of other methodologic issues. *Environ Health Perspect* 115: 455–462

164 American Academy of Pediatrics Committee on Environmental Health (2005) Lead exposure in children: Prevention, detection, and management. *Pediatrics* 116: 1036–1046

165 Yeoh B, Woolfenden S, Wheeler D, Alperstein G, Lanphear B (2008) Household interventions for prevention of domestic lead exposure in children. *Cochrane Database Syst Rev*: CD006047

166 Rogan WJ, Dietrich KN, Ware JH, Dockery DW, Salganik M, Radcliffe J, Jones RL, Ragan NB, Chisolm JJ Jr, Rhoads GG (2001) The effect of chelation therapy with succimer on neuropsychological development in children exposed to lead. *N Engl J Med* 344: 1421–1426

167 De Groot G, van Heijst AN, van Kesteren RG, Maes RA (1985) An evaluation of the efficacy of charcoal haemoperfusion in the treatment of three cases of acute thallium poisoning. *Arch Toxicol* 57: 61–66

168 Besunder JB, Super DM, Anderson RL (1997) Comparison of dimercaptosuccinic acid and calcium disodium ethylenediaminetetraacetic acid *versus* dimercaptopropanol and ethylenediaminetetraacetic acid in children with lead poisoning. *J Pediatr* 130: 966–971

169 Brown MJ, Willis T, Omalu B, Leiker R (2006) Deaths resulting from hypocalcemia after administration of edetate disodium: 2003–2005. *Pediatrics* 118: e534–536

170 Lehmann PA, Favari L (1984) Parameters for the adsorption of thallium ions by activated charcoal and Prussian blue. *J Toxicol Clin Toxicol* 22: 331–339

171 De Backer W, Zachee P, Verpooten GA, Majelyne W, Vanheule A, De Broe ME (1982) Thallium intoxication treated with combined hemoperfusion-hemodialysis. *J Toxicol Clin Toxicol* 19: 259–264

172 Hologgitas J, Ullucci P, Driscoll J, Grauerholz J, Martin H (1980) Thallium elimination kinetics in acute thallotoxicosis. *J Anal Toxicol* 4: 68–75

173 Clifton JC 2nd, Sigg T, Burda AM, Leikin JB, Smith CJ, Sandler RH (2002) Acute pediatric lead poisoning: Combined whole bowel irrigation, succimer therapy, and endoscopic removal of ingested lead pellets. *Pediatr Emerg Care* 18: 200–202

174 James FA (1984) Of 'Medals and Muddles' the context of the discovery of thallium: William Crookes's early spectro-chemical work. *Notes Rec R Soc Lond* 39: 65–90

175 Douglas KT, Bunni MA, Baindur SR (1990) Thallium in biochemistry. *Int J Biochem* 22: 429–438

176 Gehring PJ, Hammond PB (1967) The interrelationship between thallium and potassium in animals. *J Pharmacol Exp Ther* 155: 187–201

177 Melnick RL, Monti LG, Motzkin SM (1976) Uncoupling of mitochondrial oxidative phosphorylation by thallium. *Biochem Biophy Res Commun* 69: 68–73

178 Mulkey JP, Oehme FW (1993) A review of thallium toxicity. *Vet Hum Toxicol* 35: 445–453

179 Lund A (1956) Distribution of thallium in the organism and its elimination. *Acta Pharmacol Toxicol* 12: 251–259

180 Malbrain ML, Lambrecht GL, Zandijk E, Demedts PA, Neels HM, Lambert W, De Leenheer AP, Lins RL, Daelemans R (1997) Treatment of severe thallium intoxication. *J Toxicol Clin Toxicol* 35: 97–100

181 Reed D, Crawley J, Faro SN, Pieper SJ, Kurland LT (1963) Thallotoxicosis. *J Am Med Assoc* 183:

516–522

182 Rusyniak DE, Furbee RB, Kirk MS (2002) Thallium and arsenic poisoning in a small midwest town. *Ann Emerg Med* 39: 307–311

183 Meggs WJ, Hoffman RS, Shih RD, Weisman RS, Goldfrank LR (1994) Thallium poisoning from maliciously contaminated food. *J Toxicol Clin Toxciol* 32: 723–730

184 Misra UK, Kalita J, Yadav RK, Ranjan P (2003) Thallium poisoning: Emphasis on early diagnosis and response to haemodialysis. *Postgrad Med J* 79: 103–105

185 Chamberlain PH, Stavinoha WB, Davis H, Kniker WT, Panos TC (1958) Thallium poisoning. *Pediatrics* 22: 1170–1182

186 Desenclos JC, Wilder MH, Coppenger GW, Sherin K, Tiller R, van Hook RM (1992) Thallium poisoning: An outbreak in Florida, 1988. *South Med J* 85: 1203–1206

187 Prick JJG, Sillevis Smitt WG, Muller L (1955) *Thallium Poisoning.* Elsevier Publishing, Amsterdam

188 Cavanagh JB, Fuller NH, Johnson HRM (1974) The effects of thallium salts, with particular reference to the nervous system changes. A report of three cases. *Q J Med* 170: 293–319

189 Davis LE, Standefer JC, Kornfeld M, Abercrombie DM, Butler C (1980) Acute thallium poisoning: Toxicological and morphological studies of the nervous system. *Ann Neurol* 10: 38–44

190 Hoffman RS (2003) Thallium toxicity and the role of Prussian blue in therapy. *Toxicol Rev* 22: 29–40

191 Tabandeh H, Crowston JG, Thompson GM (1994) Ophthalmologic features of thallium poisoning. *Am J Ophthal* 117: 243–245

192 Feldman J, Levisohn DR (1993) Acute alopecia: Clue to thallium toxicity. *Pediatr Dermatol* 10: 29–31

193 Heyl T, Barlow RJ (1989) Thallium poisoning: A dermatological perspective. *Br J Dermatol* 121: 787–791

194 Moeschlin S (1980) Thallium poisoning. *Clin Toxicol* 17: 133–146

195 Koblenzer PJ, Weiner LB (1969) Alopecia secondary to thallium intoxication. *Arch Dermatol* 99: 777

196 Cavanagh JB, Gregson M (1978) Some effects of a thallium salt on the proliferation of hair follicle cells. *J Pathol* 125: 179–191

197 Tromme I, van Neste D, Dobbelaere F, Bouffioux B, Courtin C, Dugernier T, Pierre P, Dupuis M (1998) Skin signs in the diagnosis of thallium poisoning. *Br J Dermatol* 138: 321–325

198 Saha A, Sadhu HG, Karnik AB, Patel TS, Sinha SN, Saiyed HN (2004) Erosion of nails following thallium poisoning: A case report. *Occup Environ Med* 61: 640–642

199 Bank WJ, Pleasure DE, Suzuki K, Nigro M, Katz R (1972) Thallium poisoning. *Arch Neurol* 26: 456–464

200 Roby DS, Fein AM, Bennett RH, Morgan LS, Zatuchni J, Lippmann ML (1984) Cardiopulmonary effects of acute thallium poisoning. *Chest* 85: 236–240

201 Moore D, House I, Dixon A (1993) Thallium poisoning. Diagnosis may be elusive but alopecia is the clue. *BMJ* 306: 1527–1529

202 Cavanagh JB (1979) The 'dying back' process. A common denominator in many naturally occurring and toxic neuropathies. *Arch Pathol Lab Med* 103: 659–664

203 Cavanagh JB (1991) What have we learnt from Graham Frederick Young? Reflections on the mechanism of thallium neurotoxicity. *Neuropathol Appl Neurobiol* 17: 3–9

204 Metter D, Vock R (1984) [Structure of the hair in thallium poisoning]. *Zeitschr Rechtsmed J Leg Med* 91: 201–214

205 Wecht C, Saitz G (2007) *Mortal Evidence: The Forensics Behind Nine Shocking Cases.* Prometheus Books, New York

206 Barroso-Moguel R, Villeda-Hernandez J, Mendez-Armenta M, Rios C, Monroy-Noyola A (1994) Combined D-penicillamine and Prussian blue as antidotal treatment against thallotoxicosis in rats: Evaluation of cerebellar lesions. *Toxicology* 89: 15–24

207 Heydlauf H (1969) Ferric-cyanoferrate (II): An effective antidote in thallium poisoning. *Eur J Pharmacol* 6: 340–344

208 Kamerbeek HH, Rauws AG, ten Ham M, van Heijst AN (1971) Dangerous redistribution of thallium by treatment with sodium diethyldithiocarbamate. *Acta Med Scand* 189: 149–154

209 Manninen V, Malkonen M, Skulskii IA (1976) Elimination of thallium in rats as influenced by Prussian blue and sodium chloride. *Acta Pharmacol Toxicol* 39: 256–261

210 Meggs WJ, Cahill-Morasco R, Shih RD, Goldfrank LR, Hoffman RS (1997) Effects of Prussian

blue and N-acetylcysteine on thallium toxicity in mice. *J Toxicol Clin Toxicol* 35: 163–166

211 Rauws AG (1974) Thallium pharmacokinetics and its modification by Prussian blue. *Naunyn Schmiedebergs Arch Pharmacol* 284: 295–306.

212 Rios C, Monroy-Noyola A (1992) D-Penicillamine and Prussian blue as antidotes against thallium intoxication in rats. *Toxicology* 74: 69–76

213 Rusyniak DE, Kao LW, Nanagas KA, Kirk MA, Furbee RB, Brizendine EJ, Wilmot PE (2003) Dimercaptosuccinic acid and Prussian blue in the treatment of acute thallium poisoning in rats. *J Toxicol Clin Toxicol* 41: 137–142

214 Pearce J (1994) Studies of any toxicological effects of Prussian blue compounds in mammals – A review. *Food Chem Toxicol* 32: 577–582

215 Lund A (1956) The effect various substances on the excretion and the toxicity of thallium in the rat. *Acta Pharmacol Toxicol* 12: 260–268.

216 Mulkey JP, Oehme FW (2000) Are 2,3-dimercapto-1-propanesulfonic acid or Prussian blue beneficial in acute thallotoxicosis in rats? *Vet Hum Toxicol* 42: 325–329

217 Van der Stock J, Schepper J (1978) The effect of Prussian blue and sodium-ethylenediaminetetraacetic acid on the faecal and urinary elimination of thallium by the dog. *Res Vet Sci* 25: 337–342

218 Hoffman RS, Stringer JA, Feinberg RS, Goldfrank LR (1999) Comparative efficacy of thallium adsorption by activated charcoal, Prussian blue, and sodium polystyrene sulfonate. *J Toxicol Clin Toxicol* 37: 833–837

Molecular, Clinical and Environmental Toxicology. Volume 2: Clinical Toxicology
Edited by A. Luch

Drugs and pharmaceuticals: management of intoxication and antidotes

Silas W. Smith

New York City Poison Control Center, New York University School of Medicine, New York, USA

Abstract. The treatment of patients poisoned with drugs and pharmaceuticals can be quite challenging. Diverse exposure circumstances, varied clinical presentations, unique patient-specific factors, and inconsistent diagnostic and therapeutic infrastructure support, coupled with relatively few definitive antidotes, may complicate evaluation and management. The historical approach to poisoned patients (patient arousal, toxin elimination, and toxin identification) has given way to rigorous attention to the fundamental aspects of basic life support – airway management, oxygenation and ventilation, circulatory competence, thermoregulation, and substrate availability. Selected patients may benefit from methods to alter toxin pharmacokinetics to minimize systemic, target organ, or tissue compartment exposure (either by decreasing absorption or increasing elimination). These may include syrup of ipecac, orogastric lavage, activated single- or multi-dose charcoal, whole bowel irrigation, endoscopy and surgery, urinary alkalinization, saline diuresis, or extracorporeal methods (hemodialysis, charcoal hemoperfusion, continuous venovenous hemofiltration, and exchange transfusion). Pharmaceutical adjuncts and antidotes may be useful in toxicant-induced hyperthermias. In the context of analgesic, anti-inflammatory, anticholinergic, anticonvulsant, antihyperglycemic, antimicrobial, antineoplastic, cardiovascular, opioid, or sedative-hypnotic agents overdose, *N*-acetylcysteine, physostigmine, ʟ-carnitine, dextrose, octreotide, pyridoxine, dexrazoxane, leucovorin, glucarpidase, atropine, calcium, digoxin-specific antibody fragments, glucagon, high-dose insulin euglycemia therapy, lipid emulsion, magnesium, sodium bicarbonate, naloxone, and flumazenil are specifically reviewed. In summary, patients generally benefit from aggressive support of vital functions, careful history and physical examination, specific laboratory analyses, a thoughtful consideration of the risks and benefits of decontamination and enhanced elimination, and the use of specific antidotes where warranted. Data supporting antidotes effectiveness vary considerably. Clinicians are encouraged to utilize consultation with regional poison centers or those with toxicology training to assist with diagnosis, management, and administration of antidotes, particularly in unfamiliar cases.

Introduction

The challenges to effective evaluation and management of a patient poisoned by drugs and pharmaceuticals are diverse. The circumstances surrounding exposure are often incompletely accessible. Poisoning signs or symptoms may be subtle or delayed. Patient-specific factors – pharmacogenetics and unique susceptibilities, drug-drug interactions, cultural or geographic practices, and underlying comorbidities – may complicate presentation, response to treatment, and outcome. Polypharmacy or mixed exposures may confuse the clinical presentation. Compared to the near-inexhaustible list of products and possible combinations, few specific antidotes exist. The toxicological profiles of newly introduced pharmaceuticals may be incompletely characterized or unfamiliar to the treating practitioner. Finally, medical infrastructure may offer inconsistent support for diagnosis (*via* monitoring, radiological, or laboratory equipment) or treatment (through clinical service capacities or specific antidotes' availability). This chapter seeks to provide a rational approach to treatment of the poisoned patient and the use of specific antidotes where warranted.

General approach to the poisoned patient

The historical approach to poisoned patients placed undue emphasis on three areas – patient arousal, toxin elimination, and toxin identification. Beginning in the early 1900s in the setting of increased barbiturate poisonings and the limitations of airway management of the time, a sense of compulsion to "awaken" patients resulted in administration of various analeptics (from the Greek *analeptikos* – restorative, strengthening). These arousal agents included proconvulsants (picrotoxin, strychnine, pentylenetetrazol, and camphor), as well as sympathomimetics (amphetamines and methylphenidate), xanthines (caffeine, ethamivan), and nonspecific stimulants such as nikethamide, bemegride, prethcamide, and amiphenazole [1–6]. More recent "coma cocktails" have variously included dextrose or glucagon, thiamine, naloxone, flumazenil, and physostigmine [7–9]. This concept of the utility of nonselective "coma cocktails" persists despite efforts to educate on the risks of this paradigm [10].

Aggressive efforts to antagonize central nervous system (CNS) and respiratory depression were joined with similarly forceful measures aimed at detoxification, with the conviction that as much of any toxin should be removed as possible. Prehospital or in-hospital administration of apomorphine or emetics of ipecac, saltwater, mustard water, copper sulfate, zinc sulfate, antimony or potassium tartrate were once routinely recommended [11–13]. Binding agents such as Fullers earth and later, activated charcoal, kayexalate, and cholestyramine were introduced into clinical practice, and orogastric lavage and evacuants such as mercurials, saline, magnesium salts, sorbitol and whole bowel irrigation were enthusiastically endorsed [14].

Lastly, excessive emphasis was placed on determining the type, nature, and quantity of the drug ingested. Indeed, according to the "principles of therapy" of the time, toxin identification, removal, and dilution (in order of importance) *preceded* support of vital functions [15].

A more rational approach to poisoning (specifically by barbiturates) began in Denmark and Sweden in the late 1940s [16]. This "Scandinavian method" emphasized "close and constant attention to the support of vital functions" – i.e., cardiovascular and pulmonary support – as opposed to aggressive gastrointestinal decontamination and stimulant administration. Mortality consequently decreased precipitously from upwards of 20% to 1–2%. Initially derided as "pharmacotherapeutic nihilism", it was ultimately accepted that "intensive supportive therapy alone" sufficed for the vast majority of patients [17].

Thus, most poisoned patients can be treated in a straightforward manner that focuses on the patient, as opposed to the poison. Rigorous attention to the fundamental aspects of basic life support – airway management, oxygenation and ventilation, circulatory competence, thermoregulation, and substrate (glucose) availability – ensures good outcome in the vast majority of poisoned patients. An algorithmic strategy is summarized in Figure 1, realizing that many actions may occur simultaneously.

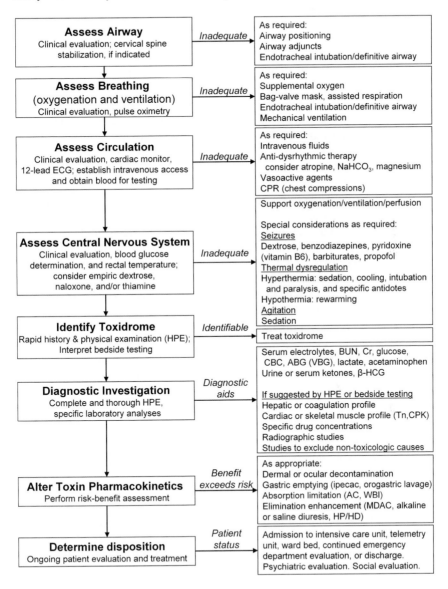

Figure 1. An algorithmic approach to the poisoned patient.

The specific details of the following maneuvers are explained in detail in emergency medicine, critical care, and anesthesiology textbooks and reviews. The patient is first assessed for airway patency and adequacy, with cervical spine stabilization if required. An inadequate airway mandates attention with airway positioning *via* head-tilt chin-lift or jaw thrust, airway adjuncts (nasopharyngeal or oropharyngeal airways), or endotracheal intubation (or surgical airway), depending upon circumstances. Inadequate breathing from either an oxygenation or ventilation standpoint is rectified with supplemental oxygen, assisted mask ventilation, or endotracheal intubation and mandatory mechanical ventilation.

Circulation is then assessed by clinical evaluation and adjuncts such as continuous cardiac monitoring and a 12-lead ECG, and intravenous (i.v.) access is obtained with simultaneous retrieval of blood for testing. Hypotension may necessitate resuscitation with i.v. fluids, colloids, or blood products, inotropic or chronotropic agents, anti-dysrhythmic therapy, or active chest compressions (CPR, cardio-pulmonary resuscitation). Conversely, life-threatening hypertension (from sympathomimetics, monoamine oxidase inhibitors, clonidine withdrawal, etc.) may require vasodilatory agents. In general, easily titratable, short-acting, direct agonists or antagonists that do not require metabolic conversion for activation are preferred – e.g., norepinephrine, phenylephrine, or epinephrine for hypotension, and nitroprusside, nitroglycerine, or phentolamine for hypertension. In the setting of a poisoned patient with a wide-complex dysrhythmia, empiric administration of sodium bicarbonate should be considered given the number of agents with cardiac sodium channel antagonism (cyclic antidepressants, Vaughan-Williams class IA and IC agents, cocaine, diphenhydramine, bupropion, propoxyphene, venlafaxine, carbamazepine, amantidine, lamotrigine, etc.). Similarly, as numerous medications are capable of inducing QT prolongation (citalopram, methadone, antipsychotics, etc.), in the setting of polymorphic ventricular tachycardia, torsade de pointes, or significantly abnormal QT interval, administration of magnesium might be advisable.

CNS manifestations of pharmaceutical intoxication are broad and may include depression or coma (e.g., benzodiazepines, barbiturates, opioids, and lithium), agitation with or without delirium (e.g., sympathomimetics, anticholinergics, and salicylates), apparent cerebrovascular accident (e.g., hypoglycemia secondary to sulfonylureas, propranolol, quinine, or salicylates), or frank seizures (e.g., bupropion, isoniazid, methylxanthines, sedative-hypnotic withdrawal, and sympathomimetics). The primary consideration is maintenance of an appropriate homeostatic milieu with adequate oxygenation, ventilation, and perfusion. During the assessment of a patient's mental status, a core (rectal) temperature should be obtained as well as bedside determination of blood glucose. Hyperthermia may be secondary to the drug itself, agitation, seizure activity, failure of feedback mechanisms, or reflect an environmental contribution. It must be immediately addressed by rapid cooling to below 38.9 °C. Failure to do so may result in irreversible cerebral injury, seizure, rhabdomyolysis, myoglobin-associated renal failure, coagulopathy, or other organ injury. Specific management of toxicant-induced hyperthermias follows later. Hypothermia may require active or passive rewarming techniques. Clinical hypoglycemia, which implies neuroglycopenia, must be rapidly reversed with administration of 0.5–1.0 g/kg of age-appropriate dextrose-containing solutions (D50 in adults, D25 in children, and D10 in neonates). Benzodiazepines (e.g., diazepam, midazolam, and lorazepam) are generally well tolerated and are first line agents for drug- and withdrawal-induced seizures and agitation. Persistent or refractory seizures should prompt consideration of empiric administration of pyridoxine and barbiturates (phenobarbital, pentobarbital), propofol, or ultimately, general anesthesia. Coincident endotracheal intubation may be required. Phenytoin and non-barbiturate anticonvulsants are typically ineffective or harmful in toxin-induced seizures [18, 19]. Altered mental status should also prompt parenteral administration of 100 mg thiamine hydrochloride. Alcohol-dependent patients without clinically apparent Wernicke's encephalopathy may require at least 200 mg of parenteral thiamine to improve neurological symptoms; overt Wernicke's encephalopathy necessitates a minimum of 500 mg thiamine hydrochloride three times daily for 2–3 days [20]. Naloxone use is considered in a separate section.

Toxidromes (toxic syndromes) are characteristic signs and symptoms that correlate with exposure to certain xenobiotics. Identifying toxidromes suggests the etiology of the patient's condition and helps guide management. "Classic" class-effect toxidromes include anticholinergic, cholinergic, sedative-hypnotic, sedative-hypnotic withdrawal, opioid, and opioid withdrawal. These should be actively sought and managed if identified.

While the patient is being stabilized, diagnostic investigations including a complete and thorough history and physical examination, laboratory analyses, and radiological studies may be undertaken to further characterize the exposure and effect. For significantly compromised patients, a typical "chemistry panel" (providing electrolytes, blood urea nitrogen, creatinine, and indirectly the anion gap), a complete blood count, arterial (or venous) blood gas, and lactate are reasonable studies. Urine or serum ketones may be required to determine the etiology of acidemia. Female patients benefit from an assessment of pregnancy status. It is useful to determine a serum acetaminophen concentration in suicidal patients or those with altered consciousness, as patients with significant acetaminophen poisoning may present without a toxidrome. Serum acetaminophen is detectable in 2–3% of patients without a reported history of ingestion; treatable concentrations are found slightly less frequently [21, 22]. Toxin-specific studies and other serum determinations are often not rapidly returned and should be obtained only if suggested by the history, physical examination, or bedside testing. Urine drug screening (UDS) is of minimal use in the acute management of intoxication. Results are not typically returned for hours; a reported "positive" substance may not be the proximate cause of the presenting condition (as the measured metabolites may persist in urine for days to weeks); and the UDS lacks sensitivity and specificity (particularly for opioids, benzodiazepines and other sedative-hypnotics, and amphetamines).

Selected patients may benefit from methods to alter toxin pharmacokinetics – limiting exposure. A discussion of these modalities and their risks and benefits occurs in the following section. Ultimately, patients will require disposition depending of severity of presentation and anticipated sequelae, which may range from admission to intensive care units, cardiac monitoring (telemetry) units, ward beds, continued emergency department evaluation, to discharge. A psychiatric assessment and social assessment, when appropriate, should precede release from medical care. Appropriate and early consultation with medical toxicologists or regional poison centers may also assist with diagnosis and management. In the U.S., this has been simplified by a uniform telephone number (1.800.222.1222) for regional poison center consultation. The International Programme on Chemical Safety (IPCS) maintains a world directory of poison centers (http://www.who.int/ipcs/poisons/centre/directory/en/).

Adjuncts to alter toxicant pharmacokinetics

Adjuncts to alter toxicant pharmacokinetics aim to minimize systemic exposure (either by decreasing absorption or increasing elimination) or to minimize exposure of a target organ or tissue compartment. In practice, this is achieved by expulsion or removal from the upper gastrointestinal tract (induced emesis, gastric lavage, or endoscopy); intraluminal binding to adsorptive materials (activated charcoal); or increasing intestinal transit time (cathartics and whole bowel irrigation). Endogenous elimination may be improved by more effective urinary clearance (urinary alkalinization and forced diuresis), improved hepatobiliary clearance, or "gut dialysis" with multiple-dose activated charcoal. Rarely, hepatic metabolism is altered to preclude ultimate toxicant formation (e.g., cimetidine to mitigate production of dapsone's methemoglobinemia inducing metabolite). Exogenous clearance utilizes hemodialysis, charcoal hemoperfusion, continuous renal replacement therapies, and exchange transfusion. All the adjuncts attempt to shift where a patient lies upon a particular dose-response curve (Fig. 2).

Drug recovery following gastrointestinal emptying techniques has been inconsistent; human studies attempting to demonstrate a survival benefit of any decontamination modality are inconclusive. Randomized trials in which a control group might not receive any decontamination could be considered unethical; volunteer studies using sublethal doses of xenobiotic cannot show mortality benefit. As might be anticipated from the fact that supportive care suffices for the majority of poisoned patients, a typical study of routine administration of charcoal following oral overdose of primarily benzodiazepines, acetaminophen, and selective serotonin reuptake inhibitors could not demonstrate benefit [16, 17, 23]. Past studies have suffered from significant exclusions. Recommendations are based both on theoretical grounds (animal and *in vitro* studies demonstrating lower peak serum concentration or faster serum

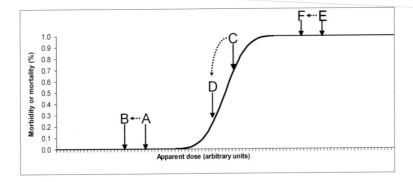

Figure 2. Adjuncts to alter toxicant pharmacokinetics attempt to shift where a patient lies upon a particular (idealized) dose-response curve. Risk will likely outweigh benefit if the patient begins at point A (negligible morbidity and mortality) and systemic exposure is reduced to B. This is the case for many drug poisonings which are managed effectively by supportive care alone. Decontamination might provide significant benefit if the patient lies upon the steep aspect of the curve [reduction from C to D – the same fixed amount as from A to B (although a percentage reduction could also be envisaged)]. With overwhelming overdose (point E), despite decontamination, benefit would be unlikely (point F).

clearance) and human studies with surrogate endpoints such as marker studies or area under the curve of plasma concentration *versus* time (AUC) improvement. Aggressive detoxification may be required for certain lethal toxins for which few antidotal options exist.

Most gastric emptying techniques are thought to be relatively ineffective beyond 1 hour. These constraints diminish possible benefit. For example, the median time from ingestion to arrival at a health care facility is on the order of 2 hours, and only about 10% of patients can be lavaged within the idealized 1-hour time frame [24]. Although in ideal situations (patients presenting early to experienced health care providers with readily available ipecac syrup) pill retrieval averages 45–55%, ipecac's benefits can be completely negated when administration is delayed as briefly as 30 min [25–28]. When orogastric lavage is performed by experienced providers within 5 min of ingestion, clinical manifestations of ingested xenobiotics have been prevented [29]. Practically, efficacy of tablet retrieval rates reduces to 45% in some cases and improvements in AUC vary from zero to 60% (averaging ~35%) [27, 30–32]. Similarly, restricting activated charcoal (AC) administration to patients presenting to health care within the first hour post ingestion would exclude up to 90% of poisoned patients from the potential benefits of AC when administered beyond an hour [24, 33]. Earlier administration of AC is more efficacious [34]. However, home and prehospital use of AC decreases the time to treatment, but has not improved clinical outcomes [35]. Drugs with opioid or anticholinergic properties that decrease peristalsis or particularly large ingestions, which independently decrease intestinal motility, may modify decision making in delayed presentations [36, 37].

Independent of side effects, the efficacy of one modality over another or combination therapy is debated. Some studies rate ipecac syrup more efficacious than orogastric lavage, but most studies have found little or no difference, and neither has been shown to be more effective than spontaneous emesis [26, 27, 31, 38]. AC has demonstrated ~50% better reductions in AUC than ipecac, which may improve or worsen its efficacy [31, 39, 40]. Gastric lavage adds no benefit to AC, except for the most critically ill patients [34, 41, 42]. Compared directly, AC has better impact than lavage on AUC and clinical effect [29, 31, 43]. Data are equivocal regarding whole bowel irrigation's ability to function similar to multiple-dose AC (MDAC) as a medium for "gut dialysis" [44, 45].

Syrup of ipecac

Syrup of ipecac is obtained from a root extract of the Amazonian flowering plant *Psychotria ipecacuanha* [46]. Its active alkaloid components, cephaeline and emetine, induce emesis *via* local irritation and central stimulation of 5-hydroxytryptamine (serotonin) 5-HT$_3$ receptors [47]. Following appropriate dose (10 mL for infants, 15–20 mL for children under 12, and 30 mL otherwise), roughly 90% of patients have a first episode of emesis within 20 min [48, 49]. Patients average three episodes in 30 min [50]. However, since ipecac's removal from most homes, the median time to administration in the acute care setting is delayed on the order of an hour, with only one-third of patients successfully vomiting within the first hour post ingestion [51].

Indications for ipecac are limited. A routinely cited example is a patient known to have taken multiple lithium tablets, which do not bind AC and may not fit through a lavage tube, who presents early to health care [50]. The American Academy of Pediatrics no longer recommends ipecac syrup for home use; ipecac use does not impact outcomes or decrease utilization of emergency services [52, 53]. Ipecac may or may not have a role in other rare ingestions that mandate gastrointestinal decontamination, but are not amenable to orogastric lavage, AC, whole bowel irrigation, or an antidote; the patient must present alert and early (<60 min post ingestion) to medical care [50].

Unsurprisingly, ipecac's most common side effect is persistent emesis. As many as eight emetic episodes occurring more than 60 min after ipecac administration have been reported [54]. This impairs administration of oral therapeutic agents, as induced emesis can last up to several hours [55]. Prolonged vomiting associated with induced sedation or absent airway reflexes increases the risk of aspiration bronchospasm, pneumonitis, and pneumonia [28, 50]. Other life-threatening side effects have been reported, including bradycardia, CNS depression, Mallory-Weiss esophageal tears, pneumomediastinum, pneumoretroperitoneum, and intracranial hemorrhage [50]. Emesis of caustics reexposes damaged esophageal mucosa to the caustic agent. Analogous pulmonary aspiration concerns accompany induced emesis of hydrocarbons.

Orogastric lavage

Orogastric lavage is performed *via* a large bore orogastric tube (adults, 36–40 French; children, 24–28 French) with fenestrae large enough to accommodate whole tablets [32]. Serial 500-mL aliquots (100–250 mL in pediatric patients) of normal saline or lactated Ringer's solution are administered and suctioned until retrieved liquid is clear. Orogastric lavage can be expected to have its best risk-to-benefit ratio when patients present early enough to have a significant gastric burden, and when severe toxicological effects are manifest or expected to become manifest [32, 42]. Because advancement of stomach contents does occur despite proper left lateral decubitus positioning [26], AC (see below) is sometimes provided prior to crystalline lavage [32, 43].

Introduction of a large, relatively rigid tube requires a cooperative patient with a protected airway (typically an endotracheal tube if the patient is ill enough to warrant gastric lavage). Orogastric lavage risks hypoxia, dysrhythmia, laryngospasm, hypothermia, gastrointestinal or pharyngeal traumatic laceration or perforation, fluid and electrolyte abnormalities, and vomiting with subsequent aspiration pneumonia [32, 56, 57].

Activated charcoal and multiple-dose activated charcoal

AC is a convoluted macromolecule created *via* pyrolysis of carbonaceous material and subsequently "activated" with steam to further increase surface area [58]. The multiple pores of various size on the surface of each macromolecule of AC account for its high adsorptive affinity for a multitude of xenobiotics – particularly chemical species that are nonionized, aromatic, and/or branched [34, 53, 59]. Maximal xenobiotic binding occurs in 10–25 min [60].

AC decreases AUC by as much as 60%, seems to improve clinical outcomes for critically ill patients, and may benefit in certain poisonings such as acetaminophen [31, 40, 61, 62]. It also increases the rate of endogenous clearance of drugs with long half-lives and some degree of entero-enteric or enterohepatic circulation [59, 63, 64]. Those findings suggested the use of MDAC as a "gut dialysis" for toxins with slow pharmacokinetics [65, 66]. A meta-analysis of volunteer studies demonstrated increased clearance of xenobiotics with longer half-lives, but not necessarily improved clinical outcome [67, 68]. MDAC has enhanced amitriptyline, carbamazepine, dapsone, dextromethorphan, phenobarbital, phenytoin, quinine, and theophylline elimination, although without definitive clinical benefit in controlled trials [63, 64, 69]. Two studies provided conflicting results for survival benefit of MDAC for yellow oleander poisoning [70, 71].

The fraction of unbound xenobiotic decreases as the charcoal-to-toxin ratio increases from 2.5:1 up to 50:1, although the yield curve levels off near 10:1 [59, 72]. In theory, the dose of AC administered to a poisoned patient would be ten times the mass of ingested xenobiotic, but those values are unknown in most clinical situations [73]. AC is practically dosed based on the patient's weight (1 g/kg), which can be divided into multiple smaller doses to be administered every 2–4 hours [59]. Although optimum dosing is unclear, MDAC is administered hourly, every 2 hours, or every 4 hours at a dose equivalent to 12.5 g/hour [66]. Pediatric charcoal doses are lower due to generally smaller ingestions and gut capacity. The total dose administered is the major determinant of efficacy particularly for larger overdoses, and can be administered continuously [74].

Emesis occurs in up to 12% of patients receiving AC; patients receiving AC *via* nasogastric tube or who vomited previously are at greater risk for emesis [75, 76]. Rarer complications include aspiration and intestinal obstruction or perforation [55, 59, 77, 78]. Aspirated AC may produce bronchiolitis obliterans, acute respiratory distress syndrome (ARDS), and death [79]. AC adheres to mucosa and obscures endoscopy; mineral acids and bases will not adhere to charcoal. AC poorly adsorbs short chain alcohols and metals such as iron, lead, and lithium [80]. AC administration requires an intact mental status or protected airway. Flavoring agents increase the palatability of AC for volunteers, but poisoned patients do not show increased compliance/tolerance with flavored AC [81].

Cathartics

Cathartics induce watery evacuation of bowel within a few hours. Hyperosmotic cathartic agents such as sorbitol are non-absorbed, osmotically active substances that draw water into the lumen, where increased intestinal volume and pressure promote peristalsis. So-called "saline" cathartic agents such as magnesium salts also directly stimulate smooth muscle to induce peristalsis [82]. Cathartics alone are not recommended for ingested poisons [83]. Cathartics have many adverse effects, including volume depletion, hypernatremia, hypermagnesemia, hyperphosphatemia, hypocalcemia, metabolic alkalosis, pain, nausea, emesis, and flatus [84, 85]. Sorbitol or laxatives are sometimes used in conjunction with the first dose of AC. While theoretically beneficial – minimizing the possible constipation of AC or promptly delivering AC to the duodenum, they do not increase the efficacy of AC [74, 86, 87]. Sorbitol is implicated in the fluid/electrolyte changes that occur with MDAC: hypermagnesemia, hypernatremia, and volume depletion [55, 84, 88]. Repetitive cathartic doses have been associated with rectal prolapse and death [89, 90].

Whole bowel irrigation

Whole bowel irrigation (WBI) employs polyethylene glycol (PEG), a large, non-absorbable organic polymer and an electrolyte lavage solution (ELS) isosmotic to serum. Large PEG-ELS volumes are introduced into the alimentary canal with less risk for fluid and electrolyte shifts caused by traditional cathartics. PEG-ELS provides non-viscous bulk for rapid transit of material in a normally functioning gastrointestinal tract. WBI should induce evacuation within 60 min, but requires 6 hours on average for complete effect. Reported improvements in AUC are modest given the more rapid absorption time for most pharmaceuticals [91]. However, reduction in AUC can be as high as 30% with poorly absorbed products or modified release preparations [92]. WBI might be considered for slowly absorbed significant ingestions such as iron, lead, and lithium, as well as modified-release preparations of β-adrenergic antagonists, bupropion, calcium-channel antagonists, carbamazepine, and theophylline [93–96]. WBI is also employed to rid patients of enterally transported illicit substances which produce toxicity upon packet rupture or leakage (e.g., cocaine, heroin, and methamphetamine) [97].

Standard dosing protocols are 1.5–2 L/h (25 mL/kg per h) enterally until rectal effluent is clear [92]. At this point, intestinal contents are assumed to have been displaced, although this is not always true [91, 98]. Nasogastric tube placement is generally required to sustain compliance with the large volume requirements, and pretreatment with an antiemetic is prudent [98]. WBI may produce nausea, vomiting, cramping, and flatus. PEG-ELS for colonoscopy has precipitated colonic perforation [99]. Unintentional bronchial administration of PEG-ELS can produce acute lung injury [100]. Ileus, obstruction, perforation or threatened perforation should preclude WBI; a protected airway is required. Desorption of toxins from AC by PEG has been demonstrated *in vitro* and *in vivo* [93, 101].

Endoscopy and surgery

Support for endoscopic therapy consists of limited case reports of retrieval in ingestions of cocaine packets, lead pellets, and medication such as sustained release calcium channel antagonists, clomipramine, iron, and meprobamate [102–106]. The procedure might be warranted for certain ingestions or cases of pharmacobezoar formation of toxic substances. Complications include perforation, aspiration, hemorrhage, and anesthetic-associated hemodynamic changes. When endoscopy fails, surgery may be required for definitive removal [107, 108]. Surgery may be required in patients with enterally transported illicit substances either due to failure of passage (with or without WBI), obstruction, or severe toxicity upon packet rupture or leakage [109, 110].

Urinary alkalinization

Weak acids in an alkaline environment exist predominantly in ionized form. Biological membranes are relatively impermeable to these charged molecules.

Alkaline serum thus inhibits the diffusion of acidic toxins (low pK_a) across cellular membranes. Similarly, an alkaline urinary pH promotes renal sequestration (or "ion-trapping") of acidic species from the systemic circulation. The relative intolerance of biological systems to acidosis limits the effectiveness of converse urinary acidification (*via* ascorbic acid or diluted HCl solutions) for renal sequestration of weak bases.

Critically ill patients may have reduced drug clearances due to decreased hepatic and renal perfusion, and thus interventions that increase clearance/elimination have the potential to significantly reduce toxicity [111]. Alkalinization improves renal elimination of chlorpropamide, 2,4-dichlorophenoxyacetic acid, diflunisal, fluoride, mecoprop, methotrexate, phenobarbital, and salicylate [112]. Urine alkalinization is considered first line therapy in patients with moderate salicylism who do not meet hemodialysis indications.

Dosing of 1–2 mEq/kg of 7.5–8.4% bicarbonate provided over 1–2 min is followed by "normal" bicarbonate infused at double the standard rate of i.v. fluid maintenance. The "normal" bicarbonate solution is prepared by adding three ampules of sodium bicarbonate (totaling 132–150 mEq) in 1 L 5% dextrose in water (D5W). The rate is titrated to maintain an alkaline urinary pH, without exceeding a serum pH of 7.55 [112].

Alkalemia decreases ionized calcium. Volume overload may occur, particularly in patients with congestive heart failure, acute renal failure, or end-stage liver disease. Bicarbonate treatment induces hypokalemia. As the proximal renal tubular cells conserve serum potassium by exchanging protons for urinary potassium, this defeats urinary alkalinization. Therefore, maintaining a normal serum potassium, with frequent monitoring and supplemental administration and/or inclusion in the bicarbonate solution, are important components of urine alkalinization.

Saline diuresis

Saline diuresis is utilized to improve excretion and minimize toxicity of overdose of ions such as magnesium, calcium, and lithium in patients who do not meet hemodialysis indications [113–115]. Hypermagnesemia may occur with excessive antacid use, gargling or ingesting magnesium sulfate compounds, and iatrogenic error [113, 116]. Hypercalcemia can result from excess calcium (in antacid tablets) or vitamin D ingestion or parenteral administration [117, 118]. Renal lithium toxicity presumably results from cytotoxic accumulation of lithium entering *via* the apical epithelial sodium channel [119]. Ensuing nephrogenic diabetes insipidus, characterized by increased water and sodium diuresis, can result in dehydration, hyperchloremic metabolic acidosis, and renal tubular acidosis. In volume depletion, activation of the renin-angiotensin-aldosterone axis leads to active resorption of sodium, and thus lithium, from the distal convoluted tubules. Therefore, adequate volume repletion with saline is prerequisite for effective renal elimination of lithium.

Boluses of 0.9% sodium chloride are administered until the patient is clinically euvolemic. Saline infusion is then provided at 1.5–2 times a standard maintenance rate. Throughout treatment renal function, urine output, and electrolytes are monitored. Congestive heart failure, renal failure, or end-stage liver disease moderate volume administration and make saline diuresis less attractive than hemodialysis in significant ingestions. Loop diuretics such as furosemide inhibit sodium resorption in the proximal convoluted tubules, and would theoretically promote elimination of lithium as natriuretics. However, these effects are countered by the action of the renin-angiotensin-aldosterone axis on the distal convoluted tubules, and diuretics do not seem to improve outcomes in lithium overdose or radiographic contrast exposure [120, 121].

Hemodialysis, charcoal hemoperfusion, and continuous renal replacement therapies

In hemodialysis (HD) the patient's blood is pumped through a circuit that includes a cartridge consisting of thousands of semi-permeable, membrane-lined capillary tubes. The blood traverses the cartridge counter-current to a circulating buffered salt solution (a.k.a. dialysate) before returning to the patient's venous circulation. Diffusible molecules flow down their electrochemical gradient from the serum to the dialysate. Hemoperfusion (HP) employs a similar circuit, but the cartridge is enveloped with AC (rather than a circulating dialysate) to adsorb xenobiotics regardless of plasma protein binding, and leave serum electrolytes largely unchanged. Continuous arteriovenous or venovenous hemofiltration (CAVH or CVVH) employ lower pressures and flow rates than HD over longer sessions for patients unable to tolerate HD or to remove xenobiotics with slow tissue redistribution [122, 123]. Peritoneal dialysis (PD) is ineffective in poisoning management, given its inherently slow kinetics and the availability of HD [124].

Extracorporeal therapies may be warranted when criteria are met for both the xenobiotic and the patient [125]. Favorable dialyzable toxin properties include low volume of distribution (V_d), relatively low molecular weight, and poor serum protein binding (or binding that worsens in overdose, as is the case for salicylate and valproate) [126]. Patient characteristics suggesting extracorporeal therapy include signs or symptoms of significant end organ toxicity; impaired elimination secondary to baseline comorbidities or critical illness-induced hypoperfusion; inability to tolerate or refractory to antidotal strategies (such as bicarbonate or saline); inadequate response to supportive care measures; concurrent electrolyte derangements (e.g., metformin-associated lactic acidosis); or serum drug concentrations historically associated with severe outcome [127]. Traditionally, charcoal HP was used for xenobiotics significantly bound to plasma proteins, but its use is declining while (high-flux membrane) HD increases.

Methanol, ethylene glycol, salicylates, lithium, halides, theophylline, and metformin-associated lactic acidosis are commonly treated with dialysis [125].

HD is used for valproate and carbamazepine poisoning; however, in the absence of high-flux dialysis membranes, the characteristics of charcoal HP may more appropriately address the larger V_d and protein binding [128].

Common side effects of extracorporeal elimination include hypotension, bleeding, and infection. Enhanced clearance of therapeutic medications and antidotes (e.g., antibiotics, fomepizole, N-acetylcysteine, water-soluble vitamins) may occur. The need for dialysis must be anticipated early; several hours of preparation time may be required to secure vascular access, equipment, and personnel.

Exchange transfusion

Exchange transfusion is a total blood volume exchange administered in small aliquots. Serial frequent phlebotomy of a small amount of circulating blood occurs with simultaneous transfusion of equivalent donor blood. This process is repeated until two to four vascular volumes have been exchanged. While the procedure is very rarely used for toxin removal, exchange transfusion is more familiar to clinicians treating severe hemolytic diseases of the newborn, hyperbilirubinemia without hemolysis, and sickle cell crisis.

Exchange transfusion removes xenobiotics that are large or bound to plasma proteins, such as thyroxine, iron, or theophylline [129, 130]. For lifethreatening ingestions, exchange transfusion is a viable option for neonates and infants whose immature vasculature cannot tolerate extracorporeal elimination modalities or in institutions lacking pediatric dialysis capacity. Exchange transfusion has been successfully employed in pediatric iron, isoniazid, phenobarbital, salicylate, theophylline, and vincristine overdose [129–134]. It has also been suggested for refractory drug-induced methemoglobinemia [135]. Whole blood exchange was utilized in an adult with a 50-fold cyclosporine dosing error [136]. Anticipated complications arise from vascular access, bleeding, hypoglycemia, hypotension, and blood product administration (immune-mediated reactions, blood incompatibility, and infections).

Toxicant-induced hyperthermia

Several hyperthermic syndromes are caused by xenobiotics. These are generally spectrum disorders, whose features may overlap with other conditions such as CNS infection, agitated delirium, and sepsis. Malignant hyperthermia (MH) occurs in patients with an autosomal-dominant defect in genes encoding the skeletal muscle ryanodine receptor (RyR-1) or the voltage-gated calcium channel (Cav1.1) who are exposed to volatile anesthetics or depolarizing muscle relaxants (succinylcholine) [137]. Hypomagnesemia may increase the probability and possibly severity of an MH event [138]. The subsequent rapid increase in myoplasmic calcium concentration increases muscle metabolism and heat production and produces muscle contractures and hyperthermia. Neuroleptic malignant syndrome (NMS) is characterized by high fever, autonomic instability, altered mental status, and muscle rigidity. Potent antipsychotics (neuroleptics) such as haloperidol and other medications (metoclopramide, droperidol, and promethazine) with significant dopamine antagonism, as well as abrupt cessation of dopaminergic agents such as those used in Parkinsonism, can precipitate this life-threatening syndrome [139]. NMS typically develops over several days and is characterized by ''lead-pipe'' rigidity [139]. Drugs that impair serotonin breakdown or re-uptake, those that act as serotonin precursors or enhance its release, or those that are serotonin agonists may lead to serotonin syndrome. Like NMS, serotonin syndrome is a spectrum disorder for which various signs and symptoms have been proposed to establish diagnosis (e.g., Sternbach and Hunter criteria) [140, 141]. In its most severe form it consists of high fever, autonomic instability, altered mental status, and may have associated diaphoresis, shivering, tremor, diarrhea, or spontaneous clonus. In serotonin syndrome, onset of symptoms is usually rapid, with 60% of patients with the serotonin syndrome presenting within 6 hours of drug exposure, and tremor and hyperreflexia predominant in the lower extremities may be a prominent feature [142]. Sympathomimetic-associated hyperthermia, seen with acute intoxication with cocaine, amphetamines, substituted amphetamines, and phencyclidine, may be clinically indistinguishable from serotonin syndrome [143]. Additionally, the agitated delirium engendered by these agents may be difficult to distinguish from that induced by hyperthermia itself. Patients with anticholinergic-associated hyperthermia will generally present with a compatible "toxidrome" – agitation; mydriasis; dry, hot, and erythematous skin; hypoactive bowel sounds; and urinary retention. While rare, thyrotoxicosis factitia, the ingestion of excess thyroid hormones due to inadvertent intake (pharmaceutical or food contamination), misuse (dieting), or significant intentional ingestion may produce hyperthermia [144, 145]. Hyperthermia may accompany toxicity with agents that uncouple oxidative phosphorylation (e.g., salicylates, dinitrophenol, pentachlorophenol) [146].

Multiple medications can also complicate or contribute to environmental hyperthermia. Several reviews and epidemiological data from major heat waves have demonstrated that anticholinergics, antiepileptics, antihistamines, antihypertensives in general and diuretics in particular, antipsychotics, and others contribute to excess morbidity and mortality [147, 148]. Conversely, exogenous heat stress can increase mortality from specific xenobiotics. In an urban setting at ambient temperatures above 31.1 °C, the mean daily number of fatal cocaine overdoses increased markedly [149].

Regardless of the cause for the hyperthermic syndrome, cessation of any possible offending or contributing agents and rapid cooling is critical. The degree of hyperthermia produced correlates with death and neurotoxicity in animal models, and temperature normalizing intervention is critically important in attenuating CNS injury and mortality [150]. Studies from the Chicago and France heat waves show that this is rarely done in a timely manner (if at all) in cases of environmental hyperthermia, with devastating results [147, 148]. The benefits of rapid cooling by ice water immersion were demonstrated over 80 years ago [151]. A large review concluded that cooling methods based on evaporative heat loss are less efficient than immersion in ice water in dissipating heat [152]. Additional studies demonstrate that cooling rates of up to 0.15–0.20 °C/min can be achieved with immersion, two to three times that of evaporation [153, 154]. Regardless of the method used, effectiveness should be repeatedly assessed.

Sedation with benzodiazepines and rigorous supportive care are necessary adjuncts in significant cases. This is primarily accomplished with titrated doses of benzodiazepines to inhibit muscle rigidity and control agitation. Animal models have demonstrated the benefit of benzodiazepines in prolonging survival, preventing seizure, and attenuating agitation in the toxicological hyperthermias [155, 156]. Phenytoin is ineffective in animal models [157]. Phenothiazines and butyrophenones, while reported, may have delayed onset and compromise mental status, lower seizure threshold, impair heat dissipation, and worsen hypotension [143].

Neuromuscular paralysis may be required to limit further heat generation in cases of NMS, serotonin syndrome, and sympathomimetic-associated hyperthermia. As the pathophysiology of MH is beyond the neuromuscular junction, paralytics are unlikely to provide benefit. Rapid i.v. administration of dantrolene, a direct-acting skeletal muscle relaxant, is the only drug proven effective for prevention and treatment of MH. Dantrolene disrupts the pathogenic excitation-contraction coupling by acting at RyR-1 to suppress depolarization-induced sarcoplasmic reticulum calcium release and normalize the voltage dependence of contractile activation [158]. Reversal of increased myotube sensitivity may also play a role [159]. Intravenous 2–3 mg/kg dantrolene is repeated until symptoms are controlled or 10 mg/kg (or more) has been administered. Following initial treatment, 1–2 mg/kg i.v. or per os is given every 6 hours for 24–72 hours to prevent recurrence. Dantrolene is packaged in vials containing 20 mg dantrolene sodium; thus, multiple vials are needed for treatment of adult patients. A large review of NMS cases did not suggest a beneficial role for dantrolene, although one case-controlled analysis found benefit [160, 161]. Bromocriptine, a dopamine agonist, has been used (off-label) to treat NMS at doses ranging from 5 to 20 mg every 6 hours [143]. Common side effects include hypotension, dyskinesia, erythromelalgia, and hallucinations. Cyproheptadine, developed as an antihistamine, additionally antagonizes 5-HT$_2$ receptors. Cyproheptadine for serotonin syndrome (off-label) is initially used in a dose range of 4–12 mg, followed by 2 mg every 2 hours for persistent symptoms; upon symptom control, 8 mg maintenance dosing is provided every 6 hours [142]. The tablet form necessitates administration orally or crushed *via* nasogastric tube.

Analgesic and anti-inflammatory antidotes

N-Acetylcysteine

N-Acetylcysteine (NAC) provides an effective means of prevention and treatment of acetaminophen (N-acetyl-p-aminophenol, APAP; paracetamol)-induced hepatotoxicity. NAC is also employed to preclude radiographic contrast-induced nephropathy [162]. The ultimate toxicant of APAP, N-acetyl-p-benzoquinone imine (NAPQI) generated primarily by CYP2E1 and CYP3A4, depletes glutathione (GSH), binds intracellular components, and, through an incompletely understood process, produces hepatic injury, centrilobular necrosis, or hepatic failure [163, 164]. NAC works by multiple mechanisms. It augments APAP sulfation to a nontoxic metabolite, it acts as a glutathione precursor or glutathione substitute to detoxify NAPQI, and possibly reverses NAPQI oxidation [165, 166]. NAC provides substantial benefit even in cases of delayed presentation following overdose [167]. Extra-hepatic benefits of NAC include improving cardiac index and systemic mean oxygen delivery despite decreasing systemic vascular resistance [168]. In a range of hepatic disorders, NAC improved baseline oxygen delivery, oxygen consumption, and dye clearance in a majority of patients [169]. Liver blood flow and cardiac index improved in septic shock patients provided NAC [170]. Only L-NAC is beneficial. Animal experiments demonstrate that the L-isomer, derived from physiological L-cysteine, prevents hepatotoxicity and provides prolonged elevations of hepatic glutathione [171]. Nonphysiological D-NAC cannot increase glutathione stores or prevent hepatotoxicity, despite increasing acetaminophen sulfation [172].

According to Rumack [163], the oral NAC dosing strategy was reached by estimating the absorption and turnover rate of glutathione at 6 mg/kg per h and an FDA safety factor of 3, to yield 70 mg/kg every 4 hours [6 (mg/kg per h) × 4 (h) × 3 (safety factor) = 72 ≈ 70 mg/kg every 4 h]. There were several assumptions as to "normal" hepatic glutathione levels and APAP to NAPQI conversion. A 140 mg/kg loading dose was added to provide an early high hepatic dose. The 72-hour duration of oral therapy was based on previous observations of multiple patients with prolonged APAP half-lives and a desire to implement a protocol that would accommodate those with half-lives longer than 12 hours (anticipating disappearance after five half-lives). While many have suggested that the 72-hour oral course is excessive, particularly after APAP has disappeared from the serum, the optimal duration of therapy is unclear. Studies assessing a shortened or "patient-tailored" approach have been small or methodologically limited [173, 174].

The Rumack-Matthew nomogram guides initiation of NAC therapy in single acute ingestions. The "treatment line" is anchored at an APAP serum concentration of either 200 µg/mL ("200 line") or 150 µg/mL ("150 line") at 4 hours post ingestion and decreased by 50% every 4 hours. The slope of the treatment line does not reflect APAP kinetics. The "150 line" is utilized in all patients in the U.S. and Australia; in the U.K. and elsewhere the "200 line" is employed, with a "100 line" modification for an array of individuals deemed at "high-risk": ethanol tolerant, those at risk for glutathione depletion (malnutrition, HIV, eating disorders, cystic fibrosis), pregnancy, and those prescribed enzyme-inducing drugs (carbamazepine, phenytoin, phenobarbitone rifampacin, isoniazid, etc.) [165, 175]. The U.S. multicenter study substantiated the safety and efficacy of its approach [176]. Proponents of the "150 line" point to the fact that 3.45–12.9% of patients above the "150 line" but below the "200 line" developed biochemical hepatotoxicity (aspartate aminotransferase, AST >1000 IU/L at any time during their course) in the U.S. multicenter trial and that patient deaths have occurred in untreated patients "between the lines" [177, 178]. In patients presenting near 8 hours after ingestion, or if a level is not available before 8 hours post ingestion, NAC is begun while awaiting APAP results and then continued or stopped once the results are available and have been plotted on the nomogram. If the time of ingestion is unknown or more than 24 hours has passed, NAC is administered. When APAP concentration and transaminase results are obtained, if transaminases are elevated or if measurable APAP exists, a full course of treatment is provided. With normal aminotransferases and without detectable APAP, treatment is not required. Concentrations obtained less than 4 hours post ingestion are not useful except to completely exclude ingestion (i.e., it is useful only if the APAP concentration is undetectable). Ongoing absorption may place individuals above the line at 4 hours, or metabolism or charcoal administration may result in a patient falling below the nomogram at 4 hours. In cases of chronic ingestion (>7.5 g/day in adult), laboratory evaluation and treatment are provided as for an unknown time of ingestion. With elevated transaminases or measurable APAP, NAC is provided.

Oral NAC is cheap and familiar to clinicians. It has minimal side effects (other than vomiting and odor) and is preferred in patients with bronchospastic disease. Its use can become problematic in cases where oral delivery is compromised, e.g., in patients with depressed mental status, significant vomiting, or impaired gastric motility. Use of an anti-emetic is encouraged.

Intravenous NAC appears to be similarly efficacious to oral NAC and eliminates many delivery issues. It has a much shorter therapy course (21 hours), expediting medical and psychiatric disposition. It avoids first pass metabolism in cases where the liver is not the only target or interest, such as those with cerebral edema or pregnancy. While i.v. NAC is slightly more expensive, total hospital charges may be less due to decreased treatment time. Histamine-mediated anaphylactoid reactions are more commonly seen with rapid i.v. loading and in patients with lower APAP levels [179]. Mild reactions have been treated by slowing the infusion rate and providing i.v. diphenhydramine, although this might alter NAC and APAP kinetics. Dosing complexity – 150 mg/kg in 200 mL of 5% dextrose over 1 hour, followed by 50 mg/kg in 500 mL of 5% dextrose over 4 hours (12.5 mg/kg per h), and then 100 mg/kg in 1000 mL of 5% dextrose over 16 hours (6.25 mg/kg per h) – yields frequent administration errors [180]. The supplied 20% solution was too concentrated for children, and dilution according to adult guidelines resulted in excess free water, and cases of hyponatremia and seizures [181]. The current U.S. package prescribing information (http://www.acetadote.net/PI_Acetadote_Revised_Apr09.pdf) and dosage calculator website (http://www.acetadote.net/dosecalc.shtml) provide dosing and administration guidelines in patients of less than 40 kg.

In a study limited by different comparison groups, data acquisition methodology, treatment location and several other factors, 20-hour only i.v. NAC was favored in patients with early presentation (<12 hours), whereas late presentation favored oral 72-hour NAC [182]. However, continuous i.v. infusion in delayed presentations with APAP-induced fulminant hepatic failure showed clear benefit in a prospective study [167]. Whatever the route, prior to cessation of NAC therapy, negative APAP concentrations and normal transaminases must be ensured, particularly in cases of massive ingestion; hepatotoxicity may follow premature cessation of therapy [183, 184]. The 16-hour maintenance dose is continued in patients receiving i.v. NAC until APAP is undetectable and transaminases are normal (or at baseline). Experimental evidence and human case reports demonstrate both delayed absorption, delayed increase following initial decline, and "crossing the nomogram" with extended-relief, opioid- or anticholinergic-containing APAP products, or co-ingestants [185, 186]. In cases of hepatic failure, i.v. NAC is continued until resolution, transplant, or death.

Anticholinergic antidotes

Physostigmine

Historically, physostigmine (eserine), a reversible carbamate inhibitor derived from the seed (Calabar bean) of the vine *Physostigma venenosum* Balfour, was used in the ancient trial by ordeal [187]. Medicinal use of physostigmine was first reported in 1864 to reverse severe atropine poisoning [188]. Naturally available (–)-physostigmine is over 100 times more effective in inhibiting acetylcholinesterase and butylcholinesterase in tissue, erythrocytes, and serum in humans and animal models than its stereoisomer [189, 190]. This activity depends upon interactions within the hydrophobic pocket of the acetylcholinesterase active center, which is distinct from the catalytic site [191]. Additionally, physostigmine binds nicotinic receptors close to, but distinct from, the acetylcholine binding site on the α-subunit [192]. At low doses, physostigmine functions as an ineffective nicotinic receptor agonist, while at higher doses it produces marked channel blockade.

Physostigmine's nonspecific analeptic properties [8] are no longer considered useful in overdose, given the clear benefits of supportive care. Indiscriminate use of physostigmine and an incomplete understanding of the pathophysiology of tricyclic antidepressant (TCA) poisoning was associated with bradydysrhythmias including asystole, seizure, and several deaths [193, 194]. In animal models, physostigmine is ineffective in attenuating TCA-induced seizures [195]. It failed to abolish dysrhythmias, decreased blood pressure, and at high doses enhanced TCA toxicity [196]. Physostigmine is currently recommended as a diagnostic and therapeutic agent for antimuscarinic poisoning [197]. Patients should have clear peripheral or central manifestations of the anticholinergic toxidrome. As a tertiary amine, physostigmine can cross the blood-brain barrier to reverse the central effects. An ECG should exclude sodium or potassium channel blockade (QRS or QT prolongation). Excessive physostigmine will produce a cholinergic syndrome, with muscarinic and nicotinic effects. As the adverse effects of bradycardia and bronchorrhea can produce significant morbidity, continuous cardiac monitoring and immediate access to atropine are recommended during physostigmine administration. Physostigmine, 1–2 mg in adults and 0.02 mg/kg (maximum 1.0 mg) in children is infused slowly over at least 5 min [198]. Repeat doses every 10–15 min can be provided if an adequate response does not occur and adverse effects are absent. Re-bolusing may be required in the setting of antimuscarinics with a prolonged duration of action.

Anticonvulsant antidotes

L-Carnitine

The anticonvulsants include carbamazepine, ethosuximide, felbamate, gabapentin, lacosamide, lamotrigine, levetiracetam, oxcarbazepine, phenobarbital, phenytoin, pregabalin, primidone, tiagabine, topiramate, valproic acid (VPA), vigabatrin, and zonisamide. These drugs enjoy widespread approved and off-label use for additional conditions, e.g., fibromyalgia (pregabalin); neuropathy and neuropathic pain (carbamazepine, gabapentin, lamotrigine, levetiracetam, and pregabalin); panic disorder (tiagabine); migraine prophylaxis and treatment of obesity, ethanol dependence, and depression (topiramate); and bipolar disorder (carbamazepine, lamotrigine, and VPA). Treatment of anticonvulsant overdose is largely supportive, with particular attention to the CNS-depressant and cardiovascular effects of some of these agents. L-(R)-Carnitine exists as the sole specific antidote in this class for significant VPA (di-n-dipropylacetic acid, 2-propylpentanoic acid) poisoning. Patients with drug-associated mitochondrial toxicity (particularly from nucleoside analogs) and anthracycline cardiotoxicity might also benefit from its administration [199, 200].

The anticonvulsant properties of VPA derive from its ability to increase γ-aminobutyric acid (GABA) availability *via* inhibition of GABA transaminase and succinic semialdehyde dehydrogenase, to attenuate N-methyl-D-aspartate (NMDA)-type glutamate receptor excitatory effects, and to slow the rate of recovery from sodium channel inactivation [201–203]. Additionally, VPA appears to affect inositol levels similar to lithium. Therapeutic concentrations are 50–100 mg/L. Potentially toxic concentrations are greater than 120 mg/L. Oral absorption of VPA is excellent [204]. Peak plasma concentrations are generally seen in 1–4 hours, although this may be markedly delayed by overdose, enteric coating, or meals [205]. Manifestations of significant VPA toxicity include CNS effects (lethargy, seizure, coma, cerebral edema), respiratory depression, metabolic derangement (hypernatremia, hyperammonemia, hypocalcemia, metabolic acidosis, carnitine deficiency), gastrointestinal effects (nausea, vomiting, and abdominal pain), pancytopenia, pancreatitis, and hepatotoxicity [206, 207]. Valproate toxicity is seen both in intentional acute overdose and in those on chronic therapy, either without adequate carnitine supplementation or on complex regimes.

Cells attempt to metabolize the VPA that is not directly excreted or glucuronidated in a manner similar to other fatty acids (Fig. 3). Thus, VPA is conjugated with coenzyme A (CoA). Carnitine enters *via* an ATP-dependent transporter. VPA is then transferred to carnitine, the normal mechanism for fatty acids entry into the mitochondrion. However, VPA-carnitine both inhibits the carnitine transporter and also diffuses out of the cell to be lost *via* renal excretion [208]. Renal resorption of carnitine is also impaired [209]. These factors contribute to intracellular carnitine depletion. Once VPA-carnitine is shuttled into the mitochondrion, it is reattached to CoA. It then undergoes β-oxidation, in an attempt to generate 2-carbon molecules for entry into the Krebs cycle. The 2-en-VPA-CoA product is neurotoxic with a prolonged half-life. The terminal 3-keto-VPA product traps CoA, leading to its mitochondrial depletion. Decreased mitochondrial CoA yields decreased ATP production, diminishing usable cellular energy currency and further limiting carnitine entry into the cell (*via* an ATP-dependent carnitine transporter). Once carnitine is depleted, normal fatty acid metabolism cannot occur [206]. Fatty acid build up is thought to underlie the Reye's-like steatohepatitis, which can be seen in toxicity [210]. CoA is also needed to make *N*-acetylglutamate, an activator of carbamoylphosphate synthetase I (CPS I), a critical enzyme in the urea cycle. When its effectiveness is limited due to inadequate activator, ammonia cannot be incorporated, and consequently, its concentrations increase. Furthermore, as CoA is depleted, β-oxidation shifts to omega (ω), or terminal carbon oxidation. This creates (among others) the hepatotoxic 4-en-VPA product. 4-en-VPA additionally inhibits CPS I, further preventing nitrogen elimination and contributing to hyperammonemia.

L-Carnitine (levocarnitine) supplementation has been recommended to reverse the adverse metabolic effects of VPA in cases of VPA-induced hepatotoxicity, VPA overdose, and primary carnitine-transporter defects [211, 212]. Hyperammonemia and serum and muscle carnitine deficiency are well described in patients chronically taking VPA [213–215]. Several studies and case reports demonstrate that carnitine supplementation reverses clinical symptoms, hypocarnitinemia, hyperammonemia, and VPA half-life prolongation in patients with toxicity due to chronic administration [216–218]. In patients with acute VPA overdose, limited clinical and laboratory data derived

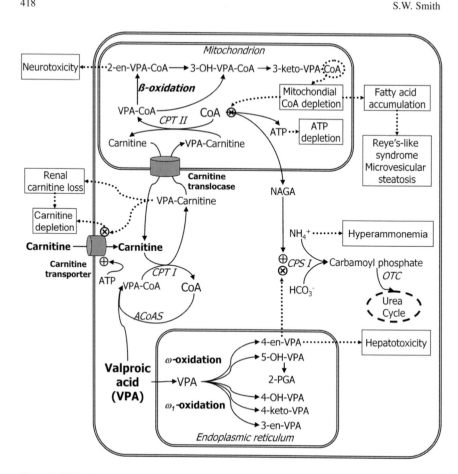

Figure 3. Valproic acid (VPA) metabolism and toxic mechanisms (see text for details). Several additional valproate metabolites are omitted. Enzymes (*italicized*): ACoAS, acyl-CoA synthetase; CPS I, carbamoyl-phosphate synthetase 1; CPT I, carnitine palmitoyltransferase I (reaction occurs on mitochondrial outer membrane); CPT II, carnitine palmitoyltransferase II (reaction occurs on mitochondrial inner membrane); and OTC, ornithine transcarbamylase. Substances: ATP, adenosine triphosphate; 2-, 3-, or 4-en-VPA, 2-propyl-2-, 3-, or 4-pentenoic acid; 3-, 4- or 5-OH-VPA, 3-, 4- or 5-hydroxy-2-propylpentanoic acid; 3-keto-VPA, 3-oxo-2-propylpentanoic acid; 2-PGA, 2-polyglutaric acid; 4-keto-VPA, 4-oxo-2-propylpentanoic acid; and NAGA, N-acetylglutamate. Symbols: ⊕, agonism or co-factor; ⊗, antagonism. Data used can be found in [201, 202, 204, 212, 482].

from case reports also suggest that reversal of metabolic derangements and improvement in clinical symptoms occurs when carnitine is provided [219–221]. A single large retrospective analysis showed a significant survival benefit with i.v. carnitine supplementation (with VPA cessation) in patients with valproate-induced hepatotoxicity [222].

L-Carnitine dosing for cases of overdose is not currently evidence based. An oral or i.v. dose of 100 mg/kg per day, divided and given every 6 hours (maximum daily dose 3 g), is provided to those patients with acute overdose and asymptomatic hyperammonemia or hepatotoxicity in the absence of CNS depression or metabolic derangement [211]. Symptomatic patients with hyperammonemia or symptomatic hepatotoxicity should receive 100 mg/kg L-carnitine i.v. over 30 min (maximum 6 g), followed by 15 mg/kg every 4 hours over 10–30 min until clinical improvement occurs [211, 223]. Others have supplemented at the higher dosing strategy when VPA concentrations exceed 450 mg/L [224]. In addition, given the decrease in protein binding that occurs, hemodialysis or hemoperfusion is recommended for patients with VPA concentrations exceeding 850–1000 mg/L or with severe clinical symptoms [202].

L-Carnitine is generally well tolerated. Side effects associated with carnitine supplementation are nausea, abdominal discomfort, dose-related diarrhea, and fishy body odor [223]. A small retrospective chart review found no adverse effects or allergic reactions in VPA overdose patients administered carnitine [225]. The current L-carnitine package inserts have no warnings or contraindications, but note that seizures have been reported to occur in patients, with or without pre-existing seizure activity, who received either oral or i.v. L-carnitine [226]. Up to 600 mg/kg per day for 5 days has been provided without complications [227]. The D-isomer and the racemate (D,L-carnitine) are contraindicated. Historic use of racemic D,L-carnitine was associated with myasthenia-like syndromes and cardiac dysrhythmias, which disappeared after L-carnitine administration [228]. D-Carnitine also competitively depletes cardiac and skeletal muscles and kidneys of L-carnitine [229].

Antihyperglycemic antidotes

Dextrose

Dextrose (D-glucose) is indicated to rapidly reverse organic or toxin-induced hypoglycemia (e.g., from sulfonylureas, insulin, ethanol, salicylates, β-adrenergic antagonists, quinolines, pentamidine, ritodrine, and disopyramide) [230, 231]. Hypoglycemia onset may be significantly delayed with certain agents (e.g., long-acting insulin or sulfonylureas). Limited CNS glycogen stores (in astrocytes) and the inability to acutely use free fatty acids make the CNS particularly vulnerable to hypoglycemia [232]. Patients (and providers) may be unaware of hypoglycemia in the absence of objective testing; both the counter-regulatory autonomic response and overt neurological deficit may be absent [233, 234]. Additionally, significant neuroglycopenia and hypoglycemia-associated delirium (particularly in salicylism) may occur despite a "normal" peripheral blood glucose [235]. A wide range of clinical presentations have been described, including diaphoresis, nausea, tachycardia, tremor, hypothermia, focal neurological deficits, and CNS agitation, confusion, or depression. These are generally reversible upon prompt treatment. Untreated hypoglycemia may result in seizure, coma, and death. Hypoglycemic seizures increase cerebral metabolic rate, contribute to ATP depletion, and produce irreversible brain damage [236, 237]. For these reasons, when bedside testing is unavailable, a risk-benefit calculation has generally favored empiric dextrose administration in the absence of a very clear alternative history or explanation for altered mental status.

Following a determination of absolute or relative hypoglycemia, 0.5– 1.0 g/kg i.v of age-appropriate dextrose containing solutions should be provided immediately – D50W (50 g/100 mL) in adults, D25W (25 g/100 mL) in children, and D10W (10 g/100 mL) in neonates. Frequent re-evaluation of response to therapy is required. Glucose uptake and distribution, hyperglycemia-induced insulin secretion in those with a competent pancreas, and ongoing toxin exposure may cause recurrent hypoglycemia and necessitate repeat dosing. Feeding, which provides significantly more calories than each 50 mL ampule of D50W (85 kcal according to one manufacturer [238]), should be commenced as soon as practicable. While D10W "maintenance" solutions may be subsequently required, at an infusion rate of 100 mL/h, this concentration only provides 34 kcal per hour. Continuous infusion of more concentrated solutions (e.g., D20W) requires a central venous catheter for administration. Only the D-isomer is clinically useful. Most glucose transporters (GLUTs) and the specific transporter required for facilitated diffusion of glucose across the blood-brain barrier, GLUT1 (SLC2A1), have a high affinity for D-glucose and negligible affinity for L-glucose [236, 239]. D-Glucose is also generally favored over other D-glucose epimers such as D-mannose or D-galactose.

D50W is hypertonic and may cause phlebitis or thrombosis at the site of injection. Extravasations of solutions containing as low as 10% dextrose have caused significant tissue injury and necrosis, particularly in young children [240]. Pseudoagglutination of red blood cells may occur if concentrated dextrose solutions without electrolytes are administered simultaneously with blood through the same infusion set [238]. Hypertonic dextrose administration may also induce generally clinically irrelevant hypophosphatemia [241].

Octreotide

Octreotide acetate, a synthetic somatostatin analogue, is now favored in cases of refractory hypoglycemia due to sulfonylureas or quinine. It is FDA approved for treatment of acromegaly, carcinoid tumors, and vasoactive intestinal peptide tumors [242]. It is a more potent inhibitor of insulin secretion than the natural hormone [242]. In pancreatic β-islet cells, ATP generated from glucose uptake and subsequent metabolism normally induces closure of the ATP-dependent potassium channel by binding to its pore subunit (Fig. 4). Sulfonylureas similarly induce channel closure after binding to a regulatory (SUR1) subunit. Increased intracellular potassium triggers calcium entry through voltage-dependent calcium channels, leading to increased cytosolic calcium and insulin exocytosis [243, 244]. Additionally, ATP contributes to

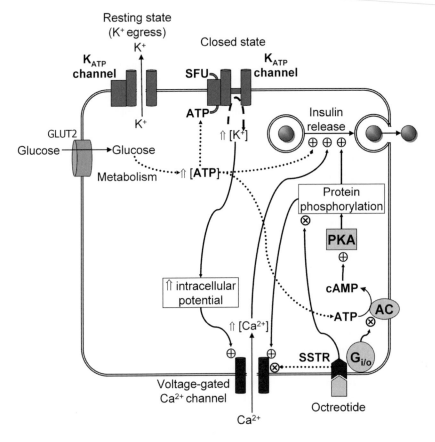

Figure 4. Pancreatic β-islet cell mechanisms of insulin release and octreotide action (see text for details). Enzymes and substances: AC, adenylyl cyclase; ATP, adenosine triphosphate; cAMP, cyclic adenosine monophosphate; GLUT2, glucose transporter 2; PKA, protein kinase A; SFU, sulfonylurea; SSTR, somatostatin receptor. Symbols: ⊕, agonism or co-factor; ⊗, antagonism. Data used can be found in [243–246].

insulin vesicles movement and provides a substrate for protein kinase A (PKA)-mediated phosphorylation. Octreotide binds to the somatostatin receptor (primarily SSTR₅) [243]. The subsequent effects continue to be explored and include inhibitory calcium channel effects, inhibition of adenylyl cyclase, and dephosphorylation of specific proteins required for movement and/or docking of vesicles [243, 245, 246]. Octreotide effectively suppresses endogenous insulin release in controlled studies in diabetics and in cases of sulfonylurea overdose, but does not (and would not be expected to have) an effect on exogenously administered insulin [247–249].

Several factors support octreotide usage following failure of initial dextrose administration and feeding. Bolused dextrose may produce hyperglycemia and thus subsequently stimulate an exaggerated insulin response, particularly when

sulfonylureas persist. This contributes to recurrent (sometimes more significant) hypoglycemia. A vicious cycle of serum glucose concentrations is described in case reports and controlled trials following dextrose administration
after sulfonylurea exposure [249–251]. Additionally, as has been demonstrated, classic neuroglycopenic symptoms may not be present, and patients may
need to be admitted during periods when circadian sleep patterns would complicate assessment. Octreotide administration also obviates the concern of excess water administration in pediatric patients receiving i.v. dextrose solutions.

Relatively few trials are available to judge the efficacy of octreotide for sulfonylurea-induced hypoglycemia. In one study, glipizide was used to induce
induced hypoglycemia (50 mg/dL) in eight healthy volunteers, who were then
resuscitated with dextrose infusion, diazoxide, or octreotide [251]. Dextrose
requirements were markedly less in patients provided octreotide and hypoglycemic events were markedly attenuated after all therapies were stopped.
One retrospective chart review of nine patients demonstrated that octreotide
significantly reduced the number of recurrent hypoglycemic events and dextrose requirement [252]. One prospective randomized controlled trial in 40
poisoned patients, despite a failure to control for carbohydrate intake and having an unusual dosing strategy (a single octreotide 75 µg dose subcutaneously), demonstrated consistently higher glucose values for the duration for which
octreotide would be expected to be effective (6–8 hours) [253]. Controlled animal studies with 25–100 µg octreotide demonstrated a similar decrease in
hypoglycemic events [254]. The remainder of human clinical experience of the
effectiveness of octreotide in sulfonylurea overdose comes from abstracts, case
reports, and case series (e.g., [249, 250, 255–257]).

Pediatric experience in sulfonylurea overdose comes only in the form of
limited abstracts and case reports in children aged 12 months to 17 years [248,
258–260]. However, octreotide has been used for prolonged periods to treat
persistent hyperinsulinemic hypoglycemia of infancy [261, 262].

Two human studies examined the effectiveness of octreotide in quinine-
induced hypoglycemia. In one study of nine healthy volunteers, 50 µg/hour
octreotide as a continuous i.v. infusion abolished quinine-induced insulin
release [263]. The authors reported resolution of hypoglycemia in an additional patient being treated with quinine for *Plasmodium falciparum* malaria. A
subsequent study in eight patients with *P. falciparum* malaria confirmed
octreotide suppression of quinine-induced hyperinsulinemia [264].

Optimal dosing of octreotide has not been definitively determined. Initial
doses of 40–100 µg subcutaneously in adults have been reported, although
50 µg every 6–8 hours is commonly provided [256, 265]. In children, an initial dose of 1.0–1.25 µg/kg is used, although up to 2.5 µg/kg (or more) has
been reported [258, 260]. Peak serum concentrations are achieved within
30 min after subcutaneous administration and within 4 min after a short
(3 min) i.v. infusion [266]. The elimination half-life (by either route of administration) is approximately 1.5 hours. In patients with severe renal impairment
(which may have contributed to sulfonylurea-induced hypoglycemia in the

first place), the plasma clearance is reduced by 50% [266]. The subcutaneous route is recommended due to longer duration of effect, as i.v. administration has resulted in treatment failure [267]. Side effects are generally minimal. Octreotide does inhibit gallbladder contractility and decreases bile secretion in normal volunteers [242]. When octreotide has been used to reverse sulfonyl-urea-induced hypoglycemia, bradycardia, hypokalemia, anaphylactoid reaction, and hypertension and apnea have been reported [257, 259]. Other adverse events include nausea, abdominal cramps, diarrhea, fat malabsorption and flatulence [268]. Octreotide also suppresses glucagon release, although hypoglycemia has been a concern only in patients on long-term therapy for organic hyperinsulinemia [269].

Glucagon is not generally recommended to correct hypoglycemia. Glycogen stores are frequently depleted by the time toxin-induced hypoglycemia manifests; glucagon's half-life (less than 20 min) is inadequate given the prolonged duration of the effect of sulfonylureas; and glucagon may exacerbate hyperinsulinemia [258]. Diazoxide, an antihypertensive agent, which reduces insulin release by opening the ATP-dependent potassium channel, is now of historical interest due to associated hypotension, reflex tachycardia, nausea and vomiting, and fluid retention [243, 265].

Antimicrobial antidotes

Pyridoxine

Since its introduction in 1952, isoniazid (INH, isonicotinic hydrazide, pyridine-4-carbohydrazide) has remained a mainstay for treatment and prophylaxis of mycobacterial infections [270]. The adult single tablet, 300 mg daily dose (4.3 mg/kg in a 70 kg individual) targets a peak plasma concentration of 3–5 µg/mL [271]. Acute INH toxicity may occur following ingestion of 20 mg/kg INH; it is common above 35–40 mg/kg [272]. The relatively narrow therapeutic window poses a significant risk for those with suicidal intent and for those who ingest extra pills to "catch up" after a brief period of incomplete compliance [273]. Historically, death rates of 21% were reported [274]. Seizures refractory to typical therapy, severe metabolic lactic acidosis, and coma may occur as early as 30 min post ingestion due to the rapid and nearly complete absorption of INH from the gastrointestinal tract. Seizures may occur at lower doses in those with pre-existing susceptibility. Associated respiratory failure, hypotension, and rhabdomyolysis may ensue. In patients provided 2.1–3.9 g (64–83 mg/kg) INH due to medication error, all experienced nausea or vomiting, vertigo, and coma within 30 min to 6 hours after ingestion [275]. Abnormal generalized discharges as sharp and slow waves were seen on EEG in all patients. Chronic INH toxicity may present with nausea, vomiting, hepatitis, hemolytic anemia, and neurological findings (restlessness, neuropathy, cerebellar findings, and psychosis).

The acute clinical effects are a product of the multiple biochemical actions of INH, which lead to pyridoxine depletion and subsequent neuronal hyperexcitability (Fig. 5) [272, 276–278]. INH hydrazones inhibit pyridoxine phosphokinase, which activates pyridoxine. INH hydrazines and hydrazides inactivate active pyridoxal 5-phosphate. INH metabolites also complex with pyridoxal 5-phosphate, leading to increased urinary elimination. Glutamic acid decarboxylase (GAD) and GABA transaminase (GABA-T) both require pyridoxal 5-phosphate as a co-factor. Inhibition of GAD exceeds that of GABA-T [279]. The resulting GABA depletion and loss of neuronal inhibition is thought to underlie seizure activity. Metabolic acidosis may be profound – survival has been reported with a pH of 6.49 [280]. Seizure-associated lactate generation is substantial; INH-induced metabolic acidosis does not develop in paralyzed dogs (despite EEG evidence of seizure) [281]. Importantly, merely correcting the acidosis (e.g., by bicarbonate) does not prevent additional seizures or terminate INH toxicity [281, 282]. INH also impairs lactate conversion to pyruvate (Fig. 5). Increased metabolism of fatty acids due to impaired glucose metabolism with hyperglycemia and ketonuria has been reported [272, 283]. INH also impairs cellular reduction-oxidation capacity *via* competitive inhibition of NAD [284, 285]. Pyridoxine deficiency also appears to play a role in INH-induced mental status changes (coma and lethargy) [275, 282, 286].

Appropriately dosed pyridoxine (vitamin B6) has been the mainstay of antidotal therapy for INH intoxication since the early reports of benefit *versus* his-

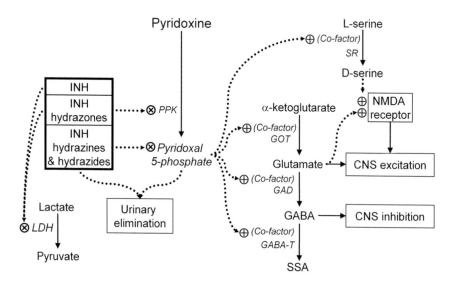

Figure 5. Mechanisms of isoniazid (INH) toxicity (see text for details). Enzymes (*italicized*): GABA-T, GABA transaminase; GAD, glutamic acid decarboxylase; GOT, glutamic-oxaloacetic transaminase; LDH, lactate dehydrogenase; PPK, pyridoxine phosphokinase; and SR, serine racemase. Substances: GABA, γ-aminobutyric acid; and SSA, succinic semi-aldehyde. Symbols: ⊕, agonism or co-factor; ⊗, antagonism. Data used can be located in [272, 276–278, 483].

torical controls [282]. Exogenous vitamin B6 provides the necessary precursor for the co-factor for GABA regeneration. Clinical experience with pyridoxine comes from case series, case reports, and animal data [273, 275, 281, 282, 287–289]. Clinical trials are absent due to ethical considerations. Vitamin B6 (as pyridoxine hydrochloride) is provided on a gram per gram basis for each gram of INH ingested, to a maximum of 5 g or 70 mg/kg (the empiric dose in ingestions of unknown quantity) [272, 282, 287]. A repeat dose can be provided if necessary. Due to the large amount of pyridoxine required, inadequate stocking and depletion of institutional and entire regional supplies have been widely reported [287, 290, 291]. In the convulsing patient, pyridoxine is administered i.v. at 0.5 g/min (5 g maximum) until seizure termination, with the remainder over 4–6 hours. Pediatric dosing should not exceed 70 mg/kg (5 g maximum). Large doses of pyridoxine have been safely administered; however, sensory neuropathy may occur with massive acute doses (>100 g) or chronic large daily doses [292]. Co-administration of benzodiazepines is synergistic in controlling seizures [288, 289]. Massive INH ingestion may require additional sedative hypnotics or anesthetic agents to suppress seizures [293]. INH is dialyzable, and hemodialysis has been used successfully in cases refractory to antidotal treatment, in those with extremely high plasma INH concentrations, and in patients with renal failure [283, 293].

Pyridoxine also appears to rapidly reverse the impaired consciousness seen in INH overdose [282, 286]. The CNS excitatory neurotransmitters include glutamate and D-serine, which with glutamate is a co-agonist of the NMDA receptor [278]. Examination of the metabolic pathways affected by pyridoxal 5-phosphate depletion (Fig. 5) suggests that inadequate stores of these neurotransmitters (due to inadequate co-factors for glutamic-oxaloacetic transaminase and serine racemase) might be contributory, in addition to general substrate or catecholamine deficiency.

Pyridoxine therapy is also recommended for poisoning through other hydrazines or hydrazine precursors (e.g., *Gyrometra* mushrooms, monomethylhydrazine, and unsymmetrical dimethylhydrazine fuel). Pyridoxine is effective in treating the chronic INH-associated neuropathy, particularly in patients with renal failure. Doses of 10–50 mg pyridoxine/day have typically been used in the chronic setting [271]. Pyridoxine has no effect in prevention or treatment of INH-associated hepatic injury.

Antineoplastic antidotes

Antineoplastic agents are used for the treatment of a variety of benign and malignant neoplasms. Some antineoplastic agents (such as the antifolates) have an expanded spectrum that includes use in rheumatology, dermatology, and obstetrics and gynecology. Toxicity may be due to the agent itself or delivery of the agent to an unintended target (e.g., extravasation). Several antidotes are used in a prophylactic fashion or on chronic basis. Amifostine (WR-2721) –

which is dephosphorylated by alkaline phosphatase to an activated, protective thiol form – is approved to decrease toxicity associated with radiotherapy and renal injury associated with cisplatin [294]. It has also been used to reduce chemotherapy-induced neutropenia; genitourinary injury associated with cyclophosphamide; and transfusion requirements, gastrointestinal and hepatic toxicity in pediatric patients [295, 296]. Cyclophosphamide and ifosfamide induce bladder toxicity (hemorrhagic cystitis) *via* their metabolite acrolein. Mesna (2-mercaptoethane sulfonate), a thiol agent that complexes with and inactivates acrolein, is provided orally or i.v. as prophylaxis [294]. Diethyldithiocarbamate (DDTC), the major metabolite of disulfiram, is an investigational agent for prevention of neuropathy from cisplatin and its analogs; it increased nephrotoxicity in one study [297]. Granulocyte colony-stimulating factor (G-CSF), granulocyte-macrophage colony-stimulating factor (GM-CSF), erythropoietin (hemopoietin) and its derivatives, oprelvekin (recombinant interleukin-11), and other stimulating factors are employed as adjuvants to reconstitute various hematopoietic lines damaged by chemotherapy and radiation [298, 299]. Palifermin (recombinant truncated human keratinocyte growth factor) is used to prevent severe mucositis in patients receiving stem-cell transplantation with a total body irradiation conditioning regimen [294]. The remaining section focuses on antineoplastic antidotes used in the acute setting.

Dexrazoxane

A dreaded complication of administration of vesicant chemotherapeutic agents is extravasation. Risk factors for extravasation include small, fragile, or sclerosed veins, obesity, comorbid conditions (diabetes, circulatory disorders, impaired sensory perception), use of rigid i.v. catheters, and clinicians' lack of knowledge and skills [300]. Redness, burning pain, and swelling may portend later blistering, ulceration, and necrosis. Dexrazoxane is U.S. FDA approved for treatment of extravasation resulting from i.v. anthracycline chemotherapy, to diminish tissue damage and the need for surgical excision of necrotic tissue [301]. Clinical efficacy data comes from two simultaneously reported open-label, single-arm, prospective multicenter studies in which only 1 out of 54 patients with biopsy-proven extravasation required surgical debridement [302]. Additional instances of successful dexrazoxane treatment of anthracycline extravasation are provided as case reports ([303] and others). Dexrazoxane is provided once daily for 3 consecutive days, with the first infusion initiated as soon as possible. Daily doses are as follows: day 1, 1000 mg/m^2 (maximum 2000 mg); day 2, 1000 mg/m^2 (maximum 2000 mg); day 3, 500 mg/m^2 (maximum 1000 mg) [301]. The dose is reduced by 50% in patients with creatinine clearance of less than 40 mL/min. In mice, efficacy rapidly decreased when dexrazoxane was provided beyond 6 hours after extravasation [304]. Dexrazoxane's mechanism of action appears to involve reversible inhibition of topoisomerase II and inhibition by its metabolite, an ethylenediamintetraacetic acid (EDTA) analogue, of free radical formation *via* iron removal from the iron-doxorubicin complex [305]. Topoisomerase II-independent effects have also been described [306]. In contrast, some authors have encouraged the non-concurrent, off-label use of topical dimethyl sulfoxide (DMSO) for anthracycline extravasation because of the risk of infection, neutropenia, and thrombocytopenia associated with dexrazoxane [307]. Dexrazoxane is also used prophylactically to limit anthracycline-associated cardiomyopathy [294].

Leucovorin

In 1950, methotrexate (MTX) joined the oncological armamentarium for leukemia [308]. MTX treatment of solid cancers was reported in 1956, and it gained FDA approval for psoriasis in 1971 [309, 310]. MTX is now used intramuscularly, intrathecally, i.v., and orally for a range of dermatological, rheumatological, obstetric, and gynecological conditions. The dose ranges from 7.5–30 mg orally once weekly for psoriasis or rheumatoid arthritis to 8–12 g/m^2 or more for osteosarcoma, leukemia, and lymphoma [311–313]. MTX poisoning may result from intentional overdose; unintentional ingestion, prescription, dispensing, administration, and patient errors; or renal insufficiency leading to persistent MTX in patients receiving high-dose chemotherapy regimens [314, 315]. MTX antagonizes folate metabolism (and rapidly proliferating cells) *via* multiple mechanisms. Dihydrofolate reductase inhibition by MTX and its polyglutamated metabolites ensures that neither dihydrofolate nor active tetrahydrofolate can be generated from folate, nor can existing dihydrofolate be recycled. Thymidylate synthase inhibition compromises thymidine synthesis. Purine ring synthesis is impaired by inhibition of the participating enzymes amidophospho-ribosyltransferase (PPAT) and 5-aminoimidazole-4-carboxamide ribonucleotide transformylase (AICART) [316, 317].

Maintenance of brisk urinary elimination with i.v. hydration and urinary alkalinization are standard therapies for patients receiving MTX. MTX is ten times more soluble in alkalinized urine (i.e., pH 7.5) than at pH 5.5 [318]. Folate (folic acid) is an ineffective therapy for MTX poisoning. While folate will inhibit renal resorption of MTX, persistent dihydrofolate reductase inhibition by MTX inhibits folate's activation. Leucovorin (folinic acid, 5-formyltetrahydrofolic acid, citrovorum factor) sustains the folate cycle by bypassing the blocked dihydrofolate reductase pathways. Addition of leucovorin "rescue" permitted the administration of very-high-dose MTX chemotherapy [319]. However, in patients receiving MTX chemotherapy, 24-hour MTX concentrations greater than 1×10^{-5} M (10 µmol/L), 48-hour concentrations greater than 1×10^{-6} M (1 µmol/L), or 72-hour concentrations greater than 1×10^{-7} M (0.1 µmol/L, 100 nM), or those with evidence of renal dysfunction are considered at high risk for toxicity [320]. In the setting of MTX persistence or toxicity, leucovorin i.v. doses are increased to 100 mg/m^2 or 1000 mg/m^2 every 6 hours according to established nomograms; doses and as high as 10 g/day have been used [319, 321]. Leucovorin therapy continues until MTX concentration are less than 0.5×10^{-7}–1.0×10^{-7} M (0.05–0.1 µmol/L, 50–100 nM) [319]. However, adequate leucovorin concentrations cannot be achieved for competitive reversal of MTX toxicity when MTX concentrations are persistently above 10–100 µmol/L; other antidotal strategies are then considered [313].

Treatment of patients ingesting MTX should not be delayed pending MTX concentrations. Inhibition of DNA synthesis is nearly complete when MTX plasma concentrations are greater than 1×10^{-8} M (0.01 µmol/L, 10 nmol/L) [322]. Therefore, leucovorin is provided until MTX concentrations are less than 1×10^{-8} M in patients receiving MTX for non-oncological indications or in patients not receiving MTX therapeutically [311]. Only leucovorin's S-form [levoleucovorin, (6S)-leucovorin] is active and rapidly metabolized to usable, reduced folates; the inactive isomer is slowly eliminated by renal excretion during i.v. administration [323]. Leucovorin was available in the U.S. only as a racemate until 2008, when levoleucovorin received FDA approval. Levoleucovorin at one-half of the usual racemic dose (as it is entirely active) appears to provide similar rescue therapy in high-dose MTX chemotherapy [324]. Oral rescue is not routinely recommended as leucovorin's bioavailability is poor above 40 mg due to saturation of active intestinal transport [323]. The calcium content of leucovorin (0.004 mEq calcium/mg leucovorin) mandates that infusion should not exceed 160 mg/min. Intrathecal administration of leucovorin is contraindicated, as death may result [325].

Glucarpidase

Glucarpidase (carboxypeptidase G_2, $CPDG_2$) is undergoing evaluation as an additional antidote for MTX toxicity. U.S. or European marketing approval for glucarpidase has not been granted at the time of writing. Competitive and complete reversal of MTX toxicity by leucovorin may not be possible at MTX concentrations above 100 µmol/L (and perhaps even lower) [313, 326, 327]. Patients with systemic MTX toxicity (significant mucositis, gastrointestinal distress, myelosuppression, hepatitis, or neurotoxicity), persistent serum MTX, and renal impairment following high-dose MTX have been considered for glucarpidase therapy in addition to leucovorin. Recommendations for glucarpidase above certain MTX concentrations have varied by malignancy, degree of renal impairment, initial MTX dose, and serum MTX concentration (e.g., Clinical Trials NCT00424645, NCT00481559, and [313, 328–330]).

Purification of "carboxypeptidase G", a pseudomonad zinc-dependent enzyme capable of MTX cleavage, was reported in 1967 [331]. Its antidotal potential was suggested in 1972. In mice injected with lethal MTX doses, carboxypeptidase G_1 rapidly decreased MTX concentrations and improved survival [332]. $CPDG_1$ selectively eliminated systemic MTX in patients treated with high dosages targeting CNS malignancy, and rescued a patient receiving MTX with renal failure in 1978 [333, 334]. After the original enzyme source of CPDG$_1$ was lost, a revived recombinant CPDG$_2$ product demonstrated success in both i.v. and intrathecal rescue of MTX overdose in non-human primates [335–337]. Successful use in multiple case reports and human trials in adult and pediatric patients with i.v. and intrathecal MTX overdose emerged [313, 315, 328, 329, 337–339].

Glucarpidase is a dimerized protein with two domains – a zinc-dependent catalytic domain that removes C-terminal glutamate residues of folate and folate analogues and a β-sheet interaction site [340]. Glucarpidase splits MTX and its 7-hydroxy-MTX metabolite into inactive 4-{[2,4-diamino-6-(pteridinyl)methyl]-methylamino}-benzoic acid (DAMPA) and hydroxy-DAMPA plus glutamate [341, 342]. MTX serum concentrations decline by 71–99% within minutes after glucarpidase [313, 315, 326, 330, 343, 344]. Intracellular, intraluminal (gastrointestinal tract) and intracerebral MTX is unaffected, creating the potential for rebound concentrations and persistent cytotoxicity [317, 328, 332, 345–347]. Leucovorin therapy must continue after carboxypeptidase administration. DAMPA's poor urinary solubility also requires ongoing alkalinization and saline diuresis to prevent renal precipitation [315, 348].

Anti-glucarpidase antibodies have been detected in patients receiving glucarpidase, although patients have been successfully treated with additional doses of glucarpidase for persistently elevated MTX concentrations [313, 326, 328, 337, 339, 342, 345]. HPLC must be used to determine actual MTX concentrations after glucarpidase as both MTX metabolites, 7-hydroxy-MTX and DAMPA, interfere with immunoassay techniques [349]. Glucarpidase has an affinity for MTX approximately 10- to 15-fold higher than it does for leucovorin; however, its affinity for folate and 5-methyltetrahydrofolate are similar [350, 351]. Glucarpidase eliminates active *levo*-(6S)-leucovorin about 50% faster than nonphysiological *dextro*-(6R)-leucovorin [348]. A study to address the clinical consequence is ongoing. Because of the stereoselective destruction of active leucovorin and its metabolites, many protocols attempt to separate leucovorin administration from glucarpidase administration by 2–4 hours. Administration of glucarpidase more proximate to leucovorin administration, and which antidote to provide should glucarpidase become available at a leucovorin dosing interval, requires a thoughtful benefit-risk assessment. Country-specific information on obtaining glucarpidase, institutional review board protocol, and consent issues have been made available online (www.btgplc.com/BTGPipeline/273/Voraxaze.html; and www.fda.gov/cder/cancer/singleIND.htm).

Cardiovascular antidotes

Cardiovascular pharmaceuticals comprise a wide variety of agents including anti-dysrhythmics, β-adrenergic antagonists (β-blockers, BBs), angiotensin antagonists, calcium channel antagonists (CCBs), cardioactive glycosides, and imidazoline derivatives. Overdose of these agents alone or in combination can generate potentially lethal combinations of impaired conduction, dysrhythmia, vasodilatation, and negative inotropy. Management of severe cases may necessitate diagnostic adjuncts such as echocardiography and right heart catheterization (Swan-Ganz measurements). In cases refractory to routine supportive care, vigorous gastrointestinal decontamination, and pharmacological intervention, aggressive measures including cardiac pacing, intra-aortic balloon counter-pulsation, or extracorporeal circulation (cardiopulmonary bypass) may be required until toxin elimination can be achieved [352]. Cardiac pacing may improve heart rate without increasing cardiac output if inotropy is compromised. Use of naloxone in the management of overdose of clonidine and angiotensin receptor antagonists and angiotensin converting enzyme inhibitors is provided in the opioid antagonists section. Strategies to mitigate the anticoagulant toxicity of vitamin K antagonists (i.e., coumadin) including exogenous oral or i.v. vitamin K, fresh frozen plasma, prothrombin concentrates, and recombinant factor VII are detailed in the 2008 American College of Chest Physicians Evidence-Based Clinical Practice Guidelines [353]. The Guidelines also address protamine sulfate for reversal of heparin anticoagulation and use of nonheparin anticoagulants for treatment and prevention of heparin-induced thrombocytopenia [354, 355].

Atropine

Atropine (D,L-hyoscyamine) is familiar to clinicians due to its use in several advanced cardiac life support (ACLS) algorithms [356]. Atropine is a central-acting, competitive antagonist of muscarinic acetylcholine receptors (M_1–M_5) [357]. It is used to counteract bradycardia from BBs, CCBs, cardioactive glycosides, and clonidine. Atropine increases basal heart rate; it does not affect the basal force of contraction [357]. Positive chronotropy alone may not produce systemic benefit in severe poisoning, and conduction system poisoning may limit responsiveness to atropine [358]. For symptomatic bradycardia, atropine 0.5–1.0 mg (pediatric dose: 0.02 mg/kg) i.v. is provided every 2–3 min to a maximum dose of 3 mg. Paradoxical parasympathetic response may occur during slow infusions or doses less then 0.5 mg (0.1 mg minimum in children) [356]. In slowing gastrointestinal motility, atropine may impair decontamination with WBI or AC.

Calcium

CCBs antagonize L-type calcium channels, slowing entry of calcium ions during myocyte depolarization; however, intracellular calcium release is not directly affected. This disrupts calcium-mediated excitation-contraction coupling, action potential generation and conduction, and vascular smooth muscle tone [359]. Exogenous i.v. calcium is indicated in cases of CCB and BB toxicity [352]. In animal models, calcium salts reverse CCB-induced deficits in contractility, blood pressure, and cardiac output [352]. Multiple uncontrolled cases reports document the effectiveness of calcium salts; however, interpretation of effectiveness is complicated by the co-administration of other modalities. Some authors advocate aggressive high-dose calcium therapy, providing large amounts of calcium without apparent ill effect [358]. This approach does carry a risk of death from hypercalcemia [reported concentration, 32.3 mg/dL (8.07 mmol/L) after 38 g calcium] [360]. Others recommend a bolus dose followed by continuous infusion to maintain physiological calcium levels [361]. Peripheral administration as calcium gluconate decreases the risk of extravasation and tissue necrosis. A standard container of 10 mL of 10% calcium gluconate provide 4.65 mEq (93 mg) elemental Ca^{2+}; 10 mL of 10% calcium chloride (1 g total $CaCl_2$) yields 13.6 mEq elemental Ca^{2+} [362]. A suggested approach is to initially administer a 0.6 mL/kg (0.28 mEq/kg) bolus of 10% calcium gluconate (0.2 mL/kg 10% $CaCl_2$) over 5–10 min [359, 361]. Empirically, this is roughly one vial (1 g) of 10% $CaCl_2$ or three vials (3 g) of 10% calcium gluconate i.v. The bolus may be repeated several times. Due to bolus dissipation, most patients are placed on an infusion of 10% calcium gluconate at 0.6–1.5 mL/kg per hour (0.28–0.7 mEq/kg per hour) or 0.2–0.5 mL/kg per hour [359, 361]. Serum phosphate, calcium, and hydration status should be closely monitored. Calcium administration for hyperkalemia has been generally contraindicated in cases of cardioactive glycoside toxicity, out of concern for dysrhythmias or systolic arrest (also known as "stone heart") [363]. While more recent studies have challenged this assertion, it is advisable to withhold calcium until the definitive cardiac glycoside antidote, digoxin-specific Fab fragments, has been provided [364].

Digoxin-specific antibody fragments (Fab)

Digoxin and cardioactive glycosides inhibit the cardiac sodium-potassium ATPase. The subsequent accumulation of sodium in the cytoplasm dissipates the driving force for calcium expulsion *via* the sodium-calcium exchanger. Increased intracellular calcium enhances actin-myosin coupling, myocyte contraction, and inotropy. In overdose, the excess calcium may result in membrane hyperexcitability and delayed after-depolarizations. Increased vagal tone decreases conduction through the AV node. The combination of increased automaticity and vagotonicity may yield lethal ventricular escape rhythms.

Digoxin-specific antibody fragments bind free digoxin in serum to decrease digoxin serum concentrations to undetectable levels within minutes [365]. Successful reversal of digoxin toxicity with digoxin-specific Fab was first reported in 1976 [366]. The results of a prospective multicenter study demonstrated significant effectiveness in reversing life-threatening digitalis toxicity, and more recent studies confirm ongoing Fab fragment utility [367, 368]. Digoxin-specific Fab were also shown to be effective in children [369].

Digoxin-specific Fab are produced from purified ovine-derived immunoglobulin G. Cleaving the Fc antibody portion significantly improves renal excretion of the complex, decreases immunogenicity, and facilitates diffusion of remaining free Fab into tissue [370]. Reflecting digoxin redistribution from target organs of toxicity, the initial response to digoxin-specific Fab was 19 min (0–60 min), and complete reversal of systemic toxicity occurred on average by 88 min (30–360 min) [367].

Indications for therapy include life-threatening or progressive dysrhythmia or shock; potassium greater than 5.0 mEq/L (acute poisoning); chronic poisoning with other end-organ manifestations such as altered mental status, significant gastrointestinal symptoms or renal impairment; or serum digoxin concentration >15 ng/mL or greater than 10 ng/mL beyond 6 hours after ingestion. Hyperkalemia is rapidly reversed by digoxin-specific Fab [365]. One vial neutralizes approximately 0.5 mg of digoxin (or digitoxin). Dosing is based either on amount ingested [number of vials = amount ingested (in mg) × 0.8 (oral bioavailability) / 0.5], or a serum concentration [number of vials = serum digoxin concentration (ng/mL) × patient weight (kg) / 100]. The number of vials is rounded up and administered i.v. over 30 min. Empiric therapy is 10–20 vials for adult or pediatric patients in acute poisoning or 3–6 vials (1–2 vials in children) in chronic poisoning. Partial reversal is recommended by some authors [371], but is not common U.S. practice due in part to concern for recrudescent toxicity with inadequate therapy [370].

Following treatment, free digoxin concentrations may rebound upwards within 12–24 hours, most likely reflecting tissue redistribution into the vascular space [372]. This provides a measure of protection against development of significant congestive heart failure (CHF) in patients dependent upon digoxin for inotropy, although exacerbation of CHF may occur [370]. Clinically significant late rebound of digoxin concentrations and toxicity have occurred in patients with marked renal dysfunction [373]. Immunogenicity from repeat digoxin-specific Fab has generally not been significant, although allergic reactions have been infrequently reported with administration [374]. Digoxin-specific Fab has been used clinically or experimentally to treat poisoning by other cardiac glycosides – yellow oleander (*Thevetia peruviana*), *Nerium oleander*, *Chan Su* and "Love Stone" (extract of the *Bufo bufo gargarizans* toad) [375, 376]. Higher dosing may be required due to poor binding affinity.

Glucagon

BBs competitively antagonize catecholamine effects at cardiac β-receptors, leading to decreased inotropy and slowed conduction through the AV node. Bradycardia, conduction delay, hypotension, and decreased cardiac output may accompany significant poisoning. BB interference with gluconeogenesis and glycogenolysis may lead to hypoglycemia, as well as blunt the catecholamine response that is important in its recognition.

Glucagon, a 29-amino acid peptide hormone secreted by pancreatic α-cells, counteracts hypoglycemia and the actions of insulin; regulates gastrointestinal motility; and mediates the rate of renal filtration, urea excretion, and water resorption [377]. The current glucagon product is now produced in non-pathogenic *E. coli* by recombinant techniques [378]. Myocardial binding occurs at a distinct glucagon receptor (GCGR) coupled with the β-agonist binding site. Antidotal (off-label) use of glucagon thus bypasses β-receptor blockade to directly induce G-protein-mediated stimulation of adenylate cyclase to convert ATP to cAMP [379]. cAMP, in turn, activates protein kinase A (PKA), which promotes the phosphorylation and opening of dormant L-type calcium channels to improve calcium-dependent excitation-contraction coupling [361]. Another proposed mechanism is C-terminal cleavage of glucagon to miniglucagon, which has a direct effect on sarcoplasmic reticulum calcium stores *via* arachidonic acid [380].

In human volunteers evaluated by cardiac catheterization, glucagon increased heart rate, cardiac index, and mean atrial pressure, but not left ventricular end-diastolic pressure (EDP) or systemic vascular resistance (SVR) [381]. Clinical experience in overdose consists primarily of case reports [382, 383]. Due to the complex nature of overdose, glucagon is often used in combination with other agents in severe BB overdose. Additionally, several *ex vivo* experiments, controlled animal studies, and uncontrolled case reports have demonstrated that glucagon can be beneficial in CCB exposure [384–386]. The recommended initial bolus dose of glucagon is 50–150 μg/kg, which may be repeated after 3–5 min [359]. A continuous infusion corresponding to the total effective bolus reversal dose is then provided per hour (e.g., if clinical response was observed following administration of 2 mg, 3 mg, and finally 5 mg, the hourly infusion would be 10 mg/hour). The effects of glucagon administered i.v. begin within 1–3 min, peak at 5–7 min and last for approximately 15 min [381]. Nausea and vomiting are common and should be anticipated. This may complicate management of patients with depressed mental status or airway concerns. Flushing, transient hyperglycemia, and smooth muscle relaxation, and ileus may also occur.

High-dose insulin euglycemia therapy

Since CCBs antagonize the L-type calcium channel in pancreatic islet cells, a subsequent decreased insulin production can produce hyperglycemia [361]. Animals poisoned by CCBs have impaired myocardial fatty acid uptake (leaving them dependent upon carbohydrate metabolism), impaired uptake of glucose, and myocardial insulin resistance [387, 388]. In humans, intracoronary verapamil increased glucose release and altered myocardial lactate use from consumption to release [389].

Decades ago, glucose-insulin-potassium (GIK) was proposed as adjuvant therapy for acute myocardial infarction, with the intent of suppressing uptake of free fatty acids, improve myocardial energy production, and stabilize intra-cellular potassium [390]. Randomized trials of GIK therapy in patients with acute myocardial infarction (AMI) have not shown benefit, although the insulin doses tend to be low (in general, ≤0.075 U/kg) [390]. Experience in the surgical literature in cases where much higher insulin doses have been used has been somewhat different [391]. Patients undergoing aortic valve replace-ment and coronary artery bypass who received high-dose insulin at 1 unit/kg per hour demonstrated more rapid lactate clearance, lower glucose, lower dobutamine requirements, a trend for improved cardiac indices, and potential anti-inflammatory benefit (lower C-reactive protein and free fatty acid levels) [392]. Insulin doses of 2.5 units/kg were tolerated without excess increase of insulin-induced potassium elimination [393]. In combination with dopamine, insulin 7 units/kg was used to significantly augment cardiac output and decrea-se systemic vascular resistance in post-coronary artery bypass graft (CABG) patients without generating excess in oxygen demand [394]. Additional bene-fits of high-dose insulin included overcoming insulin resistance, increased expression of glucose transporters, and improved turnover of sodium-potassi-um-ATPases [391].

The basis for high-dose insulin euglycemia therapy (HIET) (off-label) in overdose has been explored in a series of animal models of CCB and BB tox-icity [387, 388, 395–397]. HIET increased myocardial lactate uptake and improved systolic and diastolic heart function. Insulin outperformed epineph-rine and glucagon [395–397]. Multiple human cases of successful manage-ment of CCB overdose with HIET have been described [359, 398]. Because the beneficial cardiovascular effects of HIET are not seen for 15–60 min after initiation, it must be considered early, before patients become unsalvageable [359]. A proposed dosing scheme includes a bolus dose of regular insulin of 1.0 units/kg, followed by an infusion of 0.5–1.0 units/kg per hour, titrated upwards as necessary [359]. A dextrose bolus is also provided unless signifi-cant hyperglycemia exists, followed by an infusion of 0.5–1.0 g/kg per hour to maintain blood glucose between 100 and 250 mg/dL.

Persistent physician reticence to utilizing the high-dose insulin out of con-cern for excess hypoglycemia presents an obstacle for implementation of ade-quate HIET [399]. This ignores a body of physiological data that demonstrate that the insulin transport follows saturation kinetics [400, 401]. Alternatively, it has also been demonstrated that insulin-stimulated glucose clearance reach-es a maximum in both lean and obese subjects [402]. Taken together, this sug-gests that, from a therapeutic standpoint, since insulin effect *via* insulin recep-tors appears saturable, additional mechanisms must be at work. The effects of HIET may include counteracting CCB-mediated insulin impairment or shock-induced hyperglycemia, improving myocardial substrate utilization, and improving myocardial metabolism [359]. From an adverse-effects standpoint, once adequate and ongoing glucose has been provided, hypoglycemia should not present an excessive risk [398], although frequent serum glucose and potassium evaluation are obvious components of HIET therapy. Due to the high dosing, insulin may persist after the infusion cessation and necessitate ongoing supplemental dextrose beyond insulin infusion. As hypokalemia is an intracellular result of shift, it is supplemented cautiously.

Lipid emulsion (20%)

During administration of local anesthetics, severe toxicity may result from systemic absorption or unintended intravascular administration. Loss of consciousness, dysrhythmia, cardiovascular collapse, seizures, and lactate-associated acidemia may rapidly ensue [403]. Furthermore, in animal models, for some of the local anesthetics (bupivacaine, levobupivacaine, and ropivacaine), treatment with "standard" advanced cardiac life support (ACLS) drugs such as epinephrine may precipitate ventricular dysrhythmia [404].

Following a serendipitous observation that pretreatment with a lipid emulsion altered the dose-response to bupivacaine-induced asystole, murine and canine studies provided evidence of survival benefit with lipids in bupivacaine toxicity [405, 406]. Case reports of successful resuscitation of patients severely affected by bupivacaine, levobupivacaine, mepivacaine, prilocaine and ropivacaine (alone or in combination) followed [403, 407–409]. Pediatric experience is limited to a case of successful resuscitation following lidocaine/ropivacaine toxicity from a posterior lumbar plexus block [410]. Lipid therapy has been successfully applied in human bupropion toxicity and combined quetiapine and sertraline overdose [411, 412]. Animal models have suggested a possible benefit in clomipramine, propranolol, thiopentone, and verapamil poisoning [413–416]. An understanding of lipid's mechanism of action is incomplete. It may act as a "circulating lipid sink" in which excess lipophilic drug may dissolve; modulate intracellular processes; or provide an alternative myocardial energy supply [411]. Presumably due to central sympathetic activation, human volunteers given a 4-hour lipid emulsion (20%) infusion had increased systemic vascular resistance, blood pressure, muscle sympathetic nerve activity, and concentrations of insulin and aldosterone, without increased cardiac output [417]. Lipid emulsion increased inotropy in both spontaneously beating and paced isolated rat hearts poisoned with levobupivacaine [418].

Dosing guidelines for the off-label use of lipid emulsion in resuscitation are provisional, as optimal bolus and continuous infusion therapy and timing are still being explored. The Association of Anaesthetists of Great Britain and Ireland recommends an i.v. bolus of 1.5 mL/kg Intralipid® (20%) over 1 min, which may be repeated twice at 5-min intervals if an adequate circulation has not been restored [419]. Following the initial bolus, an infusion is commenced at 0.25 mL/kg per min (which may be increased to 0.5 mL/kg per min in inadequate circulation). Propofol is an inadequate substitute [419, 420]. Ongoing lipid therapy may be required as recrudescence may occur [421]. Hyperamylasemia may be anticipated. Additional concerns include pancreatitis, allergic reactions, acute myocardial infarction, fat embolism, and altered coagulation [420]. In lapine and porcine models of asphyxial cardiac collapse (pulseless electrical activity or arrest), lipid emulsion was markedly ineffective [422, 423]. *In vitro*, lipid affinity for both bupivacaine and ropivacaine is also adversely affected by low pH (by a factor of 1.68 in a pH drop from 7.40 to 7.00) [424]. These data suggest that ventilatory status must be aggressively addressed early in toxicity.

Magnesium

Due to their physicochemical characteristics and structure, many non-antiarrhythmic drugs are able to antagonize or alter expression of the myocardial potassium delayed rectifier channel (hERG, KCNH2, LQT2). With channel block, potassium efflux is compromised, and the repolarizing cardiac I_{Kr} current is impaired. The surface ECG reflects this as QT prolongation. Age, female gender, comorbidities such as structural heart disease, electrolyte disturbances such as hypokalemia, and heart rate (bradycardia) may provide additional risk. Certain antibiotics, antihistamines, antipsychotics, antidepressants, and methadone are prone to induce QT prolongation. QT prolongation is associated with torsade de pointes, a polymorphic ventricular arrhythmia that can degenerate into ventricular fibrillation, cardiac arrest and sudden death [425]. If significant QT prolongation (QTc >500 ms) is detected, administration of 1–2 g magnesium sulfate i.v. (pediatric dose, 25–50 mg/kg) over 5 to 60 min (depending on urgency of presentation), followed by an infusion of 2–4 mg/min is suggested [426]. Rapid infusion may cause hypotension, and magnesium should be administered cautiously in renal failure. A second bolus can be provided 5–15 min later [427]. Magnesium sulfate i.v. is effective in arrhythmias occurring due to early or delayed depolarization-induced triggered activity [427]. Acceleration of the heart rate with isoproterenol or transvenous pacing (overdrive pacing) may be needed to preclude recurrence of torsade de pointes while correction of underlying risk factors (hypokalemia and hypocalcemia) ensues. Immediate non-synchronized defibrillation is required for unstable polymorphic ventricular tachycardia or ventricular fibrillation.

Sodium bicarbonate

Severe cardiovascular toxicity may result from blockade of cardiac sodium channels by tricyclic antidepressants (TCAs) – leading to conduction delays, dysrhythmias, and myocardial depression. TCAs adversely affect maximum upstroke velocity (V_{max}), which approximates the magnitude of sodium entry [428]. The sodium channel blockade displays rate dependence. At slow rates the TCA has time to disassociate, allowing channel recovery. At faster rates, block progressively worsens. Given the anticholinergic effects of TCAs that speed the heart rate, this is a significant concern. However, attempts to decrease heart rate with propranolol produced hypotension and lethality in canine studies [429, 430].

With progressive sodium channel block, ventricular impulse propagation becomes delayed. Sodium channel blockade manifests on the surface ECG as QRS widening. A QRS equal or greater than 100 ms is a significant predictor of seizure; a QRS ≥160 ms predicts ventricular dysrhythmia [431]. The right bundle branch has a relatively longer refractory period, and it is affected disproportionately by impaired intraventricular conduction delay. Rightward terminal axis shift or outright bundle branch block may be present [432]. These rightward terminal forces may also produce terminal R waves in leftward-directed leads [433]. Acidemia secondary to hypoperfusion or seizure may generate progressively worsened block. In an acidemic environment, free TCA concentrations increase as binding to α-1 acid glycoprotein decreases, the TCA ionized fraction increases, and sodium channel blockade worsens [434]. Seizures are severe and consequential, leading to QRS widening and hypotension [435].

Administration of sodium bicarbonate improves V_{max} and action potential amplitude by increasing extracellular pH and sodium concentration [428]. Consequentially, compromised myocardial inotropy, conduction aberrations, and dysrhythmia are reversed. Several animal studies have demonstrated these beneficial effects [429, 430]. Both the sodium and alkalemia induced by sodium bicarbonate improve cardiac performance [429]. The enhanced inotropy with sodium bicarbonate is independent of and additive to vasopressor treatment [436]. Hyperventilation-induced alkalinization similarly narrows the QRS [437]. Sodium bicarbonate outperformed hyperventilation in a swine model, although hypertonic saline was superior to both [438]. This approach has been reported clinically [439]. While sodium bicarbonate is recommended for QRS widening in TCA evidence-based consensus guidelines for out-of-hospital management, actual human studies are not as extensive as one might suspect [440, 441].

Initially, hypertonic sodium bicarbonate 1–2 mEq/kg i.v. is provided, preferably with continued ECG monitoring of the QRS. Institutions usually stock either an 8.4% solution (1 mEq/mL sodium and bicarbonate ions) or a 7.5% solution (0.892 mEq/mL sodium and bicarbonate ions). Rarely, a 5% solution may be encountered (0.595 mEq/mL). A "standard" 50-mL ampule of 8.4% or 7.5% solutions would deliver 50 or 44.6 mEq of $NaHCO_3$. Several boluses may be required, either initially or as the bolus effect declines due to redistribution [429]. Ongoing alkalinization should be provided as discussed previously, with a goal of serum pH 7.55. If sodium bicarbonate administration is problematic due to fluid load, hyperventilation and/or hypertonic saline may be required [437, 439].

Due to mechanistic similarities, sodium bicarbonate has been recommended for QRS widening seen in poisoning by Vaughn-Williams Class IA and IC antidysrhythmics, cocaine, diphenhydramine, carbamazepine, and propoxyphene [442–445]. Treatment of bupropion-induced QRS widening with sodi-um bicarbonate has met with both success and failure [446]. Sodium bicar-bonate has also been suggested to treat QRS widening from venlafaxine; sim-ilar effects seen with lamotrigine might also be amenable [447, 448]. Sodium bicarbonate therapy may have a role in *Taxus* species (yew berry) toxicity [449]. Treatment of amantadine-induced QRS widening with sodium bicar-bonate may be complicated by concurrent profound hypokalemia [450].

Opioid antidotes

Naloxone

Naloxone is a competitive opioid antagonist at all receptor subtypes [451]. It can prevent or reverse the effects of opioids, notably CNS and respiratory depression. Massive doses of naloxone (5.4 mg/kg with 4.0 mg/kg per hour infusion) have been administered safely in non-opioid tolerant individuals suf-fering from spinal cord injury [452]. However, indiscriminate use of naloxone in opioid-tolerant individuals can precipitate acute opioid withdrawal, with attendant acute lung injury, seizure, hypertension, or cardiac dysrhythmia [453]. These are likely associated with the abrupt, significant, and sustained increases in plasma catecholamine concentrations (epinephrine and norepi-nephrine) that accompany narcotic reversal, particularly in the setting of hypercapnia [454]. Withdrawal-induced vomiting may compromise the airway in patients with concomitant sedative-hypnotic ingestion. Precipitated with-drawal-associated agitation and violent behavior may require chemical restraint, leading to a vicious cycle of compromised CNS and cardiopul-monary function as naloxone wears off. Self-release and relapse following naloxone administration is also a concern in opioids with prolonged duration of effect (methadone, controlled-release oxycodone hydrochloride, etc.). Naloxone is no longer recommended as the initial resuscitation of newborns with respiratory depression in the delivery room; precipitation of acute neona-tal opioid withdrawal may produce severe consequences [455]. Sudden cardiac arrest has occurred in preterm neonates given naloxone to reverse opioid over-dose [456].

Naloxone is utilized in those individuals with clear evidence of the opioid toxidrome. Those with a respiratory rate ≤12 or hypopnea are likely to benefit [457]. The goal of therapy is titration to adequate ventilatory status without withdrawal. After normocapnia is achieved by supported ventilation, this can be done with i.v. administration of 0.04–0.05 mg initially (e.g., 1 mL of 0.4 mg naloxone in 10 mL diluent or 1 mg naloxone in 20 mL diluent). Due to rapid onset, effectiveness can be assessed, and if required, the dose can be titrated upwards incrementally to 0.4 mg, 2 mg, or even 10 mg. Patients without response to 10 mg naloxone are unlikely to have opioid-induced respiratory depression. Nonopioid-dependent adults are administered 0.4–2 mg i.v.

Pediatric dosing for infants and children from birth to 5 years of age or less than 20 kg body weight is 0.1 mg/kg; children older than 5 years of age or weighing more than 20 kg are provided 2 mg [455]. For longer acting opioids, following adequate initial opioid antagonism, two-thirds of the initial naloxone reversal bolus is provided as a continuous i.v. infusion [458].

Naloxone can successfully antagonize buprenorphine overdose in children, although prolonged therapy and monitoring may be required [459]. Higher doses may be required due to reverse buprenorphine effects because of its high affinity for opioid receptors [460]. Naloxone has also been used to reverse clonidine toxicity, although this is not always the case [461]. It has been postulated that patients with higher hyperadrenergic tone (who have higher concentrations of endogenous opioids) or those in whom clonidine induces more endogenous opioid release may respond best to naloxone [462]. Mental status, blood pressure, and heart rate may respond differently.

Naloxone has been employed in angiotensin converting enzyme inhibitor overdose. One author reported that a 1.6 mg bolus of naloxone followed by repeat 2 mg bolus reversed hypotension due to overdose with 500 mg captopril [463]. Naloxone has been ineffective in reversing hypotension in other cases complicated by co-ingestants [464]. The mechanism may relate to antagonism of endogenous opioids [465]. Co-administration of 0.2 mg/kg naloxone mitigated captopril-related decreases in systolic and diastolic blood pressure in healthy volunteers [465]. A placebo-controlled study of healthy men found that naloxone pretreatment with 10 mg followed by 2.46 mg/hour infusion precluded systolic blood pressure decrease induced by captopril (50 mg) [466]. Under different experimental conditions [naloxone, 0.4 mg bolus and a 2-hour continuous infusion (4.0 mg/hour), and captopril (25 mg)], no difference was observed [467].

Sedative-hypnotic antidotes

Flumazenil

Analogous to naloxone antagonism at opioid receptors, flumazenil competitively antagonizes benzodiazepine receptors – allosteric sites located at the macromolecular $GABA_A$ receptor complex, which regulate chloride ion flux within the associated ion channel [468]. Flumazenil reverses the sedative, psychomotor, and amnestic effects of benzodiazepines [469]. Flumazenil's effectiveness depends upon the number of benzodiazepine receptors that can be occupied according to the mass-action law, the affinity of a particular benzodiazepine for the receptor, and the free benzodiazepine concentration near the receptor [470]. In contrast, antagonism of benzodiazepine-induced respiratory depression is inconsistent, and acute tolerance may develop to large doses [471–473]. Flumazenil administration can reverse bispectral index (BIS) depression and permit earlier emergence from anesthesia in patients provided non-benzodiazepine anesthesia (propofol/remifentanil) [474]. Postulated mechanisms included intrinsic CNS stimulant activity or antagonism of endogenous benzodiazepine-like ligands (endozepines). Under certain experimental conditions, flumazenil may also demonstrate partial agonist or even inverse agonist activity [475, 476].

The appropriate utilization of flumazenil as an antidote in patients with benzodiazepine overdose is still a matter of debate. Patients who ingest benzodiazepines alone or in combination generally have acceptable outcomes with supportive care alone. Proponents argue that awakening is therapeutic and diagnostic, obviates requirements for investigatory procedures, and limits complications of sedation. Opponents point to the low risk of mortality with benzodiazepine ingestion, frequent co-ingestants for which flumazenil is ineffective or contraindicated, relapse, and risks of reversal. While flumazenil can be administered safely, indiscriminate flumazenil administration may produce an acute withdrawal syndrome in benzodiazepine-dependent patients, seizures, dysrhythmias, vomiting, and agitation [477–480].

Flumazenil is not recommended in cases complicated by co-ingestants capable of inducing seizures or dysrhythmias (e.g., bupropion, carbamazepine, chloral hydrate, chlorinated hydrocarbons, chloroquine, cocaine, cyclic antidepressants, cyclosporine, isoniazid, lithium, methylxanthines, monoamine oxidase inhibitors, phenothiazines, and propoxyphene) [477, 479, 481]. As might be anticipated with an antidote of lesser half-life than many benzodiazepines, clinical condition may deteriorate following initial improvement, mandating ongoing monitoring. In one study, patients with primarily benzodiazepines ingestion remained awake for 72 ± 37 min following flumazenil; this was markedly decreased to 18 ± 7 min with co-ingestants [478]. This may be problematic in patients who, once aroused, demand release from medical care. After excluding co-ingestants of concern, vital sign abnormalities, and an aberrant ECG, and considering the risk-benefit ratio, flumazenil is administered slowly i.v., titrated to clinical effect (0.1 mg/min, max ≤ 1 mg) [481]. Off-label continuous infusions of 0.3–0.5 mg/hour have been provided to preclude relapse.

Conclusions

Patients poisoned by pharmaceuticals present many challenges to the treating clinicians. They generally benefit from aggressive support of vital functions, a careful history and physical examination, specific laboratory analyses, and a thoughtful consideration of the risks and benefits of decontamination and enhanced elimination. Data on the effectiveness of certain antidotes ranges from isolated case reports to robust clinical trials. Clinicians are encouraged to liberally utilize consultation with regional poison centers or those with toxicology training to assist with diagnosis, management, and administration of antidotes, particularly in unfamiliar cases.

Declarations

No outside funding or support was received. The author has no financial interest in any products mentioned or the companies that produce them. Use of trade names is for identification purposes only and does not constitute endorsement by the author, the NYU School of Medicine, the New York City Poison Control Center, or the New York City Department of Health and Mental Hygiene. Within the medical literature, pharmaceuticals, pharmaceutical combinations, and other products are used off-label as antidotal therapies; off-label uses are referred to in this review. This is for discussion purposes only and does not constitute endorsement of off-label use by the author, the NYU School of Medicine, the New York City Poison Control Center, or the New York City Department of Health and Mental Hygiene. As medicine is an ever-changing science, readers are encouraged to confirm the information contained in this review – by consulting product and safety information sheets, regional Poison Centers, those with toxicological expertise, and other resources – particularly in the case of new or infrequently used drugs.

Acknowledgments
The author is indebted to Lewis S. Nelson, MD, FACEP, FACMT for manuscript review.

References

1 Wax PM (1997) Analeptic use in clinical toxicology: A historical appraisal. *J Toxicol Clin Toxicol* 35: 203–209
2 Jones AW, Dooley J, Murphy JR (1950) Treatment of choice in barbiturate poisoning; series of twenty-nine cases of barbiturate poisoning treated with pentylenetetrazole (metrazol) and supportive therapy. *J Am Med Assoc* 143: 884–888
3 Orwin A, Sim M, Waterhouse JAH (1965) A study of the anti-barbiturate effects of bemegride. *Br J Psychiatry* 111: 531–533
4 Hirsh K, Wang SC (1975) Respiratory stimulant effects of ethamivan and picrotoxin. *J Pharmacol Exp Ther* 193: 657–663
5 Bickerman HA, Chusid EL (1970) The case against the use of respiratory stimulants. *Chest* 58: 53–56
6 Wolfson B, Siker ES, Ciccarelli HE (1965) A double blind comparison of doxapram, ethamivan and methylphenidate. *Am J Med Sci* 249: 391–398
7 Rappolt RT S, Gay GR, Decker WJ, Inaba DS (1980) NAGD regimen for the coma of drug-related overdose. *Ann Emerg Med* 9: 357–363
8 Nattel S, Bayne L, Ruedy J (1979) Physostigmine in coma due to drug overdose. *Clin Pharmacol Ther* 25: 96–102
9 Zvosec DL, Smith SW, Litonjua R, Westfal RE (2007) Physostigmine for γ-hydroxybutyrate coma: Inefficacy, adverse events, and review. *Clin Toxicol* 45: 261–265
10 Hoffman RS, Goldfrank LR (1995) The poisoned patient with altered consciousness. Controversies in the use of a 'coma cocktail'. *J Am Med Assoc* 274: 562–569
11 Anonymous (1915) Practical pharmacology. XXIV. *J Am Med Assoc* 64: 2063–2067
12 Temple WA, Smith NA, Beasley M (1991) Management of oil of citronella poisoning. *J Toxicol Clin Toxicol* 29: 257–262
13 Sheffield P (2008) Emetics, cathartics, and gastric lavage. *Pediatr Rev* 29: 214–215
14 Fantus B (1915) Fullers earth; its absorptive power, and its antidotal value for alkaloids. *J Am Med Assoc* 64: 1838–1845
15 Alpert JJ, Lovejoy FH Jr (1971) Management of acute childhood poisoning. *Curr Probl Pediatr* 1: 1–40
16 Clemmesen C, Nilsson E (1961) Therapeutic trends in the treatment of barbiturate poisoning. The Scandinavian method. *Clin Pharmacol Ther* 2: 220–229
17 Lawson AA, Mitchell I (1972) Patients with acute poisoning seen in a general medical unit (1960–71). *Br Med J* 4: 153–156
18 Beaubien AR, Carpenter DC, Mathieu LF, MacConaill M, Hrdina PD (1976) Antagonism of imipramine poisoning by anticonvulsants in the rat. *Toxicol Appl Pharmacol* 38: 1–6
19 Callaham M, Schumaker H, Pentel P (1988) Phenytoin prophylaxis of cardiotoxicity in experimental amitriptyline poisoning. *J Pharmacol Exp Ther* 245: 216–220

20 Sechi G, Serra A (2007) Wernicke's encephalopathy: New clinical settings and recent advances in diagnosis and management. *Lancet Neurol* 6: 442–455

21 Sporer KA, Khayam-Bashi H (1996) Acetaminophen and salicylate serum levels in patients with suicidal ingestion or altered mental status. *Am J Emerg Med* 14: 443–446

22 Ashbourne JF, Olson KR, Khayam-Bashi H (1989) Value of rapid screening for acetaminophen in all patients with intentional drug overdose. *Ann Emerg Med* 18: 1035–1038

23 Cooper GM, Le Couteur DG, Richardson D, Buckley NA (2005) A randomized clinical trial of activated charcoal for the routine management of oral drug overdose. *QJM* 98: 655–660

24 Karim A, Ivatts S, Dargan P, Jones A (2001) How feasible is it to conform to the European guidelines on administration of activated charcoal within one hour of an overdose? *Emerg Med J* 18: 390–392

25 Krenzelok EP, McGuigan M, Lheur P (1997) Position statement: Ipecac syrup. *J Toxicol Clin Toxicol* 35: 699–709

26 Saetta JP, March S, Gaunt ME, Quinton DN (1991) Gastric emptying procedures in the self-poisoned patient: Are we forcing gastric content beyond the pylorus? *J R Soc Med* 84: 274–276

27 Saetta JP, Quinton DN (1991) Residual gastric content after gastric lavage and ipecacuanha-induced emesis in self-poisoned patients: An endoscopic study. *J R Soc Med* 84: 35–38

28 Saincher A, Sitar DS, Tenenbein M (1997) Efficacy of ipecac during the first hour after drug ingestion in human volunteers. *J Toxicol Clin Toxicol* 35: 609–615

29 Lapatto-Reiniluoto O, Kivisto KT, Neuvonen PJ (2000) Gastric decontamination performed 5 min after the ingestion of temazepam, verapamil and moclobemide: Charcoal is superior to lavage. *Br J Clin Pharmacol* 49: 274–278

30 Grierson R, Green R, Sitar DS, Tenenbein M (2000) Gastric lavage for liquid poisons. *Ann Emerg Med* 35: 435–439

31 Tenenbein M, Cohen S, Sitar DS (1987) Efficacy of ipecac-induced emesis, orogastric lavage, and activated charcoal for acute drug overdose. *Ann Emerg Med* 16: 838–841

32 Vale JA, Kulig K (2004) Position paper: Gastric lavage. *J Toxicol Clin Toxicol* 42: 933–943

33 Sato RL, Wong JJ, Sumida SM, Marn RY, Enoki NR, Yamamoto LG (2003) Efficacy of superactivated charcoal administered late (3 hours) after acetaminophen overdose. *Am J Emerg Med* 21: 189–191

34 Christophersen AB, Levin D, Hoegberg LC, Angelo HR, Kampmann JP (2002) Activated charcoal alone or after gastric lavage: A simulated large paracetamol intoxication. *Br J Clin Pharmacol* 53: 312–317

35 Alaspaa AO, Kuisma MJ, Hoppu K, Neuvonen PJ (2005) Out-of-hospital administration of activated charcoal by emergency medical services. *Ann Emerg Med* 45: 207–212

36 Adams BK, Mann MD, Aboo A, Isaacs S, Evans A (2004) Prolonged gastric emptying half-time and gastric hypomotility after drug overdose. *Am J Emerg Med* 22: 548–554

37 Green R, Sitar DS, Tenenbein M (2004) Effect of anticholinergic drugs on the efficacy of activated charcoal. *J Toxicol Clin Toxicol* 42: 267–272

38 Auerbach PS, Osterloh J, Braun O, Hu P, Geehr EC, Kizer KW, McKinney H (1986) Efficacy of gastric emptying: Gastric lavage *versus* emesis induced with ipecac. *Ann Emerg Med* 15: 692–698

39 Albertson TE, Derlet RW, Foulke GE, Minguillon MC, Tharratt SR (1989) Superiority of activated charcoal alone compared with ipecac and activated charcoal in the treatment of acute toxic ingestions. *Ann Emerg Med* 18: 56–59

40 Kulig K, Bar-Or D, Cantrill SV, Rosen P, Rumack BH (1985) Management of acutely poisoned patients without gastric emptying. *Ann Emerg Med* 14: 562–567

41 Comstock EG, Boisaubin EV, Comstock BS, Faulkner TP (1982) Assessment of the efficacy of activated charcoal following gastric lavage in acute drug emergencies. *J Toxicol Clin Toxicol* 19: 149–165

42 Pond SM, Lewis-Driver DJ, Williams GM, Green AC, Stevenson NW (1995) Gastric emptying in acute overdose: A prospective randomised controlled trial. *Med J Aust* 163: 345–349

43 Bosse GM, Barefoot JA, Pfeifer MP, Rodgers GC (1995) Comparison of three methods of gut decontamination in tricyclic antidepressant overdose. *J Emerg Med* 13: 203–209

44 Kirshenbaum LA, Mathews SC, Sitar DS, Tenenbein M (1989) Whole-bowel irrigation *versus* activated charcoal in sorbitol for the ingestion of modified-release pharmaceuticals. *Clin Pharmacol Ther* 46: 264–271

45 Mayer AL, Sitar DS, Tenenbein M (1992) Multiple-dose charcoal and whole-bowel irrigation do

not increase clearance of absorbed salicylate. *Arch Intern Med* 152: 393–396

46 Lee MR (2008) Ipecacuanha: The South American vomiting root. *J R Coll Physicians Edinb* 38: 355–360

47 Manno BR, Manno JE (1977) Toxicology of ipecac: A review. *Clin Toxicol* 10: 221–242

48 Krenzelok EP, Dean BS (1987) Effectiveness of 15-mL *versus* 30-mL doses of syrup of ipecac in children. *Clin Pharm* 6: 715–717

49 Yamashita M, Yamashita M, Azuma J (2002) Urinary excretion of ipecac alkaloids in human volunteers. *Vet Hum Toxicol* 44: 257–259

50 Anonymous (2004) Position paper: Ipecac syrup. *J Toxicol Clin Toxicol* 42: 133–143

51 Garrison J, Shepherd G, Huddleston WL, Watson WA (2003) Evaluation of the time frame for home ipecac syrup use when not kept in the home. *J Toxicol Clin Toxicol* 41: 217–221

52 American Academy of Pediatrics Committee on Injury, Violence, and Poison Prevention (2003) Poison treatment in the home. *Pediatrics* 112: 1182–1185

53 Bond GR (2003) Home syrup of ipecac use does not reduce emergency department use or improve outcome. *Pediatrics* 112: 1061–1064

54 MacLean WC Jr (1973) A comparison of ipecac syrup and apomorphine in the immediate treatment of ingestion of poisons. *J Pediatr* 82: 121–124

55 Dorrington CL, Johnson DW, Brant R (2003) The frequency of complications associated with the use of multiple-dose activated charcoal. *Ann Emerg Med* 41: 370–377

56 Caravati EM, Knight HH, Linscott MS Jr, Stringham JC (2001) Esophageal laceration and charcoal mediastinum complicating gastric lavage. *J Emerg Med* 20: 273–276

57 Mofredj A, Rakotondreantoanina JR, Farouj N (2000) Severe hypernatremia secondary to gastric lavage. *Ann Fr Anesth Reanim* 19: 219–220

58 Roberts JR, Gracely EJ, Schoffstall JM (1997) Advantage of high-surface-area charcoal for gastrointestinal decontamination in a human acetaminophen ingestion model. *Acad Emerg Med* 4: 167–174

59 Chyka PA, Seger D, Krenzelok EP, Vale JA (2005) Position paper: Single-dose activated charcoal. *Clin Toxicol* 43: 61–87

60 Neuvonen PJ (1982) Clinical pharmacokinetics of oral activated charcoal in acute intoxications. *Clin Pharmacokinet* 7: 465–489

61 Spiller HA, Winter ML, Klein-Schwartz W, Bangh SA (2006) Efficacy of activated charcoal administered more than four hours after acetaminophen overdose. *J Emerg Med* 30: 1–5

62 Buckley NA, Whyte IM, O'Connell DL, Dawson AH (1999) Activated charcoal reduces the need for *N*-acetylcysteine treatment after acetaminophen (paracetamol) overdose. *J Toxicol Clin Toxicol* 37: 753–757

63 Berg MJ, Berlinger WG, Goldberg MJ, Spector R, Johnson GF (1982) Acceleration of the body clearance of phenobarbital by oral activated charcoal. *N Engl J Med* 307: 642–644

64 Berlinger WG, Spector R, Goldberg MJ, Johnson GF, Quee CK, Berg MJ (1983) Enhancement of theophylline clearance by oral activated charcoal. *Clin Pharmacol Ther* 33: 351–354

65 Levy G (1982) Gastrointestinal clearance of drugs with activated charcoal. *N Engl J Med* 307: 676–678

66 American Academy of Clinical Toxicology; European Association of Poisons Centres and Clinical Toxicologists (1999) Position statement and practice guidelines on the use of multi-dose activated charcoal in the treatment of acute poisoning. *J Toxicol Clin Toxicol* 37: 731–751

67 Campbell JW, Chyka PA (1992) Physicochemical characteristics of drugs and response to repeat-dose activated charcoal. *Am J Emerg Med* 10: 208–210

68 Pond SM, Olson KR, Osterloh JD, Tong TG (1984) Randomized study of the treatment of phenobarbital overdose with repeated doses of activated charcoal. *J Am Med Assoc* 251: 3104–3108

69 Swartz CM, Sherman A (1984) The treatment of tricyclic antidepressant overdose with repeated charcoal. *J Clin Psychopharmacol* 4: 336–340

70 De Silva HA, Fonseka MM, Pathmeswaran A, Alahakone DG, Ratnatilake GA, Gunatilake SB, Ranasinha CD, Lalloo DG, Aronson JK, de Silva HJ (2003) Multiple-dose activated charcoal for treatment of yellow oleander poisoning: A single-blind, randomised, placebo-controlled trial. *Lancet* 361: 1935–1938

71 Eddleston M, Juszczak E, Buckley NA, Senarathna L, Mohamed F, Dissanayake W, Hittarage A, Azher S, Jeganathan K, Jayamanne S, Sheriff MR, Warrell DA (2008) Multiple-dose activated charcoal in acute self-poisoning: A randomised controlled trial. *Lancet* 371: 579–587

72 Olkkola KT (1985) Effect of charcoal-drug ratio on antidotal efficacy of oral activated charcoal in

man. *Br J Clin Pharmacol* 19: 767–773

73 Hoegberg LC, Angelo HR, Christophersen AB, Christensen HR (2003) The effect of food and ice cream on the adsorption capacity of paracetamol to high surface activated charcoal: *In vitro* studies. *Pharmacol Toxicol* 93: 233–237

74 McLuckie A, Forbes AM, Ilett KF (1990) Role of repeated doses of oral activated charcoal in the treatment of acute intoxications. *Anaesth Intensive Care* 18: 375–384

75 Pollack MM, Dunbar BS, Holbrook PR, Fields AI (1981) Aspiration of activated charcoal and gastric contents. *Ann Emerg Med* 10: 528–529

76 Osterhoudt KC, Durbin D, Alpern ER, Henretig FM (2004) Risk factors for emesis after therapeutic use of activated charcoal in acutely poisoned children. *Pediatrics* 113: 806–810

77 Mariani PJ, Pook N (1993) Gastrointestinal tract perforation with charcoal peritoneum complicating orogastric intubation and lavage. *Ann Emerg Med* 22: 606–609

78 Watson WA, Cremer KF, Chapman JA (1986) Gastrointestinal obstruction associated with multiple-dose activated charcoal. *J Emerg Med* 4: 401–407

79 Menzies DG, Busuttil A, Prescott LF (1988) Fatal pulmonary aspiration of oral activated charcoal. *BMJ* 297: 459–460

80 Gades NM, Chyka PA, Butler AY, Virgous CK, Mandrell TD (2003) Activated charcoal and the absorption of ferrous sulfate in rats. *Vet Hum Toxicol* 45: 183–187

81 Rangan C, Nordt SP, Hamilton R, Ingels M, Clark RF (2001) Treatment of acetaminophen ingestion with a superactivated charcoal-cola mixture. *Ann Emerg Med* 37: 55–58

82 Stewart JJ (1983) Effects of emetic and cathartic agents on the gastrointestinal tract and the treatment of toxic ingestion. *J Toxicol Clin Toxicol* 20: 199–253

83 Barceloux D, McGuigan M, Hartigan-Go K (1997) Position statement: Cathartics. *J Toxicol Clin Toxicol* 35: 743–752

84 Smilkstein MJ, Smolinske SC, Kulig KW, Rumack BH (1988) Severe hypermagnesemia due to multiple-dose cathartic therapy. *West J Med* 148: 208–211

85 Beloosesky Y, Grinblat J, Weiss A, Grosman B, Gafter U, Chagnac A (2003) Electrolyte disorders following oral sodium phosphate administration for bowel cleansing in elderly patients. *Arch Intern Med* 163: 803–808

86 McNamara RM, Aaron CK, Gemborys M, Davidheiser S (1988) Sorbitol catharsis does not enhance efficacy of charcoal in a simulated acetaminophen overdose. *Ann Emerg Med* 17: 243–246

87 al-Shareef AH, Buss DC, Allen EM, Routledge PA (1990) The effects of charcoal and sorbitol (alone and in combination) on plasma theophylline concentrations after a sustained-release formulation. *Hum Exp Toxicol* 9: 179–182

88 Allerton JP, Strom JA (1991) Hypernatremia due to repeated doses of charcoal-sorbitol. *Am J Kidney Dis* 17: 581–584

89 Martin RR, Lisehora GR, Braxton M Jr, Barcia PJ (1987) Fatal poisoning from sodium phosphate enema. Case report and experimental study. *J Am Med Assoc* 257: 2190–2192

90 Korkis AM, Miskovitz PF, Yurt RW, Klein H (1992) Rectal prolapse after oral cathartics. *J Clin Gastroenterol* 14: 339–341

91 Ly BT, Schneir AB, Clark RF (2004) Effect of whole bowel irrigation on the pharmacokinetics of an acetaminophen formulation and progression of radiopaque markers through the gastrointestinal tract. *Ann Emerg Med* 43: 189–195

92 Tenenbein M (1997) Position statement: Whole bowel irrigation. *J Toxicol Clin Toxicol* 35: 753–762

93 Lapatto-Reiniluoto O, Kivisto KT, Neuvonen PJ (2001) Activated charcoal alone and followed by whole-bowel irrigation in preventing the absorption of sustained-release drugs. *Clin Pharmacol Ther* 70: 255–260

94 Everson GW, Bertaccini EJ, O'Leary J (1991) Use of whole bowel irrigation in an infant following iron overdose. *Am J Emerg Med* 9: 366–369

95 Smith SW, Ling LJ, Halstenson CE (1991) Whole-bowel irrigation as a treatment for acute lithium overdose. *Ann Emerg Med* 20: 536–539

96 Roberge RJ, Martin TG (1992) Whole bowel irrigation in an acute oral lead intoxication. *Am J Emerg Med* 10: 577–583

97 Hendrickson RG, Horowitz BZ, Norton RL, Notenboom H (2006) "Parachuting" meth: A novel delivery method for methamphetamine and delayed-onset toxicity from "body stuffing". *Clin Toxicol* 44: 379–382

98 Scharman EJ, Lembersky R, Krenzelok EP (1994) Efficiency of whole bowel irrigation with and without metoclopramide pretreatment. *Am J Emerg Med* 12: 302–305

99 Langdon DE (1996) Colonic perforation with volume laxatives. *Am J Gastroenterol* 91: 622–623

100 Narsinghani U, Chadha M, Farrar HC, Anand KS (2001) Life-threatening respiratory failure following accidental infusion of polyethylene glycol electrolyte solution into the lung. *J Toxicol Clin Toxicol* 39: 105–107

101 Hoffman RS, Chiang WK, Howland MA, Weisman RS, Goldfrank LR (1991) Theophylline desorption from activated charcoal caused by whole bowel irrigation solution. *J Toxicol Clin Toxicol* 29: 191–201

102 Ng HW, Tse ML, Lau FL, Chu W (2008) Endoscopic removal of iron bezoar following acute overdose. *Clin Toxicol* 46: 913–915

103 Hojer J, Personne M (2008) Endoscopic removal of slow release clomipramine bezoars in two cases of acute poisoning. *Clin Toxicol* 46: 317–319

104 Wells CD, Luckritz TC, Rady MY, Zornik JM, Leighton JA, Patel BM (2006) Bezoar formation requiring endoscopic removal after intentional overdose of extended-release nifedipine. *Pharmacotherapy* 26: 1802–1805

105 Choudhary AM, Taubin H, Gupta T, Roberts I (1998) Endoscopic removal of a cocaine packet from the stomach. *J Clin Gastroenterol* 27: 155–156

106 Clifton JC 2nd, Sigg T, Burda AM, Leikin JB, Smith CJ, Sandler RH (2002) Acute pediatric lead poisoning: Combined whole bowel irrigation, succimer therapy, and endoscopic removal of ingested lead pellets. *Pediatr Emerg Care* 18: 200–202

107 Foxford R, Goldfrank L (1985) Gastrotomy – A surgical approach to iron overdose. *Ann Emerg Med* 14: 1223–1226

108 Lapostolle F, Finot MA, Adnet F, Borron SW, Baud FJ, Bismuth C (2000) Radiopacity of clomipramine conglomerations and unsuccessful endoscopy: Report of 4 cases. *J Toxicol Clin Toxicol* 38: 477–482

109 de Prost N, Lefebvre A, Questel F, Roche N, Pourriat JL, Huchon G, Rabbat A (2005) Prognosis of cocaine body-packers. *Intensive Care Med* 31: 955–958

110 Schaper A, Hofmann R, Bargain P, Desel H, Ebbecke M, Langer C (2007) Surgical treatment in cocaine body packers and body pushers. *Int J Colorectal Dis* 22: 1531–1535

111 Bodenham A, Shelly MP, Park GR (1988) The altered pharmacokinetics and pharmacodynamics of drugs commonly used in critically ill patients. *Clin Pharmacokinet* 14: 347–373

112 Proudfoot AT, Krenzelok EP, Vale JA (2004) Position Paper on urine alkalinization. *J Toxicol Clin Toxicol* 42: 1–26

113 Jaing TH, Hung IJ, Chung HT, Lai CH, Liu WM, Chang KW (2002) Acute hypermagnesemia: A rare complication of antacid administration after bone marrow transplantation. *Clin Chim Acta* 326: 201–203

114 Scharman EJ (1997) Methods used to decrease lithium absorption or enhance elimination. *J Toxicol Clin Toxicol* 35: 601–608

115 Kleinman GE, Rodriquez H, Good MC, Caudle MR (1991) Hypercalcemic crisis in pregnancy associated with excessive ingestion of calcium carbonate antacid (milk-alkali syndrome): Successful treatment with hemodialysis. *Obstet Gynecol* 78: 496–499

116 Birrer RB, Shallash AJ, Totten V (2002) Hypermagnesemia-induced fatality following epsom salt gargles. *J Emerg Med* 22: 185–188

117 Bailey CS, Weiner JJ, Gibby OM, Penney MD (2008) Excessive calcium ingestion leading to milk-alkali syndrome. *Ann Clin Biochem* 45: 527–529

118 Chatterjee M, Speiser PW (2007) Pamidronate treatment of hypercalcemia caused by vitamin D toxicity. *J Pediatr Endocrinol Metab* 20: 1241–1248

119 Grunfeld JP, Rossier BC (2009) Lithium nephrotoxicity revisited. *Nat Rev Nephrol* 5: 270–276

120 Majumdar SR, Kjellstrand CM, Tymchak WJ, Hervas-Malo M, Taylor DA, Teo KK (2009) Forced euvolemic ciuresis with mannitol and furosemide for prevention of contrast-induced nephropathy in patients with CKD undergoing coronary angiography: A randomized controlled trial. *Am J Kidney Dis, in press*

121 Eyer F, Pfab R, Felgenhauer N, Lutz J, Heemann U, Steimer W, Zondler S, Fichtl B, Zilker T (2006) Lithium poisoning: Pharmacokinetics and clearance during different therapeutic measures. *J Clin Psychopharmacol* 26: 325–330

122 Van Bommel EF, Kalmeijer MD, Ponssen HH (2000) Treatment of life-threatening lithium toxicity with high-volume continuous venovenous hemofiltration. *Am J Nephrol* 20: 408–411

123 Bressolle F, Kinowski JM, de la Coussaye JE, Wynn N, Eledjam JJ, Galtier M (1994) Clinical pharmacokinetics during continuous haemofiltration. *Clin Pharmacokinet* 26: 457–471

124 Meyer LM, Miller FR, Rowen MJ, Bock G, Rutzky J (1950) Treatment of acute leukemia with amethopterin (4-amino, 10-methyl pteroyl glutamic acid). *Acta Haematol* 4: 157–167

125 Goldfarb DS, Matalon D (2006) Principles and techniques applied to enhance elimination. In: NE Flomenbaum, LR Goldfrank, RS Hoffman, MA Howland, NA Lewin, and LS Nelson (eds): *Goldfrank's Toxicologic Emergencies*, 8th edn., McGraw-Hill, New York, 160–72.

126 Johnson LZ, Martinez I, Fernandez MC, Davis CP, Kasinath BS (1999) Successful treatment of valproic acid overdose with hemodialysis. *Am J Kidney Dis* 33: 786–789

127 Lalau JD, Andrejak M, Moriniere P, Coevoet B, Debussche X, Westeel PF, Fournier A, Quichaud J (1989) Hemodialysis in the treatment of lactic acidosis in diabetics treated by metformin: a study of metformin elimination. *Int J Clin Pharmacol Ther Toxicol* 27: 285–288

128 Tapolyai M, Campbell M, Dailey K, Udvari-Nagy S (2002) Hemodialysis is as effective as hemoperfusion for drug removal in carbamazepine poisoning. *Nephron* 90: 213–215

129 Carlsson M, Cortes D, Jepsen S, Kanstrup T (2008) Severe iron intoxication treated with exchange transfusion. *Arch Dis Child* 93: 321–322

130 Shannon M, Wernovsky G, Morris C (1992) Exchange transfusion in the treatment of severe theophylline poisoning. *Pediatrics* 89: 145–147

131 Manikian A, Stone S, Hamilton R, Foltin G, Howland MA, Hoffman RS (2002) Exchange transfusion in severe infant salicylism. *Vet Hum Toxicol* 44: 224–227

132 Katz BE, Carver MW (1956) Acute poisoning with isoniazid treated by exchange transfusion. *Pediatrics* 18: 72–76

133 Sancak R, Kucukoduk S, Tasdemir HA, Belet N (1999) Exchange transfusion treatment in a newborn with phenobarbital intoxication. *Pediatr Emerg Care* 15: 268–270

134 Kosmidis HV, Bouhoutsou DO, Varvoutsi MC, Papadatos J, Stefanidis CG, Vlachos P, Scardoutsou A, Kostakis A (1991) Vincristine overdose: Experience with 3 patients. *Pediatr Hematol Oncol* 8: 171–178

135 Coleman MD, Coleman NA (1996) Drug-induced methaemoglobinaemia. Treatment issues. *Drug Saf* 14: 394–405

136 Kwon SU, Lim SH, Rhee I, Kim SW, Kim JK, Kim DW, Jeon ES (2006) Successful whole blood exchange by apheresis in a patient with acute cyclosporine intoxication without long-term sequelae. *J Heart Lung Transplant* 25: 483–485

137 Camerino DC, Desaphy JF, Tricarico D, Pierno S, Liantonio A (2008) Therapeutic approaches to ion channel diseases. *Adv Genet* 64: 81–145

138 Diaz-Sylvester PL, Porta M, Copello JA (2008) Halothane modulation of skeletal muscle ryanodine receptors: Dependence on Ca^{2+}, Mg^{2+}, and ATP. *Am J Physiol Cell Physiol* 294: C1103–1112

139 Smith FA, Wittmann CW, Stern TA (2008) Medical complications of psychiatric treatment. *Crit Care Clin* 24: 635–656

140 Dunkley EJ, Isbister GK, Sibbritt D, Dawson AH, Whyte IM (2003) The Hunter serotonin toxicity criteria: Simple and accurate diagnostic decision rules for serotonin toxicity. *QJM* 96: 635–642

141 Sternbach H (1991) The serotonin syndrome. *Am J Psychiatry* 148: 705–713

142 Boyer EW, Shannon M (2005) The serotonin syndrome. *N Engl J Med* 352: 1112–1120

143 Rusyniak DE, Sprague JE (2005) Toxin-induced hyperthermic syndromes. *Med Clin North Am* 89: 1277–1296

144 Ioos V, Das V, Maury E, Baudel JL, Guechot J, Guidet B, Offenstadt G (2008) A thyrotoxicosis outbreak due to dietary pills in Paris. *Ther Clin Risk Manag* 4: 1375–1379

145 Redahan C, Karski JM (1994) Thyrotoxicosis factitia in a post-aortocoronary bypass patient. *Can J Anaesth* 41: 969–972

146 Hsiao AL, Santucci KA, Seo-Mayer P, Mariappan MR, Hodsdon ME, Banasiak KJ, Baum CR (2005) Pediatric fatality following ingestion of dinitrophenol: Postmortem identification of a "dietary supplement". *Clin Toxicol* 43: 281–285

147 Argaud L, Ferry T, Le QH, Marfisi A, Ciorba D, Achache P, Ducluzeau R, Robert D (2007) Short- and long-term outcomes of heatstroke following the 2003 heat wave in Lyon, France. *Arch Intern Med* 167: 2177–2183

148 Dematte JE, O'Mara K, Buescher J, Whitney CG, Forsythe S, McNamee T, Adiga RB, Ndukwu IM (1998) Near-fatal heat stroke during the 1995 heat wave in Chicago. *Ann Intern Med* 129:

173–181

149 Marzuk PM, Tardiff K, Leon AC, Hirsch CS, Portera L, Iqbal MI, Nock MK, Hartwell N (1998) Ambient temperature and mortality from unintentional cocaine overdose. *J Am Med Assoc* 279: 1795–1800

150 Bowyer JF, Davies DL, Schmued L, Broening HW, Newport GD, Slikker W Jr, Holson RR (1994) Further studies of the role of hyperthermia in methamphetamine neurotoxicity. *J Pharmacol Exp Ther* 268: 1571–1580

151 Ferris EB, Blankenhorn MA, Robinson HW, Cullen GE (1938) Heat stroke: Clinical and chemical observations on 44 cases. *J Clin Invest* 17: 249–262

152 Bouchama A, Dehbi M, Chaves-Carballo E (2007) Cooling and hemodynamic management in heatstroke: Practical recommendations. *Crit Care* 11: R54

153 Armstrong LE, Crago AE, Adams R, Roberts WO, Maresh CM (1996) Whole-body cooling of hyperthermic runners: Comparison of two field therapies. *Am J Emerg Med* 14: 355–358

154 Costrini A (1990) Emergency treatment of exertional heatstroke and comparison of whole body cooling techniques. *Med Sci Sports Exerc* 22: 15–18

155 Nisijima K, Shioda K, Yoshino T, Takano K, Kato S (2003) Diazepam and chlormethiazole attenuate the development of hyperthermia in an animal model of the serotonin syndrome. *Neurochem Int* 43: 155–164

156 Derlet RW, Albertson TE, Rice P (1990) Antagonism of cocaine, amphetamine, and methamphetamine toxicity. *Pharmacol Biochem Behav* 36: 745–749

157 Laorden ML, Carrillo E, Miralles FS, Puig MM (1990) Effects of diltiazem on hyperthermia induced seizures in the rat pup. *Gen Pharmacol* 21: 313–315

158 Kobayashi S, Bannister ML, Gangopadhyay JP, Hamada T, Parness J, Ikemoto N (2005) Dantrolene stabilizes domain interactions within the ryanodine receptor. *J Biol Chem* 280: 6580–6587

159 Cherednichenko G, Ward CW, Feng W, Cabrales E, Michaelson L, Samso M, Lopez JR, Allen PD, Pessah IN (2008) Enhanced excitation-coupled calcium entry in myotubes expressing malignant hyperthermia mutation R163C is attenuated by dantrolene. *Mol Pharmacol* 73: 1203–1212

160 Reulbach U, Dutsch C, Biermann T, Sperling W, Thuerauf N, Kornhuber J, Bleich S (2007) Managing an effective treatment for neuroleptic malignant syndrome. *Crit Care* 11: R4

161 Sakkas P, Davis JM, Janicak PG, Wang ZY (1991) Drug treatment of the neuroleptic malignant syndrome. *Psychopharmacol Bull* 27: 381–384

162 Massicotte A (2008) Contrast medium-induced nephropathy: Strategies for prevention. *Pharmacotherapy* 28: 1140–1150

163 Rumack BH (2002) Acetaminophen hepatotoxicity: The first 35 years. *J Toxicol Clin Toxicol* 40: 3–20

164 Laine JE, Auriola S, Pasanen M, Juvonen RO (2009) Acetaminophen bioactivation by human cytochrome P450 enzymes and animal microsomes. *Xenobiotica* 39: 11–21

165 Heard KJ (2008) Acetylcysteine for acetaminophen poisoning. *N Engl J Med* 359: 285–292

166 Lauterburg BH, Corcoran GB, Mitchell JR (1983) Mechanism of action of *N*-acetylcysteine in the protection against the hepatotoxicity of acetaminophen in rats *in vivo. J Clin Invest* 71: 980–991

167 Keays R, Harrison PM, Wendon JA, Forbes A, Gove C, Alexander GJ, Williams R (1991) Intravenous acetylcysteine in paracetamol induced fulminant hepatic failure: A prospective controlled trial. *BMJ* 303: 1026–1029

168 Harrison PM, Wendon JA, Gimson AE, Alexander GJ, Williams R (1991) Improvement by acetylcysteine of hemodynamics and oxygen transport in fulminant hepatic failure. *N Engl J Med* 324: 1852–1857

169 Devlin J, Ellis AE, McPeake J, Heaton N, Wendon JA, Williams R (1997) *N*-Acetylcysteine improves indocyanine green extraction and oxygen transport during hepatic dysfunction. *Crit Care Med* 25: 236–242

170 Rank N, Michel C, Haertel C, Lenhart A, Welte M, Meier-Hellmann A, Spies C (2000) *N*-Acetylcysteine increases liver blood flow and improves liver function in septic shock patients: Results of a prospective, randomized, double-blind study. *Crit Care Med* 28: 3799–3807

171 Wong BK, Chan HC, Corcoran GB (1986) Selective effects of *N*-acetylcysteine stereoisomers on hepatic glutathione and plasma sulfate in mice. *Toxicol Appl Pharmacol* 86: 421–429

172 Wong BK, Galinsky RE, Corcoran GB (1986) Dissociation of increased sulfation from sulfate replenishment and hepatoprotection in acetaminophen-poisoned mice by *N*-acetylcysteine

stereoisomers. *J Pharm Sci* 75: 878–880
173 Tsai CL, Chang WT, Weng TI, Fang CC, Walson PD (2005) A patient-tailored *N*-acetylcysteine protocol for acute acetaminophen intoxication. *Clin Ther* 27: 336–341
174 Betten DP, Cantrell FL, Thomas SC, Williams SR, Clark RF (2007) A prospective evaluation of shortened course oral *N*-acetylcysteine for the treatment of acute acetaminophen poisoning. *Ann Emerg Med* 50: 272–279
175 Daly FF, Fountain JS, Murray L, Graudins A, Buckley NA (2008) Guidelines for the management of paracetamol poisoning in Australia and New Zealand – Explanation and elaboration. *Med J Aust* 188: 296–301
176 Smilkstein MJ, Knapp GL, Kulig KW, Rumack BH (1988) Efficacy of oral *N*-acetylcysteine in the treatment of acetaminophen overdose. Analysis of the national multicenter study (1976 to 1985) *N Engl J Med* 319: 1557–1562
177 Bridger S, Henderson K, Glucksman E, Ellis AJ, Henry JA, Williams R (1998) Deaths from low dose paracetamol poisoning. *BMJ* 316: 1724–1725
178 Rumack BH (2004) Acetaminophen misconceptions. *Hepatology* 40: 10–15
179 Pakravan N, Waring WS, Sharma S, Ludlam C, Megson I, Bateman DN (2008) Risk factors and mechanisms of anaphylactoid reactions to acetylcysteine in acetaminophen overdose. *Clin Toxicol* 46: 697–702
180 Hayes BD, Klein-Schwartz W, Doyon S (2008) Frequency of medication errors with intravenous acetylcysteine for acetaminophen overdose. *Ann Pharmacother* 42: 766–770
181 Sung L, Simons JA, Dayneka NL (1997) Dilution of intravenous *N*-acetylcysteine as a cause of hyponatremia. *Pediatrics* 100: 389–391
182 Yarema MC, Johnson DW, Berlin RJ, Sivilotti ML, Nettel-Aguirre A, Brant RF, Spyker DA, Bailey B, Chalut D, Lee JS, Plint AC, Purssell RA, Rutledge T, Seviour CA, Stiell IG, Thompson M, Tyberg J, Dart RC, Rumack BH (2009) Comparison of the 20-hour intravenous and 72-hour oral acetylcysteine protocols for the treatment of acute acetaminophen poisoning. *Ann Emerg Med* 54: 606–614
183 Doyon S, Klein-Schwartz W (2009) Hepatotoxicity despite early administration of intravenous *N*-acetylcysteine for acute acetaminophen overdose. *Acad Emerg Med* 16: 34–39
184 Smith SW, Howland MA, Hoffman RS, Nelson LS (2008) Acetaminophen overdose with altered acetaminophen pharmacokinetics and hepatotoxicity associated with premature cessation of intravenous *N*-acetylcysteine therapy. *Ann Pharmacother* 42: 1333–1339
185 Halcomb SE, Sivilotti ML, Goklaney A, Mullins ME (2005) Pharmacokinetic effects of diphenhydramine or oxycodone in simulated acetaminophen overdose. *Acad Emerg Med* 12: 169–172
186 Cetaruk EW, Dart RC, Hurlbut KM, Horowitz RS, Shih R (1997) Tylenol extended relief overdose. *Ann Emerg Med* 30: 104–108
187 Fraser TR (1863) On the characters, actions, and therapeutic uses of the bean of Calabar. *Edin Med J* 9: 36–56; 123–132; 235–248
188 Nickalls RW, Nickalls EA (1988) The first use of physostigmine in the treatment of atropine poisoning. A translation of Kleinwachter's paper entitled 'Observations on the effect of Calabar bean extract as an antidote to atropine poisoning'. *Anaesthesia* 43: 776–779
189 Atack JR, Yu QS, Soncrant TT, Brossi A, Rapoport SI (1989) Comparative inhibitory effects of various physostigmine analogs against acetyl- and butyrylcholinesterases. *J Pharmacol Exp Ther* 249: 194–202
190 Brossi A, Schonenberger B, Clark OE, Ray R (1986) Inhibition of acetylcholinesterase from electric eel by (–)- and (+)-physostigmine and related compounds. *FEBS Lett* 201: 190–192
191 Barak D, Ordentlich A, Stein D, Yu QS, Greig NH, Shafferman A (2009) Accommodation of physostigmine and its analogues by acetylcholinesterase is dominated by hydrophobic interactions. *Biochem J* 417: 213–222
192 Pereira EF, Hilmas C, Santos MD, Alkondon M, Maelicke A, Albuquerque EX (2002) Unconventional ligands and modulators of nicotinic receptors. *J Neurobiol* 53: 479–500
193 Pentel P, Peterson CD (1980) Asystole complicating physostigmine treatment of tricyclic antidepressant overdose. *Ann Emerg Med* 9: 588–590
194 Suchard JR (2003) Assessing physostigmine's contraindication in cyclic antidepressant ingestions. *J Emerg Med* 25: 185–191
195 Ago J, Ishikawa T, Matsumoto N, Ashequr Rahman M, Kamei C (2006) Mechanism of imipramine-induced seizures in amygdala-kindled rats. *Epilepsy Res* 72: 1–9
196 Fleck C, Braunlich H (1982) Failure of physostigmine in intoxications with tricyclic antidepres-

sants in rats. *Toxicology* 24: 335–344

197 Burns MJ, Linden CH, Graudins A, Brown RM, Fletcher KE (2000) A comparison of physostigmine and benzodiazepines for the treatment of anticholinergic poisoning. *Ann Emerg Med* 35: 374–381

198 Frascogna N (2007) Physostigmine: Is there a role for this antidote in pediatric poisonings? *Curr Opin Pediatr* 19: 201–205

199 Claessens YE, Cariou A, Monchi M, Soufir L, Azoulay E, Rouges P, Goldgran-Toledano D, Branche F, Dhainaut JF (2003) Detecting life-threatening lactic acidosis related to nucleoside-analog treatment of human immunodeficiency virus-infected patients, and treatment with L-carnitine. *Crit Care Med* 31: 1042–1047

200 Delaney CE, Hopkins SP, Addison CL (2007) Supplementation with L-carnitine does not reduce the efficacy of epirubicin treatment in breast cancer cells. *Cancer Lett* 252: 195–207

201 Lheureux PE, Penaloza A, Zahir S, Gris M (2005) Science review: Carnitine in the treatment of valproic acid-induced toxicity – What is the evidence? *Crit Care* 9: 431–440

202 Katiyar A, Aaron C (2007) Case files of the Children's Hospital of Michigan Regional Poison Control Center: The use of carnitine for the management of acute valproic acid toxicity. *J Med Toxicol* 3: 129–138

203 Loscher W (2002) Basic pharmacology of valproate: A review after 35 years of clinical use for the treatment of epilepsy. *CNS Drugs* 16: 669–694

204 Silva MF, Aires CC, Luis PB, Ruiter JP, Ijlst L, Duran M, Wanders RJ, Tavares de Almeida I (2008) Valproic acid metabolism and its effects on mitochondrial fatty acid oxidation: A review. *J Inherit Metab Dis, in press*

205 Ingels M, Beauchamp J, Clark RF, Williams SR (2002) Delayed valproic acid toxicity: A retrospective case series. *Ann Emerg Med* 39: 616–621

206 Eyer F, Felgenhauer N, Gempel K, Steimer W, Gerbitz KD, Zilker T (2005) Acute valproate poisoning: Pharmacokinetics, alteration in fatty acid metabolism, and changes during therapy. *J Clin Psychopharmacol* 25: 376–380

207 Sztajnkrycer MD (2002) Valproic acid toxicity: Overview and management. *J Toxicol Clin Toxicol* 40: 789–801

208 Riva R, Albani F, Gobbi G, Santucci M, Baruzzi A (1993) Carnitine disposition before and during valproate therapy in patients with epilepsy. *Epilepsia* 34: 184–187

209 Okamura N, Ohnishi S, Shimaoka H, Norikura R, Hasegawa H (2006) Involvement of recognition and interaction of carnitine transporter in the decrease of L-carnitine concentration induced by pivalic acid and valproic acid. *Pharm Res* 23: 1729–1735

210 Spahr L, Negro F, Rubbia-Brandt L, Marinescu O, Goodman K, Jordan M, Frossard JL, Hadengue A (2001) Acute valproate-associated microvesicular steatosis: Could the [^{13}C]methionine breath test be useful to assess liver mitochondrial function? *Dig Dis Sci* 46: 2758–2761

211 Russell S (2007) Carnitine as an antidote for acute valproate toxicity in children. *Curr Opin Pediatr* 19: 206–210

212 De Vivo DC, Bohan TP, Coulter DL, Dreifuss FE, Greenwood RS, Nordli DR Jr, Shields WD, Stafstrom CE, Tein I (1998) L-carnitine supplementation in childhood epilepsy: Current perspectives. *Epilepsia* 39: 1216–1225

213 Anil M, Helvaci M, Ozbal E, Kalenderer O, Anil AB, Dilek M (2009) Serum and muscle carnitine levels in epileptic children receiving sodium valproate. *J Child Neurol* 24: 80–86

214 Zelnik N, Isler N, Goez H, Shiffer M, David M, Shahar E (2008) Vigabatrin, lamotrigine, topiramate and serum carnitine levels. *Pediatr Neurol* 39: 18–21

215 Verrotti A, Greco R, Morgese G, Chiarelli F (1999) Carnitine deficiency and hyperammonemia in children receiving valproic acid with and without other anticonvulsant drugs. *Int J Clin Lab Res* 29: 36–40

216 Bohles H, Sewell AC, Wenzel D (1996) The effect of carnitine supplementation in valproate-induced hyperammonaemia. *Acta Paediatr* 85: 446–449

217 Gidal BE, Inglese CM, Meyer JF, Pitterle ME, Antonopolous J, Rust RS (1997) Diet- and valproate-induced transient hyperammonemia: Effect of L-carnitine. *Pediatr Neurol* 16: 301–305

218 Van Wouwe JP (1995) Carnitine deficiency during valproic acid treatment. *Int J Vitam Nutr Res* 65: 211–214

219 Ishikura H, Matsuo N, Matsubara M, Ishihara T, Takeyama N, Tanaka T (1996) Valproic acid overdose and L-carnitine therapy. *J Anal Toxicol* 20: 55–58

220 Romero-Falcon A, de la Santa-Belda E, Garci-Contreras R, Varela JM (2003) A case of valproate-

associated hepatotoxicity treated with L-carnitine. *Eur J Intern Med* 14: 338–340

221 Wadzinski J, Franks R, Roane D, Bayard M (2007) Valproate-associated hyperammonemic encephalopathy. *J Am Board Fam Med* 20: 499–502

222 Bohan TP, Helton E, McDonald I, Konig S, Gazitt S, Sugimoto T, Scheffner D, Cusmano L, Li S, Koch G (2001) Effect of L-carnitine treatment for valproate-induced hepatotoxicity. *Neurology* 56: 1405–1409

223 Raskind JY, El-Chaar GM (2000) The role of carnitine supplementation during valproic acid therapy. *Ann Pharmacother* 34: 630–638

224 Beauchamp J, Olson K (1999) Valproic acid overdoses: A retrospective study comparing serum drug levels and the incidence of adverse outcomes. *J Toxicol Clin Toxicol* 37: 637–638

225 LoVecchio F, Shriki J, Samaddar R (2005) L-Carnitine was safely administered in the setting of valproate toxicity. *Am J Emerg Med* 23: 321–322

226 Sigma-Tau Pharmaceuticals Inc (2006) CARNITOR® (levocarnitine) Tablets (330 mg). CARNITOR® (levocarnitine) Oral Solution (1 g per 10 mL multidose). CARNITOR® SF (levocarnitine) Sugar-Free Oral Solution (1 g per 10 mL multidose). Sigma-Tau Pharmaceuticals Inc., Gaithersburg, MD

227 Jung J, Eo E, Ahn KO (2008) A case of hemoperfusion and L-carnitine management in valproic acid overdose. *Am J Emerg Med* 26: 388.e3–4

228 Rossini PM, Marchionno L, Gambi D, Pirchio M, Del Rosso G, Albertazzi A (1981) EMG changes in chronically dialyzed uraemic subjects undergoing D,L-carnitine treatment. *Ital J Neurol Sci* 2: 255–262

229 Tsoko M, Beauseigneur F, Gresti J, Niot I, Demarquoy J, Boichot J, Bezard J, Rochette L, Clouet P (1995) Enhancement of activities relative to fatty acid oxidation in the liver of rats depleted of L-carnitine by D-carnitine and a γ-butyrobetaine hydroxylase inhibitor. *Biochem Pharmacol* 49: 1403–1410

230 Seltzer HS (1989) Drug-induced hypoglycemia. A review of 1418 cases. *Endocrinol Metab Clin North Am* 18: 163–183

231 Chan JC, Cockram CS, Critchley JA (1996) Drug-induced disorders of glucose metabolism. Mechanisms and management. *Drug Saf* 15: 135–157

232 Wender R, Brown AM, Fern R, Swanson RA, Farrell K, Ransom BR (2000) Astrocytic glycogen influences axon function and survival during glucose deprivation in central white matter. *J Neurosci* 20: 6804–6810

233 Boyle PJ, Kempers SF, O'Connor AM, Nagy RJ (1995) Brain glucose uptake and unawareness of hypoglycemia in patients with insulin-dependent diabetes mellitus. *N Engl J Med* 333: 1726–1731

234 Dalan R, Leow MK, George J, Chian KY, Tan A, Han HW, Cheow SP (2009) Neuroglycopenia and adrenergic responses to hypoglycaemia: Insights from a local epidemic of serendipitous massive overdose of glibenclamide. *Diabet Med* 26: 105–109

235 Kuzak N, Brubacher JR, Kennedy JR (2007) Reversal of salicylate-induced euglycemic delirium with dextrose. *Clin Toxicol (Phila)* 45: 526–529

236 Abdelmalik PA, Shannon P, Yiu A, Liang P, Adamchik Y, Weisspapir M, Samoilova M, Burnham WM, Carlen PL (2007) Hypoglycemic seizures during transient hypoglycemia exacerbate hippocampal dysfunction. *Neurobiol Dis* 26: 646–660

237 Auer RN, Wieloch T, Olsson Y, Siesjo BK (1984) The distribution of hypoglycemic brain damage. *Acta Neuropathol* 64: 177–191

238 Hospira, Inc (2004) Concentrated Dextrose for Intravenous Administration. Hospira Inc., Lake Forest, IL

239 Cunningham P, Afzal-Ahmed I, Naftalin RJ (2006) Docking studies show that D-glucose and quercetin slide through the transporter GLUT1. *J Biol Chem* 281: 5797–5803

240 Yosowitz P, Ekland DA, Shaw RC, Parsons RW (1975) Peripheral intravenous infiltration necrosis. *Ann Surg* 182: 553–556

241 MacLeod DB, Montoya DR, Fick GH, Jessen KR (1994) The effect of 25 grams i.v. glucose on serum inorganic phosphate levels. *Ann Emerg Med* 23: 524–528

242 Novartis Pharma Stein AG (2008) Sandostatin® octreotide acetate Injection Prescribing Information. Novartis Pharma Stein AG, Stein, Switzerland

243 Doyle ME, Egan JM (2003) Pharmacological agents that directly modulate insulin secretion. *Pharmacol Rev* 55: 105–131

244 Gerich JE (1989) Oral hypoglycemic agents. *N Engl J Med* 321: 1231–1245

245 Hansen JB, Arkhammar PO, Bodvarsdottir TB, Wahl P (2004) Inhibition of insulin secretion as a new drug target in the treatment of metabolic disorders. *Curr Med Chem* 11: 1595–1615

246 Lahlou H, Guillermet J, Hortala M, Vernejoul F, Pyronnet S, Bousquet C, Susini C (2004) Molecular signaling of somatostatin receptors. *Ann NY Acad Sci* 1014: 121–131

247 Di Mauro M, Papalia G, Le Moli R, Nativo B, Nicoletti F, Lunetta M (2001) Effect of octreotide on insulin requirement, hepatic glucose production, growth hormone, glucagon and c-peptide levels in type 2 diabetic patients with chronic renal failure or normal renal function. *Diabetes Res Clin Pract* 51: 45–50

248 Mordel A, Sivilotti MLA, Old AC, Ferm RP (1998) Octreotide for pediatric sulfonylurea poisoning. *J Toxicol Clin Toxicol* 36: 437

249 Skugor M, Siraj ES (2003) A diabetic woman with worsening heart failure, hunger, and tremor. *Cleve Clin J Med* 70: 882–888

250 Green RS, Palatnick W (2003) Effectiveness of octreotide in a case of refractory sulfonylurea-induced hypoglycemia. *J Emerg Med* 25: 283–287

251 Boyle PJ, Justice K, Krentz AJ, Nagy RJ, Schade DS (1993) Octreotide reverses hyperinsulinemia and prevents hypoglycemia induced by sulfonylurea overdoses. *J Clin Endocrinol Metab* 76: 752–756

252 McLaughlin SA, Crandall CS, McKinney PE (2000) Octreotide: An antidote for sulfonylurea-induced hypoglycemia. *Ann Emerg Med* 36: 133–138

253 Fasano CJ, O'Malley G, Dominici P, Aguilera E, Latta DR (2008) Comparison of octreotide and standard therapy *versus* standard therapy alone for the treatment of sulfonylurea-induced hypoglycemia. *Ann Emerg Med* 51: 400–406

254 Gul M, Cander B, Girisgin S, Ayan M, Kocak S, Unlu A (2006) The effectiveness of various doses of octreotide for sulfonylurea-induced hypoglycemia after overdose. *Adv Ther* 23: 878–884

255 Fleseriu M, Skugor M, Chinnappa P, Siraj ES (2006) Successful treatment of sulfonylurea-induced prolonged hypoglycemia with use of octreotide. *Endocr Pract* 12: 635–640

256 Carr R, Zed PJ (2002) Octreotide for sulfonylurea-induced hypoglycemia following overdose. *Ann Pharmacother* 36: 1727–1732

257 Tenenbein MS, Tenenbein M (2006) Anaphylactoid reaction to octreotide. *Clin Toxicol* 44: 707

258 Calello DP, Kelly A, Osterhoudt KC (2006) Case files of the Medical Toxicology Fellowship Training Program at the Children's Hospital of Philadelphia: A pediatric exploratory sulfonylurea ingestion. *J Med Toxicol* 2: 19–24

259 Curtis JA, Greenberg MI (2006) Bradycardia and hyperkalemia associated with octreotide administration. *Clin Toxicol* 44: 498

260 Rath S, Bar-Zeev N, Anderson K, Fahy R, Roseby R (2008) Octreotide in children with hypoglycaemia due to sulfonylurea ingestion. *J Paediatr Child Health* 44: 383–384

261 Al-Shanafey S, Habib Z, AlNassar S (2009) Laparoscopic pancreatectomy for persistent hyperinsulinemic hypoglycemia of infancy. *J Pediatr Surg* 44: 134–138

262 Ferraz DP, Almeida MA, Mello BF (2005) Octreotide therapy for persistent hyperinsulinemic hypoglycemia of infancy. *Arq Bras Endocrinol Metabol* 49: 460–467

263 Phillips RE, Warrell DA, Looareesuwan S, Turner RC, Bloom SR, Quantrill D, Moore AR (1986) Effectiveness of SMS 201–995, a synthetic, long-acting somatostatin analogue, in treatment of quinine-induced hyperinsulinaemia. *Lancet* 1: 713–716

264 Phillips RE, Looareesuwan S, Molyneux ME, Hatz C, Warrell DA (1993) Hypoglycaemia and counterregulatory hormone responses in severe falciparum malaria: Treatment with sandostatin. *Q J Med* 86: 233–240

265 Lheureux PE, Zahir S, Penaloza A, Gris M (2005) Bench-to-bedside review: Antidotal treatment of sulfonylurea-induced hypoglycaemia with octreotide. *Crit Care* 9: 543–549

266 Harris AG (1994) Somatostatin and somatostatin analogues: Pharmacokinetics and pharmacodynamic effects. *Gut* 35: S1–4

267 Kalman SD, Rogers R, Barrueto F Jr (2006) Glyburide sold as "Street Steroid" causes hypoglycemia complicated by inappropriate IV administration of octreotide. *Clin Toxicol* 44: 713–714

268 Lamberts SW, van der Lely AJ, de Herder WW, Hofland LJ (1996) Octreotide. *N Engl J Med* 334: 246–254

269 Mohnike K, Blankenstein O, Pfuetzner A, Potzsch S, Schober E, Steiner S, Hardy OT, Grimberg A, van Waarde WM (2008) Long-term non-surgical therapy of severe persistent congenital hyperinsulinism with glucagon. *Horm Res* 70: 59–64

270 Garibaldi RA, Drusin RE, Ferebee SH, Gregg MB (1972) Isoniazid-associated hepatitis. Report

of an outbreak. *Am Rev Respir Dis* 106: 357–365

271 Peloquin CA (2002) Therapeutic drug monitoring in the treatment of tuberculosis. *Drugs* 62: 2169–2183

272 Lheureux P, Penaloza A, Gris M (2005) Pyridoxine in clinical toxicology: A review. *Eur J Emerg Med* 12: 78–85

273 Sullivan EA, Geoffroy P, Weisman R, Hoffman R, Frieden TR (1998) Isoniazid poisonings in New York City. *J Emerg Med* 16: 57–59

274 Brown CV (1972) Acute isoniazid poisoning. *Am Rev Respir Dis* 105: 206–216

275 Agrawal RL, Dwivedi NC, Agrawal M, Jain S, Agrawal A (2008) Accidental isoniazid poisoning – A report. *Indian J Tuberc* 55: 94–96

276 Handbook of Anti-Tuberculosis Agents (2008) Isoniazid *Tuberculosis* 88: 112–116

277 Dunlop DS, Neidle A (1997) The origin and turnover of D-serine in brain. *Biochem Biophys Res Commun* 235: 26–30

278 Mustafa AK, van Rossum DB, Patterson RL, Maag D, Ehmsen JT, Gazi SK, Chakraborty A, Barrow RK, Amzel LM, Snyder SH (2009) Glutamatergic regulation of serine racemase *via* reversal of PIP2 inhibition. *Proc Natl Acad Sci USA* 106: 2921–2926

279 Wood JD, Peesker SJ (1972) The effect on GABA metabolism in brain of isonicotinic acid hydrazide and pyridoxine as a fuction of time after administration. *J Neurochem* 19: 1527–1537

280 Hankins DG, Saxena K, Faville RJ Jr, Warren BJ (1987) Profound acidosis caused by isoniazid ingestion. *Am J Emerg Med* 5: 165–166

281 Chin L, Sievers ML, Herrier RN, Picchioni AL (1979) Convulsions as the etiology of lactic acidosis in acute isoniazid toxicity in dogs. *Toxicol Appl Pharmacol* 49: 377–384

282 Wason S, Lacouture PG, Lovejoy FH Jr (1981) Single high-dose pyridoxine treatment for isoniazid overdose. *J Am Med Assoc* 246: 1102–1104

283 Terman DS, Teitelbaum DT (1970) Isoniazid self-poisoning. *Neurology* 20: 299–304

284 Jen M, Shah KN, Yan AC (2008) Cutaneous changes in nutritional disease. In: K Wolff, LA Goldsmith, SI Katz, BA Gilchrest, AS Paller, DJ Leffell (eds): *Fitzpatrick's Dermatology in General Medicine*, 7th edn., The McGraw-Hill Companies Inc. (http://www.accessmedicine.com/content.aspx?aID=2964061, accessed April 6, 2009)

285 Miller J, Robinson A, Percy AK (1980) Acute isoniazid poisoning in childhood. *Am J Dis Child* 134: 290–292

286 Brent J, Vo N, Kulig K, Rumack BH (1990) Reversal of prolonged isoniazid-induced coma by pyridoxine. *Arch Intern Med* 150: 1751–1753

287 Shah BR, Santucci K, Sinert R, Steiner P (1995) Acute isoniazid neurotoxicity in an urban hospital. *Pediatrics* 95: 700–704

288 Alvarez FG, Guntupalli KK (1995) Isoniazid overdose: Four case reports and review of the literature. *Intensive Care Med* 21: 641–644

289 Chin L, Sievers ML, Laird HE, Herrier RN, Picchioni AL (1978) Evaluation of diazepam and pyridoxine as antidotes to isoniazid intoxication in rats and dogs. *Toxicol Appl Pharmacol* 45: 713–722

290 Morrow LE, Wear RE, Schuller D, Malesker M (2006) Acute isoniazid toxicity and the need for adequate pyridoxine supplies. *Pharmacotherapy* 26: 1529–1532

291 Scharman EJ, Rosencrane JG (1994) Isoniazid toxicity: A survey of pyridoxine availability. *Am J Emerg Med* 12: 386–388

292 Schaumburg H, Kaplan J, Windebank A, Vick N, Rasmus S, Pleasure D, Brown MJ (1983) Sensory neuropathy from pyridoxine abuse. A new megavitamin syndrome. *N Engl J Med* 309: 445–448

293 Bredemann JA, Krechel SW, Eggers GW Jr (1990) Treatment of refractory seizures in massive isoniazid overdose. *Anesth Analg* 71: 554–557

294 Hensley ML, Hagerty KL, Kewalramani T, Green DM, Meropol NJ, Wasserman TH, Cohen GI, Emami B, Gradishar WJ, Mitchell RB, Thigpen JT, Trotti A 3rd, von Hoff D, Schuchter LM (2009) American Society of Clinical Oncology 2008 clinical practice guideline update: Use of chemotherapy and radiation therapy protectants. *J Clin Oncol* 27: 127–145

295 Cetingul N, Midyat L, Kantar M, Demirag B, Aksoylar S, Kansoy S (2009) Cytoprotective effects of amifostine in the treatment of childhood malignancies. *Pediatr Blood Cancer* 52: 829–833

296 Batista CK, Mota JM, Souza ML, Leitao BT, Souza MH, Brito GA, Cunha FQ, Ribeiro RA (2007) Amifostine and glutathione prevent ifosfamide- and acrolein-induced hemorrhagic cystitis. *Cancer Chemother Pharmacol* 59: 71–77

297 Gandara DR, Nahhas WA, Adelson MD, Lichtman SM, Podczaski ES, Yanovich S, Homesley HD, Braly P, Ritch PS, Weisberg SR (1995) Randomized placebo-controlled multicenter evaluation of diethyldithiocarbamate for chemoprotection against cisplatin-induced toxicities. *J Clin Oncol* 13: 490–496

298 Crawford J, Armitage J, Balducci L, Bennett C, Blayney DW, Cataland SR, Dale DC, Demetri GD, Erba HP, Foran J, Freifeld AG, Goemann M, Heaney ML, Htoy S, Hudock S, Kloth DD, Kuter DJ, Lyman GH, Michaud LB, Miyata SC, Tallman MS, Vadhan-Raj S, Westervelt P, Wong MK (2009) Myeloid growth factors. *J Natl Compr Canc Netw* 7: 64–83

299 Wyeth Pharmaceuticals Inc (2009) NEUMEGA® [nu-meg<a] (oprelvekin). Wyeth Pharmaceuticals Inc., Philadelphia, PA

300 Wengstrom Y, Margulies A (2008) European Oncology Nursing Society extravasation guidelines. *Eur J Oncol Nurs* 12: 357–361

301 TopoTarget USA Inc (2007) Totect™ (Dexrazoxane) for injection. Totect™ Package Insert. Distributed by Integrated Commercialization Solutions. Manufactured by Ben Venue Laboratories Inc., and Hameln Pharmaceuticals GmbH for TopoTarget A/S. Marketed by TopoTarget USA Inc., Rockaway, NJ

302 Mouridsen HT, Langer SW, Buter J, Eidtmann H, Rosti G, de Wit M, Knoblauch P, Rasmussen A, Dahlstrom K, Jensen PB, Giaccone G (2007) Treatment of anthracycline extravasation with Savene (dexrazoxane): Results from two prospective clinical multicentre studies. *Ann Oncol* 18: 546–550

303 Frost A, Gmehling D, Azemar M, Unger C, Mross K (2006) Treatment of anthracycline extravasation with dexrazoxane – Clinical experience. *Onkologie* 29: 314–318

304 Kane RC, McGuinn WD Jr, Dagher R, Justice R, Pazdur R (2008) Dexrazoxane (Totect): FDA review and approval for the treatment of accidental extravasation following intravenous anthracycline chemotherapy. *Oncologist* 13: 445–450

305 Reeves D (2007) Management of anthracycline extravasation injuries. *Ann Pharmacother* 41: 1238–1242

306 Yan T, Deng S, Metzger A, Godtel-Armbrust U, Porter AC, Wojnowski L (2009) Topoisomerase IIα-dependent and -independent apoptotic effects of dexrazoxane and doxorubicin. *Mol Cancer Ther, in press*

307 Dexrazoxane: New indication. Anthracycline extravasation: Continue using dimethyl sulfoxide (2009) *Prescrire Int* 18: 6–8 (http://www.find-health-articles.com/rec_pub_19382398-dexrazoxane-new-indication-anthracycline-extravasation-continue-using.htm)

308 Sacks MS, Bradford GT, Schoenbach EB (1950) The response of acute leukemia to the administration of the folic acid antagonists, aminopterin and a-methopterin; Report of 14 cases. *Ann Intern Med* 32: 80–115

309 Li MC, Hertz R, Spencer DB (1956) Effect of methotrexate therapy upon choriocarcinoma and chorioadenoma. *Proc Soc Exp Biol Med* 93: 361–366

310 Abel EA (2000) Immunosuppressant and cytotoxic drugs: Unapproved uses or indications. *Clin Dermatol* 18: 95–101

311 Roenigk HH Jr, Auerbach R, Maibach H, Weinstein G, Lebwohl M (1998) Methotrexate in psoriasis: Consensus conference. *J Am Acad Dermatol* 38: 478–485

312 Borchers AT, Keen CL, Cheema GS, Gershwin ME (2004) The use of methotrexate in rheumatoid arthritis. *Semin Arthritis Rheum* 34: 465–483

313 Buchen S, Ngampolo D, Melton RG, Hasan C, Zoubek A, Henze G, Bode U, Fleischhack G (2005) Carboxypeptidase G₂ rescue in patients with methotrexate intoxication and renal failure. *Br J Cancer* 92: 480–487

314 Moisa A, Fritz P, Benz D, Wehner HD (2006) Iatrogenically-related, fatal methotrexate intoxication: A series of four cases. *Forensic Sci Int* 156: 154–157

315 Widemann BC, Balis FM, Kempf-Bielack B, Bielack S, Pratt CB, Ferrari S, Bacci G, Craft AW, Adamson PC (2004) High-dose methotrexate-induced nephrotoxicity in patients with osteosarcoma. *Cancer* 100: 2222–2232

316 Dervieux T, Furst D, Lein DO, Capps R, Smith K, Walsh M, Kremer J (2004) Polyglutamation of methotrexate with common polymorphisms in reduced folate carrier, aminoimidazole carboxamide ribonucleotide transformylase, and thymidylate synthase are associated with methotrexate effects in rheumatoid arthritis. *Arthritis Rheum* 50: 2766–2774

317 Genestier L, Paillot R, Quemeneur L, Izeradjene K, Revillard JP (2000) Mechanisms of action of methotrexate. *Immunopharmacology* 47: 247–257

318 Sasaki K, Tanaka J, Fujimoto T (1984) Theoretically required urinary flow during high-dose methotrexate infusion. *Cancer Chemother Pharmacol* 13: 9–13

319 Bleyer WA (1977) Methotrexate: Clinical pharmacology, current status and therapeutic guidelines. *Cancer Treat Rev* 4: 87–101

320 Nirenberg A, Mosende C, Mehta BM, Gisolfi AL, Rosen G (1977) High-dose methotrexate with citrovorum factor rescue: Predictive value of serum methotrexate concentrations and corrective measures to avert toxicity. *Cancer Treat Rep* 61: 779–783

321 Flombaum CD, Meyers PA (1999) High-dose leucovorin as sole therapy for methotrexate toxicity. *J Clin Oncol* 17: 1589–1594

322 Chabner BA, Young RC (1973) Threshold methotrexate concentration for *in vivo* inhibition of DNA synthesis in normal and tumorous target tissues. *J Clin Invest* 52: 1804–1811

323 Schilsky RL, Ratain MJ (1990) Clinical pharmacokinetics of high-dose leucovorin calcium after intravenous and oral administration. *J Natl Cancer Inst* 82: 1411–1415

324 Goorin A, Strother D, Poplack D, Letvak LA, George M, Link M (1995) Safety and efficacy of L-leucovorin rescue following high-dose methotrexate for osteosarcoma. *Med Pediatr Oncol* 24: 362–367

325 Jardine LF, Ingram LC, Bleyer WA (1996) Intrathecal leucovorin after intrathecal methotrexate overdose. *J Pediatr Hematol Oncol* 18: 302–304

326 Krause AS, Weihrauch MR, Bode U, Fleischhack G, Elter T, Heuer T, Engert A, Diehl V, Josting A (2002) Carboxypeptidase-G₂ rescue in cancer patients with delayed methotrexate elimination after high-dose methotrexate therapy. *Leuk Lymphoma* 43: 2139–2143

327 Pinedo HM, Zaharko DS, Bull JM, Chabner BA (1976) The reversal of methotrexate cytotoxicity to mouse bone marrow cells by leucovorin and nucleosides. *Cancer Res* 36: 4418–4424

328 Schwartz S, Borner K, Muller K, Martus P, Fischer L, Korfel A, Auton T, Thiel E (2007) Glucarpidase (carboxypeptidase G₂) intervention in adult and elderly cancer patients with renal dysfunction and delayed methotrexate elimination after high-dose methotrexate therapy. *Oncologist* 12: 1299–1308

329 Widemann BC, Balis FM, Shalabi A, Boron M, O'Brien M, Cole DE, Jayaprakash N, Ivy P, Castle V, Muraszko K, Moertel CL, Trueworthy R, Hermann RC, Moussa A, Hinton S, Reaman G, Poplack D, Adamson PC (2004) Treatment of accidental intrathecal methotrexate overdose with intrathecal carboxypeptidase G₂. *J Natl Cancer Inst* 96: 1557–1559

330 Widemann BC, Adamson PC (2006) Understanding and managing methotrexate nephrotoxicity. *Oncologist* 11: 694–703

331 Goldman P, Levy CC (1967) Carboxypeptidase G: Purification and properties. *Proc Natl Acad Sci USA* 58: 1299–1306

332 Chabner BA, Johns DG, Bertino JR (1972) Enzymatic cleavage of methotrexate provides a method for prevention of drug toxicity. *Nature* 239: 395–397

333 Abelson HT, Ensminger W, Rosowsky A, Uren J (1978) Comparative effects of citrovorum factor and carboxypeptidase G1 on cerebrospinal fluid-methotrexate pharmacokinetics. *Cancer Treat Rep* 62: 1549–1552

334 Howell SB, Blair HE, Uren J, Frei E 3rd (1978) Hemodialysis and enzymatic cleavage of methotrexate in man. *Eur J Cancer* 14: 787–792

335 Adamson PC, Balis FM, McCully CL, Godwin KS, Poplack DG (1992) Methotrexate pharmacokinetics following administration of recombinant carboxypeptidase-G₂ in rhesus monkeys. *J Clin Oncol* 10: 1359–1364

336 Adamson PC, Balis FM, McCully CL, Godwin KS, Bacher JD, Walsh TJ, Poplack DG (1991) Rescue of experimental intrathecal methotrexate overdose with carboxypeptidase-G₂. *J Clin Oncol* 9: 670–674

337 Zoubek A, Zaunschirm HA, Lion T, Fischmeister G, Vollnhofer G, Gadner H, Pillwein K, Schalhorn A, Bode U (1995) Successful carboxypeptidase G₂ rescue in delayed methotrexate elimination due to renal failure. *Pediatr Hematol Oncol* 12: 471–477

338 O'Marcaigh AS, Johnson CM, Smithson WA, Patterson MC, Widemann BC, Adamson PC, McManus MJ (1996) Successful treatment of intrathecal methotrexate overdose by using ventriculolumbar perfusion and intrathecal instillation of carboxypeptidase G₂. *Mayo Clin Proc* 71: 161–165

339 Peyriere H, Cociglio M, Margueritte G, Vallat C, Blayac JP, Hillaire-Buys D (2004) Optimal management of methotrexate intoxication in a child with osteosarcoma. *Ann Pharmacother* 38: 422–427

340 Rowsell S, Pauptit RA, Tucker AD, Melton RG, Blow DM, Brick P (1997) Crystal structure of carboxypeptidase G$_2$, a bacterial enzyme with applications in cancer therapy. *Structure* 5: 337–347

341 Widemann BC, Sung E, Anderson L, Salzer WL, Balis FM, Monitjo KS, McCully C, Hawkins M, Adamson PC (2000) Pharmacokinetics and metabolism of the methotrexate metabolite 2,4-diamino-N^{10}-methylpteroic acid. *J Pharmacol Exp Ther* 294: 894–901

342 Widemann BC, Hetherington ML, Murphy RF, Balis FM, Adamson PC (1995) Carboxy-peptidase-G$_2$ rescue in a patient with high dose methotrexate-induced nephrotoxicity. *Cancer* 76: 521–526

343 Widemann BC, Balis FM, Murphy RF, Sorensen JM, Montello MJ, O'Brien M, Adamson PC (1997) Carboxypeptidase-G$_2$, thymidine, and leucovorin rescue in cancer patients with methotrexate-induced renal dysfunction. *J Clin Oncol* 15: 2125–2134

344 Schwartz S, Müller K, Fischer L, Korfel A, Jahnke K, Auton T, Thiel E (2005) Favorable out-come in excessive methotrexate (MTX) intoxication after high-dose (HD) MTX therapy by early use of carboxypeptidase G$_2$ (CPG$_2$). *J Clin Oncol* 23(16S): 8255

345 DeAngelis LM, Tong WP, Lin S, Fleisher M, Bertino JR (1996) Carboxypeptidase G$_2$ rescue after high-dose methotrexate. *J Clin Oncol* 14: 2145–2149

346 Abelson HT, Ensminger W, Rosowsky A, Uren J (1978) Comparative effects of citrovorum fac-tor and carboxypeptidase G1 on cerebrospinal fluid-methotrexate pharmacokinetics. *Cancer Treat Rep* 62: 1549–1552

347 Widemann BC, Balis FM, Shalabi A, Boron M, O'Brien M, Cole DE, Jayaprakash N, Ivy P, Castle V, Muraszko K, Moertel CL, Trueworthy R, Hermann RC, Moussa A, Hinton S, Reaman G, Poplack D, Adamson PC (2004) Treatment of accidental intrathecal methotrexate overdose with intrathecal carboxypeptidase G$_2$. *J Natl Cancer Inst* 96: 1557–1559

348 Hempel G, Lingg R, Boos J (2005) Interactions of carboxypeptidase G$_2$ with 6S-leucovorin and 6R-leucovorin *in vitro*: Implications for the application in case of methotrexate intoxications. *Cancer Chemother Pharmacol* 55: 347–353

349 Fotoohi K, Skarby T, Soderhall S, Peterson C, Albertioni F (2005) Interference of 7-hydroxy-methotrexate with the determination of methotrexate in plasma samples from children with acute lymphoblastic leukemia employing routine clinical assays. *J Chromatogr B Analyt Technol Biomed Life Sci* 817: 139–144

350 European Medicines Agency (2008) Pre-authorisation Evaluation of Medicines for Human Use. Withdrawal Assessment Report for Voraxaze. EMEA/CHMP/171907/2008. European Medicines Agency (EMEA), London, UK

351 Sherwood RF, Melton RG, Alwan SM, Hughes P (1985) Purification and properties of car-boxypeptidase G$_2$ from *Pseudomonas* sp. strain RS-16. Use of a novel triazine dye affinity method. *Eur J Biochem* 148: 447–453

352 Albertson TE, Dawson A, de Latorre F, Hoffman RS, Hollander JE, Jaeger A, Kerns WR 2nd, Martin TG, Ross MP (2001) TOX-ACLS: Toxicologic-oriented advanced cardiac life support. *Ann Emerg Med* 37: S78–90

353 Ansell J, Hirsh J, Hylek E, Jacobson A, Crowther M, Palareti G (2008) Pharmacology and man-agement of the vitamin K antagonists: American College of Chest Physicians Evidence-Based Clinical Practice Guidelines, 8th edn. *Chest* 133: 160S–198S

354 Hirsh J, Bauer KA, Donati MB, Gould M, Samama MM, Weitz JI (2008) Parenteral anticoagu-lants: American College of Chest Physicians Evidence-Based Clinical Practice Guidelines, 8th edn. *Chest* 133: 141S–159S

355 Warkentin TE, Greinacher A, Koster A, Lincoff AM (2008) Treatment and prevention of heparin-induced thrombocytopenia: American College of Chest Physicians Evidence-Based Clinical Practice Guidelines, 8th edn. *Chest* 133: 340S–380S

356 Dager WE, Sanoski CA, Wiggins BS, Tisdale JE (2006) Pharmacotherapy considerations in advanced cardiac life support. *Pharmacotherapy* 26: 1703–1729

357 Dhein S, van Koppen CJ, Brodde OE (2001) Muscarinic receptors in the mammalian heart. *Pharmacol Res* 44: 161–182

358 Howarth DM, Dawson AH, Smith AJ, Buckley N, Whyte IM (1994) Calcium channel blocking drug overdose: An Australian series. *Hum Exp Toxicol* 13: 161–166

359 Kerns W 2nd (2007) Management of β-adrenergic blocker and calcium channel antagonist toxi-city. *Emerg Med Clin North Am* 25: 309–331

360 Sim MT, Stevenson FT (2008) A fatal case of iatrogenic hypercalcemia after calcium channel

blocker overdose. *J Med Toxicol* 4: 25–29

361 Salhanick SD, Shannon MW (2003) Management of calcium channel antagonist overdose. *Drug Saf* 26: 65–79

362 APP (2007) Calcium Gluconate Injection, USP 10%. APP Pharmaceuticals, LLC, Schaumburg, IL

363 Nola GT, Pope, S, Harrison, DC (1970) Assessment of the synergistic relationship between serum calcium and digitalis. *Am Heart J* 79: 499

364 Ericksona CP, Olson KR (2008) Case files of the medical toxicology fellowship of the California poison control system-San Francisco: Calcium plus digoxin-more taboo than toxic? *J Med Toxicol* 4: 33–39

365 Wenger TL, Butler VP Jr, Haber E, Smith TW (1985) Treatment of 63 severely digitalis-toxic patients with digoxin-specific antibody fragments. *J Am Coll Cardiol* 5: 118A–123A

366 Smith TW, Haber E, Yeatman L, Butler VP Jr (1976) Reversal of advanced digoxin intoxication with Fab fragments of digoxin-specific antibodies. *N Engl J Med* 294: 797–800

367 Antman EM, Wenger TL, Butler VP Jr, Haber E, Smith TW (1990) Treatment of 150 cases of life-threatening digitalis intoxication with digoxin-specific Fab antibody fragments. Final report of a multicenter study. *Circulation* 81: 1744–1752

368 Lapostolle F, Borron SW, Verdier C, Taboulet P, Guerrier G, Adnet F, Clemessy JL, Bismuth C, Baud FJ (2008) Digoxin-specific Fab fragments as single first-line therapy in digitalis poisoning. *Crit Care Med* 36: 3014–3018

369 Woolf AD, Wenger T, Smith TW, Lovejoy FH Jr (1992) The use of digoxin-specific Fab fragments for severe digitalis intoxication in children. *N Engl J Med* 326: 1739–1744

370 Smith TW (1991) Review of clinical experience with digoxin immune Fab (ovine). *Am J Emerg Med* 9: 1–6

371 Bateman DN (2004) Digoxin-specific antibody fragments: How much and when? *Toxicol Rev* 23: 135–143

372 Ujhelyi MR, Robert S (1995) Pharmacokinetic aspects of digoxin-specific Fab therapy in the management of digitalis toxicity. *Clin Pharmacokinet* 28: 483–493

373 Mehta RN, Mehta NJ, Gulati A (2002) Late rebound digoxin toxicity after digoxin-specific antibody Fab fragments therapy in anuric patient. *J Emerg Med* 22: 203–206

374 Bosse GM, Pope TM (1994) Recurrent digoxin overdose and treatment with digoxin-specific Fab antibody fragments. *J Emerg Med* 12: 179–185

375 Camphausen C, Haas NA, Mattke AC (2005) Successful treatment of oleander intoxication (cardiac glycosides) with digoxin-specific Fab antibody fragments in a 7-year-old child: Case report and review of literature. *Z Kardiol* 94: 817–823

376 Brubacher JR, Lachmanen D, Ravikumar PR, Hoffman RS (1999) Efficacy of digoxin specific Fab fragments (Digibind) in the treatment of toad venom poisoning. *Toxicon* 37: 931–942

377 Ali S, Drucker DJ (2009) Benefits and limitations of reducing glucagon action for the treatment of type 2 diabetes. *Am J Physiol Endocrinol Metab* 296: E415–421

378 Eli Lilly and Company (2005) Information for the Physician. Glucagon for Injection (rDNA origin). Eli Lilly and Company, Indianapolis, IN

379 Shepherd G (2006) Treatment of poisoning caused by β-adrenergic and calcium-channel blockers. *Am J Health Syst Pharm* 63: 1828–1835

380 Sauvadet A, Rohn T, Pecker F, Pavoine C (1997) Arachidonic acid drives mini-glucagon action in cardiac cells. *J Biol Chem* 272: 12437–12445

381 Parmley WW, Glick G, Sonnenblick EH (1968) Cardiovascular effects of glucagon in man. *N Engl J Med* 279: 12–17

382 Boyd R, Ghosh A (2003) Towards evidence based emergency medicine: Best BETs from the Manchester Royal Infirmary. Glucagon for the treatment of symptomatic β blocker overdose. *Emerg Med J* 20: 266–267

383 Lee J (2004) Glucagon use in symptomatic β blocker overdose. *Emerg Med J* 21: 755

384 Stone CK, May WA, Carroll R (1995) Treatment of verapamil overdose with glucagon in dogs. *Ann Emerg Med* 25: 369–374

385 Walter FG, Frye G, Mullen JT, Ekins BR, Khasigian PA (1993) Amelioration of nifedipine poisoning associated with glucagon therapy. *Ann Emerg Med* 22: 1234–1237

386 Zaritsky AL, Horowitz M, Chernow B (1988) Glucagon antagonism of calcium channel blocker-induced myocardial dysfunction. *Crit Care Med* 16: 246–251

387 Kline JA, Leonova E, Williams TC, Schroeder JD, Watts JA (1996) Myocardial metabolism dur-

ing graded intraportal verapamil infusion in awake dogs. *J Cardiovasc Pharmacol* 27: 719–726

388 Kline JA, Leonova E, Raymond RM (1995) Beneficial myocardial metabolic effects of insulin during verapamil toxicity in the anesthetized canine. *Crit Care Med* 23: 1251–1263

389 Oldenburg O, Eggebrecht H, Gutersohn A, Schaar J, Brauck K, Haude M, Erbel R, Baumgart D (2001) Myocardial lactate release after intracoronary verapamil application in humans: Acute effects of intracoronary verapamil on systemic and coronary hemodynamics, myocardial metabolism, and norepinephrine levels. *Cardiovasc Drugs Ther* 15: 55–61

390 Puskarich MA, Runyon MS, Trzeciak S, Kline JA, Jones AE (2009) Effect of glucose-insulin-potassium infusion on mortality in critical care settings: A systematic review and meta-analysis. *J Clin Pharmacol* 49: 758–767

391 Schipke JD, Friebe R, Gams E (2006) Forty years of glucose-insulin-potassium (GIK) in cardiac surgery: A review of randomized, controlled trials. *Eur J Cardiothorac Surg* 29: 479–485

392 Koskenkari JK, Kaukoranta PK, Rimpilainen J, Vainionpaa V, Ohtonen PP, Surcel HM, Juvonen T, Ala-Kokko TI (2006) Anti-inflammatory effect of high-dose insulin treatment after urgent coronary revascularization surgery. *Acta Anaesthesiol Scand* 50: 962–969

393 Doenst T, Bothe W, Beyersdorf F (2003) Therapy with insulin in cardiac surgery: Controversies and possible solutions. *Ann Thorac Surg* 75: S721–728

394 Svedjeholm R, Ekroth R, Joachimsson PO, Tyden H (1991) High-dose insulin improves the efficacy of dopamine early after cardiac surgery. A study of myocardial performance and oxygen consumption. *Scand J Thorac Cardiovasc Surg* 25: 215–221

395 Kline JA, Raymond RM, Leonova ED, Williams TC, Watts JA (1997) Insulin improves heart function and metabolism during non-ischemic cardiogenic shock in awake canines. *Cardiovasc Res* 34: 289–298

396 Kerns W 2nd, Schroeder D, Williams C, Tomaszewski C, Raymond R (1997) Insulin improves survival in a canine model of acute β-blocker toxicity. *Ann Emerg Med* 29: 748–757

397 Holger JS, Engebretsen KM, Fritzlar SJ, Patten LC, Harris CR, Flottemesch TJ (2007) Insulin *versus* vasopressin and epinephrine to treat β-blocker toxicity. *Clin Toxicol* 45: 396–401

398 Greene SL, Gawarammana I, Wood DM, Jones AL, Dargan PI (2007) Relative safety of hyperinsulinaemia/euglycaemia therapy in the management of calcium channel blocker overdose: A prospective observational study. *Intensive Care Med* 33: 2019–2024

399 Cohen V, Jellinek SP, Fancher L, Sangwan G, Wakslak M, Marquart E, Farahani C (2009) Tarka(R) (trandolapril/verapamil hydrochloride extended-release) overdose. *J Emerg Med, in press*

400 Prigeon RL, Roder ME, Porte D Jr, Kahn SE (1996) The effect of insulin dose on the measurement of insulin sensitivity by the minimal model technique. Evidence for saturable insulin transport in humans. *J Clin Invest* 97: 501–507

401 Mokshagundam SP, Peiris AN, Stagner JI, Gingerich RL, Samols E (1996) Interstitial insulin during euglycemic-hyperinsulinemic clamp in obese and lean individuals. *Metabolism* 45: 951–956

402 Natali A, Gastaldelli A, Camastra S, Sironi AM, Toschi E, Masoni A, Ferrannini E, Mari A (2000) Dose-response characteristics of insulin action on glucose metabolism: A non-steady-state approach. *Am J Physiol Endocrinol Metab* 278: E794–801

403 Foxall G, McCahon R, Lamb J, Hardman JG, Bedforth NM (2007) Levobupivacaine-induced seizures and cardiovascular collapse treated with Intralipid. *Anaesthesia* 62: 516–518

404 Groban L, Deal DD, Vernon JC, James RL, Butterworth J (2001) Cardiac resuscitation after incremental overdosage with lidocaine, bupivacaine, levobupivacaine, and ropivacaine in anesthetized dogs. *Anesth Analg* 92: 37–43

405 Weinberg G, Ripper R, Feinstein DL, Hoffman W (2003) Lipid emulsion infusion rescues dogs from bupivacaine-induced cardiac toxicity. *Reg Anesth Pain Med* 28: 198–202

406 Weinberg GL, Di Gregorio G, Ripper R, Kelly K, Massad M, Edelman L, Schwartz D, Shah N, Zheng S, Feinstein DL (2008) Resuscitation with lipid *versus* epinephrine in a rat model of bupivacaine overdose. *Anesthesiology* 108: 907–913

407 Warren JA, Thoma RB, Georgescu A, Shah SJ (2008) Intravenous lipid infusion in the successful resuscitation of local anesthetic-induced cardiovascular collapse after supraclavicular brachial plexus block. *Anesth Analg* 106: 1578–1580

408 Litz RJ, Popp M, Stehr SN, Koch T (2006) Successful resuscitation of a patient with ropivacaine-induced asystole after axillary plexus block using lipid infusion. *Anaesthesia* 61: 800–801

409 Litz RJ, Roessel T, Heller AR, Stehr SN (2008) Reversal of central nervous system and cardiac toxicity after local anesthetic intoxication by lipid emulsion injection. *Anesth Analg* 106:

1575–1577

410 Ludot H, Tharin JY, Belouadah M, Mazoit JX, Malinovsky JM (2008) Successful resuscitation after ropivacaine and lidocaine-induced ventricular arrhythmia following posterior lumbar plexus block in a child. *Anesth Analg* 106: 1572–1574

411 Finn SD, Uncles DR, Willers J, Sable N (2009) Early treatment of a quetiapine and sertraline overdose with Intralipid. *Anaesthesia* 64: 191–194

412 Sirianni AJ, Osterhoudt KC, Calello DP, Muller AA, Waterhouse MR, Goodkin MB, Weinberg GL, Henretig FM (2008) Use of lipid emulsion in the resuscitation of a patient with prolonged cardiovascular collapse after overdose of bupropion and lamotrigine. *Ann Emerg Med* 51: 412–415

413 Harvey M, Cave G (2007) Intralipid outperforms sodium bicarbonate in a rabbit model of clomipramine toxicity. *Ann Emerg Med* 49: 178–185

414 Harvey MG, Cave GR (2008) Intralipid infusion ameliorates propranolol-induced hypotension in rabbits. *J Med Toxicol* 4: 71–76

415 Bania TC, Chu J, Perez E, Su M, Hahn IH (2007) Hemodynamic effects of intravenous fat emulsion in an animal model of severe verapamil toxicity resuscitated with atropine, calcium, and saline. *Acad Emerg Med* 14: 105–111

416 Cave G, Harvey MG, Castle CD (2005) Intralipid ameliorates thiopentone induced respiratory depression in rats: Investigative pilot study. *Emerg Med Australas* 17: 180–181

417 Florian JP, Pawelczyk JA (2009) Non-esterified fatty acids increase arterial pressure *via* central sympathetic activation in humans. *Clin Sci* 118: 61–69

418 Stehr SN, Ziegeler JC, Pexa A, Oertel R, Deussen A, Koch T, Hubler M (2007) The effects of lipid infusion on myocardial function and bioenergetics in L-bupivacaine toxicity in the isolated rat heart. *Anesth Analg* 104: 186–192

419 The Association of Anaesthetists of Great Britain & Ireland (2007) Guidelines for the Management of Severe Local Anaesthetic Toxicity (http://www.aagbi.org/publications/guidelines/docs/latoxicity07.pdf, accessed May 19, 2009)

420 Felice K, Schumann H (2008) Intravenous lipid emulsion for local anesthetic toxicity: A review of the literature. *J Med Toxicol* 4: 184–191

421 Marwick PC, Levin AI, Coetzee AR (2009) Recurrence of cardiotoxicity after lipid rescue from bupivacaine-induced cardiac arrest. *Anesth Analg* 108: 1344–1346

422 Harvey M, Cave G, Kazemi A (2009) Intralipid infusion diminishes return of spontaneous circulation after hypoxic cardiac arrest in rabbits. *Anesth Analg* 108: 1163–1168

423 Mayr VD, Mitterschiffthaler L, Neurauter A, Gritsch C, Wenzel V, Muller T, Luckner G, Lindner KH, Strohmenger HU (2008) A comparison of the combination of epinephrine and vasopressin with lipid emulsion in a porcine model of asphyxial cardiac arrest after intravenous injection of bupivacaine. *Anesth Analg* 106: 1566–1571

424 Mazoit JX, Le Guen R, Beloeil H, Benhamou D (2009) Binding of long-lasting local anesthetics to lipid emulsions. *Anesthesiology* 110: 380–386

425 De Bruin ML, Langendijk PN, Koopmans RP, Wilde AA, Leufkens HG, Hoes AW (2007) In-hospital cardiac arrest is associated with use of non-antiarrhythmic QTc-prolonging drugs. *Br J Clin Pharmacol* 63: 216–223

426 Gupta A, Lawrence AT, Krishnan K, Kavinsky CJ, Trohman RG (2007) Current concepts in the mechanisms and management of drug-induced QT prolongation and torsade de pointes. *Am Heart J* 153: 891–899

427 Khan IA, Gowda RM (2004) Novel therapeutics for treatment of long-QT syndrome and torsade de pointes. *Int J Cardiol* 95: 1–6

428 Sasyniuk BI, Jhamandas V (1984) Mechanism of reversal of toxic effects of amitriptyline on cardiac Purkinje fibers by sodium bicarbonate. *J Pharmacol Exp Ther* 231: 387–394

429 Sasyniuk BI, Jhamandas V, Valois M (1986) Experimental amitriptyline intoxication: Treatment of cardiac toxicity with sodium bicarbonate. *Ann Emerg Med* 15: 1052–1059

430 Brown TC (1976) Tricyclic antidepressant overdosage: Experimental studies on the management of circulatory complications. *Clin Toxicol* 9: 255–272

431 Boehnert MT, Lovejoy FH Jr (1985) Value of the QRS duration *versus* the serum drug level in predicting seizures and ventricular arrhythmias after an acute overdose of tricyclic antidepressants. *N Engl J Med* 313: 474–479

432 Niemann JT, Bessen HA, Rothstein RJ, Laks MM (1986) Electrocardiographic criteria for tricyclic antidepressant cardiotoxicity. *Am J Cardiol* 57: 1154–1159

433 Liebelt EL, Francis PD, Woolf AD (1995) ECG lead aVR *versus* QRS interval in predicting seizures and arrhythmias in acute tricyclic antidepressant toxicity. *Ann Emerg Med* 26: 195–201

434 Pentel PR, Keyler DE (1988) Effects of high dose α-1-acid glycoprotein on desipramine toxicity in rats. *J Pharmacol Exp Ther* 246: 1061–1066

435 Taboulet P, Michard F, Muszynski J, Galliot-Guilley M, Bismuth C (1995) Cardiovascular repercussions of seizures during cyclic antidepressant poisoning. *J Toxicol Clin Toxicol* 33: 205–211

436 Knudsen K, Abrahamsson J (1997) Epinephrine and sodium bicarbonate independently and additively increase survival in experimental amitriptyline poisoning. *Crit Care Med* 25: 669–674

437 Bessen HA, Niemann JT (1985) Improvement of cardiac conduction after hyperventilation in tricyclic antidepressant overdose. *J Toxicol Clin Toxicol* 23: 537–546

438 McCabe JL, Cobaugh DJ, Menegazzi JJ, Fata J (1998) Experimental tricyclic antidepressant toxicity: A randomized, controlled comparison of hypertonic saline solution, sodium bicarbonate, and hyperventilation. *Ann Emerg Med* 32: 329–333

439 McKinney PE, Rasmussen R (2003) Reversal of severe tricyclic antidepressant-induced cardiotoxicity with intravenous hypertonic saline solution. *Ann Emerg Med* 42: 20–24

440 Brown TC (1976) Sodium bicarbonate treatment for tricyclic antidepressant arrhythmias in children. *Med J Aust* 2: 380–382

441 Woolf AD, Erdman AR, Nelson LS, Caravati EM, Cobaugh DJ, Booze LL, Wax PM, Manoguerra AS, Scharman EJ, Olson KR, Chyka PA, Christianson G, Troutman WG (2007) Tricyclic antidepressant poisoning: An evidence-based consensus guideline for out-of-hospital management. *Clin Toxicol* 45: 203–233

442 Sharma AN, Hexdall AH, Chang EK, Nelson LS, Hoffman RS (2003) Diphenhydramine-induced wide complex dysrhythmia responds to treatment with sodium bicarbonate. *Am J Emerg Med* 21: 212–215

443 Stork CM, Redd JT, Fine K, Hoffman RS (1995) Propoxyphene-induced wide QRS complex dysrhythmia responsive to sodium bicarbonate – A case report. *J Toxicol Clin Toxicol* 33: 179–183

444 Kalimullah EA, Bryant SM (2008) Case files of the medical toxicology fellowship at the toxikon consortium in Chicago: Cocaine-associated wide-complex dysrhythmias and cardiac arrest – Treatment nuances and controversies. *J Med Toxicol* 4: 277–283

445 Mailloux D, Adar E, Su M (2005) Acute carbamazepine toxicity associated with a widened QRS interval treated with intravenous sodium bicarbonate. *Clin Toxicol* 43: 505–506

446 Wills BK, Zell-Kanter M, Aks SE (2009) Bupropion-associated QRS prolongation unresponsive to sodium bicarbonate therapy. *Am J Ther* 16: 193–196

447 Bosse GM, Spiller HA, Collins AM (2008) A fatal case of venlafaxine overdose. *J Med Toxicol* 4: 18–20

448 Buckley NA, Whyte IM, Dawson AH (1993) Self-poisoning with lamotrigine. *Lancet* 342: 1552–1553

449 Pierog J, Kane B, Kane K, Donovan JW (2009) Management of isolated yew berry toxicity with sodium bicarbonate: A case report in treatment efficacy. *J Med Toxicol* 5: 84–89

450 Schwartz M, Patel M, Kazzi Z, Morgan B (2008) Cardiotoxicity after massive amantadine overdose. *J Med Toxicol* 4: 173–179

451 Clarke SF, Dargan PI, Jones AL (2005) Naloxone in opioid poisoning: Walking the tightrope. *Emerg Med J* 22: 612–616

452 Bracken MB, Shepard MJ, Collins WF, Holford TR, Young W, Baskin DS, Eisenberg HM, Flamm E, Leo-Summers L, Maroon J (1990) A randomized, controlled trial of methylprednisolone or naloxone in the treatment of acute spinal-cord injury. Results of the Second National Acute Spinal Cord Injury Study. *N Engl J Med* 322: 1405–1411

453 Buajordet I, Naess AC, Jacobsen D, Brors O (2004) Adverse events after naloxone treatment of episodes of suspected acute opioid overdose. *Eur J Emerg Med* 11: 19–23

454 Mills CA, Flacke JW, Flacke WE, Bloor BC, Liu MD (1990) Narcotic reversal in hypercapnic dogs: Comparison of naloxone and nalbuphine. *Can J Anaesth* 37: 238–244

455 International Liaison Committee on Resuscitation (2006) The ILCOR consensus on science with treatment recommendations for pediatric and neonatal patients: Neonatal resuscitation. *Pediatrics* 117: e978–988

456 Deshpande G, Gill A (2009) Cardiac arrest following naloxone in an extremely preterm neonate. *Eur J Pediatr* 168: 115–117

457 Hoffman JR, Schriger DL, Luo JS (1991) The empiric use of naloxone in patients with altered mental status: A reappraisal. *Ann Emerg Med* 20: 246–252

458 Goldfrank L, Weisman RS, Errick JK, Lo MW (1986) A dosing nomogram for continuous infusion intravenous naloxone. *Ann Emerg Med* 15: 566–570

459 Geib AJ, Babu K, Ewald MB, Boyer EW (2006) Adverse effects in children after unintentional buprenorphine exposure. *Pediatrics* 118: 1746–1751

460 Van Dorp E, Yassen A, Sarton E, Romberg R, Olofsen E, Teppema L, Danhof M, Dahan A (2006) Naloxone reversal of buprenorphine-induced respiratory depression. *Anesthesiology* 105: 51–57

461 Horowitz R, Mazor SS, Aks SE, Leikin JB (2005) Accidental clonidine patch ingestion in a child. *Am J Ther* 12: 272–274

462 Seger DL (2002) Clonidine toxicity revisited. *J Toxicol Clin Toxicol* 40: 145–155

463 Varon J, Duncan SR (1991) Naloxone reversal of hypotension due to captopril overdose. *Ann Emerg Med* 20: 1125–1127

464 Barr CS, Payne R, Newton RW (1991) Profound prolonged hypotension following captopril overdose. *Postgrad Med J* 67: 953–954

465 Millar JA, Sturani A, Rubin PC, Lawrie C, Reid JL (1983) Attenuation of the antihypertensive effect of captopril by the opioid receptor antagonist naloxone. *Clin Exp Pharmacol Physiol* 10: 253–259

466 Ajayi AA, Campbell BC, Rubin PC, Reid JL (1985) Effect of naloxone on the actions of captopril. *Clin Pharmacol Ther* 38: 560–565

467 Bernini G, Taddei S, Graziadei L, Pedrinelli R, Salvetti A (1985) Naloxone does not modify the antihypertensive effect of captopril in essential hypertensive patients. *J Hypertens Suppl* 3: S117–119

468 Lopez-Romero B, Evrard G, Durant F, Sevrin M, George P (1998) Molecular structure and stereoelectronic properties of sarmazenil – A weak inverse agonist at the omega modulatory sites (benzodiazepine receptors): Comparison with bretazenil and flumazenil. *Bioorg Med Chem* 6: 1745–1757

469 Dunton AW, Schwam E, Pitman V, McGrath J, Hendler J, Siegel J (1988) Flumazenil: US clinical pharmacology studies. *Eur J Anaesthesiol* 2: 81–95

470 Amrein R, Hetzel W, Hartmann D, Lorscheid T (1988) Clinical pharmacology of flumazenil. *Eur J Anaesthesiol Suppl* 2: 65–80

471 Mora CT, Torjman M, White PF (1995) Sedative and ventilatory effects of midazolam infusion: Effect of flumazenil reversal. *Can J Anaesth* 42: 677–684

472 Flogel CM, Ward DS, Wada DR, Ritter JW (1993) The effects of large-dose flumazenil on midazolam-induced ventilatory depression. *Anesth Analg* 77: 1207–1214

473 Shalansky SJ, Naumann TL, Englander FA (1993) Effect of flumazenil on benzodiazepine-induced respiratory depression. *Clin Pharm* 12: 483–487

474 Dahaba AA, Bornemann H, Rehak PH, Wang G, Wu XM, Metzler H (2009) Effect of flumazenil on bispectral index monitoring in unpremedicated patients. *Anesthesiology* 110: 1036–1040

475 Polc P (1988) Electrophysiology of benzodiazepine receptor ligands: Multiple mechanisms and sites of action. *Prog Neurobiol* 31: 349–423

476 Morgan MM, Levin ED, Liebeskind JC (1987) Characterization of the analgesic effects of the benzodiazepine antagonist, Ro 15-1788. *Brain Res* 415: 367–370

477 Gueye PN, Hoffman JR, Taboulet P, Vicaut E, Baud FJ (1996) Empiric use of flumazenil in comatose patients: Limited applicability of criteria to define low risk. *Ann Emerg Med* 27: 730–735

478 Weinbroum A, Rudick V, Sorkine P, Nevo Y, Halpern P, Geller E, Niv D (1996) Use of flumazenil in the treatment of drug overdose: A double-blind and open clinical study in 110 patients. *Crit Care Med* 24: 199–206

479 Spivey WH (1992) Flumazenil and seizures: Analysis of 43 cases. *Clin Ther* 14: 292–305

480 Anonymous (1992) Treatment of benzodiazepine overdose with flumazenil. The Flumazenil in Benzodiazepine Intoxication Multicenter Study Group. *Clin Ther* 14: 978–995

481 Weinbroum AA, Flaishon R, Sorkine P, Szold O, Rudick V (1997) A risk-benefit assessment of flumazenil in the management of benzodiazepine overdose. *Drug Saf* 17: 181–196

482 Nau H, Loscher W (1984) Valproic acid and metabolites: Pharmacological and toxicological studies. *Epilepsia* 25 Suppl 1: S14–22

483 Weber WW, Hein DW (1979) Clinical pharmacokinetics of isoniazid. *Clin Pharmacokinet* 4: 401–422

Molecular, Clinical and Environmental Toxicology. Volume 2: Clinical Toxicology
Edited by A. Luch

Inhalation toxicology

Amanda Hayes[1] and Shahnaz Bakand[1,2]

[1] *Chemical Safety and Applied Toxicology (CSAT) Laboratories, School of Risk and Safety Sciences, The University of New South Wales, Sydney, Australia*
[2] *Department of Occupational Health, School of Public Health, Iran University of Medical Sciences, Tehran, Iran*

Abstract. Inhalation of gases, vapors and aerosols can cause a wide range of adverse health effects, ranging from simple irritation to systemic diseases. The large number of chemicals and complex mixtures present in indoor and outdoor air coupled with the introduction of new materials such as nanoparticles and nanofibers, is an area of growing concern for human health. Animal-based assays have been used to study the toxic effects of chemicals for many years. However, even so, very little is known about the potential toxicity of the vast majority of inhaled chemicals. As well as new or refined OECD test guidelines, continuing scientific developments are needed to improve the process of safety evaluation for the vast number of chemicals and inhaled materials. Although studying the toxic effects of inhaled chemicals is more challenging, promising *in vitro* exposure techniques have been recently developed that offer new possibilities to test biological activities of inhaled chemicals under biphasic conditions at the air liquid interface. This chapter gives an overview of inhalation toxicology as well as focusing on the potential application of *in vitro* methods for toxicity testing of airborne pollutants.

Introduction

Exposure to airborne contaminants is a major contributor to human health problems, causing adverse effects ranging from simple irritation to morbidity and mortality due to acute intense or long-term low-level repeated exposures [1–3]. Inhalation exposures can occur with gases, vapors, solid and liquid aerosols and mixtures of these. While evaluating the impact of chemicals on human health requires toxicity data, in many cases, particularly for industrial chemicals, the availability of toxicity information is quite limited [4–7].

The current approach of measuring the toxic effects of airborne contaminants relies on whole animal test methods [8]. As well as ethical concerns, heavy reliance on animal data in toxicology is the subject of debate and controversy by the scientific community [9]. Moreover, the increasing number of available industrial chemicals and new products has created a demand for alternative test methods for safety evaluation [8]. Although studying the toxic effects of inhaled chemicals *in vitro* is technically more challenging, great advances in the application of these methods for investigating the toxicity of airborne contaminants have been made in recent years. This chapter presents a review of the essentials of inhalation toxicology and a focus on the potential application of *in vitro* methods for studying the toxicity of airborne contaminants.

Air pollutants

Air contaminants are exogenous substances in outdoor or indoor air, including both particulate and gaseous contaminants, that can cause adverse health effects in humans or animals, affect plant life and impact the global environment by changing the atmosphere of the earth [10, 11]. Various physical, chemical and dynamic processes may generate air pollution leading to emission of gases, particulates or mixtures of these into the atmosphere [12]. Air quality is continuously affected by emissions from stationary and mobile sources. While great attempts have been made to reduce emissions from these sources, millions of people today face excessive air pollution in both occupational and urban environments [13].

Emissions from mobile combustion sources (e.g., automobiles) are major contributors to urban air pollution, and include carbon monoxide (CO), nitrogen oxides (NO_x), sulfur oxides (SO_x), particulate matter (PM), lead and photochemical oxidants such as ozone (O_3) and ozone precursors like hydrocarbons and volatile organic compounds (VOCs) [11, 13]. Larger air pollution particulates are derived chiefly from soil and other crusty materials, whereas fine and ultra-fine particles are derived mainly from combustion of fossil fuels in transportation, manufacturing and power generation [1]. Many industrial and commercial activities release toxic contaminants in gas, vapor or particulate form. However, air contaminants are not limited to urban or industrial environments, and common indoor air pollutants can be found in offices, schools, hospitals and homes. Tobacco smoke, fuel consumption, furniture, painting, carpeting, air conditioning, and cleaning agents can be significant sources of both chemical and biological air contaminants.

Types of air pollutants

Based on their physical properties, airborne contaminants can be classified into two main types. The first category includes gases and vapors or air pollutants that exist as distinct molecules and can dissolve and form true solutions in the air and follow the fundamental gas laws. There is no practical difference between a gas and a vapor except that a vapor is the gaseous phase of a substance that is usually solid or liquid at room temperature and atmospheric pressure. For example, processes that involve high temperature, such as welding operations and exhaust from engines, can potentially generate toxic gases such as oxides of carbon, nitrogen or sulfur. Several occupational practices may produce toxic vapors such as charging and mixing liquids, painting, spraying and dry cleaning or any other activities involving VOCs.

The second category is aerosols or suspended air pollutants, which can be solid particles or liquid droplets and can vary in size, composition and origin, such as dust, fiber, smoke, mist and fog [14]. Aerosols may result from different mechanical or chemical processes in both solid or liquid forms, which may have spherical or nonspherical shapes with a wide range of size distribution from less than 100 nm to well over 100 μm. Different mechanical processes such as grinding, cutting, sawing, crushing, screening or sieving can generate solid aerosols in dust form. Mechanical dispersing of a bulk liquid such as spraying and atomizing can generate suspended liquid mist droplets. Mist droplets have the properties of the parent liquid, and have a wide range of sizes from a few to more than 100 μm. All processes involving high-pressure liquids, such as paint spraying, can potentially generate mists.

Other forms of aerosols can be generated by processes such as combustion, condensation or sublimation. For example, high-temperature operations such as arc welding, torch cutting and metal smelting can generate extremely fine metal oxide fumes, usually less than 0.1 μm, produced by combustion, sublimation or condensation of evaporated materials. Incomplete combustion of organic materials can generate smoke that is a complex mixture containing solid and liquid aerosols, gases and vapors. For example, tobacco smoke contains thousands of chemical substances, most of which are toxic or carcinogenic. Although primary smoke particles are between 0.01 and 1 μm, they can aggregate and produce extremely larger particles called soot.

Airborne chemical exposure

The three main routes of exposure to chemicals are inhalation, dermal absorption and ingestion. Inhalation is considered the most important means by which humans are exposed to airborne chemicals and forms the focus of this review.

Human respiratory tract: Structure and function

The major physiological function of the respiratory tract is to deliver O_2 (oxygen) into the blood system and to remove CO_2 (carbon dioxide) as a metabolic waste. The human respiratory tract is anatomically well structured to achieve this function given its very large surface area of approximately 140 m^2 and a high daily exchange volume of more than 10 m^3 [15–18]. In addition, the membrane between air and blood in the gas-exchange region is extremely thin, approximately 0.4–2.5 μm [19, 20]. As well as olfactory, gas exchange and blood oxygenation functions, the respiratory system has evolved to deal with xenobiotics and many airborne materials that usually occur in the air environment [21].

However, the respiratory system cannot always deal adequately with the wide range of airborne contaminants that may occur in urban and occupational environments [20]. After inhalation, airborne contaminants may enter different regions of the respiratory tract. Some chemicals such as insoluble gases and vapors can even pass through the respiratory tract efficiently and enter into the pulmonary blood supply system. As a result, the respiratory system is both a site of toxicity for pulmonary toxicants, and a pathway for inhaled chemicals to reach other organs distant from the lungs and elicit their toxic effects at these extrapulmonary sites. The human respiratory tract can be classified into three major regions: nasopharyngeal, tracheobronchial and the pulmonary regions (Fig. 1).

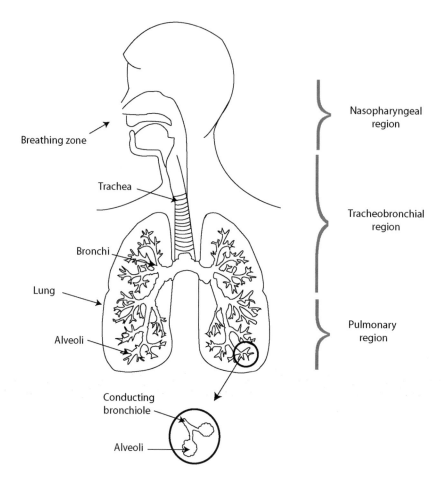

Figure 1. Anatomical regions of the respiratory tract.

Nasopharyngeal region

This part of the respiratory tract includes the nasal turbinates, epiglottis, pharynx and larynx. Air enters through the nose (and mouth), and is warmed and humidified during this passage. The nasal passages assist in collecting the coarse inhaled particles by impaction or filtration, and condition the temperature and humidity of the inhaled air. Highly water-soluble gases and vapors can also be absorbed efficiently by the nasal passages. The nasal passages are an important target area for a wide range of inhaled toxicants. For example, transitional epithelial tissue is attacked by O_3 and respiratory mucosal tissue by formaldehyde [22].

Tracheobronchial region

The tracheobronchial region includes the airways from trachea to terminal bronchioles, and delivers inhaled air to the deeper parts of the respiratory tract. Similar to the nasopharyngeal, this region is lined by mucous-secreting goblet cells and ciliated cells, which functions as a protective covering [18, 20]. Respiratory tract mucous produced by goblet cells and glandular structures can capture pollutants and cell debris. Produced mucous is continually propelled toward the pharynx by respiratory tract cilia [20, 22].

Pulmonary region

The pulmonary region is the area of gas exchange, and includes the respiratory bronchioles, alveolar ducts and alveoli. Adult human lungs consist of approximately 300 million alveoli, the gas-exchange units of the lung [23]. O_2 molecules diffuse from the inhaled air to the blood across the very thin alveolar epithelia and capillary membranes. Diffusion of CO_2 occurs in the opposite direction. The distal respiratory tract also contains several distinctive cells. For example, the alveoli are lined with two types of epithelial cells. Type I alveolar cells are very thin and cover a large surface area (approximately 90%) of the alveolar surface and bring inspired air into close contact with blood. Type II cells produce surfactant and assist in gas exchange and alveolar integrity [20, 22].

Deposition of inhaled chemicals

Apart from the physiological and anatomical characteristics of the respiratory tract, physicochemical and aerodynamic characteristics of inhaled chemicals are crucial in determining the site of deposition/absorption and the ultimate fate of inhaled contaminants.

Gases and vapors

Water solubility is the significant factor that determines the penetration site of a gas in the respiratory tract. For example, ammonia, formaldehyde, sulfur dioxide and hydrogen fluoride are extremely soluble in water and tend to be absorbed nearly completely within the nose and upper airways. While the nose acts as a scrubber for water-soluble gases to protect the lungs from potential toxic effects, the drawback of this protective action is the probability of production of toxic effects in the nose, such as formaldehyde, that may induce nasal cancer [24, 25]. Gases with low solubility such as nitrogen dioxide, O_3 and phosgene penetrate further into the pulmonary region and exert their toxicity in this region. Ultimately, very insoluble gases such as CO and hydrogen sulfide pass through the respiratory tract efficiently and are delivered throughout the body *via* the pulmonary blood supply system.

Although water solubility is a critical parameter in penetration of gaseous contaminants, other factors such as partition coefficient may also have a considerable influence. For example, when a gas penetrates to the gas-exchange region, the blood-gas partition coefficient will determine the rate of gas uptake into the blood [17, 24].

Particulate matter

While water solubility is the significant factor determining the penetration site of gaseous inhaled chemicals, particle size distribution is the most critical characteristic determining airborne behavior and deposition pattern of aerosols in the respiratory tract [26]. During inhalation, a specific volume of air from the breathing zone accelerates towards the nose (or mouth) and enters into the respiratory tract. As well as air, particles that are able to follow the air flow will enter into the respiratory tract (Fig. 1). Larger particles (5–30 µm) are usually deposited in the nasopharyngeal region by an inertial impaction mechanism. Aerosols (1–5 µm) that fail to be captured in the nasopharyngeal region will be deposited in the tracheobronchial region, and may be absorbed or removed by mucociliary clearance. Finally, the remaining particles with the smallest size distribution (<1 µm) that were not trapped in tracheobronchial region will penetrate deeply into the alveolar region, where removal mechanisms are insufficient [18, 24, 27].

The phagocytic function of alveolar macrophages to remove inhaled nano-sized particles appears to be considerably less efficient than for larger particles [28–30]. Therefore, nano-sized particles can effectively access the alveolar region of the lungs and come into intimate contact with the alveolar epithelium. Once deposited, they may enter into the blood stream and readily reach other target organs [31]. However, insoluble particles may remain in the lung indefinitely [24, 27, 30].

Transport and deposition of particles in the respiratory tract is governed by four main mechanisms: impaction, interception, sedimentation and diffusion (Fig. 1), [22, 32, 33]. Impaction occurs due to both velocity and directional change predominantly in the upper respiratory tract. When the airstream undergoes a change in direction, larger particles cannot follow the airstream

lines because of their inertial properties and hence they continue in the original direction and impact onto the surface. Interception has an important role in
the deposition of fibers, particularly for those with large aspect ratios. When
the trajectory of a particle brings it close enough to a surface to make contact,
the particle will be captured by interception.

Sedimentation refers to aerosol movement under the influence of gravity
[34, 35]. Sedimentation is a significant mechanism in the smaller bronchi, the
bronchioles and the alveolar spaces. Diffusion is a major deposition mechanism for particles smaller than 0.5 µm [36]. Diffusion is an important deposition mechanism for extremely small particles such as nanoparticles deep in the
alveoli, where the air flow is very low [31, 37].

Major responses to inhaled chemicals

Responses to inhaled chemicals range from immediate reactions to long-term
chronic effects, from specific impacts on single tissue to generalized systemic
effects [38, 39]. The severity of toxic effects of inhaled chemicals is influenced
by several factors such as type of air contaminant, airborne concentration, size
of airborne chemical (for particles), solubility in tissue fluids, reactivity with
tissue compounds, blood-gas partition coefficient (for gases and vapors), frequency and duration of exposure, interactions with other air toxicants and individual immunological status [24, 38, 39].

Exposure to air pollutants can cause different adverse effects either in the
respiratory tract or in other organs and systems distant from the lung. The site
of deposition/action of inhaled toxicants will determine, to a great extent, the
ultimate response of the respiratory tract to inhaled chemicals. Human lung
disorders involve an entire spectrum of respiratory diseases ranging from acute
irritation and sensitization to chronic pneumoconiosis, occupational asthma
and lung cancer (Tab. 1).

Acute irritant injuries

Exposure to irritants can cause acute injuries of the respiratory tract. During
inhalation, the cell lining of the respiratory tract, from the nostrils to the gas-
exchange region, is exposed to air contaminants. Penetration of the irritant gas
into the respiratory tract depends primarily on the water solubility of the gas
or vapor. For example, anhydrous ammonia is an upper respiratory irritant due
to high water solubility. In contrast, gases or vapors with low water solubility
such as nitrogen dioxide or methylene chloride that are not well absorbed in
the upper respiratory tract will penetrate deeper into the distal parts of the respiratory tract and induce tissue damage. Important respiratory irritants can be
found in Table 1.

Table 1. Air pollutants and related adverse effects

Contaminant	Toxic effects/diseases
Gases/vapors	
Chlorine (Cl_2) Ammonia (NH_3) Oxides of nitrogen (NO_x) Sulfur dioxide (SO_2) Sulfur trioxide (SO_3) Fluorine (F_2) Phosphine (PH_3) Phosgene ($COCl_2$) Acrolein	Respiratory irritation, bronchitis
Acid mists Caustic mists	Corrosion of respiratory system
Nitrogen (N_2) Hydrogen (H_2) Methane (CH_4) Helium (He_2) Ethylene (C_2H_2) Ethane (C_2H_6)	Dilution ('simple') asphyxiation
Carbon monoxide (CO) Hydrogen cyanide (HCN) Hydrogen sulfide (H_2S)	Chemical asphyxiation
Isocyanates (–N=C=O) Amines (–CR_2NH_2)	Sensitization, allergy, asthma
Particulates	
Asbestos	Asbestosis, pleural plaques, lung cancer, mesothelioma
Aluminum dust and abrasives	Aluminosis, alveolar edema, intestinal fibrosis
Beryllium	Berylliosis, pulmonary edema, pneumonia, granulomatosis, lung cancer, cor pulmonale
Cadmium (oxide)	Pneumonia, emphysema, cor pulmonale
Chromium VI	Bronchitis, fibrosis, lung cancer
Coal dust	Fibrosis, coal miner's pneumoconiosis
Cotton dust	Byssinosis
Iron oxides	Siderosis, diffuse fibrosis-like pneumoconiosis
Kaolin	Kaolinosis, fibrosis
Manganese	Manganism, manganese pneumonia
Nickel	Pulmonary edema, lung cancer, nasal cavity cancer
Silica	Silicosis, fibrosis, silicotuberculosis
Talc	Talcosis, fibrosis
Tin	Stanosis
Tungsten carbide	Hard metal disease, hyperplasia of bronchial epithelium, fibrosis
Vanadium	Irritation, bronchitis

Modified from [39].

Asphyxiation

Impaired or absence of oxygen exchange, which is characterized as asphyxia, is a toxicological hazard in various occupational and environmental settings [40]. Asphyxiant agents are classified into two groups based on their mode of action: (1) simple asphyxiants that generate tissue hypoxia by displacing oxygen from the inhaled air, e.g., CO_2, nitrogen and methane; and (2) chemical asphyxiants that generate tissue hypoxia by interfering with normal oxygen transport or utilization *via* interacting with biological molecules, e.g., CO, hydrogen cyanide and hydrogen sulfide [20, 40].

Asthma

Asthma is a pulmonary disorder characterized by mild or severe attacks of shortness of breath due to air flow limitation and/or airway hyper-responsiveness, caused by particular or unknown provoking agents [18, 41, 42]. Asthma induces bronchospasm, more production of mucus in the airways and cough due to an increasing response of the lung to the provoking agent. Even small exposures to a sensitizer may exacerbate asthma. Reactive airways dysfunction syndrome (RADS) is a separate category of asthma and can occur following acute inhalation of airborne irritants such as irritant gases, fumes and smoke [43]. Asthma is becoming an increasingly prevalent work-related respiratory disease in developed countries [44–46], and can be triggered by more than 200 chemicals including gases, vapors, particulates and allergens found in a wide variety of occupational settings [20].

Chronic obstructive pulmonary disease (COPD)

COPD is the common form of chronic lung disorder in industrialized countries, and represents the physiological abnormality resulting from long-standing, fixed, airflow obstruction; it is related to chronic bronchitis, emphysema, bronchiolitis and asthma rather than a result of a single disease [44, 47]. Smoking, air pollution, respiratory infections and genetic factors such as α_1 anti-trypsin deficiency have been identified as having causal links with COPD [20, 47].

Pneumoconiosis

Pneumoconiosis refers to any non-neoplastic lung disease caused by chronic exposure to, and hence accumulation of, airborne mineral dusts in the lung and the associated tissue reaction [20, 48]. Benign pneumoconiosis describes the presence of non-toxic materials in the lung that do not damage alveolar architecture or increase collagenous fibrosis, e.g., siderosis (iron), stannosis (tin) and baritosis (barium). In contrast, collagenous pneumoconiosis is the result of some other inorganic dusts that induce structural alterations in lung tissue and irreversible fibrosis, e.g., silicosis (silica), asbestosis (asbestos) and coal miner's pneumoconiosis (coal dust). However, in Western Europe and North America the majority of newly presenting cases of pneumoconiosis are now due to asbestos exposure rather than coal and silica exposure [49].

Lung cancer

Tobacco smoking is a well-recognized lung cancer risk factor and it has been estimated that about 80–90% of lung cancers are caused by cigarette smoking [18]. Some inhaled toxicants may induce cancer in the upper respiratory tract in nasal cavity and turbinates, e.g., formaldehyde, wood dusts, leather work and isopropyl alcohol [20]. Exposure to asbestos, arsenic or metals such as nickel, beryllium and cadmium has been associated with lung cancer. Radon gas is also a known lung carcinogen [18]. Silica, man-made fibers and welding fumes are suspected carcinogens.

Setting exposure standards

Environmental air quality standards (AQS) and occupational exposure limits (OEL) are proposed as guidelines to evaluate the health risks associated with human exposure to airborne pollutants. Although AQS are an essential part of the risk assessment process, current knowledge of toxicological potential of inhaled chemicals in relation to hazard evaluation is limited, making it difficult to establish such guidelines for a large number of airborne chemicals.

While data obtained from human experiences would be most useful in assessing the toxic effects of chemicals, human data are not always available for developing safety evaluations on airborne contaminants [8]. Moreover, after unfortunate human incidents, such as those with pharmaceutical agents like diethylstilbestrol and thalidomide, or contaminants like lead and polychlorinated biphenyls (PCBs), it is now understood that the risks of new products and technologies need to be assessed before adverse human experiences occur [2, 50, 51].

An important regulatory effort to remedy the lack of toxicity data for thousands of existing chemicals is the European Registration, Evaluation, Authorization and Restriction of Chemicals (REACH) framework, which came into effect in June 2007 [8, 52]. The major objectives of the REACH regulatory framework are to improve the knowledge associated with chemical properties and applications and to speed up the process of risk assessment. There is great interest in test systems including alternatives to animal testing that would satisfy these safety requirements.

Inhalation toxicology methods

Toxicology has, for many years, made a major contribution in providing chemical toxicity information. In general, no single method can cover the complexity of general toxicity in humans [53]. Toxicity data can be obtained from several sources including toxicological studies, epidemiological studies, quantitative structure-activity relationships (QSARs) and physiologically based toxicokinetic (PBTK) studies. While traditional toxicology methods rely on whole animal testing, *in vitro* toxicology methods, using cell culture technology in combination with the knowledge of toxicokinetics, are currently being developed and implemented in modern toxicology.

In vivo test methods

Extensive data have been generated from toxicological studies using animal models. However, most of these studies are conducted by oral and dermal exposures rather than inhalation exposure [5, 54]. While toxicology data may exist from other routes of exposure, the extrapolation of these data is most difficult to validate. To identify the lethal effects of air toxicants, inhalation toxicity tests are carried out in test animals. In brief, test animals are exposed to air toxicants dissolved or suspended in air, and the concentration that causes lethality in 50% of the dosed group (LC_{50}) is determined. In reporting an LC_{50}, both the concentration of the chemical in air that can cause death in 50% of exposed animals, and time of exposure is indicated.

Standard protocols have been adopted by regulatory agencies for both short-term and long-term inhalation tests. The OECD has initially adopted test guidelines for acute inhalation toxicity (TG 403), repeated-dose inhalation toxicity 28/14-day (TG 412) and subchronic inhalation toxicity 90-day (TG 413). Meanwhile, new guidelines for acute inhalation toxicity such as Acute Inhalation Toxicity-Fixed Dose Procedure (TG 433) and Acute Inhalation Toxicity-Acute Toxic Class (ATC) Method (TG 436) are being finalized [52, 55]. The OECD test guidelines for inhalation toxicity studies, including those in preparation, and their role in future hazard identification have been briefly discussed [52].

In inhalation studies, evaluating the dose received by the animal is more challenging due to several factors that influence the actual dose, e.g., atmospheric concentration, duration of exposure, pulmonary physiological characteristics of the test animal, and deposition/absorption patterns of the air contaminant. In a specified system, for many inhaled chemicals the actual dose is related to the product of concentration (c) and exposure time (t) by Harber's law (c × t = inhaled dose) [17, 22]. In many cases, particularly in short-time exposures to chemicals with a direct action on the respiratory system, the response is directly proportional to the product of c × t. However, many other substances, such as chemicals that exhibit systemic toxicity, do not follow

Harber's law because in such cases, several factors including absorption by the respiratory tract, tissue distribution, metabolism in potential target organs and elimination will influence the toxicity [17].

The selection of an animal species for toxicity studies is another crucial consideration that may influence the outcome of *in vivo* studies and the estimated human adverse health effects. Usually rodents such as rat, mouse, guinea pig and hamsters are used. However, different criteria should be considered in the selection of animals such as species-related physiological factors, the size of the animals, the availability of the animals, the number of animals needed, the cost of obtaining and maintaining the required number of animals and the cost of producing consistent atmospheric test concentrations [22].

The more common exposure modes to evaluate the effect of inhaled air toxicants involve whole body, head only and nose only. Whole body exposure mode is conducted most frequently for human inhalation studies. Head- and nose-only exposure modes are suitable for repeated short-time exposure for restricting the portal of entry of the test chemical to the respiratory system. Design and construction of head-only units are similar to those of nose-only units. Nose-only exposure units require an animal holder to accommodate rodents with suitable size to reduce stress and discomfort. The animal holder is normally designed to fit the general shape of the animal with a conical head-piece using polymethylmetacrylate, polycarbonate or stainless steel. The animal holder is connected to the exposure chamber that introduces the test chemical into the face or nose of the animal.

Generation of test atmospheres

Generation and characterization of known concentrations of air contaminants and reproducible exposure conditions is a more complicated and expensive procedure than that required for oral and dermal exposures. This process requires specialized equipment and techniques to generate, maintain and measure standard test atmospheres. Inhalation exposure systems involve several efficient and precise subsystems, including a conditioned air supply system, a suitable gas or aerosol generator for the test chemical, an atmosphere dilution and delivery system, exposure chamber, real-time monitoring or sampling and analytical system, and an exhaust/filter or scrubbing system (Fig. 2).

Exposure chambers can be operated in both static and dynamic systems. Usually animal inhalation toxicity studies are carried out in a dynamic system to avoid particle settling and exhaled gas complications. While the operation of the static system is relatively simple and requires comparatively less test material, this is only suitable for short exposure times due to the reliance on the air inside of the chamber. In contrast, in a dynamic system, the test atmosphere flows through the exposure chamber continuously and hence ensures atmospheric stability and no reduction in oxygen concentration due to test animal respiration [17]. This system requires accurate flow monitoring for both

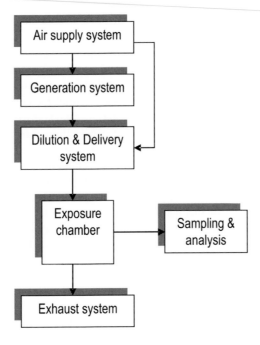

Figure 2. Components of a test atmosphere generation system (adapted from [14] with permission of the publisher Wiley-VCH).

diluent air and the primary source of contaminant in proportions that can produce the final desired concentrations.

In vitro test methods

Application of cell culture techniques in toxicological studies is referred to as *in vitro* toxicology and describes a field of study that applies technology using isolated organs, tissues and cell culture to study the toxic effects of chemicals [14]. As well as scientific advances, the development of *in vitro* toxicity test methods has been influenced by a variety of socio-economical factors. Animal welfare issues are one of the most important social concerns and have influenced the recent shift towards alternatives in toxicity testing. Each year, thousands of new cosmetics, pharmaceuticals, pesticides and consumer products are introduced into the marketplace. Considering that there are approximately 80 000 chemicals in commerce [46], as well as an extremely large number of chemical mixtures, *in vivo* testing of these numbers of chemicals requires a large number of expensive, time-consuming and in some cases non-humane tests on animal species. The necessity of determining the potential toxic effects of this large number of chemicals has provoked the need for rapid, sensitive and specific test methods.

In vitro toxicity endpoints

Different levels of organization in the human body may be affected by chemical substances from molecules to cells to tissues to organs, and to functional levels. Cytotoxicity is the adverse effect that occurs from the interaction of a toxicant with structures and/or processes essential for cell survival, proliferation and/or function [56]. Toxic chemicals can attack any of the basal cell functions, origin-specific cell functions and extracellular functions. To assess the potential cytotoxicity of chemical substances, several *in vitro* tests have been developed by measuring different biological endpoints, which are summarized in Table 2 [14, 53, 57–63]. In addition, recent research on apoptosis has enormously added to the knowledge of mechanisms involved in cell death, leading to the development of mechanistically based endpoints. Many morphological and biological changes that may occur at the cellular membrane, nucleus, specific proteases and DNA level can be used as biological endpoints for measuring apoptosis [62, 63]. Moreover, the rapid progress in genomic, transcript-

Table 2. Common biological endpoints assessed by *in vitro* toxicity tests

Biological endpoint	Detection method
Cell morphology	• Cell size and shape • Cell-cell contacts • Nuclear number, size, shape and inclusions • Nuclear or cytoplasmic vacuolation
Cell viability	• Trypan blue dye exclusion • Diacetyl fluorescein uptake • Cell counting • Replating efficiency
Cell metabolism	• Mitochondrial integrity (tetrazolium salt assays: MTT, MTS, XTT) • Lysosome and Golgi body activity (neutral red uptake) • Cofactor depletion (for example, ATP content)
Membrane leakage	• Loss of enzymes (for example, LDH), ions or cofactors (e.g., Ca^{2+}, K^+, NADPH) • Leakage of pre-labeled markers (e.g., [51]chromium or fluorescein)
Cell proliferation	• Cell counting • Total protein content (e.g., methylene blue, Coomassie blue, kenacid blue) • DNA content (e.g., Hoechst 33342) • Colony formation
Cell adhesion	• Attachment to culture surface • Detachment from culture surface • Cell-cell adhesion
Radioisotope incorporation	• Thymidine incorporation into DNA • Uridine incorporation into RNA • Amino acids incorporation into proteins

Adapted from [14]. MTT, 3-(4,5-dimethylthiazol-2-yl)-2,5-diphenyltetrazolium bromide; MTS, 3-(4,5-dimethylthiazol-2-yl)-5-(3-carboxymethoxyphenyl)-2-(4-sulfophenyl)-2*H*-tetrazolium; XTT, 3'-[1-(phenylaminocarbonyl)-3,4-tetrazolium]-*bis*-(4-methoxy-6-nitro)benzene sulfonic acid.

omic (gene expression) and proteomic technologies has created a unique, powerful tool in toxicological investigations [64].

In vitro toxicity testing of inhaled chemicals

The study of the toxic effects of inhaled chemicals is typically more challenging due to the technology required for the generation and characterization of test atmospheres, and the development of effective and reproducible techniques for exposure of cell cultures to airborne contaminants. Generation and characterization of known concentrations of air contaminants and reproducible exposure conditions require equipment and techniques to generate, maintain and measure test atmospheres comparable to those for *in vivo* studies (Fig. 2). In addition, the exposure of cells to test atmospheres requires close contact of cells and air.

A practical approach for *in vitro* inhalation toxicity testing has been proposed by the European Centre for the Validation of Alternative Methods (ECVAM) [21]. This systemic approach is initiated with the consultation of existing literature, evaluating the physicochemical characteristics of test chemicals and predicting potential toxic effects based on structure activity relationships (SARs). Physicochemical characteristics of chemicals such as molecular structure, solubility, vapor pressure, pH sensitivity, electrophilicity and chemical reactivity are important properties that may provide critical information for hazard identification and toxicity prediction [65, 66].

Initial *in vitro* tests should be conducted to identify likely target cells and toxic potency of test chemicals. Based on the obtained result, *in vitro* tests may be followed by a second phase using the following cells: nasal olfactory cells, airway epithelial cells, type II cells, alveolar macrophages, vascular endothelial cells, fibroblasts and mesothelial cells [21]. While over ten main cell types have been identified in the epithelium of the respiratory tract, for the assessment of respiratory toxicity it is important to utilize specific cell types with appropriate metabolizing activity. It has been suggested that the endpoints to be used should be selected based on the knowledge of toxic effects of test chemicals and should always include cell viability testing in at least two different cell types.

To evaluate the potential applications of *in vitro* methods for studying inhalation toxicity, more recent models developed for toxicity testing of airborne contaminants have been reviewed [14, 67, 68]. The toxic effects of air contaminants have been studied using several indirect and direct *in vitro* exposure techniques (Tab. 3).

Indirect exposure methods

Most of these, especially studies conducted on particulates are limited to exposure of cells to test chemicals solubilized or suspended in culture medium

Table 3. Indirect and direct *in vitro* exposure techniques developed for studying the toxicity of air contaminants

Exposure technique	Exposure achievement procedure
Indirect methods	
Exposure to test chemical itself	Cells are exposed to test chemicals solubilized or suspended in culture media
Exposure to collected air samples	Cells are exposed to air samples collected by filtration or impingement methods
Direct methods	
Submerged exposure condition	Test gas is introduced to cell suspension under submerged conditions using impinger or vacuum test tubes
Intermittent exposure	Cells are periodically exposed to gaseous compounds and culture medium at regular intervals using variation of techniques: rocker platforms, rolling bottles
Continuous direct exposure at the air/liquid interface	Cells are continuously exposed to airborne contaminants during the exposure period usually on their apical side, while being nourished from their basolateral side using collagen-coated or porous membranes permeable to culture media

Adapted from [14].

[69–76], which may be adequate for soluble test materials. However, this may not follow the *in vivo* exposure pattern of airborne aerosols, particularly for insoluble aerosols, due to unexpected alternation of their compositions and particle-media or particle-cell interactions [77]. Such techniques of exposure may also ignore size, which is crucial in toxicity testing of inhaled particles.

Some researchers have employed sampling of the aerosols by filtration techniques followed by the investigation of the effects of suspended and extracted particles, e.g., studies on atmospheric aerosols [78–82], or cigarette smoke condensate [83–86]. Filtration offers an advantage for on-site toxicity assessments of aerosols; however, this technique usually requires sample preparation steps, such as extraction to isolate the components of interest from a sample matrix, and ultimately, solubilization or suspension in culture media, potentially increasing experimental errors and further toxicity interactions. For example, cytotoxicity of roadside airborne particulates has been studied in rodent and human lung fibroblasts using the filtration technique [79]. Airborne particulates were sampled on glass fiber filters using a high-volume sampler. After air sampling, the filters were sonicated using benzene-ethanol solvents and to obtain a crude extract, solvents were evaporated to dryness. The crude extract was further fractionated by acid-base partitioning and all extracts were dissolved in dimethyl sulfoxide (DMSO) for cytotoxicity assays. Cytotoxicity was investigated using cell proliferation, tetrazolium salt (MTS) and lactate dehydrogenase (LDH) *in vitro* assays [79].

Indirect exposure techniques have also been developed using an impinge-
ment method where samples of airborne formaldehyde were collected in
serum-free culture media [87]. Cytotoxicity was investigated after exposing
human cells to collected air samples. The objective of this study was to develop an *in vitro* sampling and exposure technique that can be used for toxicity
testing of soluble airborne contaminants with the potential for on-site applications. An average of 96.8% was calculated for the collection efficiency of airborne formaldehyde in serum-free culture media, signifying the potential
application of this method for sampling the airborne formaldehyde and other
soluble airborne contaminants. The use of serum-free culture media as a collection solution for soluble airborne contaminants proved to be a simple technique, without any specific sample preparation or extraction steps; hence, any
potential toxic interactions of the test chemical with other toxic organic solvents during preparation were omitted.

Direct exposure methods

Several direct *in vitro* models have also been developed to deal with gas-phase
exposure of airborne contaminants using different exposure techniques.
Different features of exposure techniques developed for airborne chemicals
have been discussed in terms of their relevance, advantages and limitations
[88]. In principle, these methods include exposure of cells under submerged
conditions, intermittent exposure procedures and more recently direct exposure techniques at the air/liquid interface.

Exposure by bubbling gaseous test compounds through cells suspended in
media can easily be achieved using variations of standard laboratory processes (Fig. 3). For example, to study the *in vitro* toxic effects of O_3 on human

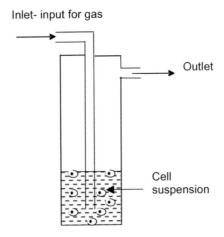

Figure 3. Exposure by bubbling test gaseous compounds through cells suspended in media.

hematic mononucleated cells (HHMC), the test gas was introduced at once to cell suspensions in vacuum test tubes [89]. However, exposure patterns *in vivo* may not be closely simulated and only a very small interface between the test gas and the target cells can be provided by the submerged exposure technique.

A variation of laboratory techniques has been developed allowing intermittent exposure of cultures to gaseous contaminants. Cell culture dishes held on chambers or platforms rotated, shaken or tilted at certain angles were exposed to gaseous compounds periodically [90, 91]. Cell culture flasks were also tilted at regular intervals to expose the cell cultures to volatile anesthetics [92]. Rolling culture bottles on roller drums were set up for *in vitro* gas exposure [93, 94]. Lung slices were alternatively fed by culture medium and exposed to diesel exhausts by rotating the culture vial on the internal wall of a flow through chamber [95]. Tissue culture flasks on a rocking platform were used to expose the cells to mainstream cigarette smoke followed by an immersion in culture media intermittently [96]. For example, a micro roller-bottle system was developed for cytotoxicity screening of volatile compounds in which primary hepatocytes attached to a collagen-coated nylon mesh (Fig. 4). The primary hepatocytes were exposed to volatile compounds injected into the roller bottle. The roller bottle was placed on a roller apparatus in an incubator at 37 °C and hepatocytes were alternatively exposed to the medium and the test atmosphere. Medium samples were then taken for measuring the cellular LDH and aspartate aminotransferase [94]. Compared to the submerged exposure, the intermittent exposure technique provided a larger interface between gaseous compound and target cells. Nevertheless, in such exposure conditions cells are always covered by an intervening layer of medium that may influence both accuracy and reproducibility of the results.

In the 1990s, technology became available that allowed cells to be cultured on permeable porous membranes in commercially available transwell or snapwell inserts (Fig. 5). In this system, once cells are established on the mem-

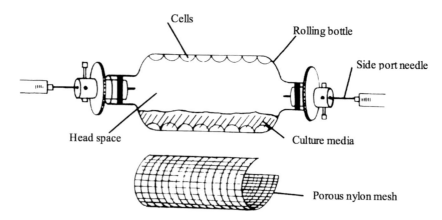

Figure 4. A micro roller bottle system (modified from [94]).

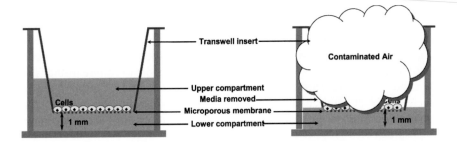

Figure 5. The culture of human cells on porous membranes. Left: Culture of cells on microporous membranes; Right: Exposure of cells to airborne contaminants following removal of media in the upper compartment (modified from [14] with permission of the publisher Wiley-VCH).

brane, the upper layer of culture media can be removed, and the cells directly exposed to air contaminants. In a direct exposure technique at the air/liquid interface target cells can be exposed to airborne contaminants continuously during the exposure time on their apical side, while being nourished from their basolateral side. Direct exposure of cells to airborne contaminants was initially achieved by growing cells on collagen-coated membranes located on special platforms [97] and more recently porous membranes in transwell inserts [77, 98, 99] or snapwell inserts [100–102]. Both static and dynamic direct exposure methods have been established for exposure purposes.

Exposure to volatile chemicals is a significant contributor to human health problems; however, toxicity testing of volatile compounds has always faced significant technological problems [60, 103–105]. Apart from high volatility, many VOCs are less water soluble or insoluble. These physicochemical properties may produce technical challenges during the course of in $vitro$ experiments. Static direct exposure methods have been developed for toxicity assessment of VOCs, in which test atmospheres of selected VOCs were generated in sealed glass chambers with known volumes [106]. Human cells including A549 pulmonary type II-like cell lines, HepG2 hepatoma cell lines and skin fibroblasts were exposed to airborne toxicants at different concentrations directly at the air/liquid interface. Cytotoxicity was investigated using the tetrazolium salt (MTS; Promega) and neutral red uptake (NRU; Sigma) assays in $vitro$. Using the static direct exposure method, the airborne IC_{50} (50% inhibitory concentration) values for selected VOCs were established, e.g., for xylene ($IC_{50} = 5350–8200$ ppm) and toluene ($IC_{50} = 10\,500–16\,600$ ppm) after 1-hour exposure. The static direct exposure method proved to be a practical and reproducible technique for in $vitro$ inhalation studies of volatile chemicals.

A typical experimental set-up for dynamic direct exposure at the air/liquid interface requires appropriate exposure chambers. Standard tissue culture incubators are used for exposure purposes [107]. Dynamic delivery and direct exposure of human cells to airborne contaminants can be achieved using specific exposure chambers [108] or horizontal diffusion chamber systems [109]. Toxic effects of individual airborne chemicals such as O_3, SO_2 and NO_2 [100, 109, 110], and complex mixtures, such as diesel motor exhaust [110], cigarette smoke [99], and combustion products [111, 112], have been studied using cultured human lung cells on porous membranes permeable to culture media. The dynamic direct exposure technique at the air/liquid interface offers a reproducible contact between chemically and physically unmodified airborne contaminants and target cells and technically may reflect more closely inhalation exposure *in vivo* [100, 101, 109].

Nanotoxicology: An emerging issue of inhalation toxicology

The pattern of human exposure to aerosols and particulates has changed enormously. Historically important pulmonary diseases (e.g., silicosis, coal miner's pneumoconiosis and asbestos-related cancer) have been significantly reduced *via* improvement of engineering and other control measures [35]. With emerging modern technologies such as nanotechnology and related material sciences, a new category of particles, nanoparticles, with unique characteristics are increasingly manufactured and introduced for commercial use. Nanoparticles are defined as primary particles with at least one dimension <100 nm [37, 113–115]. Nanoparticles have already being implemented in sunscreens, cosmetics, pharmaceuticals, food additives, self cleaning paints and glass, clothing, disinfectants, fuel additives, electronics, therapeutics, batteries and other products [115–120]. However, by increasing the application of nanoparticles, protection of the human respiratory system from exposure to nanoparticles and ultrafine particulates has become an emerging health concern [116]. While very little is known about their interactions with biological systems, the very small size distribution and tremendous large surface area of nanoparticles available for undergoing reactions may potentially play a significant role in toxicological effects of nanoparticles [37, 115, 121].

The defense mechanisms of the human body may not be able to deal adequately with such nanomaterials, smaller than common irritants and pollens. There is evidence that the human lung macrophages, which develop to remove inhaled particles, are not able to deal with nanomaterials smaller than 70 nm, enabling these particles to access deeply into the lung and perhaps enter the blood stream [29]. Microscopic examination of human monocytic cells after exposure to nanotubes demonstrated frustrated phagocytosis, suggesting that the ability of macrophages to remove nanofibers from the lung may be impaired [122]. It has been reported that combustion-derived nanoparticles (CDNP) and their components can migrate from their site of deposition in the lung, to other organs [114]. At the site of final retention in the target organs, nanomaterials may trigger mediators and hence activate inflammatory or immunological responses [123].

Apart from their local inflammatory effects, nanoparticles have the potential to translocate away from their site of deposition and into the blood circulation. Blood-borne particles may be delivered to secondary target organs such as brain, heart, spleen, kidney and liver causing numerous additional adverse health effects [37, 114].

With respect to toxicity testing of nanoparticles, several limitations have been identified that need to be addressed in future investigations [113, 115, 124–126]. Conventional exposure techniques are not able to determine the fraction of inhaled particles that ultimately cross the pulmonary epithelial barrier into the cardiovascular system; consequently, particle concentrations to which endothelial cells are exposed *in vivo* remain unknown [126]. Most current nanomaterials are extremely insoluble. Low water solubility is a major restrictive characteristic and may cause technical problems during the course of *in vitro* experimentation [106]. Therefore, future studies performed under dynamic exposure conditions can potentially provide more physiologically relevant toxicity information, leading to a better understanding of the interaction between target cells and nanoparticles.

Current knowledge of the toxicological potential of nanoparticles in relation to risk assessment is very limited, which makes it impossible to establish safety guidelines. In addition, available methods of sampling and analytical techniques are not able to adequately quantify the concentration of nanoparticles in environmental samples [37, 124, 127]. For example, due to the small size and low mass in any gravimetric method, the likely concentration of respirable particles is presumed to be very low. One of the key questions related to nanoparticle exposure is determining what potential characteristics of a nanoscale material needs to be measured, e.g., mass concentration, surface area, number concentration, size distribution, surface reactivity, particle agglomeration, chemical composition and/or morphology [37]. It is probable that the mass of a toxic concentration of nanoparticles in air will be very small, compared with conventional particles.

It has been recommended that high resolution imaging techniques, such as transmission electron microscopy (TEM) and scanning electron microscopy (SEM), may provide an efficient means by which to characterize particle size, shape and structure for a number of nanomaterials [128, 129]. Particle size distribution and shape are two crucial physicochemical characteristics in the context of exposure assessment and toxicity screening studies. TEM techniques have demonstrated how some nanomaterials such as metal oxide nanoparticles can be internalized within human cells [126]. Currently, these techniques serve as advanced research tools for toxicological investigations and qualitative structural evaluation of nanoparticles, both of which are expensive and non-quantitative. Much research is also needed to develop methods of detection and quantification that provide detection limits low enough to quantify the exposure concentration of inhaled nanoparticles and to reduce the uncertainty factors involved in their risk assessment.

Conclusion

Inhalation of airborne contaminants, e.g., gases, vapors, and aerosols, is a major contributor to human health problems, and can cause adverse effects ranging from simple irritation to morbidity and mortality through acute intense or long-term low-level repeated exposures. The large number of chemicals and complex mixtures present in indoor and outdoor air, coupled with the introduction of new materials such as nanoparticles and nanofibers, is an area of growing concern particularly in the industrial and urban environment. Animal-based assays have for many years been the preferred method to study the toxic effects of chemicals. However, very little is known about the potential toxicity of the vast majority of inhaled chemicals. As well as scientific and economic concerns, there is an increasingly strong urge to reduce animal testing on ethical grounds. The REACH regulatory framework intends to reduce the number of animal testings and speed up the risk assessment process. As well as new or improved OECD test guidelines, continuing scientific developments are needed to improve the process of safety evaluation for the vast number of chemicals. In addition, introducing a new category of chemicals/preparations to the marketplace such as nanoparticles and nanofibers, for which toxicity data is all but absent, emphasizes the demand on alternative toxicity test methods.

Development, standardization and validation of reproducible *in vitro* test methods could play a significant role in safety evaluation of chemicals and can contribute to a better understanding of the interactions between chemical exposure and toxic effects at the cellular level. The most appropriate cell systems with biotransformation activities and cellular functions comparable to the *in vivo* environment, such as a range of primary cell cultures and a battery of human cell-based assay systems, would need to be implemented. Although *in vitro* toxicology methods cannot mimic the biodynamics of the whole body, *in vitro* test systems in combination with the knowledge of QSAR and PBTK models have the potential to be considered more broadly for risk assessment of human inhalation exposures. A key molecular structure may provide some readily available information for toxicity prediction. Further, the application of PBTK models may provide a scientific basis for extrapolation of concentrations that produce cellular toxicity *in vitro*, to equivalent *in vivo* dosages.

For inhalation toxicity testing, promising *in vitro* exposure techniques have been recently developed that offer new possibilities for testing biological activities of inhaled chemicals under biphasic conditions at the air-liquid interface. The study of the toxic effects of inhaled chemicals *in vitro* requires effective and reproducible techniques for exposure of cell cultures to airborne contaminants. Direct exposure techniques may have the potential to be applied extensively to study the toxic effects of airborne contaminants, as the exposure pattern *in vivo* is more closely simulated by this method. Development and validation of appropriate *in vitro* sampling and exposure techniques may provide an advanced technology for studying the toxicity of nano- and ultrafine particles where inhalation toxicity data are much needed.

References

1 Dockery DW, Pope CA 3rd, Xu X, Spengler JD, Ware JH, Fay ME, Ferries BG Jr, Speizer FE (1993) An association between air pollution and mortality in six U.S. cities. *N Engl J Med* 329: 1753–1759

2 Greenberg MI, Phillips SD (2003) A brief history of occupational, industrial and environmental toxicology. In: MI Greenberg, RJ Hamilton, SD Phillips, GJ McCluskey (eds): *Occupational, Industrial and Environmental Toxicology,* 2nd edn., Mosby, Philadelphia, PA, 2–5

3 Winder C, Stacey NH (2004) Working examples on occupational toxicology. In: C Winder, NH Stacey (eds): *Occupational Toxicology,* 2nd edn., CRC Press, Boca Raton, FL, 549–577

4 NTP (1984) *Toxicology Testing Strategies to Determine Needs and Priorities.* National Toxicology Program, National Research Council, Washington DC

5 Agrawal MR, Winder C (1996) The frequency and occurrence of LD_{50} values for materials in the workplace. *J Appl Toxicol* 16: 407–422

6 EPA (1998) *Chemical Hazard Availability Study.* The Environmental Protection Agency, Office of Pollution Prevention and Toxics, Washington, DC

7 Faustman E, Omenn G (2001) Risk Assessment. In: CD Klaassen (ed.): *Casarett and Doull's Toxicology: The Basic Science of Poisons.* 6th edn., McGraw-Hill, New York, 83–104

8 Costa DL (2008) Alternative test methods in inhalation toxicology: Challenges and opportunities. *Exp Toxicol Pathol* 60: 105–109

9 Blaauboer BJ (2002) The applicability of *in vitro*-derived data in hazard identification and characterisation of chemicals. *Environ Toxicol Pharm* 11: 213–225

10 Raabe OG (1999) Respiratory exposure to air pollutants. In: DL Swift, WM Foster (eds): *Air Pollutants and the Respiratory Tract*, Marcel Dekker, New York, 39–73

11 Ghorbanli M, Bakand Z, Bakhshi Khaniki G, Bakand S (2007) Air pollution effects on the activity of antioxidant enzymes in *Nerium oleander* and *Robinia pseudo acacia* plants in Tehran. *Iranian J Environ Health Sci Eng* 4: 157–162

12 Lioy PJ, Zhang J (1999) Air pollution. In: DL Swift, WM Foster (eds): *Air Pollutants and the Respiratory Tract*, Marcel Dekker, New York, 1–38

13 Costa DL (2001) Air pollution. In: CD Klaassen (ed.): *Casarett and Doull's Toxicology: The Basic Science of Poisons,* 6th edn., McGraw-Hill, New York, 979–1012

14 Hayes A, Bakand S, Winder C (2007) Novel *in vitro* exposure techniques for toxicity testing and biomonitoring of airborne contaminants. In: U Marx, V Sandig (eds): *Drug Testing: In Vitro-Breakthroughs and Trends in Cell Culture Technology*, Wiley-VCH, Berlin, 103–124

15 Beckett WS (1999) Detecting respiratory tract responses to air pollutants. In: DL Swift, WM Foster (eds): *Air Pollutants and the Respiratory Tract*, Marcel, New York, 105–118

16 Boulet LP, Bowie D (1999) Acute occupational respiratory diseases. In: CE Mapp (ed.): *Occupational Lung Disorders*, European Respiratory Society, Huddersfield, UK, 320–346

17 Hext PM (2000) Inhalation toxicology. In: B Ballantyne, TC Marrs, T Syversen (eds): *General and Applied Toxicology,* Vol. 1, 2nd edn., Macmillan, London, 587–601

18 Witschi H, Last JA (2001) Toxic responses of the respiratory system. In: CD Klaassen (ed.): *Casarett and Doull's Toxicology: The Basic Science of Poisons,* 6th edn., McGraw-Hill, New York, 515–534

19 Brouder J, Tardif R (1998) Absorption. In: P Wexler (ed.): *Encyclopedia of Toxicology*, Vol. 1, Academic Press, San Diego, CA, 1–7

20 Winder C (2004) Occupational respiratory diseases. In: C Winder, NH Stacey (eds): *Occupational Toxicology,* 2nd edn., CRC Press, Boca Raton, FL, 71–114

21 Lambre CR, Aufderheide M, Bolton RE, Fubini B, Haagsman HP, Hext PM, Jorissen M, Landry Y, Morin JP, Nemery B, Nettesheim P, Pauluhn J, Richards RJ, Vickers AEM, Wu R (1996) *In vitro* tests for respiratory toxicity, the report and recommendations of ECVAM workshop 18. *Altern Lab Anim* 24: 671–681

22 Valentine R, Kennedy GL (2001) Inhalation toxicology. In: A Wallace Hayes (ed.): *Principles and Methods of Toxicology,* 4th edn., Taylor and Francis, Philadelphia, PA, 1085–1143

23 Witschi HP, Brain JD (1985) *Toxicology of Inhaled Materials: General Principles of Inhalation Toxicology. Handbook of Experimental Pharmacology,* Vol. 75, Springer, Secaucus, NJ

24 Rozman KK, Klaassen CD (2001) Absorption, distribution and excretion of toxicants. In: Klaassen CD (ed.): *Casarett and Doull's Toxicology: The Basic Science of Poisons,* 6th edn., McGraw-Hill, New York, 105–132

25 IARC (2004) *IARC Classifies Formaldehyde as Carcinogenic to Humans*. International Agency for Research on Cancer, Press Release, N 153

26 Asgharian B, Wood R, Schlesinger RB (1995) Empirical modelling of particle deposition in the alveolar region of the lungs: A basis for interspecies extrapolation. *Fundam Appl Toxicol* 27: 232–238

27 Siegmann K, Scherrer L, Siegmann HC (1999) Physical and chemical properties of airborne nanoscale particles and how to measure their impact on human health. *J Mol Struct* 458: 191–201

28 Lundborg M, Johard U, Lastbom L, Gerde P, Camner P (2001) Human alveolar macrophage phagocytic function is impaired by aggregates of ultrafine carbon particles. *Environ Res* 86: 244–253

29 Bergeron S, Archambault D (2005) *Canadian Stewardship Practices for Environmental Nanotechnology*. Science-Metrix, Canada (http://www.science-metrix.com/eng/reports_2005_t.htm)

30 Mühlfeld C, Gehr P, Rothen-Rutishauser B (2008) Translocation and cellular entering mechanisms of nanoparticles in the respiratory tract. *Swiss Med Wkly* 138: 387–391

31 Oberdörster G, Oberdörster E, Oberdörster J (2005) Nanotoxicology: An emerging discipline evolving from studies of ultrafine particles. *Environ Health Perspect* 113: 823–839

32 Schlesinger RB (2000) Disposition of inhaled particles and gases. In: M Cohen, J Zelikoff, RB Schlesinger (eds): *Pulmonary Immunotoxicology*. Kluwer Academic Publishers, Boston, MA, 85–106

33 Eaton DL (2005) Toxicology. In: L Rosenstock, MR Cullen, CA Brodkin, CA Redlich (eds): *Textbook of Clinical Occupational and Environmental Medicine*, 2nd edn., Elsevier Saunders, Philadelphia, PA, 83–118

34 Vincent JH (1995) *Aerosol Science for Industrial Hygienists*. Elsevier Science, Pergamon Press, Oxford

35 Johnson D, Swift D (1997) Sampling and sizing particles. In: SR DiNardi (ed.): *The Occupational Environment – Its Evaluation and Control*, American Industrial Hygienists Association, AIHA Press, Fairfax, VA, 245–261

36 William PL, Burson JL (1985) *Industrial Toxicology – Safety and Health Applications in the Workplace*. Van Nostard Reinhold, New York

37 Borm PJ, Robbins D, Haubold S, Kuhlbusch T, Fissan H, Donaldson K, Schins R, Stone V, Kreyling W, Lademann J, Krutmann J, Warheit D, Oberdörster E (2006) The potential risks of nanomaterials: A review carried out for ECETOC. *Partic Fibre Toxicol* 3: 1–35

38 David A, Wagner GR (1998) Respiratory system. In: JM Stellman (ed.): *Encyclopedia of Occupational Health and Safety*. 4th edn., Geneva, International Labour Office, 10.1–10.7

39 Winder C (2004) Toxicology of gases, vapours and particulates. In: C Winder, NH Stacey (eds): *Occupational Toxicology*, 2nd edn., CRC Press, Boca Raton, FL, 399–424

40 Shusterman D (2002) Asphyxiation. In: DJ Hendrick, PS Burge, WS Beckett, A Churg (eds): *Occupational Disorders of the Lung: Recognition, Management and Prevention*, WB Saunders, London, 279–303

41 Hendrick DJ, Burge PS (2002) Asthma. In: DJ Hendrick, PS Burge, WS Beckett, A Churg (eds): *Occupational Disorders of the Lung: Recognition, Management and Prevention*, WB Saunders, London, 33–76

42 Lizarralde SM, Wake B, Thompson V, Weisman RS (2003) Jewelers. In: MI Greenberg, RJ Hamilton, SD Phillips, GJ McCluskey (eds): *Occupational, Industrial, and Environmental Toxicology*, 2nd edn., Mosby, Philadelphia, PA, 198–215

43 Tarlo SM, Chan-Yeung M (2005) Occupational asthma. In: L Rosenstock, MR Cullen, CA Brodkin, CA Redlich (eds): *Textbook of Clinical Occupational and Environmental Medicine*, 2nd edn., Elsevier Saunders, Philadelphia, PA, 293–308

44 Koenig JQ, Luchtel DL (1997) Respiratory responses to inhaled toxicants. In: EJ Massaro (ed.): *Handbook of Human Toxicology*, CRC Press, Boca Raton, FL, 551–606

45 Mapp C (1999) *Occupational Lung Disorders*. European Respiratory Society Journals, Huddersfield, UK

46 NTP (2002) *The National Toxicology Program Annual Plan Fiscal Year 2001*. U.S. Department of Health and Human Services. Public Health Service. NIH Publication No. 02–5092

47 Stenton C (2002) Chronic obstructive pulmonary disease (COPD). In: DJ Hendrick, PS Burge, WS Beckett, A Churg (eds): *Occupational Disorders of the Lung: Recognition, Management and Prevention*, WB Saunders, London, 77–91

48 Mapel W Coultas D (2002) Disorders due to minerals other than silica, coal, and asbestos, and to

metals. In: DJ Hendrick, PS Burge, WS Beckett, A Churg (eds): *Occupational Disorders of the Lung: Recognition, Management and Prevention*, WB Saunders, London, 163–190

49 Meredith S, Blank PD (2002) Surveillance: Clinical and epidemiological perspectives. In: DJ Hendrick, PS Burge, WS Beckett, A Churg (eds): *Occupational Disorders of the Lung: Recognition, Management and Prevention*, WB Saunders, London, 7–24

50 McClellan RO (1999) Health risk assessments and regulatory considerations for air pollutants. In: DL Swift, WM Foster (eds): *Air Pollutants and the Respiratory Tract*. Marcel Dekker, New York, 289–338

51 Thorne PS (2001) Occupational toxicology. In: CD Klaassen (ed.): *Casarett and Doull's Toxicology: The Basic Science of Poisons,* 6th edn., McGraw-Hill, New York, 1123–1140

52 Arts JH, Muijser H, Jonker D, van de Sandt JJ, Bos PM, Feron VJ (2008) Inhalation toxicity studies: OECD guidelines in relation to REACH and scientific developments. *Exp Toxicol Pathol* 60: 125–133

53 Barile FA (1994) *Introduction to In Vitro Cytotoxicity, Mechanisms and Methods*. CRC Press, Boca Raton, FL

54 Miller GC, Klonne DR (1997) Occupational exposure limits. In: SR DiNardi (ed.): *The Occupational Environment – Its Evaluation and Control*, American Industrial Hygienists Association, AIHA Press, Fairfax, VA, 21–42

55 OECD (2004) *Chemicals Testing: OECD Guidelines for the Testing of Chemicals. Section 4: Health Effects*. Organisation for Economic Co-operation and Development, http://www.oecd.org/document/55/0,2340,en_2649_34377_2349687_1_1_1_1,00.html (accessed February 2009)

56 Ekwall B (1983) Screening of toxic compounds in mammalian cell cultures. *Ann NY Acad Sci* 407: 64–77

57 Balls M, Clothier RH (1992) Cytotoxicity assays for intrinsic toxicity and irritancy. In: RR Watson (ed.): *In Vitro Methods of Toxicology*. CRC Press, Boca Raton, FL, 37–52

58 Anderson D, Russell T (1995) *The Status of Alternative Methods in Toxicology*. The Royal Society of Chemistry. Cambridge, UK

59 Barile FA (1997) Continuous cell lines as a model for drug toxicology assessment. In: JV Castell, MJ Gomez-Lechon (eds): *In Vitro Methods in Pharmaceutical Research*, Academic Press, San Diego, 33–54

60 Zucco F, de Angelis I, Stammati A (1998) Cellular models for *in vitro* toxicity testing. In: M Clynes (ed.): *Animal Cell Culture Techniques,* Springer Lab Manual, Springer, Berlin, 395–422

61 Doyle A, Griffiths JB (2000) *Cell and Tissue Culture for Medical Research*. John Wiley & Sons, UK

62 Wilson AP (2000) Cytotoxicity and viability assays. In: JRW Masters (ed.): *Animal Cell Culture,* 3rd edn., Oxford University Press, New York, 175–219

63 Zucco F, de Angelis I, Testai E, Stammati A (2004) Toxicology investigations with cell culture systems: 20 years after. *Toxicol In Vitro* 18: 153–163

64 Eisenbrand G, Pool-Zobel B, Baker V, Balls M, Blaauboer BJ, Boobis A, Carere A, Kevekordes S, Lhuguenot JC, Pieters R, Kleiner J (2002) Methods of *in vitro* toxicology. *Food Chem Toxicol* 40: 193–236

65 Gad SC (2000) *In Vitro Toxicology*. Taylor and Francis, New York

66 Faustman EM, Omenn GS (2001) Risk assessment. In: CD Klaassen (ed.): *Casarett and Doull's Toxicology: The Basic Science of Poisons,* 6th edn., McGraw-Hill, New York, 83–104

67 Aufderheide M (2005) Direct exposure methods for testing native atmospheres. *Exp Toxicol Pathol* 57: 213–226

68 Bakand S, Winder C, Khalil C, Hayes A (2005) Toxicity assessment of industrial chemicals and airborne contaminants: Transition from *in vivo* to *in vitro* test methods: A review. *Inhal Toxicol* 17: 775–787

69 Nadeau D, Vincent R, Kumarathasan P, Brook J, Dufresne A (1995) Cytotoxicity of ambient air particles to rat lung macrophages: Comparison of cellular and functional assays. *Toxicol In Vitro* 10: 161–172

70 Governa M, Valentino M, Amati M, Visona I, Botta GC, Marcer G, Gemignani C (1997) Biological effects of contaminated silicon carbide particles from a work station in a plant producing abrasives. *Toxicol In Vitro* 11: 201–207

71 Goegan P, Vincent R, Kumarathasan P, Brook JR (1998) Sequential *in vitro* effects of airborne particles in lung macrophages and reporter Cat-gene cell lines. *Toxicol In Vitro* 12: 25–37

72 Baeza-Squiban A, Bonvallot V, Boland S, Marano F (1999) Diesel exhaust particles increase NF-

κB DNA binding activity and c-Fos proto-oncogene expression in human bronchial epithelial cells. *Toxicol In Vitro* 13: 817–822

73 Becker S, Soukup JM, Gallagher JE (2002) Differential particulate air pollution induced oxidant stress in human granulocytes, monocytes and alveolar macrophages. *Toxicol In Vitro* 16: 209–221

74 Takano Y, Taguchi T, Suzuki I, Balis JU, Kazunari Y (2002) Cytotoxicity of heavy metals on primary cultured alveolar type II cells. *Environ Res* 89: 138–145

75 Riley MR, Boesewetter DE, Kim AM, Sirvent FP (2003) Effects of metals Cu, Fe, Ni, V, and Zn on rat lung epithelial cells. *Toxicology* 190: 171–184

76 Okeson CD, Riley MR, Riley-Saxton E (2004) *In vitro* alveolar cytotoxicity of soluble components of airborne particulate matter: Effects of serum on toxicity of transition metals. *Toxicol In Vitro* 18: 673–680

77 Diabaté S, Mülhopt S, Paur HR, Krug HF (2002) Pro-inflammatory effects in lung cells after exposure to fly ash aerosol *via* the atmosphere or the liquid phase. *Ann Occup Hyg* 46 Suppl 1: 382–385

78 Hamers T, van Schaardenburg MD, Felzel EC, Murk AJ, Koeman JH (2000) The application of reporter gene assay for the determination of the toxic potency of diffuse air pollution. *Sci Total Environ* 262: 159–174

79 Yamaguchi T, Yamazaki H (2001) Cytotoxicity of airborne particulates sampled roadside in rodent and human lung fibroblasts. *J Health Sci* 47: 272–277

80 Alfaro-Moreno E, Martinez L, Garcia-Cuellar C, Bonner JC, Murray JC, Rosas I, Rosales SP, Osornio-Vargas AR (2002) Biologic effects induced *in vitro* by PM_{10} from three different zones of Mexico City. *Environ Health Perspect* 110: 715–720

81 Glowala M, Mazurek A, Piddubnyak V, Fiszer-Kierzkowska A, Michalska J, Krawczyk Z (2002) HSP70 overexpression increases resistance of V79 cells to cytotoxicity of airborne pollutants, but does not protect the mitotic spindle against damage caused by airborne toxins. *Toxicology* 170: 211–219

82 Baulig A, Sourdeval M, Meyer M, Marano F, Baeza-Squiban A (2003) Biological effects of atmospheric particles on human bronchial epithelial cells. Comparison with diesel exhaust particles. *Toxicol In Vitro* 17: 567–573

83 Bombick DW, Putnam KP, Doolittle DJ (1998) Comparative cytotoxicity studies of smoke condensates from different types of cigarettes and tobaccos. *Toxicol In Vitro* 12: 241–249

84 Bombick BR, Murli H, Avalos JT, Bombick DW, Morgan WT, Putnam KP, Doolittle DJ (1998) Chemical and biological studies of a new cigarette that primarily heats tobacco. Part 2. *In vitro* toxicology of mainstream smoke condensate. *Food Chem Toxicol* 36: 183–190

85 McKarns SC, Bombic DW, Morton MJ, Doolittle DJ (2000) Gap junction intercellular communication and cytotoxicity in normal human cells after exposure to smoke condensates from cigarettes that burn or primarily heat tobacco. *Toxicol In Vitro* 14: 41–51

86 Putnam KP, Bombic DW, Doolittle DJ (2002) Evaluation of eight *in vitro* assays for assessing the cytotoxicity of cigarette smoke condensate. *Toxicol In Vitro* 16: 599–607

87 Bakand S, Hayes AJ, Winder C, Khalil C, Markovic B (2005) *In vitro* cytotoxicity testing of airborne formaldehyde collected in serum-free culture media. *Toxicol Indust Health* 21: 147–154

88 Ritter D, Knebel J, Aufderheide M (2001) *In vitro* exposure of isolated cells to native gaseous compounds – Development and validation of an optimized system for human lung cells. *Exp Toxicol Pathol* 53: 373–386

89 Cardile V, Jiang X, Russo A, Casella F, Renis M, Bindoni M (1995) Effects of ozone on some biological activities of cells *in vitro*. *Cell Biol Toxicol* 11: 11–21

90 Blanquart C, Giuliani F, Houcine O, Guennou C, Marano F, Jeulin C (1995) *In vitro* exposure of rabbit trachelium to SO_2: Effects on morphology and ciliary beating. *Toxicol In Vitro* 9: 123–132

91 Rusznak C, Devalia JL, Sapsford RJ, Davies RJ (1996) Ozone-induced mediator release from human bronchial epithelial cells *in vitro* and the influence of nedocromil sodium. *Eur Respir J* 9: 2298–2305

92 Mückter H, Zwing M, Bäder S, Marx T, Doklea E, Liebl B, Fichtl B, Georgieff M (1998) A novel apparatus for the exposure of cultured cells to volatile agents. *J Pharmacol Toxicol Methods* 40: 63–69

93 Shiraishi F, Hashimoto S, Bandow H (1986) Induction of sister-chromatid exchanges in Chinese hamster V79 cells by exposure to the photochemical reaction products of toluene plus NO_2 in the gas phase. *Mutat Res* 173: 135–139

94 DelRaso NJ (1992) *In vitro* methods for assessing chemical or drug toxicity and metabolism in

primary hepatocytes. In: RR Watson (ed.): *In Vitro Methods of Toxicology*, CRC Press, Boca Raton, FL, 176–201

95 Morin JP, Fouquet F, Monteil C, Le Prieur E, Vaz E, Dionnet F (1999) Development of a new *in vitro* system for continuous *in vitro* exposure of lung tissue to complex atmospheres: Application to diesel exhaust toxicology. *Cell Biol Toxicol* 15: 143–152

96 Bombick DW, Ayres PH, Putnam K, Bombick BR, Doolittle DJ (1998) Chemical and biological studies of a new cigarette that primarily heats tobacco. Part 3. *In vitro* toxicity of whole smoke. *Food Chem Toxicol* 36: 191–197

97 Chen LC, Fang CP, Qu QS, Fine JM, Schlesinger RB (1993) A novel system for the *in vitro* exposure of pulmonary cells to acid sulfate aerosols. *Fund Appl Toxicol* 20: 170–176

98 Knebel J, Ritter D, Aufderheide M (2002) Exposure of human lung cells to native diesel motor exhaust-development of an optimized *in vitro* test strategy. *Toxicol In Vitro* 16: 185–192

99 Aufderheide M, Knebel J, Ritter D (2003) Novel approaches for studying pulmonary toxicity *in vitro*. *Toxicol Lett* 140–141: 205–211

100 Bakand S, Hayes A, Winder C (2007) Comparative *in vitro* cytotoxicity assessment of selected gaseous compounds in human alveolar epithelial cells. *Toxicol In Vitro* 21: 1341–1347

101 Bakand S, Hayes A, Winder C (2007) An integrated *in vitro* approach for toxicity testing of airborne contaminants. *J Toxicol Environ Health A* 70: 1604–1612

102 Potera C (2007) A new approach for testing airborne pollutants. *Environ Health Perspect* 115: A149–151

103 Stark DM, Shopsis C, Borenfreund E, Babich H (1986) Progress and problems in evaluating and validating alternative assays in toxicology. *Food Chem Toxicol* 24: 449–455

104 Frazier JM, Bradlaw JA (1989) *Technical problems associated with in vitro toxicity testing systems*. A Report of the CAAT Technical Workshop of May 17–18, 1989. The Johns Hopkins Center for Alternatives to Animal Testing (CAAT), Baltimore, MD

105 Dierickx PJ (2003) Evidence for delayed cytotoxicity effects following exposure of rat hepatoma-derived Fa32 cells: Implications for predicting human acute toxicity. *Toxicol In Vitro* 17: 797–801

106 Bakand S, Winder C, Khalil C, Hayes A (2006) A novel *in vitro* exposure technique for toxicity testing of selected volatile organic compounds. *J Environ Monit* 8: 100–105

107 Lang DS, Jörres RA, Mücke M, Siegfried W, Magnussen H (1998) Interactions between human bronchoepithelial cells and lung fibroblasts after ozone exposure *in vitro*. *Toxicol Lett* 96–97: 13–24

108 Aufderheide M, Mohr U (2000) CULTEX – An alternative technique for cultivation and exposure of cells of the respiratory tract to the airborne pollutants at the air/liquid interface. *Exp Toxicol Pathol* 52: 265–270

109 Bakand S, Winder C, Khalil C, Hayes A (2006) An experimental *in vitro* model for dynamic direct exposure of human cells to airborne contaminants. *Toxicol Lett* 165: 1–10

110 Knebel J, Ritter D, Aufderheide M (1998) Development of an *in vitro* system for studying effects of native and photochemically transformed gaseous compounds using an air/liquid culture technique. *Toxicol Lett* 96–97: 1–11

111 Lestari F, Markovic B, Green AR, Chattopadhyay G, Hayes AJ (2006) Comparative assessment of three *in vitro* exposure methods for combustion toxicity. *J Appl Toxicol* 26: 99–114

112 Lestari F, Green AR, Chattopadhyay G, Hayes AJ (2006) An alternative method for fire smoke toxicity assessment using human lung cells. *Fire Safe J* 41: 605–615

113 Warheit DB (2004) Nanoparticles health impacts. *Mater Today* 7: 32–35

114 Donaldson K, Tran L, Jimenez LA, Duffin R, Newby DE, Mills N, MacNee W, Stone V (2005) Combustion-derived nanoparticles: A review of their toxicology following inhalation exposure. *Partic Fibre Toxicol* 2: 10

115 Suh WH, Suslick KS, Stucky GD, Suh YH (2009) Nanotechnology, nanotoxicology, and neuroscience. *Prog Neurobiol* 87: 133–170

116 Lindberg HK, Falck GC, Suhonen S, Vippola M, Vanhala E, Catalán J, Savolainen K, Norppa H (2009) Genotoxicity of nanomaterials: DNA damage and micronuclei induced by carbon nanotubes and graphite nanofibres in human bronchial epithelial cells *in vitro*. *Toxicol Lett* 186: 166–173

117 Karn B, Masciangioli T, Zhang W, Colvin V, Alivisatos P (2005) *Nanotechnology and the Environment; Applications and Implications*. American Chemical Society, Washington, DC

118 Liu W (2006) Nanoparticles and their biological and environmental applications. *J Biosci Bioeng*

     102: 1–7
119 Nel A, Xia T, Mädler L, Li N (2006) Toxic potential of materials at the nanolevel. *Science* 311:
     622–627
120 Renn O, Roco MC (2006) *White Paper on Nanotechnology Risk Governance*. International Risk
     Governance Council, Geneva
121 Dechsakulthorn F, Hayes A, Bakand S, Joeng L, Winder C (2008) *In vitro* cytotoxicity of select-
     ed nanoparticles using human skin fibroblasts. *Altern Animal Test Exper – AATEX* 14: 397–400
122 Brown DM, Kinloch IA, Bangert U, Windle AH, Walter DM, Walker GS, Scotchford CA,
     Donaldson K, Stone V (2007) An *in vitro* study of the potential of carbon nanotubes and
     nanofibers to induce inflammatory mediators and frustrated phagocytosis. *Carbon* 45:
     1743–1756
123 Donaldson K, Stone V, Tran CL, Kreyling W, Borm PJ (2004) Nanotoxicology. *Occup Environ
     Med* 61: 727–728
124 Seaton A (2006) Nanotechnology and the occupational physician. *Occup Med* 56: 312–316
125 Tolstoshev A (2006) *Nanotechnology, Assessing the Environmental Risks for Australia*. Earth
     Policy Centre, University of Melbourne, Australia
126 Gojova A, Guo B, Kota R, Rutledge JC, Kennedy IM, Barakat AI (2007) Induction of inflamma-
     tion in vascular endothelial cells by metal oxide nanoparticles: Effects of particle composition.
     Environ Health Perspect 115: 403–409
127 Cohen BS, McCammon CS Jr (2001) *Air Sampling Instruments for Evaluation of Atmospheric
     Contaminants*. 9th edn., ACGIH, Cincinnati, OH
128 Englert CB (2007) Nanomaterials and the environment: Uses, methods and measurement. *J
     Environ Monit* 9: 1154–1161
129 Drobne D (2007) Nanotoxicology for safe and sustainable nanotechnology. *Arh Hig Rada
     Toksikol* 58: 471–478

Molecular, Clinical and Environmental Toxicology. Volume 2: Clinical Toxicology
Edited by A. Luch

Biological testing for drugs of abuse

David Vearrier, John A. Curtis and Michael I. Greenberg

Department of Emergency Medicine, Drexel University College of Medicine, USA

Abstract. Testing for drugs of abuse has become commonplace and is used for a variety of indications. Commonly employed testing methods include immunoassay and chromatography. Testing methods vary in their sensitivity, specificity, time, and cost. While urine remains the most common body fluid used for testing of drugs of abuse, over the last several decades the use of alternative matrices such as blood, sweat, oral fluids, and hair has increased dramatically. Each biological matrix offers advantages and disadvantages for drug testing, and the most appropriate matrix frequently depends on the indications for the drug test. Drugs of abuse that are most commonly tested include alcohol, amphetamines, cannabinoids, cocaine, opiates, and phencyclidine. Testing may involve detection of the parent compound or metabolites and sensitivity, specificity, and reliability of drug testing may vary depending on the drug being tested. Toxicologists have a responsibility to understand the strengths and limitations of testing techniques and matrices to be able to critically evaluate the results of a drug test.

Introduction

Testing for drugs of abuse has become commonplace in the workplace and in modern medical practice. The origins of testing for drugs of abuse can be found in the pathology laboratory when illicit drug use was suspected to be a contributing cause of death. Today, drug tests are used for a wide variety of applications. Applicants for employment must frequently undergo testing prior to securing a position. Both the federal government and the U.S. military test employees, physicians use drug testing to suggest possible diagnoses, rehabilitation programs monitor subjects for abstinence, athletes are tested for performance-enhancing drugs, authorities test persons suspected of operating a vehicle under the influence, and employees with safety sensitive or other positions or special responsibilities often undergo intermittent or random drug testing.

Testing for drugs of abuse may take a variety of forms. While urine tests are most commonly used, serum, hair, oral fluid, sweat, and meconium tests are also available. A variety of testing methods are utilized including thin-layer chromatography (TLC), immunoassays, and gas chromatography–mass spectrometry (GC-MS). The precise method used varies according to the reasons for performing the test and for a variety of applicable regulations.

Despite the rapid increase in testing for drugs of abuse, many professionals who use drug testing or interpret the results of those tests have limited understanding of the actual testing procedure and the benefits and limitations of various testing methodologies. This may result in complacency and, at times, results in misapplication of toxicological principles. This complacency may be an indirect result of misplaced trust in the infallibility of the laboratory and the belief that a laboratory report is always accurate. The goal of this chapter is to introduce the reader to testing methods widely used today, explain their benefits and drawbacks, discuss the limitations of various testing methods, and present an overview of the medicolegal milieu in which drug testing is performed.

Testing methods

A variety of methods have been developed for identifying drugs of abuse in biological matrices. Testing methodologies differ in their sensitivity, specificity, cost, availability, and time. The most appropriate testing method will depend on the specific purpose for which testing is performed.

Thin-layer chromatography

TLC is a qualitative method of testing that distinguishes compounds based on their degree of polarity. A small amount of sample is placed *via* micropipette on a testing plate that is coated with a polar substance such as silica. The base of the testing plate is placed in a non-polar solvent, e.g., benzene, cyclohexane, chloroform or others, and the solvent rises up the plate by capillary action. Compounds in the tested sample migrate up the plate along with the nonpolar solvent to varying distances depending on their polarity; more polar compounds remain stationary or travel only a short distance, while less polar compounds travel farther. The compounds can be visualized on the plate using ultraviolet light or by chemical reaction leading to a colored product. Compounds can then be identified by comparison with known values or internal standards.

The use of TLC in drug testing, while historically important, is not commonly used for drug testing today as more sensitive techniques requiring less technical expertise are available. Additionally, TLC is limited in that it cannot quantify the amount of drug identified in the body fluid in question. While TLC has been used as a confirmatory test in the past, today it has largely been abandoned in favor of gas (GC) or liquid chromatography (LC).

Immunoassay

Immunoassays depend on an antigen-antibody reaction to detect drugs of abuse in body fluids. A variety of specific techniques have been developed that vary in how the antigen-antibody reaction occurs in the sample. The presence of the drug and the antigen-antibody reaction can be measured using radioactivity or an enzymatic reaction.

Radioimmunoassays (RIA) utilize radioactivity to identify the presence of drugs of abuse in body fluids. In RIA, a known quantity of the drug of abuse is labeled with a radioactive atom, commonly iodine-125. For example, to detect cocaine use, benzoylecgonine can be labeled with iodine-125 [1]. Then the body fluid being tested, a known quantity of the radioactive drug of abuse, and antibodies directed against the drug of abuse are combined. The radioactive antigen competes with antigen in the body fluid, if present, to bind with antibodies. Antibody-antigen complexes are removed by centrifugation and the radioactivity of the supernatant is measured. If there is no drug of abuse present in the body fluid, more of the radioactive antigen will bind to antibodies and be removed, and the radioactivity of the supernatant will be decreased. If the drug of interest is present in the body fluid it will bind the antibody, leaving more of the radioactive antigen unbound and retained in the supernatant, and the radioactivity of the supernatant will be increased. The radioactivity of the supernatant can be compared to standard curves to determine the concentration of the drug of abuse in the body fluid tested.

When RIA was first developed in the 1950s it was hailed as an innovative technique allowing the measurement of minute quantities of a particular substance (e.g., insulin) in the blood. Although RIA has historically been used in testing for drugs of abuse, today it has largely been supplanted by enzyme immunoassays. Enzyme immunoassays are considered superior to RIA in that they do not require the sophisticated equipment or use of radioactive materials inherent to RIA.

Enzyme immunoassays, also known as enzyme-linked immunosorbent assays (ELISA), identify an antigen, such as a drug of abuse, present in body fluid by means of a colorimetric or fluorescent signal. ELISA uses enzymes that have been covalently attached to antibodies. These enzymes act on substrate to produce a colored or fluorescent product that can be qualitatively or quantitatively measured.

Several specific ELISA techniques exist and the exact steps involved vary depending on the ELISA being performed, although the tests are all similar. Samples of the body fluid, along with positive and negative controls, are added to wells on a microtiter plate. Drugs of abuse present in the body fluid nonspecifically adsorb to the sides of the well. Antibodies against the drug being tested are added to each well. An enzyme-linked antibody is then added that binds specifically to the initial antibodies added. After an incubation period, the well is emptied and washed. Lastly, the substrate for the enzyme is added. If the drug being tested was present in the body fluid, the drug/antibody/enzyme-linked antibody complex will adhere to the wall of the well and the substrate will be metabolized to a fluorescent or colorimetric signal. The strength of the signal can be compared to standard curves for quantification. If no drug was present, the antibody/enzyme-linked antibody complex will be washed away and no fluorescent or colorimetric product will be produced.

ELISA is currently the method of choice in most clinical laboratories and clinically related testing situations. ELISA testing is fast, inexpensive, highly sensitive, and widely available. The major drawback to ELISA is its limited specificity. The test uses antibody-antigen interaction to determine the presence of drugs of abuse in the body fluid being tested. If a compound that is structurally similar to the drug of abuse is present in the body fluid, it may interact with the antibody, causing a false-positive result (Tab. 1).

Point-of-care immunoassays are becoming increasingly available. These tests use many of the same principles of ELISA but require minimal equipment or expertise. Specific testing apparatuses are available from various companies. The tests generally depend on a competitive immunoassay in which a drug-pigment conjugate in the test competes with the drug of abuse in the body fluid, if present, for a limited amount of antibody. If the drug of abuse is present at sufficient concentration in the body fluid, it occupies the antibody binding sites, and the drug-conjugate remains free. The drug-conjugate is then able to bind to other antibodies immobilized on a solid support where it will cause a visible line, signifying a positive result. In the absence of drug of abuse in the body fluid, the drug-conjugate will bind to the antibody and will be unavailable to bind to the antibodies on the solid support, no line will be generated, signifying a negative result. Unlike laboratory immunoassay tests which are frequently quantitative determinations, point-of-care immunoassays are qualitative tests in which only a positive or negative reading may be obtained. The tests are frequently designed to be read as negative if the drug concentration is below an arbitrarily set limit of detection.

Gas chromatography–mass spectroscopy

GC, also known as gas-liquid chromatography or gas-liquid partition chromatography, is a technique used to separate compounds present in a mixture based on their polarity and vapor pressure. A gas chromatograph contains a glass or metal column that is either coated with a polymer or contains polymer-coated beads. An inert gas such as helium or nitrogen is pumped through the column at a specific rate and the temperature inside the column is kept constant.

The body fluid to be tested is introduced, usually *via* an autosampler, into a heated headspace. The mixture volatilizes and is advanced through the column by the inert gas. As the mixture travels through the column, the individual compounds are retained in the column for different lengths of time depending on the strength of interaction with the polymer (polarity) and their tendency to remain in a gaseous state. For example, a compound with a higher boiling point will remain in the column for a longer period of time because it condenses onto the solid support (stationary phase) and spends less time being advanced through the column by the inert gas (mobile phase). Individual compounds in the mixture have characteristic retention times depending on the solid support used, length of the column, and temperature.

Table 1. Characteristics of biological testing for drugs of abuse

Drug of abuse	Characteristics of biological testing	Testing limitations
Amphetamines	• Available immunoassays are directed against amphetamine or amphetamine/d-methamphetamine • A modified immunoassay directed against MDMA is commercially available	• Amphetamine immunoassays have low sensitivities for MDMA and numerous other "designer" amphetamines and may yield false-negative results • The MDMA immunoassay has poor sensitivity for amphetamine and methamphetamine • Similar chemical structures and metabolic pathways may lead to false-positive results in patients taking a variety of licit medications • Amphetamine salts may be legally prescribed • GC-MS may yield false-positive amphetamine or methamphetamine results if a chiral derivatizing agent is not used to distinguish between levoamphetamine/levomethamphetamine (metabolites of licit medications) from dextroamphetamine/dextromethamphetamine (drugs of abuse)
Barbiturates	• Immunoassays are directed against secobarbital or a number of barbiturate compounds	• Barbiturate immunoassays generally have high sensitivities and specificities
Benzodiazepines	• Most commercially available immunoassays are directed against diazepam, nordiazepam, or oxazepam • Several other benzodiazepines are metabolized to one of those compounds resulting in their detection	• Clonazepam, lorazepam, and alprazolam are not metabolized to one of those compounds and may not be detected by available immunoassays resulting in substantial false-negative rates
Cannabinoids	• Most commercially available immunoassays are directed against THC or THC-COOH • THC and THC-COOH ratios may be useful for determining the timing of marijuana use	• Cannabinoid immunoassays generally have high sensitivities and specificities • THC-COOH is unstable in urine over time and prolonged storage prior to testing may lead to false negative results • Cannabinoids have low incorporation rates into hair leading to false-negative results if hair is used as the testing substrate
Cocaine	• Immunoassays are directed against benzoylecgonine • Detection of anhydroecgonine or anhydroecgonine methyl ester suggests crack cocaine use	• Cocaine immunoassays generally have high sensitivities and specificities

(continued on next page)

Table 1. (continued)

Drug of abuse	Characteristics of biological testing	Testing limitations
	• Detection of substantial concentrations of cocaethylene suggests concomitant cocaine and ethanol use	
Ethanol	• Portable breath analyzers use electrochemical cell technology while infrared spectroscopy breath analyzers are typically used as a confirmatory test • Serum ethanol levels are higher than whole blood ethanol levels and corrections must be applied to compare the testing methods • Testing for fatty acid ethyl esters (FAEEs) allows determination of recent ethanol use in the absence of acute intoxication	• Electrochemical cell breath analyzers cannot distinguish between ethanol, methanol, and isopropyl alcohol • Oral fluid testing for ethanol may be falsely elevated after recent ethanol consumption due to residual drug in the oral cavity • Testing for FAEEs in hair may be confounded by cosmetic hair treatments, use of alcohol containing hair care products, and inter-individual variability
Opioids	• Most commercially available immunoassays are directed against morphine • Immunoassays directed against buprenorphine, methadone, 6-monoacetylmorphine (6-MAM), oxycodone, and propoxyphene are available • Detection of 6-MAM in serum or urine indicates heroin use • A serum morphine:codeine ratio of >1 and urine morphine: codeine ratio >2 is suggestive of heroin use	• Opiate immunoassays directed against morphine have intermediate sensitivity for oxycodone and oxymorphone and low sensitivity for buprenorphine, fentanyl, meperidine, methadone, and propoxyphene • If low cut-off values are used, poppy seed ingestion may result in false positive results • False negative results for 6-MAM are common due to its short half-life
PCP	• Immunoassays are directed against phencyclidine	• False positive immunoassays may be caused by dextromethorphan and venlafaxine

MDMA, 3,4-methylenedioxymethamphetamine; THC, Δ^9-tetrahydrocannabinol; THC-COOH, 11-nor-9-carboxy-Δ^9-tetrahydrocannabinol; PCP, phencyclidine.

As the individual compounds exit the gas chromatograph, they are further analyzed by MS. The mass spectrometer showers the emitted compound with high-energy electrons. These electrons fragment and ionize the compound and the fragments are driven into a detector by an electromagnetic field, which separates fragments based on their mass and charge. The particular fragments produced by bombardment of the compound and the proportional abundance of the fragments are unique to its chemical structure. In the lay media, MS has been called "molecular fingerprinting" because of the unique fragmentation patterns produced by each molecule. Comparison of the fragmentation pattern produced by MS to a computer database can then identify the drug present in the body fluid.

GC-MS is widely considered the "gold standard" for specific drug identification and is therefore used in laboratory confirmation of suspected positive results. It is highly sensitive and specific in identifying drugs present in biological matrices. The major drawback to GC-MS is that it requires expert technicians to perform the assays and it is relatively costly. In addition, samples must often be sent to a reference laboratory and results may not be available for several days. GC-MS only effectively analyzes drugs that are volatile or that can be made volatile by derivatization, and that will not be decomposed at the temperatures used by the gas chromatograph. Drugs of abuse that cannot be volatilized, such as benzodiazepines, must instead be analyzed using LC-MS.

High-performance liquid chromatography–mass spectroscopy

As mentioned above, compounds that cannot be volatilized either in their parent form or through derivatization are more appropriately studied using high-performance liquid chromatography (HPLC). Like GC, HPLC uses a column containing a stationary phase. In the case of HPLC, the stationary phase is typically coated onto small (approximately 5-μm) silica beads. While in GC the mobile phase is an inert gas, in HPLC a liquid solvent is used. A high degree of pressure (approximately 400 atm) is necessary in HPLC to push the solvent through the micro-beads.

To test body fluids for drugs of abuse, a sample is introduced into the column. The solvent carries the sample through the column and individual compounds are separated by their tendency to move with the solvent (mobile phase) or interact with the stationary phase on the micro-beads. As the solvent, now containing only one compound at a time due to the above separation process, exits the column it is aerosolized, sprayed with high-energy electrons, and analyzed using MS. The function of the mass spectrometer in HPLC-MS is the same as in GC-MS, described in the section above.

As with GC-MS, HPLC-MS is considered a "gold standard" technique. It is both highly sensitive and highly specific for testing of drugs of abuse in body fluids. The primary drawbacks of HPLC-MS are its limited availability, often only being performed in reference laboratories, and the cost and time of performing the test.

Testing substrates

Testing for drugs of abuse can be performed on a variety of substrates. Common substrates include urine, blood, oral fluids, sweat, and hair. The most appropriate substrate for testing depends on the goals of the testing program. Commonly tested substrates vary in their sensitivity, length of time after drug use that the test will remain positive (window of detection), invasiveness of obtaining a sample, ability of the subject to falsify a sample, and cost.

Urine

Urine is the most widely used substrate for testing of drugs of abuse [2]. Urine collection is painless though considered by some to be invasive of privacy, especially when directly observed urine collection is used.

The window of detection for urine testing depends on the drug being tested, whether the testing method detects parent drug or metabolite, the method of drug use, the pattern and intensity of drug use, the cut-off values used, and the concentration of urine. Typically, urine tests will turn positive within hours of abuse of a drug [2]. The concentration of drug and/or metabolites in the urine generally peaks within 6 hours of administration and typically remains positive for several days [2]. In cases of heavy or daily drug use, urine tests may remain positive for longer periods, up to several weeks in cases of daily marijuana use [3]. As a result, urine tests cannot determine intoxication. Unlike hair or sweat tests, the risk of false positives due to environmental contamination is low. Stated another way, external skin or hair contamination from ambient smoke or drug particulates is unlikely to cause a false-positive urine test [2].

The risk of false negatives, conversely, is relatively high. Subjects may seek to avoid a positive drug test result by adulteration, substitution, or dilution of their urine or by ingesting "masking" agents. Urine adulteration is the addition of a substance to the urine sample that is designed to interfere with the accuracy of the test. Common urine adulterants include oxidizing agents like nitrites, peroxides, or bleach and immunoglobulin interferants like gluteraldehyde. Some adulterants are sold commercially specifically for the purpose of producing false-negative drug tests. Urine substitution is the submission of synthetic urine or the urine of another person. Imaginative products such as "The Whizzinator", a prosthetic penis that came in various skin tones with synthetic urine, have been, and in some cases continue to be, sold over the internet. Subjects may drink excessive quantities of water or add water to their urine specimen to dilute the concentration of drug in their urine to below the cut-off for positivity. Finally, they may ingest products, e.g., goldenseal, that are designed to mask drug use, with varying degrees of efficacy. Numerous websites and several books are devoted to helping drug users obtain "clean" test results. The risk of sample adulteration, dilution, or substitution can be minimized, but not eliminated, by directly observed urine collection and by specimen validity testing. Specimen validity testing may detect the presence of adulterants or abnormally acidic, basic, or dilute urine.

Point-of-care urine tests for drugs of abuse are widely available, both for testing facilities and retail sale to the public. Sales of retail drugs of abuse testing kits are generally marketed to parents wishing to test their children.

Blood

Blood testing for drugs of abuse is frequently used in forensic toxicology for scenarios where there is a question of criminal behavior. Blood tests are ideal for situations in which testing accuracy is paramount and the cost and degree of invasiveness are considered justified. Blood tests are considered to be most resilient to judicial review. A significant body of literature has accumulated investigating testing for drugs of abuse in whole blood, plasma, or serum because of the importance of this testing modality for legal/forensic applications [4, 5].

Drugs of abuse appear in the blood immediately after injection or inhalation and within hours of ingestion of the drug. Drug tests that target the parent compound will report negative results once the serum level of the drug is below an arbitrary cut-off value. In some cases, assays for drug metabolites may remain positive longer, allowing detection of recent drug use.

Blood tests are invasive in that phlebotomy must be performed for sample collection. A sample collector such as a phlebotomist or nurse must be involved in sample collection. As with urine testing, risk of false positives due to environmental contamination is low. The risk of false-negative results is also low – because the sample is actively obtained, risk of adulteration or substitution of the sample is minimal. False-negative results may occur if collection of the sample is significantly delayed because a phlebotomist or nurse is not immediately available.

Testing methodologies that allow quantification of the concentration of drug of abuse are frequently utilized in blood testing because serum drug levels may correlate with the degree of intoxication. Additionally, quantification of the drug concentration is useful for cases in which legal limits exist, e.g., for driving under the influence of alcohol [4]. It is generally considered standard practice in forensic toxicology to perform both a screening test and confirmatory test for the drug in question. With blood or serum testing, the most common tests used for screening and confirmation are GC-MS and LC-MS or LC-MS/MS because of their high degrees of sensitivity, specificity, and accuracy at determining drug concentration [4].

Various commercially available immunoassay kits for testing for drugs of abuse in blood have been validated. Historically, a significant amount of sample preparation was necessary to avoid interference of endogenous proteins (e.g., hemoglobin) with testing results, although some currently available microtiter immunoassays require minimal to no sample processing. These tests also offer excellent sensitivity and specificity, but quantification of drug concentration is not reliable [6]. The inability to reliably quantify the concentration of drug in the blood limits the usefulness of immunoassay testing in forensic scenarios, although the significant time advantage over GC or LC may be useful as a screening procedure when obtaining rapid results is critical. While positive test results should be confirmed using a second testing method, e.g., GC or LC, as mentioned above, in some cases a negative immunoassay result may be sufficient and obviate the need for more expensive and time-consuming GC or LC testing [7].

Blood tests for drugs of abuse are frequently more expensive than other testing modalities, even more so when the cost of specimen collection is considered. There are no commercially available point-of-care tests for testing for drugs of abuse in blood.

Oral fluids

Oral fluid is a relatively new substrate for testing of drugs of abuse. Traditionally, blood and urine were the only bodily fluids used in drug testing. However, recent studies have shown oral fluid to be a reasonable substrate for testing for very recent drug use and its use in post-incident workplace testing and roadside testing continues to increase [8].

Drugs of abuse partition between blood and oral fluids with the salivary concentrations depending on the pH of saliva, pH of the blood, pKa of the drug, and degree of serum protein binding [9]. Because of the ongoing partitioning of drugs of abuse between blood and oral fluids, concentrations of drugs in oral fluids largely follow the same pharmacokinetics as in the blood. Therefore, as with blood testing for drugs of abuse, drug levels in oral fluids rapidly decline and drug concentrations will decline below detectable levels within hours after last drug use [9]. Therefore, oral fluid testing is useful only for detecting very recent drug use.

Sample collection can be performed by direct expectoration or by use of a commercial collection device. Direct expectoration is useful in that concentrations in oral fluid can be measured, whereas with commercial devices the use of a diluent makes accurate measurement of drug concentrations impossible [10]. The two main drawbacks to oral fluid collection by direct expectoration are issues of hygiene and the ability of the subject to produce an adequate sample volume. Commercially available collection devices typically use a swab or absorbent pad to collect oral fluids. The sensitivity and specificity of collection devices for specific drugs of abuse is variable and depends on the individual device used [11–13].

Oral fluid has both benefits and drawbacks as a testing substrate. The major benefit to testing of oral fluid over other bodily fluids is the ease and non-invasiveness of sample collection. Sample collection can occur in the presence of another person without invasion of their privacy. Lay personnel can easily collect oral fluid samples with minimal training unlike phlebotomy for blood collection or even the training necessary in urine collection to minimize the chance of sample adulteration or substitution. The main drawbacks in oral fluid as a testing substrate are the variability in saliva volume and acidity. Saliva volume can be affected by xenobiotics, including both licit and illicit drugs. Illicit drugs that decrease saliva production include amphetamines and cannabis, while numerous therapeutic medications have similar effects [10, 14, 15]. Additionally, salivary volume is affected by a number of disease states including diabetes mellitus, alcoholic liver cirrhosis, and renal dysfunction, among others [14].

Saliva acidity varies with salivary gland stimulation and the rate of saliva production. The acidity of oral fluids can be seen as a balance between bacterial metabolic activities producing acid and lowering the salivary pH and the buffering capacity of bicarbonate present in oral secretions. Salivary gland stimulation increases oral fluid pH by two mechanisms: in addition to increased dilution of acidic bacterial metabolic byproducts, salivary stimulation also produces a higher concentration of bicarbonate in secreted fluids, further increasing its buffering capacity [14].

The acidity of oral fluids influences the concentration of drugs of abuse in the saliva by altering the partition of drugs between blood and saliva. Oral secretions generally have a lower pH than that of the blood. As a result, basic drugs (amphetamines, methamphetamine, MDMA, opiates), tend to concentrate within the saliva, while acidic drugs (benzodiazepines) tend to concentrate within the blood [10]. As an example, the ratio of concentration in oral fluid to blood for methamphetamine is 25, while for diazepam it is 0.015 [10]. As oral fluid pH decreases, the oral fluid:blood concentration ratios will change even further favoring the concentration of basic drugs into the saliva and of acidic drugs into the blood. The concentration of protein in the saliva also changes with salivary gland stimulation, although this is not thought to be an important consideration in testing for drugs of abuse.

Another factor that influences the concentration of illicit drugs in oral fluids is residual drug in the oral cavity or local absorption during inhalation or ingestion of the drug. For example, smoking marijuana and amphetamines may temporarily result in high concentrations of these drugs in oral fluid [16, 17]. This may be seen as an advantage in that positive results suggest very recent drug use and, by extension, may imply intoxication.

Sweat

Testing for drugs of abuse using sweat remains an uncommon practice. There are two general types of sweat patches. Fast patches are designed to be applied for up to 30 minutes and rely on heating to induce sweating for specimen collection [18, 19]. Patches designed for prolonged use are commercially available and may be worn for a period of up to 2 weeks [20]. The patch accumulates both drugs and their metabolites *via* a semi-permeable membrane that adheres to the skin [2]. Drugs are thought to accumulate in sweat from total body water *via* passive diffusion [21]. Following patch removal, drugs are eluted from the patch using a solvent and then may be tested in the same manner as bodily fluids using immunoassays, GC-MS, LC-MS, and other techniques. Sweat testing has been validated for heroin and other opioids, cocaine, benzodiazepines, marijuana, and amphetamines, although the sensitivity of sweat testing has not been well described [19, 22–25].

The premise of sweat testing for drugs of abuse is that any illicit drug use by the subject while wearing a patch will result in a positive test result. The advantages of sweat as a matrix for drug testing, therefore, is that a single sweat patch test can continuously monitor a subject for up to 2 weeks, whereas monitoring a subject for 2 weeks using urine testing would necessitate multiple tests. Additionally, testing is less invasive than urine or blood collection and little training is required for test administrators. Commercially available sweat patches are tamper evident.

Sweat does have its drawbacks as a matrix for drug testing. As a relatively new medium, the admissibility of sweat tests results as evidence in legal proceedings remains problematic [26]. Additionally, concerns remain about contamination resulting in false-positive results [27]. Illicit drug on the skin at the time of patch application that is not adequately removed by an isopropyl alcohol wipe may result in a false-positive result [26, 27]. The sweat patch is relatively resistant to external contamination, although if the sweat patch becomes soaked with a basic solution, such as may occur with profuse sweating, external contamination with illicit drug may cause a false-positive result [26, 27]. Finally, there is concern that chronic illicit drug users may continue to release drugs or drug metabolites through the skin from subcutaneous adipose tissue for prolonged periods after their last use resulting in a false-positive sweat patch test despite no recent drug use [28]. In one report, measureable levels of cocaine, morphine, and methadone were found in stimulated sweat samples from drug users after 6 drug-free days [29].

Hair/nails

Hair sampling is performed by cutting a bundle of hair 60 to 120 strands thick (approximately the thickness of a pencil), usually from the vertex of the head. The hair is cut as close to the scalp as possible with a single-use or properly cleaned cutting instrument [30, 31]. If head hair is unavailable, then pubic or axillary hair may be used. To minimize the risk of false positives due to environmental contamination, hair must be thoroughly washed prior to analysis. An initial wash with ethanol may be performed to remove oils and loosely adhering drugs, followed by washing with phosphate buffer or ethanol/water mixtures [32]. Following washing, the drugs are released from the hair by solvent extraction or, preferably, by protein digestion [32, 33]. The drug testing may then be performed using immunoassay, GC-MS, LC-MS, or other techniques.

The greatest benefit conferred by using hair in drug testing is the ability to detect illicit drug use over an extended period of time. While the rate of hair growth is variable, it is assumed to average approximately 1 cm per month with the least variation in hair growth rate occurring on the posterior vertex of the head [31]. Therefore, a hair sample that is a few centimeters in length will yield information on illicit drug use over several months. Additionally, segmentation of the hair sample and comparison of testing results of the various segments may distinguish between occasional or single drug exposures and habitual drug use [30].

As a matrix for testing for drugs of abuse, hair has several drawbacks. False-positive results due to external contamination are of concern. This risk may be minimized by using cut-off values, validated washing procedures, comparing drug concentrations in washes to that of a digested specimen, and testing for drug metabolites that would not be present from external contamination [32]. Despite adoption of these techniques, some studies have reported that external contamination may still result in false-positive tests [34, 35].

Also of concern is that concentrations of some illicit drugs, such as cocaine and codeine, are higher in darker hair because of binding to melanin [36, 37]. By extension, races or ethnicities with a propensity for darker hair would, on a population basis, be more likely to exceed cut-off values when tested for those drugs. This potential bias is of concern in using hair in screening tests, such as pre-employment screening, because it may result in unfair discrimination against those races/ethnicities with darker hair. Porosity of hair, as well as chemical treatment of hair can affect results and may vary with ethnicity and cultural norms. Several methods have been described to minimize testing bias as a result of hair color and porosity including measuring and adjusting for increased drug uptake and use of digestion techniques that leave melanin-drug complexes intact [32, 38].

Drugs of abuse

While the spectrum of xenobiotics with the potential for abuse is limited only by the human imagination, current testing for drugs of abuse focuses on a few classes of commonly used drugs with high abuse potentials (Fig. 1, Tab. 1). Pre-employment and occupational drug tests frequently include amphetamines, cannabinoids, cocaine, opiates, and phencyclidine. These drugs are sometimes referred to as the NIDA 5 because they are the five drugs that the U.S. National Institute of Drug Abuse (NIDA) recommended for inclusion in pre-employment drug testing in 1988. More comprehensive tests may also include barbiturates and benzodiazepines, among others.

Alcohol

Alcohol is the most widely used drug of abuse and a leading cause of morbidity and mortality. In the United States, the prevalence of alcohol dependence is approximately 6% for men and 2% for women and alcohol-dependent individuals are much more likely to suffer legal or occupational difficulties as a result of their alcohol use [39]. Although the consumption of alcohol among adults is legal in many countries, those same countries generally have laws prohibiting driving motor vehicles while intoxicated and mandatory alcohol

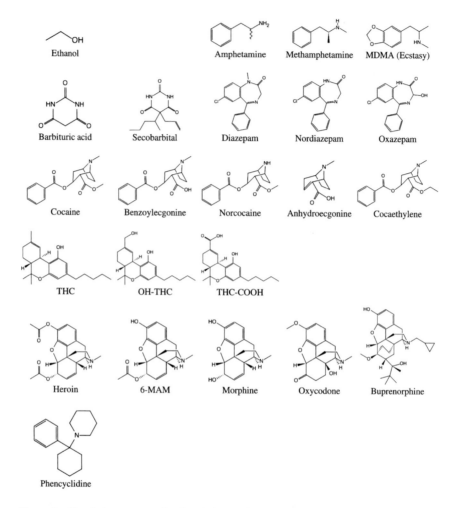

Figure 1. Chemical structures of selected drugs of abuse and relevant metabolites. 6-MAM, 6-monoacetylmorphine; MDMA, 3,4-methylenedioxymethamphetamine; THC, Δ^9-tetrahydrocannabinol; OH-THC, 11-hydroxy-Δ^9-tetrahydrocannabinol; THC-COOH, 11-nor-9-carboxy-Δ^9-tetrahydrocannabinol.

testing for prospective employees in sensitive positions, e.g., commercial drivers. Therefore, alcohol testing is frequently performed in both forensic and pre-employment settings.

Ethanol is an odorless, colorless liquid that is miscible with water (Fig. 1). It diffuses across lipid membranes and modulates activity at a variety of neuroreceptors and ion channels including voltage-gated calcium channels, glutamate receptors, γ-aminobutyric acid A (GABA$_A$) receptors, glycine receptors, and 5-hydroxytryptamine (5-HT$_3$, serotonin) receptors [40]. It has adverse effects on a variety of organs, although its effects on the central nervous system (CNS) are most relevant to the legal restrictions on its use. Ethanol is a CNS depressant that may cause slowed reaction times and impaired judgment. Ethanol is rapidly absorbed from the gastrointestinal tract, although the speed of absorption varies with the time of day, drinking pattern, alcoholic drink consumed, and fasting state of the individual. Under ideal conditions alcohol is almost completely absorbed within 60 minutes from ingestion though the above factors may delay alcohol absorption by several hours. Following absorption, ethanol is primarily metabolized into acetaldehyde by alcohol dehydrogenase, but small amounts are excreted unchanged in urine, sweat, or exhaled breath. Alcohol dehydrogenase has a low Michaelis constant, resulting in predominantly zero-order metabolism, and displays polymorphism, resulting in ethnic and racial differences in pharmacokinetics [41]. Increased metabolism in people who consume alcohol regularly is largely due to induction of cytochrome P450 2E1, which also metabolizes ethanol to acetaldehyde [41]. Acetaldehyde is subsequently metabolized to acetate by aldehyde dehydrogenase, which also displays ethnic and racial polymorphisms [42].

Testing for ethanol is most commonly performed by breath analyzer or blood test (Tab. 1). Breath analyzers estimate the blood ethanol concentration by measuring the amount of volatilized ethanol present in exhaled breath. There is a well-established mean blood-to-breath ratio for ethanol, although there is considerable variation in the ratio depending on the stage of ethanol absorption/elimination and individual factors necessitating the use of conservative calculations and confidence intervals [43, 44]. Additionally, falsely elevated test results may be obtained if ethanol has been recently ingested and residual ethanol is in the mouth, if there has been recent vomiting containing ethanol, or with recent use of multi-dose inhalers or mouthwash [45].

Breath ethanol analyzers typically rely on one of two technologies: electrochemical cells or infrared spectroscopy. Electrochemical cells (EC) use a fuel-cell sensor that detects volatilized ethanol. Advantages to EC breath analyzers are their high sensitivity, longevity, stable performance, and portability [44]. Handheld breath ethanol analyzers used by law enforcement in the field typically use EC technology. While EC breath analyzers are not biased by acetone, they are unable to distinguish between ethanol, methanol, and isopropyl alcohol.

Infrared spectroscopy (IR) breath analyzers are not portable, but are considered more resistant to legal challenges than EC breath analyzers. The primary advantage of IR technology is a real-time continuous measurement of ethanol concentration throughout sample delivery allowing determination of true ethanol breath concentration that is not biased by residual mouth ethanol [44]. Frequently, therefore, a field screening test using an EC breath analyzer is performed and, if positive, a confirmatory IR breath analysis or blood test is then performed. A major drawback of IR breath analyzers is their lack of portability; a driver with a breath ethanol concentration above the legal limit in the field may be below the legal limit by the time they are transported to a law enforcement facility for IR breath analysis.

Blood tests for ethanol may be performed using immunoassay or GC-MS. Typically, GC-MS is used in forensic ethanol testing, while immunoassay tests are more commonly performed at healthcare facilities for medical reasons. While forensic ethanol concentrations are defined for whole blood, healthcare facilities typically measure ethanol in serum or, rarely, in plasma. Serum ethanol concentrations are typically higher than whole blood concentrations (serum is composed of a greater percent water than whole blood) with a mean ratio of serum-to-whole blood ethanol concentration of 1.15, although there is interpersonal variability requiring the use of confidence intervals [46]. Therefore, a correction must be applied to serum ethanol concentrations to estimate whole blood ethanol concentration.

Oral fluid testing for ethanol has been suggested to be a rapid, noninvasive method for evaluating persons who are unable to comply with breath testing; however, residual alcohol in the mouth after recent consumption may result in falsely elevated results [47].

Testing for fatty acid ethyl esters (FAEEs) allows the determination of recent ethanol use in the absence of ongoing intoxication. FAEEs are non-oxidative metabolites of ethanol that may detected in serum for days after last ethanol use [48]. Testing for FAEEs in hair may allow the determination of alcohol use over a period of weeks to months, although this method is confounded by cosmetic hair treatments, use of alcohol containing hair care products, and inter-individual variability in FAEE concentrations in hair [30].

Amphetamines

The amphetamine class of drugs includes amphetamine, methamphetamine, 3,4-methylenedioxymethamphetamine (MDMA), and numerous other "designer" amphetamines (Fig. 1). Amphetamines are chemically synthesized, although in some cases they are derived from a natural substance, e.g., methcathinone is derived from a plant (Khat). Abuse of amphetamines, including methamphetamine and MDMA, remains a concern worldwide. Methamphetamine abuse is particularly prevalent in rural Midwestern and Western United States [49]. MDMA abuse is prevalent among young partygoers and college students in Australia, England, and the United States among whom it is called "ecstasy" or "E" and is associated with dance parties called "raves" [50].

Amphetamines exert their effects primarily through release of dopamine, norepinephrine, and other monoamines from presynaptic terminals. The exact mode of action is more complex and also varies among members of the class. As would be expected, the clinical manifestations of amphetamine intoxication vary with the drug that was used and may include a sympathomimetic toxidrome, perceptual changes, psychosis, and anorexia among others. Amphetamines are generally lipophilic with large volumes of distribution [51]. Bioavailability and time to peak effects are variable depending on the drug and the method of use. Elimination occurs both *via* hepatic metabolism and renal excretion with the relative importance of each pathway and half-lives varying with the members of the class [51].

Testing for amphetamines can be performed on urine, blood, oral fluids, and hair (Tab. 1). The amphetamine immunoassay remains problematic as false-positive and false-negative results may arise. Despite attempts by manufacturers to develop a reagent with greater specificity for amphetamines, false-positive results remain an issue. False-positive results may stem from structural similarities or from common metabolic pathways between amphetamines and numerous prescription medications, over-the-counter cold preparations, and dietary aids [52, 53]. False-positive results from interfering substances may be more common than true-positives, depending on the population being studied [53].

Additionally, amphetamine immunoassays may report false-negative results in subjects using methamphetamine, MDMA, or designer amphetamine compounds due to limited cross-reactivity between these compounds and amphetamine immunoassay reagents. Despite modified amphetamine immunoassays developed by manufacturers to have improved cross-reactivity with the above compounds, false-negative results remain problematic and immunoassays with greater cross-reactivities may suffer from greater false-positive results with licit non-amphetamine compounds (see above) [54].

GC-MS is typically used for confirmatory testing for amphetamines following positive screening immunoassays. Although GC-MS does not suffer the same lack of specificity as immunoassays with compounds with structural similarities to amphetamines, it can still deliver false-positive results due to the stereoisomerism of amphetamines. Some nasal decongestants contain levomethamphetamine while selegiline, a monoamine-oxidase inhibitor, is metabolized into levoamphetamine and levomethamphetamine, both of which have low abuse potentials, while the stereoisomer dextromethamphetamine is an illicit drug with high abuse potential. To confirm the presence of dextromethamphetamine, a chiral derivatizing agent must be used to result in chromatographically separable diastereomers. Several methods of derivatization have been described [55]. Even with the confirmation of dextromethamphetamine *via* derivatization and GC-MS, it must be confirmed that the patient is not being legally prescribed dextroamphetamine.

Barbiturates and benzodiazepines

Barbiturates and benzodiazepines have long histories of both licit and illicit use (Fig. 1). Barbiturates were developed in the early 20th century and were the predominant sedative-hypnotics for the first half of that century. Use of barbiturates was plagued by a low therapeutic index, resulting in a number of unintentional overdoses as well as completed suicides. Benzodiazepines were developed over the last half of the 20th century and rapidly replaced barbiturates as the sedative-hypnotic of choice due to their improved safety profile. Both classes of medications have a high abuse potential, although benzodiazepine abuse is far more common today due to their extensive availability.

Barbiturate immunoassays are typically directed against a number of barbiturate compounds (Tab. 1). Barbiturate immunoassays have high sensitivities and specificities due to similar structures between members of the barbiturate class (minimizing false negatives) and a lack of structural similarities to medications outside the barbiturate class (minimizing false positives) [56]. Benzodiazepine immunoassays are more problematic. Most currently marketed benzodiazepine immunoassays target diazepam, nordiazepam, or oxazepam. A number of benzodiazepines are metabolized to these compounds making the benzodiazepine immunoassay useful for most benzodiazepines. However, clonazepam, lorazepam, and alprazolam are not metabolized through those pathways and are frequently not detected by standard benzodiazepine immunoassays. These are currently popularly prescribed, resulting in substantial false-negative rates for immunoassays at detecting benzodiazepine use or abuse [56].

Testing for benzodiazepines may be performed on serum, urine, oral fluid, and hair. Windows of detection time are variable depending on the benzodiazepine ingested and their considerable variability in half-life and metabolism as well as other factors such as route of administration, chronicity and extent of use, and individual pharmacokinetic differences. Benzodiazepine concentrations in oral fluid are lower than in serum due to extensive serum protein binding, but detectable concentrations of benzodiazepines are present in oral fluid for hours after the last use. The concentration-time profile for benzodiazepines in oral fluid appears to mimic that of the blood [57]. Sweat testing for benzodiazepines has also been found to be effective at determining benzodiazepine use [58]. Urine is also effective for determining benzodiazepine use with a window of detection as long as several weeks, depending on the benzodiazepine ingested and laboratory technique used [59, 60]. As with other drugs of abuse, hair testing for benzodiazepines has a particularly long window of detection, on the order of months, which makes it particularly suitable for detecting the administration of benzodiazepines in drug-facilitated assault when there may be substantial delay between administration of the drug and sample collection [61]. Again, because of the variety of compounds present in the benzodiazepine class, their variable metabolism, and their variable urinary excretion or incorporation into hair, different testing substrates may be most appropriate for detecting the use of specific class members.

Cannabinoids

Cannabinoids are obtained from the plant *Cannabis sativa* and are the active ingredient in marijuana and hashish. Cannabinoids is the most widely produced and most widely consumed illicit drug worldwide. In 2006, more cannabis was produced worldwide than opium, heroin, and cocaine combined. While more cannabis is grown in North America than on any other continent (31% of global production in 2006), cannabis resin (hashish) production is largely concentrated in Morocco and Afghanistan [62].

Hashish (cannabis resin) consumption is largely focused in Western and Central Europe, while marijuana (dried flowers and leaves of cannabis) use is more popular in North America. The United Nations Office on Drugs and Crime estimated that 166 million people worldwide, or 3.9% of the global population age 15–64 used cannabis in the year 2006. Prevalence of cannabis use is highest in Oceania (14.5% of population age 15–64), followed by North America (10.5%), Africa (8%), and West and Central Europe (6.9%) [62]. Persons who try cannabis at least once have a 9% risk of cannabis dependency, usually within the first 10 years after onset of cannabis use [63]. Marijuana use is the second most common reason for admission to a drug treatment program, accounting for 16% of admissions in 2005, and was reported in 23% of emergency department visits related to drug abuse in the United States [64].

Cannabis sativa contains a total of 66 cannabinoids, with the major psychoactive cannabinoid being Δ^9-tetrahydrocannabinol (THC, Fig. 1). THC is rapidly absorbed following smoking with a bioavailability of approximately 18% and a peak plasma concentration in 3–10 minutes. Ingestion of THC results in slower absorption and longer lasting effects with a bioavailability of approximately 6% and peak plasma concentrations in 1–2 hours [65, 66]. Following absorption, THC quickly distributes into tissues and accumulates in adipose tissue, liver, lung, and spleen. It is then slowly released back into the blood stream, resulting in a long terminal half-life [66]. THC is primarily metabolized by CYP3A and CYP2C into numerous metabolites. Major metabolites include the equipotent psychoactive 11-hydroxy-Δ^9-THC (OH-THC) and subsequently the non-active 11-nor-9-carboxy-Δ^9-THC (THC-COOH, Fig. 1) [4]. Approximately 80–90% of THC metabolites are excreted over the 5-day period after use with 20–35% being glucuronidated and eliminated in the urine and 65–80% eliminated in feces [4, 64].

Various validated methods of determination of THC, OH-THC, THC-COOH in urine, blood, oral fluid, sweat, and hair have been developed (Tab. 1) [67–69]. THC-COOH is the most important metabolite for testing because of its long half-life. Measurement of THC and THC-COOH ratios has also been proposed to determine the timing of marijuana use [70, 71].

Blood testing for THC should specify whether serum or whole blood was used as concentrations between whole blood and plasma/serum may be significantly different due to poor distribution of THC and its metabolites into red blood cells and therefore a higher concentration of THC and its metabolites in serum rather than whole blood [72, 73]. The window of detection for THC in plasma ranges from 3 to 27 hours after last use, while the window of detection for THC-COOH in plasma ranges from 2 to 7 days, although a detection time of 25 days has been reported in a chronic heavy user [66, 74]. In Germany, the cannabis influence factor (CIF) is used to interpret acute cannabis intoxication in cases of driving under the influence; however, the accuracy of the CIF remains questionable [66]. Additionally, a THC-COOH above 75 ng/mL suggests regular cannabinoid consumption and is the basis for disqualification from driving in some parts of Germany [66].

Urine testing for THC and its metabolites has a substantially longer window of detection time. Infrequent users generally have detection periods of 1–6 days, depending on testing method and cut-off values, with some immunoassays detecting cannabinoids up to 2 weeks after last use [3, 66]. Detection periods are substantially longer in frequent or heavy users, lasting from weeks up to 3 months [66, 75]. Because of the prolonged detection period for THC-COOH in urine, abstinence can be determined by serially declining THC-COOH urine levels. To avoid false-positive increases in THC-COOH levels caused by urine concentration, THC-COOH/creatinine ratios should be used for monitoring [76]. Various ratios have been developed to minimize false-positive and false-negative results [77]. Detectable THC in the urine suggests marijuana use within the last 8 hours and therefore is useful for suggesting impairment or intoxication [78]. An important consideration in urine testing for cannabinoids is their instability in that medium over time. THC-COOH is degraded over time and storage of samples below freezing is recommended to minimize false-negative results [79].

Hair testing for cannabinoids is of limited utility. THC and THC-COOH have very low incorporation rates into hair, probably as a result of their physicochemical properties [80]. Hair testing therefore has limited sensitivity for cannabinoids and false-negative results should be expected [81]. Use of GC-MS/MS improves the sensitivity of hair testing for cannabinoids by lowering the level of quantification of THC-COOH to 0.16 pg/mg hair, although false-negative results may still occur [82]. Additionally, environmental contamination of hair with cannabinoids from passive cannabis smoke exposure may confound hair testing, resulting in false positives. Determination of THC-COOH in the hair, which is not present in cannabis smoke and therefore cannot be present due to external contamination, implies cannabis use [66].

Oral fluid and sweat sample testing are superior to urine testing at indicating recent cannabis use as saliva concentrations mirror plasma concentrations [67]. The positive predictive value (PPV) of oral fluid analysis using GC-MS is 90%, while sweat samples have a PPV of 80% [83]. An LC-MS protocol with acceptable accuracy has also been developed [67]. Unfortunately, commercially available point-of-care oral fluid testing for cannabinoids, useful in assessing driver impairment, at this time have inadequate sensitivities and specificities for cannabinoids [84].

Cocaine

Cocaine is a natural plant alkaloid present in the leaves of *Erythroxylum coca* (Fig. 1). Historically, the indigenous peoples of South America used the leaves for their psychoactive properties. Procedures to isolate cocaine from the coca leaf were developed in Europe in the 1800s and cocaine became a popular medication and recreational drug. Over the course of the 20th century, cocaine was illegalized in industrialized nations.

Cocaine remains a very popular drug of abuse in the United States and Western Europe and abuse of cocaine in these regions is second only to cannabis abuse [85]. In the United States, 2.5% of persons aged 12 years or older have used cocaine in the last year and cocaine accounts for a disproportionate number of admissions to substance abuse treatment services [85, 86].

Cocaine may be abused in several forms including cocaine powder, freebase, and crack cocaine. Cocaine powder is composed of a cocaine salt, frequently cocaine hydrochloride, that is obtained from the coca leaf by maceration of the leaf followed by treatment with an acidic solution. The acidic solution results in the protonation of cocaine, which increases its aqueous solubility. Following extraction of cocaine from the leaf into the aqueous solution, the water is allowed to dry yielding powdered cocaine. Powdered cocaine is frequently insufflated or injected, but not smoked as the temperatures necessary for volatilization of the cocaine salt frequently results in pyrolysis of the drug.

Freebase cocaine is produced by dissolution of cocaine salt into aqueous solution followed by treatment with a weak base such as ammonia. The weak base deprotonates the cocaine decreasing its solubility in water. An organic phase is added, such as diethyl ether, into which the cocaine dissolves. Tobacco or marijuana cigarettes can be dipped into the diethyl ether or evaporation of the solvent yields freebase cocaine. Freebase cocaine is unsuitable for insufflation or injection, but volatilizes at a lower temperature than cocaine powder making it ideal for smoking. Because of the dangers of producing freebase cocaine and the advent of the more popular and more easily produced crack cocaine, freebase cocaine use is no longer prevalent.

Production of crack cocaine is similar to freebase cocaine except that the addition of the organic phase is skipped and the weak base used is frequently sodium bicarbonate rather than ammonia. Because of the residual water present in crack cocaine, when heated the rock makes a cracking sound as the water cooks off lending crack cocaine its name. As with freebase cocaine, crack cocaine is suitable for smoking and not for insufflation or injection.

Cocaine is rapidly and extensively metabolized in the liver and plasma by esterases to a number of metabolites. Because of its short half-life, testing for cocaine as a drug of abuse frequently focuses on detection of cocaine metabolites, most notably benzoylecgonine (BE), although norcocaine and ecgonine methyl ester may also be used in drug testing (Fig. 1). Two other byproducts, anhydroecgonine methyl ester and anhydroecgonine, are pyrolysis products of cocaine and are only produced when cocaine is smoked, allowing differentiation between insufflation or injection of cocaine powder and smoking of crack cocaine [87–89]. Another metabolite, cocaethylene, is formed from the transesterification of alcohol with cocaine and can be measured during drug testing to assess for the concomitant abuse of cocaine and ethanol.

Testing for cocaine may be performed on serum, urine, oral fluids, and hair (Tab. 1). BE and other cocaine metabolites are rapidly cleared from the serum with a mean half-life of 3.6 hours. Therefore, although serum testing for cocaine and its metabolites will yield frequent false-negatives due to BE levels having fallen below the limit of detection, a positive serum test for BE is suggestive of acute cocaine intoxication [90]. BE can be detected in the urine within a few hours of cocaine use and concentrations may remain above the cut-off concentrations for approximately 2–3 days following last use [91]. Oral fluid testing for cocaine and its metabolites can be performed whether the cocaine is injected or smoked and gives an intermediate window of detection of hours to days depending on the chronicity and intensity of use [9]. Sweat testing for cocaine may detect cocaine, BE, or ecgonine methyl ester up to 2–3 weeks after last cocaine use, giving sweat testing a substantially longer window of detection than serum, oral fluid, or urine testing [18, 23]. Additionally, sweat patches can detect anhydroecgonine methyl ester which specifically demonstrates smoking of cocaine in the subject [19]. As with other drugs of abuse, hair testing can detect cocaine use within the past 3 months [92]. Presence of cocaine metabolites such as BE and ecgonine methyl ester suggest that external contamination was not a cause for a positive test [30].

Opioids

The dried sap of the poppy plant *Papaver somniferum*, known as opium, has been used by humans for thousands of years. The 19th century saw the isolation of morphine from opium, the synthesis of heroin, and exponential increases in the abuse of this highly addictive class of drugs. Recreational use of opioids was banned in the early 20th century, although derivatization of semisynthetic opiates and development of novel synthetic opioids for medicinal uses continues today. The abuse of heroin and diversion of prescription opioids remains a considerable problem for the United States and Western Europe today.

Opioids generally undergo extensive metabolism leading to a number of metabolites that are of variable importance in drug testing. Heroin (diacetylmorphine) is the only opioid that is metabolized to 6-monoacetylmorphine (6-MAM, Fig. 1). Therefore, presence of 6-MAM definitively indicates heroin use as opposed to use of legitimate prescription opioids and testing for 6-MAM may be an important component of testing for opioids. Another laboratory measurement used to determine heroin use is the morphine-to-codeine ratio. A serum morphine-to-codeine ratio greater than unity is suggestive of heroin use while a morphine-to-codeine ratio less than unity is consistent with codeine use [93]. Similarly, a urine morphine-to-codeine ratio greater than two is suggestive of heroin use [94]. Acetylcodeine and codeine may also be used as markers of illicit heroin use as they are common adulterants of street heroin [95]. Chromatography procedures are frequently designed to test for the morphine metabolites morphine-3-glucuronide and morphine-6-glucuronide as well as other parent opioid compounds [4].

The broad range of compounds considered opioids, and their considerable variety in molecular structure, make immunoassay testing of these compounds problematic (Fig. 1). Commercially available immunoassays for opiates are targeted against morphine. They are therefore effective at detecting opiates with similar structures to morphine such as codeine, heroin, 6-MAM, and hydromorphone [56]. However, opiates with less structural similarity to morphine, such as oxycodone and oxymorphone may yield a negative screening immunoassay especially when taken in lower doses. This is especially problematic because of the popularity of oxycodone as a prescription medication and as a drug of abuse [96]. Additionally, buprenorphine, fentanyl, meperidine, methadone, and propoxyphene all have insufficient structural similarity to morphine to be detected by commercially available immunoassays targeted against morphine, and special immunoassays specific to each drug must be used [56].

Depending on the cut-off values used, as well as the amount ingested, false-positive tests for opiates may result from consumption of poppy seeds. Poppy seeds are used in cooking and in bakery products and contain small amounts of morphine and codeine. Positive oral fluid and urine screening immunoassays have been documented following the ingestion of poppy seeds or poppy seed bagels by volunteers [97].

Testing for opiates as a drug of abuse may be performed using serum, oral fluid, sweat, urine, or hair (Tab. 1). Serum testing for opiates is most useful for determining opiate intoxication. Due to the short half-life of 6-MAM in the serum (on the order of 10–12 min), 6-MAM is frequently below the level of detection and the serum morphine-to-codeine ratio may be more practical for determining heroin use when using serum testing [98]. 6-MAM has a substantially longer detection time in the urine and urine testing for 6-MAM is frequently used to determine heroin use. Sweat patches have shown to be useful for detecting heroin, 6-MAM, morphine, codeine, methadone, and buprenorphine [18, 23, 25]. Hair testing is effective in detecting opiates and 6-MAM accumulates in hair, allowing the long-term determination of heroin use, although careful sample preparation must be undertaken to preserve the metabolite [33]. External contamination is particularly of concern with hair testing for opiates as the presence of heroin metabolites 6-MAM and morphine does not exclude external contamination as the cause of a positive hair test due to spontaneous heroin hydrolysis [99]. Controversy remains on the most appropriate decontamination procedure to minimize false-positives results due to external contamination [100].

Phencyclidine

Phencyclidine (PCP, Fig. 1) was initially developed as a general anesthetic; however, a high frequency of dysphoric reactions and postanesthesia psychosis resulted in the discontinuation of its use. PCP has been a common drug of abuse in the United States since the 1970s and is commonly known as angel dust, crystal, and ice. Tobacco or marijuana cigarettes laced with PCP may be referred to as wet, fry, or supergrass. PCP may be smoked, insufflated, ingested, or injected intravenously or subcutaneously. PCP use is frequently combined with other drugs of abuse, with marijuana, alcohol, and cocaine being the most frequently co-abused drugs [101].

The popularity of PCP as a drug of abuse waxes and wanes. Between 1993 and 2003, the popularity of PCP as a primary substance of abuse or a secondary substance of abuse among patients entering drug treatment programs increased, although the proportion of treatment program admissions due to PCP remained constant at 0.2% of all admissions [101]. PCP use is most common among adults aged 25–34 years, males, and Blacks. While historically, PCP use has been largely confined to urban areas, recent data show increasing prevalence in more rural areas [101]. PCP remains an uncommon drug of abuse outside the United States, although it is encountered in Europe.

PCP undergoes both hepatic metabolism and renal elimination. PCP is a weak base and therefore acidic urine increases renal clearance, although urine acidification is not routinely recommended due to an increased risk of myoglobinuric renal failure. Several medications have structural characteristics that may result in false-positive results for PCP by immunoassay, including dextromethorphan and venlafaxine among others [102–104]. In settings, where PCP use is uncommon, false-positive results due to dextromethorphan use or abuse may be more common than true-positive results [56]. Some commercially available PCP immunoassay reagents have lower cross-reactivity with dextromethorphan than others.

Testing for PCP can be performed on urine, serum, oral fluids, sweat, and hair (Tab. 1). Smoking PCP results in detectable PCP in the serum for 5–15 minutes and in the urine for up to 8 days [104]. Techniques for determining PCP in oral fluid have been developed and validated [105]. Hair testing allows determination of PCP use over a longer period of time. Simultaneous measurement of PCP and its metabolites in hair gives evidence that the subject used PCP and that external contamination of the hair was not responsible for the positive test result [106].

Conclusion

Testing for drugs of abuse is regularly utilized in a number of practical situations today and the use of drug testing continues to increase. Several testing techniques are available, including immunoassay and chromatography, each with their benefits and drawbacks. While historically, urine and blood testing have been most frequently utilized in testing for drugs of abuse, the use of alternative matrices such as sweat, oral fluid, and hair has greatly expanded over the last 20 years. Continuing research into the performance of these alternative matrices for specific testing indications or the testing of specific drugs promises to further refine the ability to select a matrix and testing technique that is most appropriate in a given situation.

Toxicologists have a responsibility to understand the strengths and limitations of testing techniques and matrices to be able to critically evaluate the results of a drug test. As discussed above, false-positive and false-negative results are not unexpected in certain testing situations and a thorough familiarity with testing for drugs of abuse will enable the toxicologist to knowledgeably assess the probability of such a result. Additionally, the failure of many clinicians and laypersons to adequately understand the limitations inherent to drug testing underlines the importance of the toxicologist being able to serve in an educational role to others in interpreting the results of drug testing.

References

1 Mulé, SJ, Jukofsky D, Kogan M, De Pace A, Verebey K (1977) Evaluation of the radioimmunoassay for benzoylecgonine (a cocaine metabolite) in human urine. *Clin Chem* 23: 796–801
2 Dolan K, Rouen D, Kimber J (2004) An overview of the use of urine, hair, sweat and saliva to detect drug use. *Drug Alcohol Rev* 23: 213–217
3 Smith-Kielland A, Skuterud B, Mørland J (1999) Urinary excretion of 11-nor-9-carboxy-Δ^9-tetrahydrocannabinol and cannabinoids in frequent and infrequent drug users. *J Anal Toxicol* 23: 323–332
4 Kraemer T, Paul LD (2007) Bioanalytical procedures for determination of drugs of abuse in blood. *Anal Bioanal Chem* 388: 1415–1435
5 Moeller MR, Kraemer T (2002) Drugs of abuse monitoring in blood for control of driving under the influence of drugs. *Ther Drug Monit* 24: 210–221
6 Kroener L, Musshoff F, Madea B (2003) Evaluation of immunochemical drug screenings of whole blood samples. A retrospective optimization of cutoff levels after confirmation-analysis on GC-MS and HPLC-DAD. *J Anal Toxicol* 27: 205–212
7 Spiehler V, Isenschmid DS, Matthews P, Kemp P, Kupiec T (2003) Performance of a microtiter plate ELISA for screening of postmortem blood for cocaine and metabolites. *J Anal Toxicol* 27: 587–591
8 Bernhoft IM, Steentoft A, Johansen SS, Klitgaard NA, Larsen LB, Hansen LB (2005) Drugs in injured drivers in Denmark. *Forensic Sci Int* 150: 181–189
9 Drummer OH (2005) Pharmacokinetics of illicit drugs in oral fluid. *Forensic Sci Int* 150: 133–142
10 Drummer OH (2008) Introduction and review of collection techniques and applications of drug testing of oral fluid. *Ther Drug Monit* 30: 203–206
11 O'Neal CL, Crouch DJ, Rollins DE, Fatah AA (2000) The effects of collection methods on oral fluid codeine concentrations. *J Anal Toxicol* 24: 536–542
12 Crouch DJ, Walsh JM, Flegel R, Cangianelli L, Baudys J, Atkins R (2005) An evaluation of selected oral fluid point-of-collection drug-testing devices. *J Anal Toxicol* 29: 244–248
13 Walsh JM, Flegel R, Crouch DJ, Cangianelli L, Baudys J (2003) An evaluation of rapid point-of-collection oral fluid drug-testing devices. *J Anal Toxicol* 27: 429–439
14 Aps JK, Martens LC (2005) The physiology of saliva and transfer of drugs into saliva. *Forensic Sci Int* 150: 119–131
15 Teixeira H, Proenca P, Verstraete A, Corte-Real F, Vieira DN (2005) Analysis of Δ^9-tetrahydrocannabinol in oral fluid samples using solid-phase extraction and high-performance liquid chromatography–electrospray ionization mass spectrometry. *Forensic Sci Int* 150: 205–211
16 Crouch DJ (2005) Oral fluid collection: The neglected variable in oral fluid testing. *Forensic Sci Int* 150: 165–173
17 Cook CE, Jeffcoat AR, Hill JM, Pugh DE, Patetta PK, Sadler BM, White WR, Perez-Reyes M (1993) Pharmacokinetics of methamphetamine self-administered to human subjects by smoking S-(+)-methamphetamine hydrochloride. *Drug Metab Dispos* 21: 717–723

18 Huestis MA, Oyler JM, Cone EJ, Wstadik AT, Schoendorfer D, Joseph RE Jr (1999) Sweat testing for cocaine, codeine and metabolites by gas chromatography–mass spectrometry. *J Chromatogr B Biomed Sci Appl* 733: 247–264

19 Liberty HJ, Johson BD, Fortner N, Randolph D (2003) Detecting crack and other cocaine use with fastpatches. *Addict Biol* 8: 191–200

20 PharmChek® Drugs of Abuse Patch (2009) Available from: http://www.pharmchem.com/ Products/Patch_details.htm (accessed April 24, 2009)

21 Kidwell DA, Holland JC, Athanaselis S (1998) Testing for drugs of abuse in saliva and sweat. *J Chromatogr B Biomed Sci Appl* 713: 111–135

22 Kintz P (1996) Drug testing in addicts: A comparison between urine, sweat, and hair. *Ther Drug Monit* 18: 450–455

23 Cone EJ, Hillsgrove MJ, Jenkins AJ, Keenan RM, Darwin WD (1994) Sweat testing for heroin, cocaine, and metabolites. *J Analyt Toxicol* 18: 298–305

24 Kintz P, Tracqui A, Mangin P, Edel Y (1996) Sweat testing in opioid users with a sweat patch. *J Analyt Toxicol* 20: 393–397

25 Kintz P, Tracqui A, Marzullo C, Darreye A, Tremeau F, Greth P, Ludes B (1998) Enantioselective analysis of methadone in sweat as monitored by liquid chromatography/ion spray-mass spectrometry. *Ther Drug Monit* 20: 35–40

26 United States of America v. Jamie M. Snyder (2002) 5: 99-CR-528 (HGM/GJD), US District Court Northern District of New York [http://www.drugpolicy.org/docUploads/usv_snyder.pdf]

27 Kidwell DA, Smith FP (2001) Susceptibility of PharmChek drugs of abuse patch to environmental contamination. *Forensic Sci Int* 116: 89–106

28 Levisky JA, Bowerman DL, Jenkins WW, Karch SB (2000) Drug deposition in adipose tissue and skin: Evidence for an alternative source of positive sweat patch tests. *Forensic Sci Int* 110: 35–46

29 Balabanova S, Schneider E, Wepler R, Hermann B, Boschek HJ, Scheitler H (1992) [Significance of drug determination in pilocarpine sweat for detection of past drug abuse]. *Beitr Gerichtl Med* 50: 111–115

30 Curtis J, Greenberg M (2008) Screening for drugs of abuse: Hair as an alternative matrix: A review for the medical toxicologist. *Clin Toxicol (Phila)* 46: 22–34

31 Society of Hair Testing (2004) Recommendations for hair testing in forensic cases. *Forensic Sci Int* 145: 83–84

32 Baumgartner WA, Hill VA (1993) Sample preparation techniques. *Forensic Sci Int* 63: 121–143.

33 Polettini A, Stramesi C, Vignali C, Montagna M (1997) Determination of opiates in hair. Effects of extraction methods on recovery and on stability of analytes. *Forensic Sci Int* 84: 259–269

34 Romano G, Barbera N, Spadaro G, Valenti V (2003) Determination of drugs of abuse in hair: Evaluation of external heroin contamination and risk of false positives. *Forensic Sci Int* 131: 98–102

35 Blank DL, Kidwell DA (1993) External contamination of hair by cocaine: An issue in forensic interpretation. *Forensic Sci Int* 63: 145–160

36 Rollins DE, Wilkins DG, Krueger GG (2003) The effect of hair color on the incorporation of codeine into human hair. *J Anal Toxicol* 27: 545–551

37 Reid RW, O'Connor FL, Deakin AG, Ivery DM, Crayton JW (1996) Cocaine and metabolites in human graying hair: Pigmentary relationship. *J Toxicol Clin Toxicol* 34: 685–690

38 Kidwell DA, Lee EH, DeLauder SF (2000) Evidence for bias in hair testing and procedures to correct bias. *Forensic Sci Int* 107: 39–61

39 Caetano R, Cunradi C (2002) Alcohol dependence: A public health perspective. *Addiction* 97: 633–645

40 Narahashi T, Kuriyama K, Illes P, Wirkner K, Fischer W, Mühlberg K, Scheibler P, Allgaier C, Minami K, Lovinger D, Lallemand F, Ward RJ, DeWitte P, Itatsu T, Takei Y, Oide H, Hirose M, Wang XE, Watanabe S, Tateyama M, Ochi R, Sato N (2001) Neuroreceptors and ion channels as targets of alcohol. *Alcohol Clin Exp Res* 25 (5 Suppl ISBRA): 182S–188S

41 Norberg A, Jones AW, Hahn RG, Garielsson JL (2003) Role of variability in explaining ethanol pharmacokinetics: Research and forensic applications. *Clin Pharmacokinet* 42: 1–31

42 Edenberg HJ (2007) The genetics of alcohol metabolism: Role of alcohol dehydrogenase and aldehyde dehydrogenase variants. *Alcohol Res Health* 30: 5–13

43 Norberg A, Jones AW, Hahn RG (2003) Role of variability in explaining ethanol pharmacokinetics: Research and forensic applications. *Clin Pharmacokinet* 42: 1–31

44 Zuba D (2008) Accuracy and reliability of breath alcohol testing by handheld electrochemical

analysers. *Forensic Sci Int* 178: e29–33

45 Trafford DJ, Makin HL (1994) Breath-alcohol concentration may not always reflect the concentration of alcohol in blood. *J Anal Toxicol* 18: 225–228

46 Rainey PM (1993) Relation between serum and whole-blood ethanol concentrations. *Clin Chem* 39: 2288–2292

47 Smolle KH, Hofmann G, Kaufmann P (1999) Q.E.D. Alcohol test: A simple and quick method to detect ethanol in saliva of patients in emergency departments. Comparison with the conventional determination in blood. *Intensive Care Med* 25: 492–495

48 Soderberg BL, Salem RO, Best CA (2003) Fatty acid ethyl esters. Ethanol metabolites that reflect ethanol intake. *Am J Clin Pathol* 119: S94–99

49 Kraman P (2004) Drug Abuse in America - Rural Meth. Trends Alert. The Council of State Governments, Lexington, KY, March 2004

50 Weir E (2000) Raves: A review of the culture, the drugs, and the prevention of harm. *Can Med Assoc J* 162: 1829–1830

51 Chiang WK (2006) Amphetamines. In: LR Goldfrank, NE Flomenbaum, NA Lewin, MA Howland, RS Hoffman, LS Nelson (eds): *Goldfrank's Toxicologic Emergencies*, 8th edn., McGraw-Hill, New York, 1118–1132

52 Cody JT (2002) Precursor medications as a source of methamphetamine and/or amphetamine positive drug testing results. *J Occup Environ Med* 44: 435–450

53 Stout PR, Klette KL, Horn CK (2004) Evaluation of ephedrine, pseudoephedrine and phenylpropanolamine concentrations in human urine samples and a comparison of the specificity of DRI amphetamines and Abuscreen online (KIMS) amphetamines screening immunoassays. *J Forensic Sci* 49: 160–164

54 Stout PR, Klette KL, Wiegand R (2003) Comparison and evaluation of DRI methamphetamine, DRI ecstasy, Abuscreen ONLINE amphetamine, and a modified Abuscreen ONLINE amphetamine screening immunoassays for the detection of amphetamine (AMP), methamphetamine (MTH), 3,4-methylenedioxyamphetamine (MDA), and 3,4-methylenedioxymethamphetamine (MDMA) in human urine. *J Anal Toxicol* 27: 265–269.

55 Paul BD, Jemionek J, Lesser D, Jacobs A, Searles DA (2004) Enantiomeric separation and quantitation of (±)-amphetamine, (±)-methamphetamine, (±)-MDA, (±)-MDMA, and (±)-MDEA in urine specimens by GC-EI-MS after derivatization with (*R*)-(–)- or (*S*)-(+)-α-methoxy-α-(trifluoromethy)phenylacetyl chloride (MTPA). *J Anal Toxicol* 28: 449–455

56 Krasowski MD, Pizon AF, Siam MG, Giannoutsos S, Iyer M, Ekins S (2009) Using molecular similarity to highlight the challenges of routine immunoassay-based drug of abuse/toxicology screening in emergency medicine. *BMC Emerg Med* 9: 5

57 Smink BE, Hofman BJ, Dijkhuizen A, Lusthof KJ, de Gier JJ, Egberts AC, Uges DR (2008) The concentration of oxazepam and oxazepam glucuronide in oral fluid, blood and serum after controlled administration of 15 and 30 mg oxazepam. *Br J Clin Pharmacol* 66: 556–560

58 Kintz P, Tracqui A, Mangin P (1996) Sweat testing for benzodiazepines. *J Forensic Sci* 41: 851–854

59 Kintz P, Villain M, Cirimele V, Pépin G, Ludes B (2004) Windows of detection of lorazepam in urine, oral fluid and hair, with a special focus on drug-facilitated crimes. *Forensic Sci Int* 145: 131–135

60 Verstraete AG (2004) Detection times of drugs of abuse in blood, urine, and oral fluid. *Ther Drug Monit* 26: 200–205

61 Chèze M, Duffort G, Deveaux M, Pépin G (2005) Hair analysis by liquid chromatography–tandem mass spectrometry in toxicological investigation of drug-facilitated crimes: Report of 128 cases over the period June 2003-May 2004 in metropolitan Paris. *Forensic Sci Int* 153: 3–10

62 World Drug Report (2008) United Nations Office on Drugs and Crime (online available at: http://www.unodc.org/documents/wdr/WDR_2008/WDR_2008_eng_web.pdf; accessed March 28, 2009)

63 Chen CY, O'Brien MS, Anthony JC (2005) Who becomes cannabis dependent soon after onset of use? Epidemiological evidence from the United States: 2000–2001. *Drug Alcohol Depend* 79: 11–22

64 Elkashef A, Vocci F, Huestis M, Haney M, Budney A, Gruber A, el-Guebaly N (2008) Marijuana neurobiology and treatment. *Subst Abus* 29: 17–29

65 Ohlsson A, Lindgren JE, Wahlen A, Agurell S, Hollister LE, Gillespie HK (1980) Plasma Δ^9-tetrahydrocannabinol concentrations and clinical effects after oral and intravenous administration

and smoking. *Clin Pharmacol Ther* 28: 409–416

66 Musshoff F, Madea B (2006) Review of biologic matrices (urine, blood, hair) as indicators of recent or ongoing cannabis use. *Ther Drug Monit* 28: 155–163

67 Teixeira H, Verstraete A, Proenca P, Corte-Real F, Monsanto P, Vieira DN (2007) Validated method for the simultaneous determination of Δ^9-THC and Δ^9-THC-COOH in oral fluid, urine and whole blood using solid-phase extraction and liquid chromatography–mass spectrometry with electrospray ionization. *Forensic Sci Int* 170: 148–155

68 Maralikova B, Weinmann W (2004) Simultaneous determination of Δ^9-tetrahydrocannabinol, 11-hydroxy-Δ^9-tetrahydrocannabinol and 11-nor-9-carboxy-Δ^9-tetrahydrocannabinol in human plasma by high-performance liquid chromatography/tandem mass spectrometry. *J Mass Spectrom* 39: 526–531

69 Huestis MA, Cone EJ (2004) Relationship of Δ^9-tetrahydrocannabinol concentrations in oral fluid and plasma after controlled administration of smoked cannabis. *J Anal Toxicol* 28: 394–399

70 Cone EJ, Huestis MA (1993) Relating blood concentrations of tetrahydrocannabinol and metabolites to pharmacologic effects and time of marijuana usage. *Ther Drug Monit* 15: 527–532

71 Huestis MA, Henningfield JE, Cone EJ (1992) Blood cannabinoids. II. Models for the prediction of time of marijuana exposure from plasma concentrations of Δ^9-tetrahydrocannabinol (THC) and 11-nor-9-carboxy-Δ^9-tetrahydrocannabinol (THCCOOH). *J Anal Toxicol* 16: 283–290

72 Giroud C, Ménétrey A, Augsburger M, Buclin T, Sanchez-Mazas P, Mangin P (2001) Δ^9-THC, 11-OH-Δ^9-THC and Δ^9-THCCOOH plasma or serum to whole blood concentrations distribution ratios in blood samples taken from living and dead people. *Forensic Sci Int* 123: 159–164

73 Skopp G, Pötsch L, Mauden M, Richter B (2002) Partition coefficient, blood to plasma ratio, protein binding and short-term stability of 11-nor-Δ^9-carboxy tetrahydrocannabinol glucuronide. *Forensic Sci Int* 126: 17–23

74 Huestis MA, Henningfield JE, Cone EJ (1992) Blood cannabinoids. I. Absorption of THC and formation of 11-OH-THC and THCCOOH during and after smoking marijuana. *J Anal Toxicol* 16: 276–282

75 Kielland KB (1992) [Urinary excretion of cannabis metabolites]. *Tidsskr Nor Laegeforen* 112: 1585–1586

76 Lafolie P, Beck O, Blennow G, Boréus L, Borg S, Elwin CE, Karlsson L, Odelius G, Hjemdahl P (1991) Importance of creatinine analyses of urine when screening for abused drugs. *Clin Chem* 37: 1927–1931

77 Fraser AD, Worth D (1999) Urinary excretion profiles of 11-nor-9-carboxy-Δ^9-tetrahydrocannabinol: a Δ^9-THCCOOH to creatinine ratio study. *J Anal Toxicol* 23: 531–534

78 Manno JE, Manno BR, Kemp PM, Alford DD, Abukhalaf IK, McWilliams ME, Hagaman FN, Fitzgerald MJ (2001) Temporal indication of marijuana use can be estimated from plasma and urine concentrations of Δ^9-tetrahydrocannabinol, 11-hydroxy-Δ^9-tetrahydrocannabinol, and 11-nor-Δ^9-tetrahydrocannabinol-9-carboxylic acid. *J Anal Toxicol* 25: 538–549

79 Golding Fraga S, Diaz-Flores Estevez J, Diaz Romero C (1998) Stability of cannabinoids in urine in three storage temperatures. *Ann Clin Lab Sci* 28: 160–162

80 Nakahara Y, Takahashi K, Kikura R (1995) Hair analysis for drugs of abuse. X. Effect of physicochemical properties of drugs on the incorporation rates into hair. *Biol Pharm Bull* 18: 1223–1227

81 Musshoff F, Driever F, Lachenmeier K, Lachenmeier DW, Banger W, Madea B (2006) Results of hair analyses for drugs of abuse and comparison with self-reports and urine tests. *Forensic Sci Int* 156: 118–123

82 Uhl M (2000) Tandem mass spectrometry: A helpful tool in hair analysis for the forensic expert. *Forensic Sci Int* 107: 169–179

83 Samyn N, De Boeck G, Verstraete AG (2002) The use of oral fluid and sweat wipes for the detection of drugs of abuse in drivers. *J Forensic Sci* 47: 1380–1387

84 Crouch DJ, Walsh JM, Cangianelli L, Quintela (2008) Laboratory evaluation and field application of roadside oral fluid collectors and drug testing devices. *Ther Drug Monit* 30: 188–195

85 World situation with regard to drug abuse - Report by the secretariat. United Nations Economic and Social Council Commission on Narcotic Drugs (online available at: http://daccess-ods.un.org/TMP/648688.html; accessed May 19, 2009)

86 The NSDUH Report - Cocaine Use: 2002 and 2003. Substance Abuse and Mental Health Services Administration (SAMHSA) (online available at: http://www.oas.samhsa.gov/2k5/cocaine/cocaine.pdf; accessed May 19, 2009)

87 Jacob P 3rd, Jones RT, Benowitz NL, Shulgin AT, Lewis ER, Elias-Baker BA (1990) Cocaine

smokers excrete a pyrolysis product, anhydroecgonine methyl ester. *J Toxicol Clin Toxicol* 28: 121–125

88 Toennes SW, Fandino AS, Kauert G (1999) Gas chromatographic-mass spectrometric detection of anhydroecgonine methyl ester (methylecgonidine) in human serum as evidence of recent smoking of crack. *J Chromatogr B Biomed Sci Appl* 735: 127–132

89 Paul BD, McWhorter LK, Smith ML (1999) Electron ionization mass fragmentometric detection of urinary ecgonidine, a hydrolytic product of methylecgonidine, as an indicator of smoking cocaine. *J Mass Spectrom* 34: 651–660

90 Linder MW, Bosse GM, Henderson MT, Midkiff G, Valdes R (2000) Detection of cocaine metabolite in serum and urine: frequency and correlation with medical diagnosis. *Clin Chim Acta* 295: 179–185

91 Cone EJ, Sampson-Cone AH, Darwin WD, Huestis MA, Oyler JM (2003) Urine testing for cocaine abuse: Metabolic and excretion patterns following different routes of administration and methods for detection of false-negative results. *J Anal Toxicol* 27: 386–401

92 Felli M, Martello S, Marsili R, Chiarotti M (2005) Disappearance of cocaine from human hair after abstinence. *Forensic Sci Int* 154: 96–98

93 Shah JC, Mason WD (1990) Plasma codeine and morphine concentrations after a single oral dose of codeine phosphate. *J Clin Pharmacol* 30: 764–766

94 Moriya F, Chan KM, Hashimoto Y (1999) Concentrations of morphine and codeine in urine of heroin abusers. *Leg Med* (Tokyo) 1: 140–144

95 Rook EJ, Huitema AD, van den Brink W, Hillebrand MJ, van Ree JM, Beijnen JH (2006) Screening for illicit heroin use in patients in a heroin-assisted treatment program. *J Anal Toxicol* 30: 390–394

96 Compton WM, Volkow ND (2006) Major increases in opioid analgesic abuse in the United States: Concerns and strategies. *Drug Alcohol Depend* 81: 103–107

97 Rohrig TP, Moore C (2003) The determination of morphine in urine and oral fluid following ingestion of poppy seeds. *J Anal Toxicol* 27: 449–452

98 Ceder G, Jones AW (2001) Concentration ratios of morphine to codeine in blood of impaired drivers as evidence of heroin use and not medication with codeine. *Clin Chem* 47: 1980–1984

99 Romano G, Barbera N, Spadaro G, Valenti V (2003) Determination of drugs of abuse in hair: Evaluation of external heroin contamination and risk of false positives. *Forensic Sci Int* 131: 98–102

100 Hill V, Cairns T, Cheng CC, Schaffer M (2005) Multiple aspects of hair analysis for opiates: Methodology, clinical and workplace populations, codeine, and poppy seed ingestion. *J Anal Toxicol* 29: 696–703

101 The DASIS Report. Trends in Admissions for PCP: 1993–2003. Substance Abuse & Mental Health Services Administration (SAMHSA) (online available at: http://www.oas.samhsa.gov/2k5/PCPtx/PCPtx.htm; accessed May 19, 2009)

102 Santos PM, López-García P, Navarro JS, Fernández AS, Sádaba B, Vidal JP (2007) False positive phencyclidine results caused by venlafaxine. *Am J Psychiatry* 164: 349

103 Schier J (2000) Avoid unfavorable consequences: Dextromethorpan can bring about a false-positive phencyclidine urine drug screen. *J Emerg Med* 18: 379–381

104 Moeller KE, Lee KC, Kissack JC (2008) Urine drug screening: practical guide for clinicians. *Mayo Clin Proc* 2008 83: 66–76

105 Kala SV, Harris SE, Freijo TD, Gerlich S (2008) Validation of analysis of amphetamines, opiates, phencyclidine, cocaine, and benzoylecgonine in oral fluids by liquid chromatography–tandem mass spectrometry. *J Anal Toxicol* 32: 605–611

106 Nakahara Y, Takahashi K, Sakamoto T, Tanaka A, Hill VA, Baumgartner WA (1997) Hair analysis for drugs of abuse. XVII. Simultaneous detection of PCP, PCHP, and PCPdiol in human hair for confirmation of PCP use. *J Anal Toxicol* 21: 356–362

Drugs of abuse: management of intoxication and antidotes

Ivan D. Montoya and David J. McCann

Division of Pharmacotherapies and Medical Consequences of Drug Abuse, National Institute on Drug Abuse (NIDA), USA

Abstract. Illicit drug intoxications are an increasing public health problem for which, in most cases, no antidotes are clinically available. The diagnosis and treatment of these intoxications requires a trained clinician with experience in recognizing the specific signs and symptoms of intoxications to individual drugs as well as polydrug intoxications, which are more the rule than the exception. To make the diagnosis, the clinical observation and a urine toxicology test are often enough. Evaluating the blood levels of drugs is frequently not practical because the tests can be expensive and results may be delayed and unavailable to guide the establishment of a treatment plan. Other laboratory tests may be useful depending on the drug or drugs ingested and the presence of other medical complications. The treatment should be provided in a quiet, safe and reassuring environment. Vital signs should be closely monitored. Changes in blood pressure, respiratory frequency and temperature should be promptly treated, particularly respiratory depression (in cases of opiate intoxication) or hyperthermia (in cases of cocaine or amphetamine intoxication). Intravenous fluids should be administered as soon as possible. Other psychiatric and medical complication should receive appropriate symptomatic treatment. Research on immunotherapies, including vaccines, monoclonal and catalytic antibodies, seems to be a promising approach that may yield specific antidotes for drugs of abuse, helping to ameliorate the morbidity and mortality associated with illicit drug intoxications.

Introduction

Drug overdose is the second leading cause of unintentional injury death in the United States (after motor vehicle injuries) and thus a great public health concern. Illicit drug intoxications may be intentional or unintentional. They may resolve in the streets, result in hospital emergency department (ED) visits, or be associated with the death of the user. Although it is often difficult to obtain a reliable picture of the incidence and/or prevalence of illicit drug intoxication, it is evident that they are on the rise. In 1999, there were 11 155 cases of unintentional drug poisoning deaths in the United States and in 2005 the number rose to 22 448 cases. This increase was largely seen in non-metropolitan counties, where the increase was of 159% *versus* 51% in metropolitan counties. It has been suggested that the dramatic increase in rural areas may be due to the increase in prescription opioid abuse [1–3].

A large proportion of overdose deaths are associated with a history of illicit drug use. In particular, suicide, which is the fourth leading cause of death in the United States, is often associated with alcohol or other drugs use. The 2004 National Violent Death Reporting System showed that alcohol and opiates were present in 33.3% and 16.4% of suicide victims, respectively, followed by cocaine (9.4%), marijuana (7.7%), and amphetamines (3.9%). Rates of ED visits for illicit drug overdose are high and appear to be increasing. According to the Drug Abuse Warning Network (DAWN) report of 2006, central nervous system (CNS) and psychotherapeutic agents were the most frequent drugs reported in the nonmedical-use category of ED visits (50% and 44% of non-medical-use visits, respectively). Among the CNS agents, opiate/opioid analgesics were the most frequently found (33%); and among the opioids, methadone alone or in combination with oxycodone and hydrocodone was the most frequently found [4, 5].

It has been estimated that, in 2006, there were almost 1.7 million ED visits that involved drug misuse or abuse. Of them, more than one half (55%) involved illicit drugs, either alone or in combination with another drug type. The most frequently reported illicit drugs (estimated number of visits) were cocaine (550 000), marijuana (290 000), heroin (190 000), stimulants (107 000) and phencyclidine (PCP, 22 000). Prescription opiates/opioids were found in 240 000 ED visits and the most commonly found were oxycodone (65 000), hydrocodone (58 000), methadone (45 000), morphine (20 000) and fentanyl (16 000). Buprenorphine was included for the first time in this report with an estimated 4400 ED visits. Between 2004 and 2006 there has been an important increase in the ED reports of amphetamine (118%) and narcotic analgesics (39%) [5]. Given the increasing public health relevance of illicit drug intoxications, appropriate early diagnosis and treatment are critical in preventing a fatal outcome. Currently, new methods to treat drug overdoses are being investigated. Active immunizations with vaccines as well as passive immunotherapies such as monoclonal or catalytic antibodies are being investigated for the treatment of drug overdose and are providing encouraging results. In this chapter we review the pharmacology/toxicology, clinical manifestation, main laboratory exams, and treatment (current and potential) of opioid, cocaine, methamphetamine, marijuana, and PCP intoxications.

Opioids

Opioid-related intoxication is a growing public health problem. Overdose associated with heroin use as well as the misuse of prescription opioid analgesics have shown an alarming increase in mortality in recent years. Between 1999 and 2004, a 62.5% increase in deaths from unintentional poisoning has been reported, which is primarily attributed to prescription opioid analgesics. According to the National Center for Health Statistics, between 1999 and 2002 the number of opioid analgesic intoxications listed on death certificates increased by 91.2%. In 2002, the number of deaths due to opioid analgesics was higher than those associated with either heroin or cocaine. Between 1997 and 2007, the *per capita* retail purchases of methadone, hydrocodone, and oxycodone in the United States increased 13-fold, 4-fold, and 9-fold, respectively. Unfortunately, opioid-related intoxications and deaths are increasingly affecting people living in rural areas where general awareness and treatment services are limited [1, 6, 7].

Opioid agonists bind to and activate at least three different types of opioid receptors, designated μ (mu), κ (kappa), and δ (delta). They interact with these binding sites in the CNS and other tissues to produce analgesia and many other effects. Long-term use can produce dependence and the abrupt interruption of their use can produce a withdrawal state [8]. The toxicity of the opioids varies with the agent and the user's vulnerability, as well as the tolerance developed from chronic use. The therapeutic dose of opioids varies depending on the intended indication and the patient's ability to tolerate the medication. Opioids can be administered *via* oral, intranasal, subcutaneous, and parenteral routes, both legally and illicitly. The time to reach peak serum concentrations varies depending on the route of administration. For example, the time to peak concentration of heroin administered intravenously is less than 1 minute, intranasally and intramuscularly is 3–5 minutes, and subcutaneously is 5–10 minutes. The metabolism is primarily in the liver and the excretion is mostly urinary [9–11].

Commonly abused opiates include heroin, oxycodone, fentanyl, opium, codeine, hydrocodone, morphine, meperidine, pentazocine, propoxyphene, and tramadol. Street preparations of some of these drugs may contain variable amounts of active drugs that may increase the risk of overdose or complicate its clinical manifestations. Opioid intoxications, particularly heroin, are frequently seen among "body packers" [12].

Clinical manifestations

The opiate intoxication syndrome is characterized by the triad of miotic pupils, respiratory depression, and depressed level of consciousness. Opioid overdose is commonly associated with hypoxia, mild hypotension, gastric hypomotility and ileus. Severe intoxication can produce apnea, acute lung injury, pulmonary edema, cardiac dysrhythmias, anoxic encephalopathy, shock, coma, and death. The "heroin-lung" is an infrequent but severe complication that is characterized by a sudden onset of non-cardiogenic pulmonary edema after intravenous heroin overdose. The presence of mydriasis in a patient with severe opioid intoxication may be due to the presence of severe acidosis, hypoxia, respiratory depression, or anticholinergic exposure. Seizures are infrequent but when they occur they may be due to severe hypoxia or the administration of proportionally high doses of naloxone [13–17]. Fentanyl can produce severe respiratory depression with muscle rigidity, spasms, and seizures [18]. The concomitant overdose of heroin and cocaine can produce hypertension, ventricular fibrillation, hyperkalemia and rhabdomyolysis [19].

Laboratory

Urine concentrations of opiates can be measured with semiquantitative and qualitative EMIT(R) (enzyme multiplied immunoassay technique) homogenous enzyme immunoassays. They can detect morphine, methadone, codeine, and hydromorphine, and high concentrations of nalorphine and meperidine. The evaluation of plasma opioid levels is not clinically useful. In patients with severe opiate intoxication, monitoring should include electrolytes, blood/urea/nitrogen (BUN) and creatinine, pulse oximetry, arterial blood gases, pulmonary function tests, and cardiac markers. Creatinine phosphokinase (CPK) may be useful when a patient experiences chest pain, seizure or coma. Treatment is based more on clinical presentation than on specific laboratory data [20–23].

Treatment

A patient with a diagnosis of opiate intoxication should be treated in the emergency room because of the high risk of respiratory depression and death. The treatment should include symptomatic treatment, psychosocial support, and close monitoring of vital signs, particularly respiratory frequency, fluids and electrolytes. Ventilation and oxygenation may be required. Pulse oximetry monitoring and/or arterial blood gases should be regularly examined. In some cases, mechanical ventilation may be needed [24, 25].

The medication of choice for the treatment of opiate overdose is the opiate antagonist naloxone. An initial dose of 0.4–2.0 mg should be administered intravenously, repeating as needed to reverse the intoxication. If an intravenous line cannot be secured, then naloxone can be administered by other routes such as subcutaneously, intralingually, or intratracheally [24, 26–30]. It has been reported that buprenorphine overdose may require doses of naloxone of 10 mg or more to reverse its overdose effects [31].

If a patient does not show clinical improvement after the administration of 10 mg naloxone, then the clinician may suspect concomitant overdose with other drugs or may question the diagnosis of opioid-induced toxicity. Pregnant women with opiate intoxication should be treated with lower doses of naloxone because this medication may induce opiate withdrawal to the fetus and result in fetal distress, meconium staining and fetal death [32, 33]. Because the effects of naloxone lasts about 20–90 minutes and the action of some opiates may last longer, intoxicated patients treated with naloxone should be closely observed given the possible return of respiratory depression. A continuous infusion of naloxone may be required in cases of intoxication with a long-acting opioid agonist [17, 34, 35].

Given the alarming increase in opiate overdose deaths, particularly in rural areas where health care resources are difficult to reach, and the fact that peers or family members are usually the actual first responders, there is considerable interest in providing such first responders with the opportunity to intervene within an hour of the onset of overdose symptoms. Studies are being conducted to evaluate the public health role that lay persons may have when trained to safely administer naloxone to individuals with opiate intoxication in the community. The advantages and limitations of the availability of over-the-counter naloxone are being evaluated [36].

Clinicians treating opiate intoxication should keep in mind the possibility of multiple drugs or adulterants that may be co-administered with opiates, in particularly cocaine and scopolamine. The administration of naloxone to patients with a mixed overdose of opiates plus cocaine may precipitate a sympathomimetic toxicity because it may remove the opioid-mediated CNS depressant effects and allow the emergence of cocaine's adrenergic effects [19].

During the course of naloxone treatment, if clinical manifestations of opiate withdrawal emerge, the medications should be stopped and clonidine and/or benzodiazepines may be administered. Naloxone should be reinstated at a dose that is enough to maintain adequate respiratory function without withdrawal. Patients may be discharged from the hospital when they can mobilize as usual, the oxygen saturation on room air is >92%, respiratory rate is between 10 and 20 breaths/min, heart rate is >50 and <100 beats/min, and there is an acceptable level of consciousness. If the patient has a history of opiate addiction, a referral for drug abuse treatment should be offered [13, 24, 37–39].

Studies conducted in the early 1970s evaluated vaccines against morphine. Recently, there is increasing interest in immunotherapies for addictions. Vaccines can elicit specific antibodies that bind to the drug in the circulation and reduce its entry into the CNS, thus preventing the neurotoxic and reinforcing effects of the drugs. One of the most interesting anti-opiate vaccines is made from 6-succinylmorphine because it generates antibodies that bind not only to morphine but also to heroin and 6-acetylmorphine. This is a desirable effect because heroin is rapidly metabolized to 6-acetylmorphine and morphine and this vaccine could prevent the CNS effects of all three substances. In 2006, a novel structural formulation of a bi-valent vaccine against morphine/heroin was developed. The antibodies produced in response to this vaccine appear equally specific for morphine and heroin and do not cross-recognize other structurally dissimilar opiate medications. This vaccine appears to block the reinforcing effects of heroin in rodents and may potentially be effective in preventing relapse to heroin use [40–45]. Further research is needed to evaluate vaccines as well as other immunotherapies as antidotes to intoxications with different types of opiates. Currently, no opiate vaccines or antibodies are available for clinical use.

Cocaine

The shrub *Erythroxylon coca* has been used for centuries by South American Indians because of its stimulant effects. The active ingredient of coca derivatives is cocaine. The most commonly used coca derivatives are coca tea, coca paste, cocaine powder, and crack. The concentration of cocaine in coca leaves is about 0.13–0.68%, in coca tea there is about 4.8–5.7 mg per tea bag, coca paste is about 40–85% cocaine sulfate, and street cocaine is about 10–60% pure. Cocaine is legally used clinically in 4–11.8% solutions for topical and nasopharyngeal anesthesia [46–48].

The metabolism of cocaine is primarily *via* plasma hydrolysis by serum cholinesterase. The two major metabolites are benzoylecgonine and ecgonine methyl ester. Benzoylecgonine has been detected in the urine of persons who use coca derivatives, including coca tea. The mechanism of action of cocaine is by blocking the reuptake of endogenous catecholamines, particularly dopamine and norepinephrine, which explains the adrenergic and dopaminergic effects of cocaine. The local anesthetic effects of cocaine are explained by the blockade of sodium channels in cell membranes [49–53].

Cocaine intoxication has been reported with most forms of coca derivatives. Its symptoms not only depend on the amount used and concentration of cocaine but also the type of impurities, adulterants and other drugs of abuse present or concomitantly abused. For example, cocaine is often used in combination with heroin (known as a "speedball") and the symptoms of intoxication are different from those of cocaine alone. Some of the most frequently found adulterants include lidocaine, caffeine, ephedrine, acetaminophen, phenacetin, theophylline, and magnesium sulfate. Additionally, other concurrently used drugs of abuse include amphetamine, methamphetamine, PCP, and opioids, as well as tobacco and alcohol. The concurrent ingestion of alcohol and cocaine produces the active metabolite cocaethylene, which has been associated with a significantly increased risk of intoxication and sudden death. Thus, it is expected that patients with cocaine intoxication are likely to have symptoms enhanced or distorted by the concomitant ingestion of other substances [54–56].

All routes of administration, including intravenous, intranasal, smoked, oral, rectal, and intravaginal, have been associated with cocaine intoxication. Intoxication may be due to the deliberate or accidental ingestion of cocaine-containing substances. Deliberate use is often associated with recreational administration of large amounts of cocaine in a brief period of time. Intoxication with cocaine for suicidal purposes is relatively infrequent. In contrast, accidental ingestion is relatively frequent. It has been reported that cocaine smugglers may transport cocaine by swallowing multiple packets of the substance ("body packers") and the rupture of a packet may produce a severe intoxication [57, 58]. Among pre-school children, cocaine intoxication may be due to accidental ingestion of cocaine left unattended at home. Additionally, although infrequent, cocaine intoxication may occur in patients receiving cocaine for local anesthesia, in particular children or debilitated patients [59].

The incidence of cocaine intoxication depends on multiple factors, including the type of coca derivative administered, the route of administration, the locale where it is surveyed, and the genetic characteristics of the population. For example, populations who have lower plasma cholinesterase levels may have a high risk of more severe cocaine toxicity, even with lower doses. Also, infants and young children have lower plasma cholinesterase levels and may be at a high risk of cocaine intoxication [60, 61].

Clinical manifestations

The signs and symptoms of intoxication develop soon after the cocaine ingestion. They can be observed within minutes (intravenous route) to a few hours (oral route), depending on the dose, purity, and route of administration. Intoxication is characterized by intense cardiovascular and psychomotor excitation. Patients with cocaine intoxication often show up at the emergency room complaining of severe psychomotor agitation, palpitations, chest pain or other cardiovascular complications, muscle twitches, diaphoresis, hyperthermia, severe headache, epistaxis, tachypnea and other respiratory symptoms, severe anxiety, delirium, or shock.

Documentation of an accurate medical history may be challenging because the patient and/or his/her contacts may try to deny illicit cocaine use. In the physical exam, the patient looks restless, with muscle twitches, particularly in the face and extremities. The vital signs may show tachycardia, hypertension, tachypnea, and hyperthermia. Hyperthermia may be due to the motor agitation, vasoconstriction, and possibly a direct effect on the hypothalamus through potentiation of dopaminergic neurotransmission in the basal ganglia [62–64].

The examination of the eyes may show mydriasis due to the sympathomimetic effect of cocaine. The nose may show remnants of cocaine in the form of white powder, as well as rhinorrhea and ulcerations. When cocaine is smoked, the intoxicated patient may show sings of lip burns and inflammation of upper respiratory airways [65–67].

The cardiovascular system is greatly affected by cocaine intoxication. In addition to the classic tachycardia and hypertension, the patient may have arrhythmias, ventricular fibrillation, myocardial ischemia and infarction. In addition, endocarditis, myocarditis, and dissection and rupture of the aorta have been reported. Respiratory signs may include upper airway burns, dyspnea, bronchospasm, wheezing, pleuritis, hemoptysis, pulmonary edema, and signs of hypoxia [68–73].

The neuropsychiatric effects of cocaine are prominent. They include restlessness, anxiety, agitation delirium, psychosis, choreiform movements, hyperreflexia, fasciculations, and tonic-clonic seizures followed by coma. Seizures may be seen in the form of generalized tonic-clonic, partial motor, or partial complex convulsions, and can progress to status epilepticus. Cocaine-induced seizures are generally brief and self-limited. There are also reports of CNS ischemia, infarction, intracranial hemorrhage, and strokes associated with cocaine intoxication [74–81].

Cocaine intoxication can be associated with vomiting and other digestive problems. Body packers who suffer a rupture of cocaine packets in the gastrointestinal (GI) tract may have severe damage, including bowel bleeding, ischemia, necrosis, and ulcers. Intravenous cocaine use has been associated with hepatic dysfunction, with high aminotransferase levels. Kidney function may be severely affected due to myoglobinuria associated with rhabdomyolysis. Metabolic acidosis can be observed and may be aggravated by the presence of seizures, which in turn may contribute to worsen cardiac dysrhythmias and other heart problems [82–88].

Given the variability in cocaine metabolism, amount of cocaine in coca derivatives, and route of administration, the lethal dose has not been well established and can be quite variable. Death is often associated with cardiovascular collapse, pulmonary edema and respiratory depression. Also, hyperthermia itself can be life threatening.

Laboratory

Patients with suspected cocaine intoxication should undergo a battery of laboratory tests. The qualitative urine toxicology using dipsticks can be easily performed and serves to confirm the diagnosis. Blood or plasma cocaine levels are often not required. An electrocardiogram (ECG) should be performed to all patients with suspected diagnosis of cocaine intoxication. A blood sample should be collected to evaluate complete blood count (CBC), electrolytes, and CPK and troponin levels. X-rays and other imaging tests may be useful to determine if the patient is a body packer. Cholinesterase plasma levels should be evaluated in a patient with severe intoxication but without a history of heavy cocaine use and/or if the clinician suspects that he or she is a poor cocaine metabolizer. Routine urinalyses are needed to monitor kidney function and the presence of myoglobin. Patients with persistent neuropsychiatric changes should have a computed tomography (CT) scan and/or lumbar puncture to rule out the nervous system hemorrhage, infarction, and/or infection. Other tests may include the evaluation of meconium (when fetal exposure to maternal cocaine use is suspected) and nasal swabs (to determine the presence of snorted cocaine), as well as other tests needed according to the clinical manifestations [60, 89–94].

Treatment

A patient with a diagnosis of mild to moderate cocaine intoxication (mild agitation, tachycardia, and/or hypertension) may be treated in the emergency room with symptomatic treatment and psychosocial support and discharged to home after 8–12 hours. A patient with delirium, severe hypertension, significant hyperthermia, chest pain suggestive of myocardial ischemia, dysrhythmias, rhabdomyolysis, renal failure, hepatic failure, seizures, and/or suspected rupture of cocaine packet should be admitted for further evaluation and symptomatic treatment [95].

Patients agitated or with delirium should be treated in a calm and quiet environment. Benzodiazepines are the medications of choice. Seizures are usually controllable with a benzodiazepine (diazepam, midazolam or lorazepam). If they persist, administration of phenobarbital or a short-acting barbiturate may be necessary. Severe hyperthermia is a serious medical emergency and should be treated aggressively. The patient should be sedated, placed unclothed in a cool room, and sponged with or immersed in cool water [95–97].

Hypertension usually improves after the administration of benzodiazepines and does not require anti-hypertensive agents. Hypertension that does not respond to benzodiazepines or with evidence of CNS, cardiac or renal damage may require treatment with nitroglycerin or phentolamine. Beta adrenergic blockers should not be used because of the possible potentiation of vasoconstriction. Dysrhythmias may be treated with calcium channel blockers, although they should be used with caution in patients at risk for seizures. For ventricular arrhythmia, lidocaine and amiodarone are generally the first choice of treatment. Amiodarone can prolong the QT interval and should be used with caution in patients intoxicated with cocaine combined with other substance that prolong the QT interval. Renal insufficiency should be treated with fluids and diuretics such as mannitol or furosemide [98–102].

Suspected body packers may require repeated radiological evaluations to document that all packets have been evacuated. They should remain in the hospital until all cocaine packets have been passed. Patients intoxicated with cocaine in combination with opioids who may require naloxone should be treated with caution because naloxone may remove the CNS depressant effects of the opioids and may exacerbate the cocaine-induced sympathomimetic toxicity. The treatment of concomitant intoxication with cocaine and alcohol should be conducted with caution, particularly in patients receiving benzodiazepines because of the risk of potentiating the CNS depressant effects of alcohol [58, 102–104].

Currently, antidotes for cocaine intoxication are not clinically available. Immunotherapies such as vaccines, monoclonal antibodies and catalytic antibodies are being investigated to block the access of cocaine to the brain and thus prevent its neurotoxic and reinforcing effects. Cocaine vaccines that produce anti-cocaine specific antibodies can reduce the amounts entering the brain and antagonize the CNS effects of cocaine. A cocaine vaccine has shown in rats that it can attenuate the behavioral effects of systemically administered cocaine. In humans, the vaccine can produce detectable levels of polyclonal anti-cocaine antibodies, which have been associated with reductions in cocaine use [105–108]. A cocaine vaccine is currently being evaluated in clinical trials.

Passive immunization with monoclonal antibodies (mAb) may be more efficacious than vaccines in preventing the access of cocaine to the brain. A murine anti-cocaine mAb appears to attenuate the behavioral effects of cocaine. A recently developed anti-cocaine mAb, designated as 2E2, has been shown to change the *in vivo* distribution of cocaine in mice by sequestering cocaine in plasma and decreasing cocaine concentrations in the brain [107, 109–111]. Catalytic antibodies enhance cocaine metabolism and may be a promising treatment strategy for cocaine overdose. Cocaine can be degraded by hydrolysis of its benzoyl ester to ecgonine methyl ester and benzoic acid, which are not reinforcing or toxic. Therefore, antibodies able to catalyze can accelerate the degradation of cocaine to products with low or no toxicity, and prevent the acute as well as possibly the long-term consequences of cocaine intoxication [111–116]. Monoclonal and catalytic antibodies may be promising antidotes for cocaine intoxications and to prevent its CNS complications.

Amphetamines

Amphetamines, including methamphetamine, are CNS stimulants with a strong noradrenergic central and peripheral effect. They are approved by the U.S. Food and Drug Administration (FDA) for the treatment of attention deficit hyperactivity disorder (ADHD). They can produce abuse and dependence and, over time, they can produce tolerance. There is a regional pattern of abuse, with higher prevalence in the west coast of the United States. Amphetamines can be used *via* oral, intravenous, smoked, and rectal routes. They are metabolized in the liver by aromatic hydroxylation, *N*-dealkylation and deamination. The metabolites of methamphetamine include amphetamine (major metabolite), *p*-hydroxymethamphetamine, and norephedrine. The excretion is primarily in the urine and the biological half-life is about 4–5 hours [117, 118].

Methamphetamine can be manufactured in clandestine laboratories using multiple compounds depending on the method of synthesis. The acute administration of large doses of methamphetamine can produce intoxication. Intoxication may be due to intentional or unintentional ingestion or accidental rupture of ingested bags by "body packers". The methamphetamine blood concentration in fatal cases is about 0.23–40 µg/mL [119–121].

Clinical manifestations

The clinical manifestations of amphetamine intoxication depend on the ingested dose and the individual vulnerability to the effects of the drug. Mild intoxication can produce motor hyperactivity, tachycardia, hypertension, fasciculations, tremors, and diaphoresis. Moderate intoxication intensifies these symptoms and stereotyped activity, compulsive behaviors, psychomotor agitation, dysrhythmias, tachypnea, and hyperthermia can be observed. Severe intoxications are characterized by vomiting, diarrhea, intense tachycardia, severe hypertension, uncontrolable psychomotor agitation, symptoms of psychosis with hallucinations, irritability, paranoia, intense headache, and severe hyperthermia (greater than 41 °C). Severe hyperthermia is often associated with a high fatality rate. The patient may develop seizures, intracerebral hemorrhage, renal and hepatic problems, coagulopathy, rhabdomyolysis, multiorgan failure, coma, and death [119–124].

Laboratory

Amphetamine and amphetamine-like compounds are readily detectable in the urine. Urine toxicology test is useful to confirm the diagnosis of amphetamine intoxication. Amphetamines are difficult to detect in the plasma and the evaluation of blood levels may not be useful to determine amphetamine intoxication. The clinical observation of toxic effects is more relevant than an estimate of the ingested dose. Serum electrolytes, CBC, coagulation profile, renal function, hepatic enzymes, CPK, and ECG should be ordered for all patients. Users who smoke methamphetamine may have a peculiar odor of ammonia or stale urine. A semi-quantitative immunoassay is available and the detection limit (sensitivity) is 0.3 µg/mL for amphetamine or methamphetamine. Some medications for the treatment of respiratory infections that contain ephedrine, pseudoephedrine, or phenylpropanolamine, as well as the antidepressant bupropion, can produce false-positive urine results for amphetamines [119, 125–127].

Treatment

Individuals intoxicated with amphetamines usually seek treatment in the ED when during psychotic episodes they are causing harm to themselves or others, or when they present trauma usually associated with violent behaviors or motor vehicle accidents. It is infrequent that amphetamine intoxicated individuals seek treatment for the medical problems associated with this intoxication. Treatment should be inpatient, particularly for patients with abnormal vital signs or moderate to severe clinical intoxications. It should include abundant fluids and electrolytes, as well as close monitoring of vital signs, including temperature. Hyperthermia above 40 °C mandates immediate cooling and sedation with benzodiazepines. If the patient has convulsions, these should be treated with benzodiazepines or phenobarbital. The hypertension is generally transient and usually responds to sedation with benzodiazepines. Nitroprusside, a short acting, titratable agent, should be considered when the hypertension is severe or unresponsive to benzodiazepines [122, 123, 128–130].

Agitated patients should be sedated with a benzodiazepine. Control of agitation is an important treatment in amphetamine overdose since agitation often leads to hyperthermia, a common cause of mortality in amphetamine overdose. Extreme agitation with severe psychotic symptoms may require additional treatment with antipsychotic medications. Sedation with benzodiazepines to control agitation is sufficient in the vast majority of cases. Oxygen and intravenous fluids should be administered as clinically indicated and hyperthermia corrected. If severe tachycardia persists and is associated with hemodynamic compromise or myocardial ischemia, additional therapy may be required, but this is unusual [122, 123, 128–130].

In the future, immunotherapies may be useful for the treatment of amphetamine overdose. Active and passive immunization to treat the toxic effects of methamphetamine and to treat methamphetamine dependence are being investigated. Monoclonal antibodies appear to reduce the toxic effects of methamphetamine. Animal studies suggest that anti-methamphetamine antibodies can reduce methamphetamine self-administration and inhibit methamphetamine-stimulated locomotor activity. Given the severe toxic effects of methamphetamine, it is hoped that immunotherapies will prove to be effective antidotes of methamphetamine overdose [131–134].

Marijuana

Marijuana refers to a mixture of crushed leaves, twigs, seeds and/or flowers of the plant called *Cannabis sativa*. Marijuana appears to contain more than 400 chemicals, including more than 60 cannabinoids. The most clinically relevant cannabinoids are cannabinol (CBN), cannabidiol (CBD), and Δ^9-tetrahydrocannabinol (THC). THC is the ingredient of marihuana that accounts for most of its physiological and psychoactive effects. It is lipid soluble and water insoluble. Some of the metabolites of THC have psychoactive or other properties [135–139].

The most common method of marijuana administration is smoking, often alone or in combination with tobacco. Marijuana is also ingested, usually in the form of brownies or candy. Intravenous use of hashish oil or an extract of marijuana obtained by boiling marijuana in water has been reported. The Δ^9-THC is available as a medication under the name dronabinol. A synthetic cannabinoid, nabilone, is also available. They have been used in clinical practice as antiemetics, analgesics, muscle relaxants, to reduce intraocular pressure, and to stimulate appetite in individuals with anorexia nervosa or acquired immunodeficiency syndrome (AIDS) [140–142].

Marijuana intoxication is usually difficult to predict because the blood concentration of THC in marijuana depends on the variety of the plant from which it is obtained, the part of the plant that is used (e.g., the flowers have a higher concentration of THC and this form of marijuana is known as hashish), and the route of administration. Additionally, the relationship between plasma THC levels and degree of intoxication is non-linear and there is great individual variability to the toxic effects of marijuana. THC is metabolized in the liver to 11-hydroxy-Δ^9-THC, which is pharmacologically active. This is then metabolized to 11-nor-Δ^9-THC carboxylic acid, which is not active. This metabolite and a small amount THC are excreted in urine. The plasma half-life of THC is about 4 days but it has been detected for up to 2 weeks [139, 143–146].

Clinical manifestations

The clinical manifestations depend on the level of intoxication. A mild intoxication is usually manifested with dry mouth, conjunctival injection, mydriasis, eyelid lag, tachycardia, mild euphoria, hyperphagia, heightened sensory awareness, and feeling of well-being. Moderate intoxication usually presents with increased tachycardia, nausea, vomiting, poor concentration, memory impairments, perceptual alterations (including the sense of time), intense mood fluctuations, and sometimes panic reactions. Severe intoxications may be associated with confusional states, ataxia, somnolence, poor concentration, slurred speech, postural hypotension, urinary retention, atrial fibrillation, and angina. Changes in the ECG, including dysrhythmias and ST segment abnormalities, can be present. Seizures may occur in patients with existing seizure disorders [141, 147–152].

The clinical manifestations of marijuana intoxication can be affected by the concomitant administration of other drugs. For example, the cardiovascular effects of marijuana can be exacerbated by the use of cocaine, amphetamines, and amoxapine, as well as anticholinergic and sympathomimetic medications. CNS depressants can increase the drowsiness and somnolence. The intravenous use of hashish oil has been reported to produce an intoxication characterized by headache, nausea, vomiting, abdominal pain, tachycardia, shortness of breath, chills, fever, shock, and, eventually, death [153–157].

Laboratory

THC is difficult to detect in plasma. A semi-quantitative EMIT homogenous enzyme immunoassay is used to measure the presence of cannabinoids in urine. Urine tests do not correlate with symptoms or degree of exposure. A positive result indicates only the likelihood of prior use or the possibility of exposure to sidestream smoke. Following a single cigarette, THC metabolites are detectable for several days. In casual users cannabinoids may be excreted for up to 2 weeks after cessation of use, and greater than 4 weeks in heavy users. Immunoassays and GC-MS procedures can detect THC and its metabolites in urine, both acutely and following chronic use. Problems with urine testing include the influence of many factors on the results: dose of the drug, time elapsed since dosing, and the amount of water the subject has drunk since dosing [139, 146, 158–161].

Treatment

Mild to moderate intoxications can be treated with supportive care and benzodiazepines. Oral intoxications may require induction of vomiting with syrup of ipecac or administration of activated charcoal to prevent the absorption of

THC, especially after accidental exposure in children. For severe intoxications with perceptual manifestations, agitation or risk of seizures, benzodiazepines are the medications of choice (usually diazepam 5–10 mg orally). Patients with hypotension may be placed in the Trendelenberg position and administered intravenous fluids [162, 163].

Phencyclidine

Phencyclidine (PCP, Sernylan®) is a potent veterinary analgesic and anesthetic that has been taken off the market because of its abuse potential and severe psychiatric side effects. It has dissociative and sympathomimetic properties and the effects are generally dose related. The prevalence of PCP abuse varies across different regions of the USA [164–167].

PCP is rapidly absorbed when ingested orally, the onset of action is in about 2–5 minutes, and the effect can last 4–6 hours. PCP is highly distributed into tissue and its concentration in the brain can be 6–9 times higher than the plasma levels. PCP is metabolized in liver and the excretion is by the kidneys [167–170]. PCP stimulates α-adrenergic receptors, potentiating the effects of norepinephrine, epinephrine and serotonin. It increases pre-frontal cortex dopamine and serotonin release, decreases γ-aminobutyric acid (GABA) release, and acts as a non-competitive antagonist at NMDA (N-methyl D-aspartate)-glutamate receptors [167, 171–173].

The effects of PCP are dose dependent. The administration of 1–5 mg produces mild euphoria and numbness. Doses of 5–10 mg produce a mild intoxication characterized by confusion, ataxia, and dysarthria. Doses higher than 20 mg can produce a severe intoxication with myoclonus, seizures, coma and eventually death. Independent of the dose, deaths may occur when the individual has psychological effects that put him/her at risk of accidents, violence or suicide. Urine PCP levels do not correlate with clinical toxicity [166, 169, 174, 175].

Clinical manifestations

PCP intoxication is characterized by bizarre behaviors, hallucinations/delusions, tachycardia, hypertension, hyperthermia, miosis, nystagmus and dystonias. More advanced intoxications may produce generalized rigidity, localized dystonias, facial grimacing, athetosis, mutism, lethargy, hyperthermia, diaphoresis, hypersalivation, bronchorrhea, bronchospasm, and urinary retention. The intoxication may progress to produce seizures, apnea, coma, hypothermia, cardiac arrest, and rhabdomyolysis that may progress to renal failure. Hypertension is present in more than half of the patients intoxicated with PCP and can produce severe complications. Hypertension usually lasts about 4 hours but sometimes it remains elevated for more than 24 hours.

Psychiatric symptoms are characteristic of PCP intoxication. Perceptual changes in the form of vivid hallucinations are common. They can be terrifying and the intoxicated patient may show paranoid behavior accompanied by withdrawn, combative, or self-destructive behaviors. These symptoms resemble a severe psychotic episode and put the patient at great risk of dying [166, 174, 176–184].

Laboratory

Qualitative urine levels of PCP may be useful to establish the diagnosis and should be interpreted with care. The cut-off for detection of PCP in urine is 25 ng/mL. PCP plasma levels are not clinically useful. Urinalysis may help to determine myoglobin levels in the event of possible rhabomyolysis. Serum CPK and electrolytes should be evaluated. ECG should be performed when cardiac dysrhythmia is suspected [168, 171, 175, 185–188].

Treatment

The treatment should be conducted in a safe and supportive environment, minimizing noise, lights, and touch. Vital signs, including temperature, should be closely monitored. If oral ingestion of PCP is suspected, syrup of ipecac to induce vomiting is not recommended because of the risk of sudden changes in mental status. Fluids and electrolytes should be provided to keep the patient well hydrated. For severe hypertension, phentolamine or nitroprusside may be required. Other cardiovascular complications, including dysrhythmias, should be monitored and adequately treated. For agitated patients or those at risk of or with seizures, benzodiazepines such as diazepam or lorazepam should be administered. Hyperthermia may improve with cooling measures and by controlling the motor agitation with benzodiazepines. In cases of severe intoxication with respiratory depression, an endotracheal intubation may be required [164, 167, 172, 181, 182, 184, 189–191].

Although not yet available for clinical use, immunotherapy for PCP intoxication is a promising approach that is under active investigation. Studies in animals have shown that anti-PCP monoclonal antibodies (mAb6B5) can prevent the access of PCP to the brain and decrease the amount of PCP available to stimulate the brain receptors. These antibodies act as peripheral pharmacokinetic antagonists by capturing and holding the PCP in the vascular compartment. A single dose of murine Ab6B5 can prevent the death of animals exposed to high doses of PCP. Thus, anti-PCP antibodies appear to prevent the toxic effects of PCP on the brain and may be useful for the treatment of PCP overdose [170, 192–197].

Although the mechanism is not clear, mAb6B5 provides long-term reductions in PCP brain concentrations and seems to confer CNS protection for up to a month after its administration. This is an important therapeutic effect because the antibody may serve to prevent relapse to PCP use after an episode of intoxication. Furthermore, the continued prevention of the brain reinforcing effect of PCP may discourage an individual from repeated use and may serve as a tool for the treatment of PCP addiction. Investigators have scaled the data from rat studies to human use and suggest that a single 1 g dose of mAb6B5 may significantly reduce the adverse effects of a 1.2 g/day binge of PCP, for up to 6 weeks [192, 193, 198, 199].

Investigators are now evaluating a chimeric murine anti-PCP antibody (Ch-mAb6B5). It appears to have the same antigen-binding profile as the original murine mAb6B5 and broader specificity for potent arylcyclohexylamines. Thus, the Ch-mAb6B5 may offer the possibility of using a single monoclonal antibody for the treatment of overdose by pharmacologically related drugs [200].

References

1 Paulozzi LJ, Xi Y (2008) Recent changes in drug poisoning mortality in the United States by urban-rural status and by drug type. *Pharmacoepidemiol Drug Saf* 17: 997–1005
2 CDC (2007) Unintentional poisoning deaths – United States, 1999–2004. *MMWR Morb Mortal Wkly Rep* 56: 93–96
3 Hall AJ, Logan JE, Toblin RL, Kaplan JA, Kraner JC, Bixler D, Crosby AE, Paulozzi LJ (2008) Patterns of abuse among unintentional pharmaceutical overdose fatalities. *J Am Med Assoc* 300: 2613–2620
4 CDC (2006) Toxicology testing and results for suicide victims – 13 states, 2004. *MMWR Morb Mortal Wkly Rep* 55: 1245–1248
5 Substance Abuse and Mental Health Services Administration, Office of Applied Studies (2008) Drug Abuse Warning Network, 2006: National Estimates of Drug-Related Emergency Department Visits. DHHS Publication No. (SMA) 08-4339. Rockville, MD. DAWN Series D-30.
6 Paulozzi LJ, Budnitz DS, Xi Y (2006) Increasing deaths from opioid analgesics in the United States. *Pharmacoepidemiol Drug Saf* 15: 618–627
7 Paulozzi LJ, Annest JL (2007) US data show sharply rising drug-induced death rates. *Inj Prev* 13: 130–132.
8 Snyder SH, Pert CB, Pasternak GW (1974) The opiate receptor. *Ann Intern Med* 81: 534–540
9 Schuster CR, Smith BB, Jaffe JH (1971) Drug abuse in heroin users. An experimental study of self-administration of methadone, codeine, and pentazocine. *Arch Gen Psychiatry* 24: 359–362
10 Jasinski DR, Preston KL (1986) Comparison of intravenously administered methadone, morphine and heroin. *Drug Alcohol Depend* 17: 301–310
11 Kuhar MJ (1978) Opiate receptors: Some anatomical and physiological aspects. *Ann NY Acad Sci* 311: 35–48
12 Utecht MJ, Stone AF, McCarron MM (1993) Heroin body packers. *J Emerg Med* 11: 33–40
13 Cullen W, Bury G., Langton D (2000) Experience of heroin overdose among drug users attending general practice. *Br J Gen Pract* 50: 546–549
14 Tagliaro F, De BZ (1999) Heroin overdose is often the truer description. *Addiction* 94: 973–974
15 Sporer KA (1999) Acute heroin overdose. *Ann Intern Med* 130: 584–590
16 Darke S, Zador D (1996) Fatal heroin 'overdose': A review. *Addiction* 91: 1765–1772
17 Duberstein JL, Kaufman DM (1971) A clinical study of an epidemic of heroin intoxication and heroin-induced pulmonary edema. *Am J Med* 51: 704–714
18 Safwat AM, Daniel D (1983) Grand mal seizure after fentanyl administration. *Anesthesiology* 59: 78
19 McCann B, Hunter R, McCann J (2002) Cocaine/heroin induced rhabdomyolysis and ventricular fibrillation. *Emerg Med J* 19: 264–265

20 Cone EJ, Darwin WD (1992) Rapid assay of cocaine, opiates and metabolites by gas chromatography–mass spectrometry. *J Chromatogr* 580: 43–61
21 Cone EJ, Caplan YH, Black DL, Robert T, Moser F (2008) Urine drug testing of chronic pain patients: Licit and illicit drug patterns. *J Anal Toxicol* 32: 530–543
22 Goldberger BA, Cone EJ, Grant TM, Caplan YH, Levine BS, Smialek JE (1994) Disposition of heroin and its metabolites in heroin-related deaths. *J Anal Toxicol* 18: 22–28
23 Yang W, Barnes AJ, Ripple MG, Fowler DR, Cone EJ, Moolchan ET, Chung H, Huestis MA (2006) Simultaneous quantification of methamphetamine, cocaine, codeine, and metabolites in skin by positive chemical ionization gas chromatography–mass spectrometry. *J Chromatogr B Analyt Technol Biomed Life Sci* 833: 210–218
24 Dixon P (2007) Managing acute heroin overdose. *Emerg Nurse* 15: 30–35
25 Strang J (2002) Looking beyond death: Paying attention to other important consequences of heroin overdose. *Addiction* 97: 927–928
26 Strang J, Kelleher M, Best D, Mayet S, Manning V (2006) Emergency naloxone for heroin overdose. *BMJ* 333: 614–615
27 Wasiak J, Clavisi O (2002) Is subcutaneous or intramuscular naloxone as effective as intravenous naloxone in the treatment of life-threatening heroin overdose? *Med J Aust* 176: 495
28 Maio RF, Gaukel B, Freeman B (1987) Intralingual naloxone injection for narcotic-induced respiratory depression. *Ann Emerg Med* 16: 572–573.
29 Wanger K, Brough L, Macmillan I, Goulding J, MacPhail I, Christenson JM (1998) Intravenous *vs* subcutaneous naloxone for out-of-hospital management of presumed opioid overdose. *Acad Emerg Med* 5: 293–299
30 O'Brien CP, Greenstein R, Ternes J, Woody GE (1978) Clinical pharmacology of narcotic antagonists. *Ann NY Acad Sci* 311: 232–240
31 Gal TJ (1989) Naloxone reversal of buprenorphine-induced respiratory depression. *Clin Pharmacol Ther* 45: 66–71
32 Umans JG, Szeto HH (1985) Precipitated opiate abstinence *in utero*. *Am J Obstet Gynecol* 151: 441–444
33 Zuspan FP, Gumpel JA, Mejia-Zelaya A, Madden J, Davis R (1975) Fetal stress from methadone withdrawal. *Am J Obstet Gynecol* 122: 43–46
34 Dowling J, Isbister GK, Kirkpatrick CM, Naidoo D, Graudins A (2008) Population pharmacokinetics of intravenous, intramuscular, and intranasal naloxone in human volunteers. *Ther Drug Monit* 30: 490–496
35 Steinberg AD, Karliner JS (1968) The clinical spectrum of heroin pulmonary edema. *Arch Intern Med* 122: 122–127
36 Kim D, Irwin KS, Khoshnood K (2009) Expanded access to naloxone: Options for critical response to the epidemic of opioid overdose mortality. *Am J Public Health* 99: 402–407
37 Brzozowski M, Shih RD, Bania TC, Hoffman RS (1993) Discharging heroin overdose patients after observation. *Ann Emerg Med* 22: 1638–1639
38 Christenson J, Etherington J, Grafstein E, Innes G, Pennington S, Wanger K, Fernandes C, Spinelli JJ, Gao M (2000) Early discharge of patients with presumed opioid overdose: Development of a clinical prediction rule. *Acad Emerg Med* 7: 1110–1118
39 Etherington J, Christenson J, Innes G, Grafstein E, Pennington S, Spinelli JJ, Gao M, Lahiffe B, Wanger K, Fernandes C (2000) Is early discharge safe after naloxone reversal of presumed opioid overdose? *Can J Emerg Med* 2: 156–162
40 Akbarzadeh A, Mehraby M, Zarbakhsh M, Farzaneh H (1999) Design and synthesis of a morphine-6-succinyl-bovine serum albumin hapten for vaccine development. *Biotechnol Appl Biochem* 30: 139–146
41 Anton B, Leff P (2006) A novel bivalent morphine/heroin vaccine that prevents relapse to heroin addiction in rodents. *Vaccine* 24: 3232–3240
42 Bonese KF, Wainer BH, Fitch FW, Rothberg RM, Schuster CR (1974) Changes in heroin self-administration by a rhesus monkey after morphine immunisation. *Nature* 252: 708–710
43 Spector S, Berkowitz B, Flynn EJ, Peskar B (1973) Antibodies to morphine, barbiturates, and serotonin. *Pharmacol Rev* 25: 281–291
44 Wainer BH, Fitch FW, Fried J, Rothberg RM (1973) A measurement of the specificities of antibodies to morphine-6-succinyl-BSA by competitive inhibition of ^{14}C-morphine binding. *J Immunol* 110: 667–673
45 Wainer BH, Fitch FW, Rothberg RM, Schuster CR (1973) *In vitro* morphine antagonism by anti-

bodies *Nature* 241: 537–538

46 Gay GR, Sheppard CW, Inaba DS, Newmeyer JA (1973) An old girl: flyin' low, dyin' slow, blinded by snow: Cocaine in perspective. *Int J Addict* 8: 1027–1042

47 Siegel RK (1984) Changing patterns of cocaine use: Longitudinal observations, consequences, and treatment. *NIDA Res Monogr* 50: 92–110

48 Siegel RK, ElSohly MA, Plowman T, Rury PM, Jones RT (1986) Cocaine in herbal tea. *J Am Med Assoc* 255: 40

49 Floren AE, Small JW (1993) Mate de coca equals cocaine. *J Occup Med* 35: 95–96

50 Jenkins AJ, Llosa T, Montoya I, Cone EJ (1996) Identification and quantitation of alkaloids in coca tea. *Forensic Sci Int* 77: 179–189

51 Jackson GF, Saady JJ, Poklis A (1991) Urinary excretion of benzoylecgonine following ingestion of Health Inca Tea. *Forensic Sci Int* 49: 57–64

52 Rump AF, Theisohn M, Klaus W (1995) The pathophysiology of cocaine cardiotoxicity. *Forensic Sci Int* 71: 103–115

53 Barnett G, Hawks R, Resnick R (1981) Cocaine pharmacokinetics in humans. *J Ethnopharmacol* 3: 353–366

54 Leri F, Bruneau J, Stewart J (2003) Understanding polydrug use: Review of heroin and cocaine co-use. *Addiction* 98: 7–22

55 Patel MB, Opreanu M, Shah AJ, Pandya K, Bhadula R, Abela GS, Thakur RK (2009) Cocaine and alcohol: A potential lethal duo. *Am J Med* 122: e5–e6

56 Renfroe CL, Messinger TA (1985) Street drug analysis: An eleven year perspective on illicit drug alteration. *Semin Adolesc Med* 1: 247–257

57 June R, Aks SE, Keys N, Wahl M (2000) Medical outcome of cocaine bodystuffers. *J Emerg Med* 18: 221–224

58 McCarron MM, Wood JD (1983) The cocaine 'body packer' syndrome. Diagnosis and treatment. *J Am Med Assoc* 250: 1417–1420

59 Mott SH, Packer RJ, Soldin SJ (1994) Neurologic manifestations of cocaine exposure in childhood. *Pediatrics* 93: 557–560

60 Hoffman RS, Henry GC, Howland MA, Weisman RS, Weil L, Goldfrank LR (1992) Association between life-threatening cocaine toxicity and plasma cholinesterase activity. *Ann Emerg Med* 21: 247–253

61 Havlik DM, Nolte KB (2000) Fatal "crack" cocaine ingestion in an infant. *Am J Forensic Med Pathol* 21: 245–248

62 Sherer MA (1988) Intravenous cocaine: Psychiatric effects, biological mechanisms. *Biol Psychiatry* 24: 865–885

63 Bauwens JE, Boggs JM, Hartwell PS (1989) Fatal hyperthermia associated with cocaine use. *West J Med* 150: 210–212

64 Callaway CW, Clark RF (1994) Hyperthermia in psychostimulant overdose. *Ann Emerg Med* 24: 68–76

65 Siegel RK (1977) Cocaine: Recreational use and intoxication. *NIDA Res Monogr* 13: 119–136

66 Zeiter JH, McHenry JG, McDermott ML (1990) Unilateral pharmacologic mydriasis secondary to crack cocaine. *Am J Emerg Med* 8: 568–569

67 Daggett RB, Haghighi P, Terkeltaub RA (1990) Nasal cocaine abuse causing an aggressive midline intranasal and pharyngeal destructive process mimicking midline reticulosis and limited Wegener's granulomatosis. *J Rheumatol* 17: 838–840

68 Ribeiro M, Dunn J, Sesso R, Dias AC, Laranjeira R (2006) Causes of death among crack cocaine users. *Rev Bras Psiquiatr* 28: 196–202

69 Blaho K, Logan B, Winbery S, Park L, Schwilke E (2000) Blood cocaine and metabolite concentrations, clinical findings, and outcome of patients presenting to an ED. *Am J Emerg Med* 18: 593–598

70 Om A, Ellahham S, Ornato JP (1992) Reversibility of cocaine-induced cardiomyopathy. *Am Heart J* 124: 1639–1641

71 Willens HJ, Chakko SC, Kessler KM (1994) Cardiovascular manifestations of cocaine abuse. A case of recurrent dilated cardiomyopathy. *Chest* 106: 594–600

72 Lora-Tamayo C, Tena T, Rodriguez A (1994) Cocaine-related deaths. *J Chromatogr A* 674: 217–224

73 Finkle BS, McCloskey KL (1977) The forensic toxicology of cocaine. *NIDA Res Monogr* 13: 153–192

74 Malbrain ML, Wauters A, Demeyer I, Demedts P, Verbraeken H, Daelemans R, Neels H (1993) Drug smuggler's delirium. *BMJ* 306: 1002

75 Nnadi CU, Mimiko OA, McCurtis HL, Cadet JL (2005) Neuropsychiatric effects of cocaine use disorders. *J Natl Med Assoc* 97: 1504–1515

76 Zagnoni PG, Albano C (2002) Psychostimulants and epilepsy. *Epilepsia* 43 Suppl 2: 28–31

77 Pudiak CM, Bozarth MA (1994) Cocaine fatalities increased by restraint stress. *Life Sci* 55: L379–L382

78 Pascual-Leone A, Dhuna A, Altafullah I, Anderson DC (1990) Cocaine-induced seizures. *Neurology* 40: 404–407

79 Kramer LD, Locke GE, Ogunyemi A, Nelson L (1990) Cocaine-related seizures in adults. *Am J Drug Alcohol Abuse* 16: 307–317

80 Lowenstein DH, Massa SM, Rowbotham MC, Collins SD, McKinney HE, Simon RP (1987) Acute neurologic and psychiatric complications associated with cocaine abuse. *Am J Med* 83: 841–846

81 Myers JA, Earnest MP (1984) Generalized seizures and cocaine abuse. *Neurology* 34: 675–676

82 Peyriere H, Mauboussin JM (2000) Cocaine-induced acute cytologic hepatitis in HIV-infected patients with nonactive viral hepatitis. *Ann Intern Med* 132: 1010–1011

83 Van der Woude FJ, Waldherr R (1999) Severe renal arterio-arteriolosclerosis after cocaine use. *Nephrol Dial Transplant* 14: 434–435

84 Merigian KS, Roberts JR (1987) Cocaine intoxication: Hyperpyrexia, rhabdomyolysis and acute renal failure. *J Toxicol Clin Toxicol* 25: 135–148

85 Menashe PI, Gottlieb JE (1988) Hyperthermia, rhabdomyolysis, and myoglobinuric renal failure after recreational use of cocaine. *South Med J* 81: 379–381

86 Ahijado F, Garcia de V, Luno J (1990) Acute renal failure and rhabdomyolysis following cocaine abuse. *Nephron* 54: 268

87 Enriquez R, Palacios FO, Gonzalez CM, Amoros FA, Cabezuelo JB, Hernandez F (1991) Skin vasculitis, hypokalemia and acute renal failure in rhabdomyolysis associated with cocaine. *Nephron* 59: 336–337

88 Herzlich BC, Arsura EL, Pagala M, Grob D (1988) Rhabdomyolysis related to cocaine abuse. *Ann Intern Med* 109: 335–336

89 Beerman R, Nunez D Jr, Wetli CV (1986) Radiographic evaluation of the cocaine smuggler. *Gastrointest Radiol* 11: 351–354

90 Hoffman RS, Thompson T, Henry GC, Hatsukami DK, Pentel PR (1998) Variation in human plasma cholinesterase activity during low-dose cocaine administration. *J Toxicol Clin Toxicol* 36: 3–9

91 Mattes CE, Lynch TJ, Singh A, Bradley RM, Kellaris PA, Brady RO, Dretchen KL (1997) Therapeutic use of butyrylcholinesterase for cocaine intoxication. *Toxicol Appl Pharmacol* 145: 372–380

92 Om A, Ellahham S, Ornato JP, Picone C, Theogaraj J, Corretjer GP, Vetrovec GW (1993) Medical complications of cocaine: Possible relationship to low plasma cholinesterase enzyme. *Am Heart J* 125: 1114–1117

93 Ostrea EM Jr, Romero A, Knapp DK, Ostrea AR, Lucena JE, Utarnachitt RB (1994) Postmortem drug analysis of meconium in early-gestation human fetuses exposed to cocaine: Clinical implications. *J Pediatr* 124: 477–479

94 Jacob P III, Lewis ER, Elias-Baker BA, Jones RT (1990) A pyrolysis product, anhydroecgonine methyl ester (methylecgonidine), is in the urine of cocaine smokers. *J Anal Toxicol* 14: 353–357

95 Lobl JK, Carbone LD (1992) Emergency management of cocaine intoxication. Counteracting the effects of today's 'favorite drug'. *Postgrad Med* 91: 161–166

96 Shanti CM, Lucas CE (2003) Cocaine and the critical care challenge. *Crit Care Med* 31: 1851–1859

97 Catravas JD, Waters IW, Walz MA, Davis WM (1977) Antidotes for cocaine poisoning. *N Engl J Med* 297: 1238

98 Lange RA, Cigarroa RG, Yancy CW Jr, Willard JE, Popma JJ, Sills MN, McBride W, Kim AS, Hillis LD (1989) Cocaine-induced coronary-artery vasoconstriction. *N Engl J Med* 321: 1557–1562

99 Lange RA, Cigarroa RG, Flores ED, McBride W, Kim AS, Wells PJ, Bedotto JB, Danziger RS, Hillis LD (1990) Potentiation of cocaine-induced coronary vasoconstriction by β-adrenergic blockade. *Ann Intern Med* 112: 897–903

100 Pitts WR, Lange RA, Cigarroa JE, Hillis LD (1997) Cocaine-induced myocardial ischemia and

infarction: Pathophysiology, recognition, and management. *Prog Cardiovasc Dis* 40: 65–76

101 McCord J, Jneid H, Hollander JE, de Lemos JA, Cercek B, Hsue P, Gibler WB, Ohman EM, Drew B, Philippides G, Newby LK (2008) Management of cocaine-associated chest pain and myocardial infarction: A scientific statement from the American Heart Association Acute Cardiac Care Committee of the Council on Clinical Cardiology. *Circulation* 117: 1897–1907

102 Williams RG, Kavanagh KM, Teo KK (1996) Pathophysiology and treatment of cocaine toxicity: Implications for the heart and cardiovascular system. *Can J Cardiol* 12: 1295–1301

103 Hoffman RS, Smilkstein MJ, Goldfrank LR (1990) Whole bowel irrigation and the cocaine body-packer: A new approach to a common problem. *Am J Emerg Med* 8: 523–527

104 Hoffman RS, Chiang WK, Weisman RS, Goldfrank LR (1990) Prospective evaluation of "crack-vial" ingestions. *Vet Hum Toxicol* 32: 164–167

105 Martell BA, Mitchell E, Poling J, Gonsai K, Kosten TR (2005) Vaccine pharmacotherapy for the treatment of cocaine dependence. *Biol Psychiatry* 58: 158–164

106 Kosten TR, Rosen M, Bond J, Settles M, Roberts JS, Shields J, Jack L, Fox B (2002) Human therapeutic cocaine vaccine: Safety and immunogenicity. *Vaccine* 20: 1196–1204

107 Fox BS, Kantak KM, Edwards MA, Black KM, Bollinger BK, Botka AJ, French TL, Thompson TL, Schad VC, Greenstein JL, Gefter ML, Exley MA, Swain PA, Briner TJ (1996) Efficacy of a therapeutic cocaine vaccine in rodent models. *Nat Med* 2: 1129–1132

108 Koetzner L, Deng S, Sumpter TL, Weisslitz M, Abner RT, Landry DW, Woods JH (2001) Titer-dependent antagonism of cocaine following active immunization in rhesus monkeys. *J Pharmacol Exp Ther* 296: 789–796

109 Norman AB, Tabet MR, Norman MK, Buesing WR, Pesce AJ, Ball WJ (2007) A chimeric human/murine anticocaine monoclonal antibody inhibits the distribution of cocaine to the brain in mice. *J Pharmacol Exp Ther* 320: 145–153

110 Paula S, Tabet MR, Farr CD, Norman AB, Ball WJ Jr (2004) Three-dimensional quantitative structure-activity relationship modeling of cocaine binding by a novel human monoclonal antibody. *J Med Chem* 47: 133–142

111 Norman AB, Norman MK, Buesing WR, Tabet MR, Tsibulsky VL, Ball WJ (2009) The effect of a chimeric human/murine anti-cocaine monoclonal antibody on cocaine self-administration in rats. *J Pharmacol Exp Ther* 328: 873–881

112 Gao D, Narasimhan DL, Macdonald J, Brim R, Ko MC, Landry DW, Woods JH, Sunahara RK, Zhan CG (2009) Thermostable variants of cocaine esterase for long-time protection against cocaine toxicity. *Mol Pharmacol* 75: 318–323

113 Gao Y, LaFleur D, Shah R, Zhao Q, Singh M, Brimijoin S (2008) An albumin-butyryl-cholinesterase for cocaine toxicity and addiction: Catalytic and pharmacokinetic properties. *Chem Biol Interact* 175: 83–87

114 Jutkiewicz EM, Baladi MG, Cooper ZD, Narasimhan D, Sunahara RK, Woods JH (2008) A bacterial cocaine esterase protects against cocaine-induced epileptogenic activity and lethality. *Ann Emerg Med, in press*

115 Mets B, Winger G, Cabrera C, Seo S, Jamdar S, Yang G, Zhao K, Briscoe RJ, Almonte R, Woods JH, Landry DW (1998) A catalytic antibody against cocaine prevents cocaine's reinforcing and toxic effects in rats. *Proc Natl Acad Sci USA* 95: 10176–10181

116 Zheng F, Zhan CG (2008) Structure-and-mechanism-based design and discovery of therapeutics for cocaine overdose and addiction. *Org Biomol Chem* 6: 836–843

117 Patrick KS, Straughn AB, Perkins JS, Gonzalez MA (2009) Evolution of stimulants to treat ADHD: Transdermal methylphenidate. *Hum Psychopharmacol* 24: 1–17

118 Sever PS, Caldwell J, Dring LG, Williams RT (1973) The metabolism of amphetamine in dependent subjects. *Eur J Clin Pharmacol* 6: 177–180

119 Takekawa K, Ohmori T, Kido A, Oya M (2007) Methamphetamine body packer: Acute poisoning death due to massive leaking of methamphetamine. *J Forensic Sci* 52: 1219–1222

120 Molina NM, Jejurikar SG (1999) Toxicological findings in a fatal ingestion of methamphetamine. *J Anal Toxicol* 23: 67–68

121 Logan BK, Fligner CL, Haddix T (1998) Cause and manner of death in fatalities involving methamphetamine. *J Forensic Sci* 43: 28–34

122 Lan KC, Lin YF, Yu FC, Lin CS, Chu P (1998) Clinical manifestations and prognostic features of acute methamphetamine intoxication. *J Formos Med Assoc* 97: 528–533

123 Chan P, Chen JH, Lee MH, Deng JF (1994) Fatal and nonfatal methamphetamine intoxication in the intensive care unit. *J Toxicol Clin Toxicol* 32: 147–155

124 McKetin R, McLaren J, Lubman DI, Hides L (2006) The prevalence of psychotic symptoms among methamphetamine users. *Addiction* 101: 1473–1478

125 Nixon AL, Long WH, Puopolo PR, Flood JG (1995) Bupropion metabolites produce false-positive urine amphetamine results. *Clin Chem* 41: 955–956

126 Segal DS, Kuczenski R (1997) An escalating dose "binge" model of amphetamine psychosis: Behavioral and neurochemical characteristics. *J Neurosci* 17: 2551–2566

127 Thurman EM, Pedersen MJ, Stout RL, Martin T (1992) Distinguishing sympathomimetic amines from amphetamine and methamphetamine in urine by gas chromatography/mass spectrometry. *J Anal Toxicol* 16: 19–27

128 Zimmerman JL (2003) Poisonings and overdoses in the intensive care unit: General and specific management issues. *Crit Care Med* 31: 2794–2801

129 Richards JR, Bretz SW, Johnson EB, Turnipseed SD, Brofeldt BT, Derlet RW (1999) Methamphetamine abuse and emergency department utilization. *West J Med* 170: 198–202

130 Richards JR, Johnson EB, Stark RW, Derlet RW (1999) Methamphetamine abuse and rhabdomyolysis in the ED: A 5-year study. *Am J Emerg Med* 17: 681–685

131 Byrnes-Blake KA, Laurenzana EM, Carroll FI, Abraham P, Gentry WB, Landes RD, Owens SM (2003) Pharmacodynamic mechanisms of monoclonal antibody-based antagonism of (+)-methamphetamine in rats. *Eur J Pharmacol* 461: 119–128

132 Gentry WB, Laurenzana EM, Williams DK, West JR, Berg RJ, Terlea T, Owens SM (2006) Safety and efficiency of an *anti*-(+)-methamphetamine monoclonal antibody in the protection against cardiovascular and central nervous system effects of (+)-methamphetamine in rats. *Int Immunopharmacol* 6: 968–977

133 Gentry WB, Rüedi-Bettschen D, Owens SM (2009) Development of active and passive human vaccines to treat methamphetamine addiction. *Hum Vaccin* 5: 206–213

134 McMillan DE, Hardwick WC, Li M, Gunnell MG, Carroll FI, Abraham P, Owens SM (2004) Effects of murine-derived *anti*-methamphetamine monoclonal antibodies on (+)-methamphetamine self-administration in the rat. *J Pharmacol Exp Ther* 309: 1248–1255

135 Hutchings DE, Brake SC, Banks AN, Nero TJ, Dick LS, Zmitrovich AC (1991) Prenatal Δ^9-tetrahydrocannabinol in the rat: Effects on auditory startle in adulthood. *Neurotoxicol Teratol* 13: 413–416.

136 Razdan RK (1986) Structure-activity relationships in cannabinoids. *Pharmacol Rev* 38: 75–149

137 Hollister LE (1974) Structure-activity relationships in man of cannabis constituents, and homologs and metabolites of Δ^9-tetrahydrocannabinol. *Pharmacology* 11: 3–11

138 Lemberger L, McMahon R, Archer R, Matsumoto K, Rowe H (1974) Pharmacologic effects and physiologic disposition of $\Delta^{6a,10a}$ dimethyl heptyl tetrahydrocannabinol (DMHP) in man. *Clin Pharmacol Ther* 15: 380–386

139 Perez-Reyes M, Owens SM, Di GS (1981) The clinical pharmacology and dynamics of marihuana cigarette smoking. *J Clin Pharmacol* 21: 201S–207S

140 Robson P (2005) Human studies of cannabinoids and medicinal cannabis. *Handb Exp Pharmacol* 719–756

141 Williamson EM, Evans FJ (2000) Cannabinoids in clinical practice. *Drugs* 60: 1303–1314

142 Mechoulam R, Carlini EA (1978) Toward drugs derived from cannabis. *Naturwissenschaften* 65: 174–179

143 Bech P, Rafaelsen L, Rafaelsen OJ (1974) Cannabis: A psychopharmacological review. *Dan Med Bull* 21: 106–120

144 Thomas R, Chesher G (1973) The pharmacology of marihuana. *Med J Aust* 2: 229–237

145 Nahas GG (1986) Cannabis: Toxicological properties and epidemiological aspects. *Med J Aust* 145: 82–87

146 Johansson EK, Hollister LE, Halldin MM (1989) Urinary elimination half-life of Δ^1-tetrahydrocannabinol-7-oic acid in heavy marijuana users after smoking. *NIDA Res Monogr* 95: 457–458

147 Leweke FM, Gerth CW, Klosterkotter J (2004) Cannabis-associated psychosis: Current status of research. *CNS Drugs* 18: 895–910

148 Johns A (2001) Psychiatric effects of cannabis. *Br J Psychiatry* 178: 116–122

149 Marcus AM, Klonoff H, Low M (1974) Psychiatric status of the marihuana user. *Can Psychiatr Assoc J* 19: 31–39

150 Hochman JS, Brill NQ (1971) Marijuana intoxication: Pharmacological and psychological factors. *Dis Nerv Syst* 32: 676–679

151 ThacoreVR, Shukla SR (1976) Cannabis psychosis and paranoid schizophrenia. *Arch Gen*

Psychiatry 33: 383–386

152 MacInnes DC, Miller KM (1984) Fatal coronary artery thrombosis associated with cannabis smoking. *J R Coll Gen Pract* 34: 575–576

153 Vaziri ND, Thomas R, Sterling M, Seiff K, Pahl MV, Davila J, Wilson A (1981) Toxicity with intravenous injection of crude marijuana extract. *Clin Toxicol* 18: 353–366

154 Nihira M, Hayashida M, Ohno Y, Inuzuka S, Yokota H, Yamamoto Y (1998) Urinalysis of body packers in Japan. *J Anal Toxicol* 22: 61–65

155 Osterwalder JJ (1995) Patients intoxicated with heroin or heroin mixtures: How long should they be monitored? *Eur J Emerg Med* 2: 97–101

156 Voytek B, Berman SM, Hassid BD, Simon SL, Mandelkern MA, Brody AL, Monterosso J, Ling W, London ED (2005) Differences in regional brain metabolism associated with marijuana abuse in methamphetamine abusers. *Synapse* 57: 113–115

157 Forney R, Martz R, Lemberger L, Rodda B (1976) The combined effect of marihuana and dex-troamphetamine. *Ann NY Acad Sci* 281: 162–170

158 Wall ME, Brine DR, Pitt CG, Perez-Reyes M (1972) Identification of Δ^9-tetrahydrocannabinol and metabolites in man. *J Am Chem Soc* 94: 8579–8581

159 DiGregorio GJ, Sterling GH (1987) Marijuana pharmacology and urine testing. *Am Fam Physician* 35: 209–212.

160 Huestis MA, Cone EJ (1998) Differentiating new marijuana use from residual drug excretion in occasional marijuana users. *J Anal Toxicol* 22: 445–454

161 Cone EJ, Johnson RE (1986) Contact highs and urinary cannabinoid excretion after passive exposure to marijuana smoke. *Clin Pharmacol Ther* 40: 247–256

162 Stuyt EB, Sajbel TA, Allen MH (2006) Differing effects of antipsychotic medications on sub-stance abuse treatment patients with co-occurring psychotic and substance abuse disorders. *Am J Addict* 15: 166–173

163 Berk M, Brook S, Trandafir AI (1999) A comparison of olanzapine with haloperidol in cannabis-induced psychotic disorder: A double-blind randomized controlled trial. *Int Clin Psycho-pharmacol* 14: 177–180

164 Baldridge EB, Bessen HA (1990) Phencyclidine. *Emerg Med Clin North Am* 8: 541–550

165 Burns RS, Lerner SE (1976) Perspectives: Acute phencyclidine intoxication. *Clin Toxicol* 9: 477–501

166 McCarron MM (1986) Phencyclidine intoxication. *NIDA Res Monogr* 64: 209–217

167 Morgan JP, Solomon JL (1978) Phencyclidine. Clinical pharmacology and toxicity. *NY State J Med* 78: 2035–2038

168 Bronner W, Nyman P, von Minden D (1990) Detectability of phencyclidine and 11-nor-Δ^9-tetrahydrocannabinol-9-carboxylic acid in adulterated urine by radioimmunoassay and fluo-rescence polarization immunoassay. *J Anal Toxicol* 14: 368–371

169 Burns RS, Lerner SE (1978) Causes of phencyclidine-related deaths. *Clin Toxicol* 12: 463–481

170 Owens SM, Gunnell M, Laurenzana EM, Valentine JL (1993) Dose- and time-dependent changes in phencyclidine metabolite covalent binding in rats and the possible role of CYP2D1. *J Pharmacol Exp Ther* 265: 1261–1266

171 Baskin LB, Morgan DL (1997) Drugs detected in patients suspected of acute intoxication. *Tex Med* 93: 50–58

172 Fallis RJ, Aniline O, Weiner LP, Pitts FN Jr (1982) Massive phencyclidine intoxication. *Arch Neurol* 39: 316

173 McCann DJ, Winter JC (1986) Effects of phencyclidine, *N*-allyl-*N*-normetazocine (SKF-10,047), and verapamil on performance in a radial maze. *Pharmacol Biochem Behav* 24: 187–191

174 Rappolt RT Sr, Gay GR, Farris RD (1980) Phencyclidine (PCP) intoxication: Diagnosis in stages and algorithms of treatment. *Clin Toxicol* 16: 509–529

175 Walker S, Yesavage JA, Tinklenberg JR (1981) Acute phencyclidine (PCP) intoxication: Quantitative urine levels and clinical management. *Am J Psychiatry* 138: 674–675

176 Barton C H, Sterling ML, Vaziri ND (1980) Rhabdomyolysis and acute renal failure associated with phencyclidine intoxication. *Arch Intern Med* 140: 568–569

177 Bessen HA (1982) Intracranial hemorrhage associated with phencyclidine abuse. *J Am Med Assoc* 248: 585–586

178 Brecher M, Wang BW, Wong H, Morgan JP (1988) Phencyclidine and violence: Clinical and legal issues. *J Clin Psychopharmacol* 8: 397–401

179 Burns RS, Lerner SE, Corrado R, James SH, Schnoll SH (1975) Phencyclidine – States of acute intoxication and fatalities. *West J Med* 123: 345–349

180 Cogen FC, Rigg G, Simmons JL, Domino, EF (1978) Phencyclidine-associated acute rhabdomyolysis. *Ann Intern Med* 88: 210–212

181 Eastman JW, Cohen SN (1975) Hypertensive crisis and death associated with phencyclidine poisoning. *J Am Med Assoc* 231: 1270–1271

182 McCarron MM, Schulze BW, Thompson GA, Conder MC, Goetz WA (1981) Acute phencyclidine intoxication: Clinical patterns, complications, and treatment. *Ann Emerg Med* 10: 290–297

183 Stein GY, Fradin Z, Ori Y, Singer P, Korobko Y, Zeidman A (2005) Phencyclidine-induced multiorgan failure. *Isr Med Assoc J* 7: 535–537

184 Stein JI (1973) Phencyclidine induced psychosis. The need to avoid unnecessary sensory influx. *Mil Med* 138: 590–591

185 ElSohly MA, Little TL Jr, Mitchell JM, Paul BD, Mell LD Jr, Irving J (1988) GC/MS analysis of phencyclidine acid metabolite in human urine. *J Anal Toxicol* 12: 180–182

186 ElSohly MA, Stanford DF (1990) Cutoff of 25 ng/mL for the EMIT d.a.u. phencyclidine assay. *J Anal Toxicol* 14: 192–193

187 McCarron MM, Walberg CB, Soares JR, Gross SJ, Baselt RC (1984) Detection of phencyclidine usage by radioimmunoassay of saliva. *J Anal Toxicol* 8: 197–201

188 Walberg CB, McCarron MM, Schulze BN (1983) Quantitation of phencyclidine in serum by enzyme immunoassay: Results in 405 patients. *J Anal Toxicol* 7: 106–110

189 Grover D, Yeragani VK, Keshavan MS (1986) Improvement of phencyclidine-associated psychosis with ECT. *J Clin Psychiatry* 47: 477–478

190 Lahmeyer HW, Stock PG (1983) Phencyclidine intoxication, physical restraint, and acute renal failure: Case report. *J Clin Psychiatry* 44: 184–185

191 Rappolt RT, Gay GR, Farris RD (1979) Emergency management of acute phencyclidine intoxication. *J Am Coll Emerg Physicians – JACEP* 8: 68–76

192 Hardin JS, Wessinger WD, Wenger GR, Proksch JW, Laurenzana EM, Owens SM (2002) A single dose of monoclonal anti-phencyclidine IgG offers long-term reductions in phencyclidine behavioral effects in rats. *J Pharmacol Exp Ther* 302: 119–126

193 Laurenzana EM, Gunnell MG, Gentry WB, Owens SM (2003) Treatment of adverse effects of excessive phencyclidine exposure in rats with a minimal dose of monoclonal antibody. *J Pharmacol Exp Ther* 306: 1092–1098

194 Proksch JW, Gentry WB, Owens SM (2000) The effect of rate of drug administration on the extent and time course of phencyclidine distribution in rat brain, testis, and serum. *Drug Metab Dispos* 28: 742–747

195 Valentine JL, Arnold LW, Owens SM (1994) Anti-phencyclidine monoclonal Fab fragments markedly alter phencyclidine pharmacokinetics in rats. *J Pharmacol Exp Ther* 269: 1079–1085

196 Valentine JL, Mayersohn M, Wessinger WD, Arnold LW, Owens SM (1996) Antiphencyclidine monoclonal Fab fragments reverse phencyclidine-induced behavioral effects and ataxia in rats. *J Pharmacol Exp Ther* 278: 709–716

197 Valentine JL, Owens SM (1996) Antiphencyclidine monoclonal antibody therapy significantly changes phencyclidine concentrations in brain and other tissues in rats. *J Pharmacol Exp Ther* 278: 717–724

198 Pitas G, Laurenzana EM, Williams DK, Owens SM, Gentry WB (2006) Anti-phencyclidine monoclonal antibody binding capacity is not the only determinant of effectiveness, disproving the concept that antibody capacity is easily surmounted. *Drug Metab Dispos* 34: 906–912

199 Proksch JW, Gentry WB, Owens, SM (2000) Anti-phencyclidine monoclonal antibodies provide long-term reductions in brain phencyclidine concentrations during chronic phencyclidine administration in rats. *J Pharmacol Exp Ther* 292: 831–837

200 Lacy HM, Gunnell MG, Laurenzana, EM, Owens, SM (2008) Engineering and characterization of a mouse/human chimeric anti-phencyclidine monoclonal antibody. *Int Immunopharmacol* 8: 1–11

Molecular, Clinical and Environmental Toxicology. Volume 2: Clinical Toxicology
Edited by A. Luch

Chemical warfare agents

Kamil Kuča and Miroslav Pohanka

Center of Advanced Studies and Department of Toxicology, University of Defense, Hradec Kralove, Czech Republic

Abstract. Chemical warfare agents are compounds of different chemical structures. Simple molecules such as chlorine as well as complex structures such as ricin belong to this group. Nerve agents, vesicants, incapacitating agents, blood agents, lung-damaging agents, riot-control agents and several toxins are among chemical warfare agents. Although the use of these compounds is strictly prohibited, the possible misuse by terrorist groups is a reality nowadays. Owing to this fact, knowledge of the basic properties of these substances is of a high importance. This chapter briefly introduces the separate groups of chemical warfare agents together with their members and the potential therapy that should be applied in case someone is intoxicated by these agents.

Introduction

Chemical warfare agents (CWA) are a group of toxic substances originally developed for military purposes. Production and storage of these compounds is prohibited by the Convention on the Prohibition of the Development, Production, Stockpiling and Use of Chemical Weapons and on Their Destruction. Although the probability of their military use is relatively low, their misuse by terrorist groups or individuals is high. This high probability is the result of the easiness of their preparation in any chemical laboratory [1].

Probably the most known misuse of these agents is the Tokyo subway sarin attack. In 1995, a Japanese religious cult Aum Shinrikyo released the nerve agent sarin in a Tokyo subway. This terrorist attack resulted in 5500 poisoned people and 12 deaths. It is known that members of the Aum Shinrikyo cult misused sarin previously in Matsumoto city (1994) and VX agent in Osaka (1994) [2].

Owing to the fact that we are living in the war against terrorism, the knowledge of the properties of the main CWA is important to those working in the field, but also to those who could be in charge in case such toxic agents are spread [3]. This chapter introduces the most known groups of CWA. They are listed according to their importance. The importance is established based on their toxicity and probability of misuse (tactical use): nerve agents > vesicants > incapacitating agents, blood agents, lung-damaging agents > riot-control agents. By contrast, toxins originate from living organisms (biological agents). They either represent macromolecules (glycoproteins) or low molecular weight chemicals of different structure (chemical agents) [4]. Toxins are considered in a special section at the end of the chapter.

Nerve agents

Nerve agents are the most toxic CWA. They belong to the class of organophosphorus compounds. They are divided into two major groups: the 'G-agents' and the 'V-agents'. Tabun (GA), sarin (GB), soman (GD) and cyclosarin (GF) belong to G-agents. The best known member of V-agents is VX. Other members are named according to the country of their origin, Russian VX and Chinese VX. Structures of all nerve agents are depicted in Figure 1 [5].

Nerve agents can be disseminated as a vapor (spray of aerosols being spontaneously evaporated) or as liquid. They range from being nonpersistent to very persistent in the environment. Sarin is a volatile liquid (high vapor pressure) and tends to be nonpersistent as it evaporates readily. Soman and tabun are also relatively volatile. VX is a relatively nonvolatile liquid (low vapor pressure) and is therefore particularly persistent [6].

Nerve agents in their pure state are colorless, but impure agents may be yellow to brown liquids depending on the level of the impurity. When dispersed, the more volatile agents constitute both a vapor and a liquid hazard (G-agents). Others (V-agents) are less volatile and represent primarily a liquid hazard. They are moderately soluble in water and have very high miscibility with fat and nonpolar solvents. A variety of odors have been described, mainly a fruity odor. The odor most likely is caused by impurities.

Nerve agents are chemicals that interfere with the action of the nervous system. Their toxic effect is based on the inhibition of the enzyme acetylcholinesterase (AChE) in the peripheral and central cholinergic nervous system. Their reaction with cholinesterases is irreversible. After the nerve agent inhibits AChE, the enzyme can no longer hydrolyze the neuromediator acetyl-

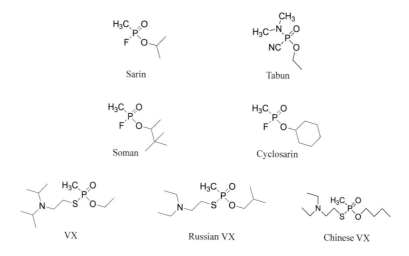

Figure 1. Nerve agents. 'G-agents': tabun (GA), sarin (GB), soman (GD), cyclosarin (GF); 'V-agents': VX, Russian VX, Chinese VX.

choline. Acetylcholine then accumulates in neurosynaptic clefts and continues to stimulate the affected organ. The clinical effects from nerve agent exposure are caused by excess of acetylcholine (cholinergic crisis) [7].

Routes of exposure differ depending on the physico-chemical properties of nerve agents (volatile or nonvolatile). Due to the solubility in both fat and water all nerve agents can be absorbed through the eyes, the respiratory tract and the skin. Vapors of volatile agents are absorbed by inhalation and they represent strong respiratory hazards. The toxic effect comes in less than 1 minute to several minutes. Liquid agents (droplets from spray or aerosol clouds) penetrate mainly through the eyes and the skin at the point of contact. If liquid nerve agents are absorbed through the eyes, their effects start immediately. If the liquid nerve agent is absorbed through the skin, the toxic effect is delayed from few minutes to several hours [3].

Lowered AChE levels in blood are indicators of nerve agent intoxication [8]. The signs and symptoms and the severity of nerve agent poisoning depend upon the amount of nerve agent absorbed and the route by which the nerve agent entered the body. Symptoms of their toxicity vary depending on the type of cholinergic receptor affected – muscarinic or nicotinic, respectively influencing of the central or peripheral nervous system (CNS, PNS). At muscarinic receptors (parasympathetic effects), nerve agents cause constricted pupils (miosis) and glandular hypersecretion (salivary, bronchial, lacrimal, bronchoconstriction, vomiting, diarrhea, urinary and fecal incontinence, bradycardia). At nicotinic receptors (motor and post-ganglionic sympathetic) nerve agents cause sweating of the skin. On the skeletal muscle, they cause initial defasciculation followed by weakness and flaccid paralysis. At CNS cholinergic receptors, nerve agents produce irritability, giddiness, fatigue, emotional lability, lethargy, amnesia, ataxia, fasciculation seizures, coma and central respiratory depression [5].

The combination of anticholinergics (symptomatic drugs), AChE reactivators (causal drugs) and anticonvulsives (symptomatic drugs) is considered as the most promising treatment of nerve agent poisonings. Atropine (acetylcholine blocker) is considered to be the most effective anticholinergic drug used in all cases of such intoxication (Fig. 2A) [7].

With regard to AChE reactivators (called 'oximes'), there are five different compounds clinically used (pralidoxime, obidoxime, trimedoxime, methoxime and HI-6) (Fig. 2B). Another group of drugs are anticonvulsives (Fig. 2A). Among them the most promising compound is diazepam followed by avizafon (pro-diazepam). There is also the option of using several drugs in advance, e.g., prophylactics. From this group, pyridostigmine is the most frequently used compound worldwide [6].

Vesicants

Vesicants are known as blister agents (chemicals that cause blisters). The most known members of the vesicants family are sulfur mustard (HD; *bis*-2-

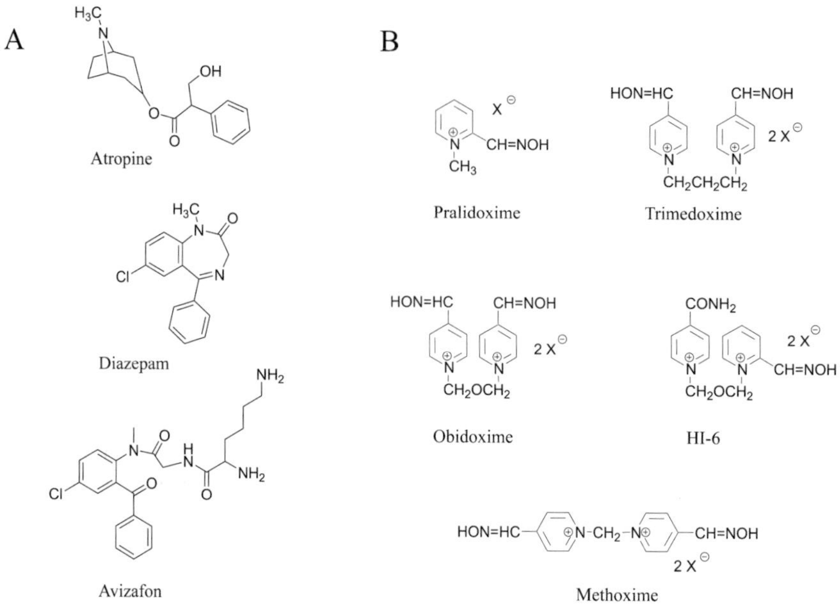

Figure 2. Atropine and anticonvulsives (A); acetylcholinesterase (AChE) reactivators ("oximes") (B).

chloroethylsulfide), nitrogen mustards (HN-1, HN-2, HN-3), lewisite (L) and phosgene oxime (CX). Chemical structures of the members of vesicants family are shown in Figure 3. Their primary target and action is on the skin. These agents produce large, painful and tissue damaging blisters [9].

Mustards together with lewisite can be disseminated in liquid form. Sulfur mustard and nitrogen mustards are similar in their physical characteristics: oily colorless liquids (purified form). Unpurified forms are brown. Mustard smells like garlic or horseradish. Some nitrogen mustards have a slightly fishy odor while others are odorless. They are poorly soluble in water. Nitrogen mustards are less volatile and more persistent than sulfur mustard. Lewisite contains arsenic in its molecule structure. It is a colorless to brown liquid depending on its purity. It has fruity to geranium-like odor. Phosgene oxime is colorless. It could be used in liquid or crystalline form. It has a disagreeable penetrating odor. All vesicants are persistent in the environment, especially in cold or wooded areas.

Mustards can impair many metabolic reactions in the intoxicated organism. They react with biomacromolecules to form covalent adducts by alkylation. The most well-known influenced biomolecules are DNA, RNA, proteins and cell membranes.

Although vesicants are considered nonlethal weapons, high concentrations of these agents can cause death. Unlike nerve agents, mustards do not manifest their symptoms within a short period of time; the latency takes several

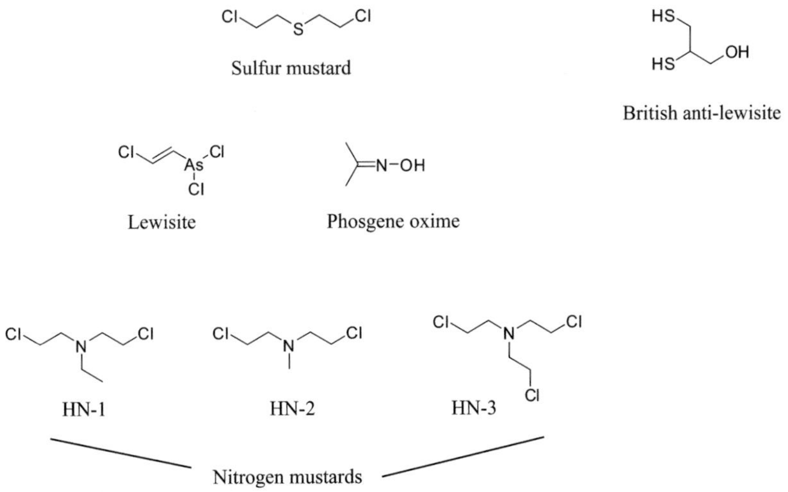

Figure 3. Vesicants and the antidote British anti-lewisite (BAL). Sulfur mustard (HD; *bis*-2-chloroethylsulfide), nitrogen mustards (HN-1, HN-2, HN-3), lewisite (L) and phosgene oxime (CX).

hours (12 hours). That means a soldier may be exposed to these agents for several hours before realizing the danger. Vesicants attack the skin, respiratory system and eyes. They can also contaminate food and water, which can be ingested by victims.

Mustards are chemically different from lewisite and phosgene oxime. Due to this difference they cause several specific symptoms. Mustards affect the skin and respiratory system. When they come into contact with skin, they produce redness at the point of contact usually followed by blistering and ulceration. Mustards cause large fluid-filled blisters on exposed skin. These blisters break, making the exposed individual susceptible to infections. The burns are most severe in warm and sweaty areas of the body such as armpits, groin and the face and neck. If mustards are inhaled they have destructive effects on lung tissue. Mucous is secreted. Lungs can be filled with mucous, causing death by 'dry land drowning'. These agents can produce inflammation of the lungs and the entire respiratory system, and finally of the whole body. However, death is rare and usually results from bacterial infection of the lungs. On the other hand, the risk of carcinoma arising is strongly elevated due to alkylation of guanine bases in DNA.

Lewisite causes intense pain and burns upon contact with the skin. Severe exposure of the eyes to lewisite can result in permanent injury or blindness. The respiratory symptoms are similar to those caused by mustards. Moreover, lewisite attacks the capillaries of the circulatory system, the liver, and the intestines, most likely due to its content of arsenic. Phosgene oxime produces immediate irritation and pain of the skin on contact. It immediately irritates the mucous membranes of the eyes or nose upon contact.

Due to the different chemical origin of vesicants, the treatment of intoxication also varies. In case of mustard poisoning, no specific antidotes are applicable. All other treatment measures are symptomatic – the relief of pain, itching and infection prevention. British anti-lewisite (BAL; dimercaprol) is generally used to treat lewisite poisoning (Fig. 3). Supportive treatment to combat infection and pain is also applied. In case of phosgene oxime poisoning supportive treatment is applied [9–11].

Incapacitating agents

Incapacitating agents are also termed psychochemical agents. These agents may be administered through contaminated food and drinks or applied as aerosols. They were designed to reduce effectiveness of soldiers by interfering with the CNS. Among the incapacitating agents, 3-quinuclidinyl benzilate (QNB or BZ agent) and D-lysergic acid diethylamide (LSD) are the most known (Fig. 4A).

The BZ compound is an odorless stable crystalline solid. It is well soluble in many solvents and extremely persistent in soil and water. LSD is a stable crystalline solid and well soluble in water. In general, these agents alter or disrupt the higher regulatory activity of the CNS. It may cause the intoxicated

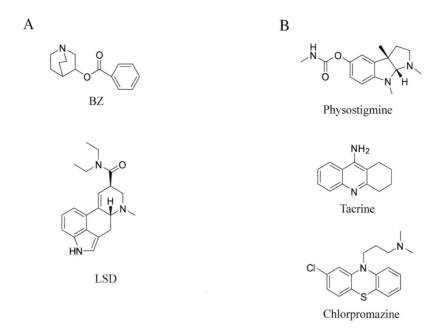

Figure 4. Incapacitating agents (A) and antidotes (B). BZ, 3-quinuclidinyl benzilate (QNB); LSD, D-lysergic acid diethylamide.

victim to ignore danger and accidentally injure himself/herself or their colleagues. The effects of incapacitating agents are temporary, but may last for hours to days. No permanent injury is sustained. These agents are not a direct cause of death.

The effects of BZ and LSD differ. BZ is a CNS depressant (cholinergic blocking agent) that interferes with the neuronal transmission of information. It impairs higher functions of the brain such as memory, problem solving and comprehension. By contrast, LSD belongs to the CNS stimulants. It causes excessive nerve activity by facilitating transmission of nerve impulses, thereby flooding the brain with too much information. The intoxicated person is unable to concentrate and no longer acts in a decisive manner.

Incapacitating agents normally enter the body *via* ingestion. However, they can also be absorbed through skin or the respiratory tract. First symptoms appear after 30 minutes to several hours and may persist for several days. Abnormal and inappropriate behavior, such as irrational statements, delusion, hallucination, dizziness, and impaired muscular coordination, dry mouth, and difficulty in swallowing, are among the general signs of intoxication. BZ can induce increases in heart rate, pupil size, and skin temperature, as well as drowsiness, dry skin, and a decrease in alertness. With increasing doses of BZ there is progressive deterioration of mental capability, ending in stupor and delirium that may last several days. The effects of LSD in the body start after 30–90 minutes. It can cause rather long-lasting psychological problems (from hours to several days), such as hallucination, depersonalization, reliving of repressed memories, and mild neuro-vegetative symptoms.

There is no specific therapy for treatment of intoxication caused by these agents. In the case of exposure to BZ, AChE inhibitors like physostigmine or tacrine derivatives are the treatment of choice (Fig. 4B). The effect of LSD can be rapidly reversed by administration of chlorpromazine [12, 13].

Blood agents

Blood agents (cyanogens) are named according to their effects on victims. They generally enter the body *via* inhalation and are distributed through blood. They interfere with the normal oxygen exchange between red blood cells and organ tissues and/or oxygen consumption within cells. Hydrogen cyanide (AC; prussic acid), cyanogen chloride (CK) and arsine (SA) are the best known members of this family (Fig. 5A).

Hydrogen cyanide and cyanogen chloride are colorless volatile liquids. Hydrogen cyanide can be disseminated in vapor or liquid form. Cyanogen chloride is disseminated as a vapor. Hydrogen cyanide smells somewhat like bitter almonds. Cyanogen chloride has a pungent biting odor. Arsine is a colorless and odorless gas. It is well soluble in solvents. All blood agents are nonpersistent in the environment. Due to a high degree of volatility, liquids of these compounds rapidly vaporize and disperse.

A   B

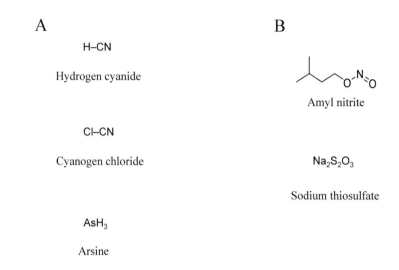

H–CN

Hydrogen cyanide

Amyl nitrite

Cl–CN

Cyanogen chloride

$Na_2S_2O_3$

Sodium thiosulfate

AsH_3

Arsine

Figure 5. Blood agents (A) and antidotes (B). Hydrogen cyanide (AC; prussic acid), cyanogen chloride (CK) and arsine (SA).

Blood agents rapidly affect essential enzyme systems that contain iron in their prosthetic group. These are, for example, enzymes that are vital in the absorption and release of oxygen or that contribute to mitochondrial electron transport chains (cytochrome c oxidase, complex IV). Since these compounds are designed to interfere with the ability of hemoglobin to carry oxygen or to block the use of oxygen by cells in the body, the poisoning primarily affects the cardiovascular and nervous systems (high oxygen demand).

Exposure to blood agents may occur by inhalation, and cyanide exposure may also occur by ingestion or absorption through skin and eyes. High concentrations of hydrogen cyanide may cause death after only a few breaths. Typical signs of intoxication by these agents are the following: increased rate and depth of breath, great difficulty of breathing (respiratory failure), dizziness, nausea, vomiting, headache, violent convulsions and cardiac symptoms (eventually leading to cardiac arrest). Arsine causes hemolysis resulting in generalized weakness, jaundice, delirium and renal failure. High doses of arsine may also result in death. In the case of blood agent intoxication, most important is the speed of the therapy. The antidotes act rapidly to reverse the toxin's action. If specific antidotes and artificial respiration/supportive care are administered soon enough, survival rates are high. There are two drugs suggested for treatment of cyanide poisoning (Fig. 5B): amyl nitrite is provided as the first measure, and then sodium thiosulfate is administered [12, 14, 15].

Lung-damaging agents

Lung-damaging agents are also known as choking agents or pulmonary agents. Their toxicity is due to their effect on lung tissue. Lung-damaging agents include phosgene (CG), chlorine (Cl) and chloropicrin (PS). The structures are shown in Figure 6.

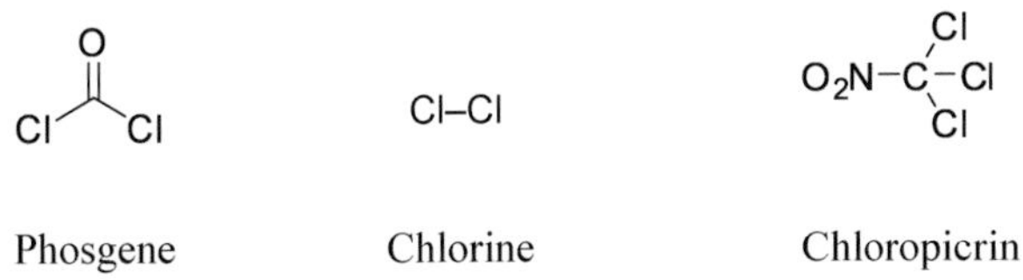

| Phosgene | Chlorine | Chloropicrin |

Figure 6. Lung-damaging agents. Phosgene (CG), chlorine (Cl) and chloropicrin (PS).

Lung-damaging agents are usually disseminated as gases. In winter conditions, phosgene is a colorless liquid (boiling point $-7.8\ ^{\circ}$C). Its odor resembles the smell of newly mowed hay or grass. Chlorine has a characteristic odor and produces immediate irritation of the respiratory system. Chloropicrin is a colorless oily liquid with high volatility. These agents are mostly present in gaseous form and do not persist in the environment.

The lung-damaging agents considered here are mainly absorbed through the respiratory system. They attack the lungs by causing extensive damage to the alveoli resulting in pulmonary edema ('dry land drowning'). This effect disables proper oxygen exchange at the air-blood vessel interface. Also other parts of the respiratory tract, trachea, bronchi, etc., may be irritated, but usually not significantly damaged. Some minor eye irritation might be observed. The damage to the lung tissue can result in secondary infection.

The most manifested signs are watering of the eyes, nausea, vomiting, uncontrollable painful coughing, choking, chest tightness, shallow and labored breathing, cyanosis, frothy sputum, clammy skin, rapid and feeble pulse, low blood pressure and delayed pulmonary edema. Possible shock can lead to death. Because no specific antidotes for poisoning by these agents are known, treatment is only symptomatic. Treatment of the resulting anoxia with oxygen is indispensible [4, 12, 16].

Riot-control agents

Riot-control agents are nonlethal compounds producing an immediate but temporary effect already at very low concentrations. These agents are divided into two groups – lacrimators (tear gases, lachrymatory gases, irritants) and vomiting agents (Fig. 7). Eyes are the main target of lacrimators. Chloracetophenone (CN), *o*-chlorobenzilidine malononitrile (CS) and dibenz[*b,f*]-1,4-oxazepine

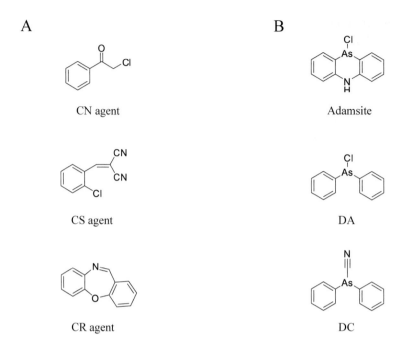

A   B

CN agent   Adamsite

CS agent   DA

CR agent   DC

Figure 7. Lacrimators (A) and vomiting agents (B). CN, chloracetophenone; CS, *o*-chlorobenzilidine malononitrile; CR, dibenz[*b,f*]-1,4-oxazepine; DM, diphenylaminochloroarsine (adamsite); DA, diphenylchloroarsine; DC, diphenylcyanoarsine.

(CR) are considered the main members of this group (Fig. 7A). Vomiting agents are the second group of riot-control agents. Main members of this group are: diphenylaminochloroarsine (adamsite, DM), diphenychloroarsine (DA), and diphenylcyanoarsine (DC) (Fig. 7B).

All lacrimators mentioned in this chapter are solids with low vapor pressure. They are dispersed as fine particles or in solutions. The vomiting agent adamsite appears as yellow to green crystals, DA as colorless crystals and DC as white solid. All compounds are poorly soluble in water.

Lacrimators and vomiting agents are mainly absorbed through the respiratory track and the eyes. The CN agent causes irritation to the upper respiratory tract and possibly also in skin. Both CS and CR induce eye pain, discomfort, excessive tearing and painful sensitivity to light. CS is considerably more potent than CN. It causes more severe respiratory symptoms. If moderate exposure occurs, signs last for minutes. In case of severe exposure, signs can take several hours. Vomiting agents cause pepper-like irritation in the upper respiratory tract, irritation of the eyes and lacrimation. Violent sneezing, coughing, nausea, vomiting, hypersalivation and malaise are also typical. The sinuses fill rapidly and violent headache occurs.

Generally, no specific therapy is required. Removal from the contaminated environment is sufficient for recovery in short time. Contaminated skin should be washed. Eyes and mouth should be rinsed with water. If headache occurs mild analgesics are recommended [3, 17, 18].

Toxins

Toxins are chemical compounds of biological origin. Following the improvement in biotechnology, the ability to produce large quantities of toxins increases. The potential misuse of toxins as CWA also increases. Toxins that are only available in small amounts in nature can be produced in large quantities using bioengineering techniques. Those toxins with high potential to be misused as warfare agents are listed below [19, 20].

Botulinum toxin and ricin

Probably the best and most widely known toxins are the macromolecules (proteins) botulinum toxin and ricin. These toxins are discussed in the next chapter of this book, 'Biological warfare agents' [20–22].

Abrin

Abrin is a phytotoxin (plant poison) that was isolated from the seeds of *Abrus precatorius* (rosary pea or jequirity pea). It is a glycoprotein with an average molecular mass of 65 kDa. It exists in two forms, abrin a and abrin b. Both are composed of two chains, i.e., A- and B-chain. Abrin can be isolated as white or yellowish-white powder or crystals. It is well soluble in water and relatively stable in the environment.

The mechanism of toxic action of abrin is identical to that of ricin. Their toxic effects are caused by entering body cells and blocking protein synthesis *via* inactivation of ribosomes. However, abrin is much more poisonous than ricin. It can be inhaled as mist or powder. Abrin particles or droplets can penetrate through skin or enter the body through the eyes. It also can be ingested as contaminant of food or water.

The symptoms of intoxication depend on the route of entry into the body and the dose received. Initial symptoms of abrin poisoning by ingestion occur within less than 6 h after exposure. If abrin is inhaled, symptoms can be recognized within 8 h. Upon ingestion abrin causes severe gastroenteritis, nausea, and vomiting, and eventually might lead to dehydration, cyanosis, circulatory collapse, hematuria, oliguria, uremia and death within 12 days. After inhalation of abrin, difficult breathing may occur, then fever, cough, nausea and tightness of the chest. Heavy sweating may follow as well as fluid accumulation in the lungs (pulmonary edema). Blood pressure and respiratory failure may cause death. Abrin is a potent irritant of skin and eyes. If skin is exposed, redness and pain will follow. Death due to abrin inhalation is mostly within 36 h after exposure.

There is no antidote available for abrin intoxication. The most important factor is getting the abrin off or out of the body as quickly as possible (flushing of stomach with activated charcoal or washing out eyes with water). Artificial ventilation, intravenous fluids and drugs treating low blood pressure can be applied [23, 24].

Aflatoxins

Aflatoxins are a group of highly toxic secondary metabolites produced mainly by certain fungi belonging to the genus *Aspergillus*, such as *A. flavus* and *A. parasiticus*. They occur mainly on cereal (maize, rice, wheat, etc.), oilseeds (soybean, sunflower, etc.), spices (chillies, black pepper, etc.), tree nuts (almonds, pistachio, etc.) and milk. *Aspergillus* contamination mostly occurs in poor and undeveloped countries.

Eighteen different types of aflatoxins are known. The types B_1, B_2, G_1, and G_2 are the most spread aflatoxins (Fig. 8). Usually, aflatoxin B_1 (AFB$_1$) is predominant. Pure AFB$_1$ is a pale-white to yellow crystalline, odorless solid. It is soluble in methanol, chloroform, acetone, and acetonitrile. The toxicity of aflatoxins decreases in the order $B_1 > G_1 > B_2$ and G_2. Aflatoxins are known as carcinogens (classified as Group 1 carcinogens), mutagens and immunosuppressants. However, they are of only limited toxicity in their original form (parent compounds). Instead, they require metabolic activation to exert toxici-

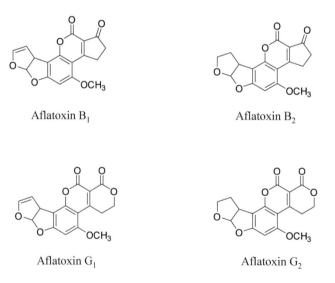

Aflatoxin B$_1$

Aflatoxin B$_2$

Aflatoxin G$_1$

Aflatoxin G$_2$

Figure 8. Aflatoxins.

ty. The product of cytochrome P450 enzyme-dependent metabolic activation can cause damage to the liver and may lead to liver cancer. Jaundice, fever, ascites, edema of the feet, and vomiting are the symptoms associated with afla-toxin intoxication (aflatoxicosis). In the case of high levels of aflatoxin inges-tion, large quantities of activated charcoal should be applied. Antioxidants may have a protective effect. Symptomatic treatment is recommended [25].

Staphylococcal enterotoxin B

Staphylococcal enterotoxins are excreted by the Gram-positive coccus *Staphylococcus aureus*, which occurs worldwide. There are seven immunologi-cally different forms of these toxins known: A, B, C_1, C_2, C_3, D and E. Staphylococcal enterotoxin B (SEB) is the most widely spread member of this family. It is one of those toxins responsible for staphylococcal food poisoning.

SEB consists of 239 amino acids and has a molecular mass of 28 kDa. It is stable in the environment and soluble in water. Moreover, it is moderately resistant to temperature. It acts by stimulating cytokine release and inflamma-tion. The onset of symptoms in staphylococcal food poisoning is usually rapid. The clinical signs include nonspecific flu-like symptoms, including fever, chills and headache. It incapacitates the intoxicated for up to 2 weeks. It can be inhaled as aerosol or ingested *via* food or water. Symptoms depend on the route of exposure. If SEB is ingested, symptoms start within several hours. Nausea, vomiting and diarrhea may occur. Since the toxin can be swallowed during mucociliary clearance, gastrointestinal signs may also occur upon exposure to aerosols. Inhalation of SEB causes nonproductive cough, chest pain and dyspnea. Signs can progress with increasing respiratory distress, hypoxia, and ultimately pulmonary edema and respiratory failure can occur. After skin contact, erythema and induration are possible. As treatment, only supportive care (artificial respiration and hydration) is possible to date [20].

T-2 toxin

Trichothecene mycotoxins are a group of secondary metabolites that are formed during growth of *Fusarium* fungi found on many crops such as corn, wheat, barley, oats, rice, etc. They are spread all over the world (Asia, Africa, South and North America, Europe). Toxin production is greatest with increased humidity and temperatures between 6 ° and 24 °C. The most known toxins of this origin are deoxynivalenol and T-2 (Fig. 9). Both compounds are sesquiterpenoids of low molecular weight.

Compared to other toxins the toxicity of trichothecenes is rather low. These compounds inhibit protein synthesis, followed by secondary disruption of DNA and RNA synthesis. Trichothecenes can enter the organism *via* inhala-tion or ingestion. They are also able to cause damage to the skin. Skin contacts

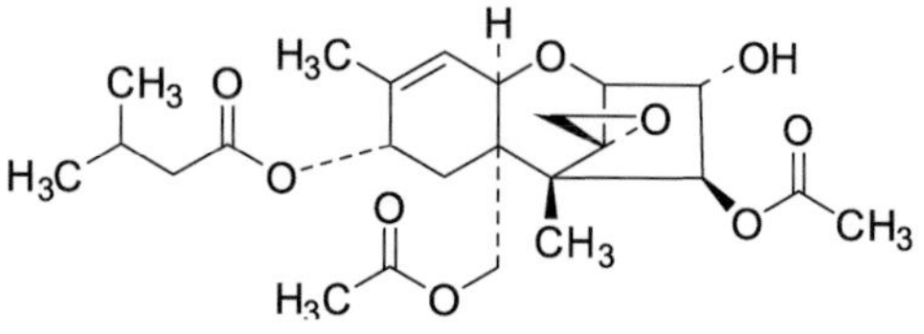

T-2 toxin

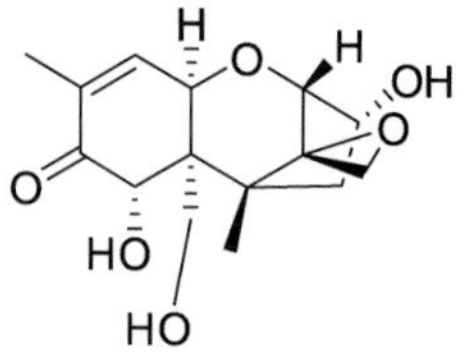

Deoxynivalenol

Figure 9. Trichothecenes.

cause redness, tenderness, blistering and necrosis. If inhaled, nasal itching and pain, sneezing, nose bleeding, watery nasal discharge, difficulty in breathing, wheezing, and coughing can occur. Nausea, vomiting, bloody diarrhea, weakness, prostration, dizziness are also possible, in some cases ending by death.

Administration of adsorbents (activated charcoal) is suggested to remove incorporated toxin. Symptomatic treatment is also recommended [26, 27].

Anatoxins

Anatoxins are toxins produced by cyanobacteria. Anatoxin-a, homoanatoxin-a and anatoxin-a(s) are the most known members of this group (Fig. 10). These toxins can enter the body *via* ingestion, inhalation and through the skin. Anatoxin-a is a small bicyclic compound, soluble in water. It binds and stimulates acetylcholine receptors and also irreversibly inhibits the enzyme AChE. Symptoms of anatoxin-a poisoning are similar to nerve agent poisoning. It acts within minutes after ingestion. Intoxication can cause twitching, muscle spasm, paralysis and respiratory arrest leading to death. The chemical structure of homoanatoxin-a is very similar to anatoxin-a, so is its mechanism of action. Anatoxin-a(s) is an AChE inhibitor of organophosphate origin. It is the only natural organophosphonate known. It has effects similar to those of nerve agents: severe cholinergic overstimulation causing salivation, lacrimation, uri-

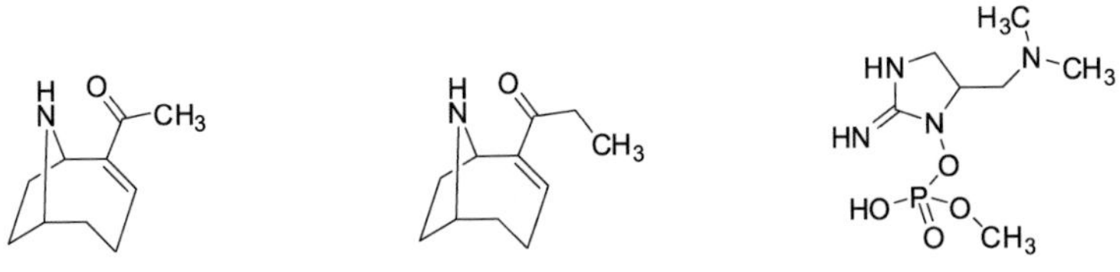

Figure 10. Anatoxins.

nary incontinence, defecation, convulsion, fasciculation and respiratory arrest. There is no specific treatment available. Only artificial respiration as supportive care is recommended [28].

Conclusion

The important groups of chemical warfare agents were introduced in this chapter. Although presented compounds are considered as tactically the most possible for terrorist misuse, many more chemicals could act as potential CWA. For example, drugs or agrochemicals originally developed for daily use could be misused as poisons in terrorist hands. Therefore, scientists working in this area of research should focus their attention to new groups of highly toxic compounds with the potential to be prepared for their pertinent misuse and to act as chemical warfare agents.

Acknowledgments
This work was supported by the Ministry of Defense (Czech Republic) – Project No. OVUOFVZ 200803.

References

1 Bajgar J (2006) *Use of Chemical Weapons and Negotiation on Their Prohibition: From History to Present Time* (In Czech), Nucleus, Hradec Kralove, Czech Republic
2 Tu AT (2002) *Chemical Terrorism: Horrors in Tokyo Subway and in Matsumoto City*, Alaken Inc., Fort Collins, CO
3 Gupta RC (2009) *Handbook of Toxicology of Chemical Warfare Agents*, Academic Press, London, UK
4 Patocka J (2004) *Military Toxicology* (In Czech), Grada, Prague, Czech Republic
5 Marrs TC (1993) Organophosphate poisoning. *Pharmacol Ther* 58: 51–66
6 Bajgar J (2004) Organophosphates/nerve agent poisoning: Mechanism of action, diagnosis, prophylaxis, and treatment. *Adv Clin Chem* 38: 151–216
7 Kassa J (2002) Review of oximes in the antidotal treatment of poisoning by organophosphorus nerve agents. *J Toxicol Clin Toxicol* 40: 803–816
8 Bajgar J, Fusek J, Kassa J, Jun D, Kuča K, Hajek P (2008) An attempt to assess functionally minimal acetylcholinesterase activity necessary for survival of rats intoxicated with nerve agents.

Chem Biol Interact 175: 281–285

9 Saladi RN, Smith E, Persaud AN (2006) Mustard: A potential agent of chemical warfare and terrorism. *Clin Exp Dermatol* 31: 1–5

10 Dacre JC, Goldman M (1996) Toxicology and pharmacology of the chemical warfare agent sulfur
mustard. *Pharmacol Rev* 48: 289–326

11 Goldman M, Dacre JC (1989) Lewisite: Its chemistry, toxicology, and biological effects. *Rev
Environ Contam Toxicol* 110: 75–115

12 Chauhan S, Chauhan S, D'Cruz R, Faruqi S, Singh KK, Varma S, Singh M, Karthik V (2008)
Chemical warfare agents. *Environ Toxicol Pharmacol* 26: 113–122

13 Passie T, Halpern JH, Stichtenoth DO, Emrich HM, Hintzen A (2008) The pharmacology of lysergic acid diethylamide: A review. *CNS Neurosci Ther* 14: 295–314

14 Lee EJ (1997) Pharmacology and toxicology of chemical warfare agents. *Ann Acad Med Singapore* 26: 104–107

15 Martin CO, Adams HP (2003) Neurological aspects of biological and chemical terrorism: A
review for neurologists. *Arch Neurol* 60: 21–25

16 Russell D, Blain PG, Rice P (2006) Clinical management of casualties exposed to lung damaging
agents: A critical review. *Emerg Med J* 23: 421–424

17 Ballantyne B (1977) The acute mammalian toxicology of dibenz[b,f]-1,4-oxazepine. *Toxicology*
8: 347–379

18 Henriksson J, Johannisson A, Bergqvist PA, Norrgren L (1996) The toxicity of organoarsenic-
based warfare agents: *In vitro* and *in vivo* studies. *Arch Environ Contam Toxicol* 30: 213–219

19 Patocka J, Hon Z, Streda L, Kuča K, Jun D (2007) Biohazard of protein biotoxins. *Def Sci J* 57:
825–837

20 Patocka J, Streda L (2006) Protein biotoxins of military significance. *Acta Medica (Hradec
Kralove)* 49: 3–11

21 Patocka J, Kuča K, Jun D (2006) Botulinum toxin: Bioterror or biomedicinal agent? *Def Sci J* 56:
189–197

22 Audi J, Belson M, Patel M, Schier J, Osterloh J (2005) Ricin poisoning: A comprehensive review.
J Am Med Assoc 294: 2342–2351

23 Dickers KJ, Bradberry SM, Rice P, Griffiths GD, Vale JA (2003) Abrin poisoning. *Toxicol Rev* 22:
137–142

24 Garber EA (2008) Toxicity and detection of ricin and abrin in beverages. *J Food Prot* 71:
1875–1883

25 Bennett JW, Klich M (2003) Mycotoxins. *Clin Microbiol Rev* 16: 497–516

26 Dohnal V, Jezkova A, Jun D, Kuča K (2008) Metabolic pathways of T-2 toxin. *Curr Drug Metab*
9: 77–82

27 Williams PP (1989) Effects of T-2 mycotoxin on gastrointestinal tissues: A review of *in vivo* and
in vitro models. *Arch Environ Contam Toxicol* 18: 374–387

28 Osswald J, Rellán S, Gago A, Vasconcelos V (2007) Toxicology and detection methods of the
alkaloid neurotoxin produced by cyanobacteria, anatoxin-a. *Environ Int* 33: 1070–1089

Molecular, Clinical and Environmental Toxicology. Volume 2: Clinical Toxicology
Edited by A. Luch

Biological warfare agents

Miroslav Pohanka and Kamil Kuča

Center of Advanced Studies and Department of Toxicology, University of Defense, Hradec Kralove, Czech Republic

Abstract. Biological warfare agents are a group of pathogens and toxins of biological origin that can be potentially misused for military or criminal purposes. The present review attempts to summarize necessary knowledge about biological warfare agents. The historical aspects, examples of applications of these agents such as anthrax letters, biological weapons impact, a summary of biological warfare agents and epidemiology of infections are described. The last section tries to estimate future trends in research on biological warfare agents.

Introduction

The threat of misuse of weapons of mass destruction has changed after termination of the Cold War. We can distinguish between nuclear, biological and chemical weapons (NBC) as the main categories of weapons of mass destruction. The first, nuclear, are typical for superpowers; the two last are bogies of asymmetric war. The term "bioterrorism" has now appeared [1]. Due to low cost of production of chemical and biological weapons, these are also referred to as "weapons of the poor".

Two terms should be clarified: Biological weapons and biological warfare agents (BWA). A biological weapon is applicable as a military device. It consists of a technical part that enables germ particles, and biological warfare and reagent-stabilizing agents to be disseminated under outdoor environmental conditions. Transmission of BWA is typically based on spraying, contamination of food or water, or dispersion through conventional explosives [2].

The present chapter summarizes the most important facts about BWA. It is divided into sections relating to common knowledge on BWA and examples of the most relevant BWA. For better evenness, non-viable BWA (toxins) such as ricin and botulotoxin are presented on a similar scale to the viable BWA (pathogens).

Some historical aspects

The application of biological weapons is not a novel idea. Attempts to use infectious diseases as a weapon were made in ancient civilizations through contamination of food or drinking water. In 1346, during the battle for the seaport city of Kaffa located in today's Ukraine, the Tatar forces catapulted plaque victims into the city in order to spread this disease [3, 4]. This event had terrible consequences when Genoese merchants escaping from Kaffa spread bubonic plague inside Europe in 1348 [5]. Misuse of plague was also perpetrated by Russian soldiers who catapulted plague-infected corpses into the Estonian town Reval held by Swedish enemies in 1710. Another method of biological warfare was carried out by the British colonial army in North America. When smallpox occurred in the crew at Fort Pitt in 1763, captain Ecuyer spread this infection among the Native American population unsympathetic to the British during the Pontiac's Rebellion using contaminated blankets and handkerchiefs. The effect of infection was amplified due to the immunological naivety of Native Americans [6].

The period of World War I is known for massive application of chemical weapons. BWA were not typical during this period. However, the potency of biological weapons was well recognized and there was attempt to prevent its use. The convention called *"Protocol for the prohibition of the use in war of asphyxiating, poisonous or other gases, and of bacteriological methods of warfare"* was result of this effort. It was signed by many countries in 1925 and entered into force in February 1928. Since the convention did not include prohibition of the development, production and storage of biological weapons, the practical impact was reduced [7].

In the period of 1930s and 1940s, some powers escalated their potency to produce biological weapons. The largest research and production facilities were built by the Japanese in the infamous Unit 731 in occupied China. The Unit 731 was localized in Manchuria from 1932 until the end of the World War II. The staff of around 3000, comprising mostly scientists and technicians, was responsible for extensive efforts in research and development. For realization of their targets they carried out trials on humans, including prisoners in the Beiyinhe jail. At least 10 000 prisoners lost their lives due to these tests [8].

The period after World War II was influenced by the hegemony of two superpowers. The United States built facilities in Fort Detrick and Pine Bluff. Development of military facilities in former Soviet Union is still unclear, partially due to the high level of security and hiding of these activities behind a screen of civilian biotechnology research [9]. Only some sporadic testimonies are known. The most complex one was given by Ken Alibek in his book: *"Biohazard: The chilling true story of the largest covert biological weapons program in the world"*. Soviet production of biological weapons continued even after the year 1972 when a new convention *"The United Nations Convention on the prohibition of the development, production, and stockpiling of bacteriological and toxin weapons and their destruction"* was ratified by many countries including Soviet Union and United States.

Another chapter of in the history of biological weapons concerns terrorist activities, such as that made by the Rajneeshee community in Oregon. The followers of Bhagwan Shree Rajneesh contaminated salad bars at two restaurants by *Salmonella* sp. inoculation. They wanted to manipulate the upcoming elections. Without this action, according to their belief, the results of the election might prevent them from developing their community into a world headquarter [10]. Unsuccessful attempts to use *Bacillus anthracis*, *Vibrio cholerae* and botulinum toxin to construct their own biological weapons were made by the Aum Shinrikyo cult in Japan. They even sent their members to Africa to collect samples of the Ebola virus [11]. Aum Shinrikyo executed nine different biological attacks. In 1993, they attempted to release aerosolized clouds of *B. anthracis* from the roof of the building of their cult headquarters in Kameido, near Tokyo. Fortunately, they were unsuccessful due to dissemination of the non-virulent strain Sterne 34F2, which is normally used for animal vaccination against anthrax [12]. After these failures they used the nerve agent sarin in the Tokyo subway system in 1995, resulting in 12 deaths and approximately 3800 injured, an event that made them notorious. Successful attempts to misuse the virulent strain of *B. anthracis* would be more horrific in their consequences. Here, the sending out of so-called "anthrax letters", i.e., letters prepared with purified spores of *B. anthracis*, has been widely recognized. This case is described in a separate section below.

Handling of BWA

Handling of BWA is very dangerous. This is partly due to complicated detection of leaked microorganisms and only gradual manifestation of disease symptoms when compared with toxic compounds. Unwanted release of BWA could lead to tragic consequences. The Sverdlovsk tragedy is an example of such a disaster: fully virulent spores of *B. anthracis* were released from a military facility in the Russian city Sverdlovsk in 1979, resulting in many deaths [13, 14].

Many devices can protect staff when handling BWA. There are laws for protection that are valid in certain countries, e.g., in the European Union: the Council Directive of 26 November 1990 on the protection of workers from risks related to exposure to biological agents at work (90/979/EEC). The main mechanism of protection comes from two kinds of barriers: the first barrier divides staff from the samples to be handled. This could be laminar boxes, special suits, and other tools separating laboratory workers from samples. An image of a laminar box is shown in Figure 1. The second barrier protects surroundings from pertinent contamination inside the laboratory. This could be special walls such as stainless steel armor, special ventilation with air disinfected by UV lamps and closed with high efficiency particulate air (HEPA) filters, and sterilizing of waste. Manipulation of unknown samples should not contain any steps producing aerosol particles or leading to sample spurt.

A common criterion for laboratory protection estimation is called the biological safety level (BSL). Four values are attributed (1–4), described as follows:

- BSL 1 is a laboratory appropriate for handling of microorganisms that are not hazardous for human life or health. Such a laboratory can be run by adhering to the rules of common microbiological safety and hygienic fundamentals.

- BSL 2 is appropriate for handling of microorganisms with limited virulence, i.e., virulent in immunologically insufficient and elderly people. These microorganisms are common in the environment and/or its virulence can be suppressed in vaccinated individuals. Hazardous manipulation of samples such as those potentially producing aerosols should be performed in digesters. Although BSL 2 is technically on a similar level as BSL 1, some safety procedures such as disinfection and wearing of gloves are necessary.
- BSL 3 is a laboratory suitable for manipulation, cultivation and analysis of causative agents of serious diseases. Vaccines or regular treatments for the disease should be available. Greater technological demands compared with BSL 2 are required, e.g., exhaust air must be filtered, the inside of laboratories is under lower pressure, laboratory staff must wear special protective clothing.
- BSL 4 is a laboratory suitable for work with all microorganisms including those causing diseases that are not curable and not protectable by vaccines. BSL 4 has further improvements in comparison with BSL 3. In particular, entrance into laboratories is through two doors with special disinfection measures. The two doors are electronically protected to suppress simultaneous opening. All material including waste, air, and cadavers leaving the

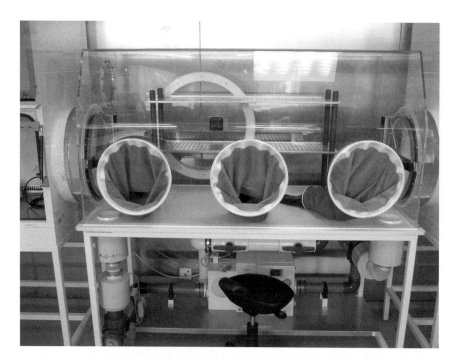

Figure 1. Special digester used in a BSL 4 lab.

laboratory have to be sterilized. Personal protection suits are supplied by air and should be slightly pressurized.

Categories of agents

In principle, all known pathogens or toxins could potentially be used for biological weapon construction. At least 1400 infectious organisms including more than 200 viral and 500 bacterial species are virulent to humans [15]. However, only few of them have been found really effective for biological weapon construction. Although we can use many of distinguishing scales, the one most frequently used comes from the Centers for Disease Control and Prevention (CDC; http://www.bt.cdc.gov). CDC divides BWA into three categories (A–C) according to its virulence and easiness of pertinent production:

- Category A: Agents that are easily disseminated or transmitted from person to person resulting in high mortality rates. Agents in this category represent serious risk when misused for military and/or criminal activities.
- Category B: Agents that exert low mortality but could be moderately easy disseminated.
- Category C: Pathogens (and toxins) that could be engineered for mass dissemination in the future; however, their actual virulence or elaborative dissemination would not allow mass application.

Another useful classification was made by the Australia Group (http://www. australiagroup.net). This organization has members from 30 countries (including EU countries, Japan, the United States, Canada etc.). The Australia Group was founded in 1985 as a reaction to the application of chemical weapons in the Iran-Iraq War. The Group has established common export controls for chemical and biological weapons for non-proliferation purposes. The control is also focused on dual-use biological equipment and related technology, such as complete BSL 3 or 4 containment facilities, fermenters having capacity greater than 20 L, centrifugal separators including decanters and flowraters greater than 100 L per hour, aerosol inhalation chambers with capacity greater than 1 m^3, devices for aerosol production, etc. The BWA are divided into biological agents (human pathogens), plant pathogens, and animal pathogens. The most important virulent organisms are:

- Viral BWA: chikungunya virus, Congo-Crimean hemorrhagic fever virus, Dengue fever virus, Eastern equine encephalitis virus, Ebola virus, Hantaan virus, Junin virus, Lassa fever virus, Lymphocytic choriomeningitis virus, Machupo virus, Marburg virus, Monkey pox virus, Rift Valley fever virus, Russian Spring-Summer encephalitis virus, Variola virus, Venezuelan equine encephalitis virus, White pox, Yellow fever virus, Japanese encephalitis virus, Kyasanur Forest virus, Louping ill virus, Murray Valley encephalitis virus, Omsk hemorrhagic fever virus, Oropouche virus, Powassan virus, Rocio virus, St Louis encephalitis virus, Hendra virus,

South American hemorrhagic fever, Pulmonary – renal syndrome – hemorrhagic fever viruses, Nipah virus.
- Rickettsial BWA: *Coxiella burnetii, Bartonella quintana, Rickettsia
  prowazeki, Rickettsia rickettsii.*
- Bacterial BWA: *Bacillus anthracis, Brucella abortus, Brucella melitensis,
  Brucella suis, Chlamydia psittaci, Clostridium botulinum, Francisella
  tularensis, Burkholderia mallei, Burkholderia pseudomallei, Salmonella
  typhi, Shigella dysenteriae, Vibrio cholerae, Yersinia pestis, Clostridium
  perfringens* (producing epsilon toxin), *Escherichia coli* serotype O157.
- Toxins: botulotoxin (botulinum toxin), *Clostridium perfringens* toxins, conotoxin, ricin, saxitoxin, shiga toxin, *Staphylococcus aureus* toxin, tetrodotoxin, verotoxin, microcystin, aflatoxins, abrin, cholera toxin, diacetoxyscirpenol toxin, T-2 toxin, HT-2 toxin, modeccin toxin, volkensin toxin, viscumin.

Diseases whose causative organisms have been considered as potential biological agents are also enlisted in Annex A of the NATO Handbook on the
Medical Aspects of NBC Defensive Operations [16]. When evaluating the
risks of BWA, military threat has to be distinguished from terrorist or criminal
acts. The most frequently known microorganisms and their normal characteristics are compiled in Table 1. According to the CDC the most serious agents
(category A) are *B. anthracis, Clostridium botulinum* toxin, *Yersinia pestis,
Variola major, F. tularensis,* and viruses causing hemorrhagic fevers (such as
Ebola, Marburg or Machupo). Other agents such as ricin toxin, *Staphylococcal*
enterotoxin B and *Brucella* sp. are often noted, but the CDC evaluated them as
less important (category B). Selected BWA are indicated in Table 1.

Table 1. Potential biological weapon agents (BWA) and resulting diseases. The most commonly noted
agents are mentioned. The entire category A and parts of category B according to CDC are listed. A
pulmonary intake of aerosol is taken for infection dose

Agent	Disease	Infection dose	Taxonomy	Category according to CDC
Bacillus anthracis	Anthrax	8000–40 000 spores	Bacterial	A
Brucella melitensis	Brucellosis	10–100 organisms	Bacterial	B
Francisella tularensis	Tularemia	10–50 organisms	Bacterial	A
Yersinia pestis	Plaque	<100 organisms	Bacterial	A
Rickettsia prowazekii	Epidemic typhus	Spreading by vector	Rickettsial	B
Variola major	Smallpox	10–100 organisms	Viral	A
Hemorrhagic fever viruses	Ebola, Marburg, Lassa, Dengue, etc	1–10 organisms	Viral	A
Botulinum toxin (from *Clostridium botulinum*)	Botulism	0.001 µg/kg (LD$_{50}$)	Bacterial toxin	A
Ricin (from *Ricinus communis*)	Ricin poisoning	3–5 µg/kg (LD$_{50}$)	Plant toxin	B

Expected impact of biological weapons

Biological weapons are easy and cheap to produce. The cost-effect of conventional, chemical and nuclear weapons has been compared with biological weapons [16]: 50% casualties/km^2 cost about $2000 for conventional, $800 for nuclear, $600 for chemical and $1 for biological weapons. Another characteristic is the mass needed for delivery: per square kilometer, 1–5 kg of a biological weapon would be capable of producing the same number of casualties as 500 kg of a chemical weapon. These parameters are only approximates but explain the inherent danger of biological weapons in the hands of terrorists and totalitarian states. Scientists from the CDC came up with a hypothetical model of a North American suburb with 100 000 inhabitants exposed in the target area [17]; attack by *B. anthracis* spores, *Francisella tularensis* and *Brucella melitensis* 5-μm aerosol particles was considered. The needed prophylaxis program was calculated approximately for 420 000–1 490 000 participants if any of these given agents were used. Per 100 000 exposed inhabitants, the following numbers were predicted: 50 000 cases of anthrax inhalation with 32 875 deaths due to *B. anthracis*; 82 500 cases of tularemia with 6188 deaths due to *F. tularensis*; and 82 500 cases of brucellosis with 413 deaths due to *B. melitensis*. The expected economic impact could reach $Mio 579.4 for brucellosis, $Mio 5402.4 for tularemia and $Mio 26 204.1 for anthrax. Kaufmann and coworkers also expressed the necessity of the fast start of prophylaxis program. For example, delaying the initiation of prophylaxis for anthrax until days 4–6 after attack would result in additional net losses of $Mio 13.4–283.1. These conclusions, among others, call attention to the military possibilities of biological weapons as well as to the importance of their timely detection.

The most important agents

In the frame of this chapter it is impossible to present all potential BWA. The best known representatives of BWA are explained in more detail below. All agents enlisted into category A according the CDC and some of category B agents are presented. The most relevant toxins enlisted as BWA are also mentioned. Instead of elaborating on the virulent organism, those that produce toxins are described by keeping the focus on the toxin itself.

When toxins are considered as biological agents, it is surprising that many of the pathogens such as *B. anthracis* are not fully virulent when the genetic information for toxin production is suppressed [18, 19]. This fact points to the complexity in infection progression. Only small changes in the genetic information could reduce or, on the other hand, heighten the virulence. *F. tularensis* represents an example. This is one of the most serious BWA; however, the mutant called light vaccine strain (LVS) would cause infection in rodents but would fail to cause serious infection in humans due to the manifestation of antigens triggering long-memory B lymphocytes [20, 21].

Bacillus anthracis

B. anthracis is a large, spore-forming, Gram-positive, non-motile bacterium [22]. It grows under aerobic conditions. The vegetative bacillus is relatively large, rod-shaped; the longest side is as much as 10 μm long [23]. *B. anthracis* forms endospores, and cultivation is quite easy. Spores are stable for a long period even under outdoor conditions. Titbal et al. [24] described their resistance to physical conditions and survival up to 200 years. Isolation of *B. anthracis* and description of their properties were carried out by two famous scientists, Robert Koch and Louis Pasteur. The life cycle of *B. anthracis* was described by Robert Koch in 1876 [25].

B. anthracis is the causative agent of anthrax disease. Anthrax is a zoonosis infecting domesticated as well as wild animals. A typical reservoir is in herbivore populations. The disease is easily transmittable to humans. With inadequate prophylaxis, a large-scale epidemic could easily arise. The well-known Plague of Athens (430–417) is suspected to have been an epidemic caused by inhalational anthrax [26], although other theories have been stated [27]. Three forms of the disease can be found. The most typical is the cutaneous form. It is caused by spores penetrating into skin and resulting in dermal ulcers. Gastrointestinal anthrax is a form that can occur after consuming poorly cooked meat contaminated with *B. anthracis* spores. Intestinal ulcers are followed by spreading of *B. anthracis* into the lymphatic system, causing septicemia. Pulmonary anthrax is the third form. This occurs after inhalation of spores. This would be the most likely form if *B. anthracis* were to be misused for military purposes. Although the first symptoms look like influenza, the fast progression of anthrax would continue. Mortality for pulmonary anthrax is very high. The disease can be treated with penicillin; however, some strains of *B. anthracis* were found being β-lactamase positive. The drugs ciprofloxacin, erythromycin, tetracyclin, doxycycline and chloramphenicol are widely recommended [28].

The virulence of *B. anthracis* is increased due to secretion of anthrax toxin [29]. The plasmid pX01 region of the bacillus is involved in the production of the anthrax toxin [30]. The anthrax toxin is composed of three proteins [31]: a edema factor necessary for causing edema, a protective antigen that supports the penetration of edema factor, and the lethal factor operating inside the cell [32]. The lethal factor proteolytically cleaves MAPK-activating enzymes [33, 34]. Both the lethal factor and the protective antigen together constitute the lethal toxin.

Brucella melitensis

In the past *B. melitensis* has undergone several taxonomic changes. The older name *Micrococcus melitensis* can still be found in the literature. *B. melitensis* belong to Gram-negative, typically rod-shaped bacilli. No spore formation has been observed. The viable cells are non-motile. *B. melitensis* as well as three other species (*B. suis*, *B. abortus* and *B. canis*) can cause the disease known as brucellosis; brucellosis caused by *B. melitensis* is the most serious form for humans. The proteome of *B. melitensis* virulent strain 16 M has been fully characterized [35].

The British Army physician David Bruce firstly isolated *B. melitensis* in 1887. Brucellosis is a zoonotic disease and for this reason it is a naturally occurring human infection caused by eating infected food products, especially by drinking infected milk, or by inhalation of aerosols containing the bacilli; low infection doses of 10–100 CFU can cause disease. Person to person spread is uncommon [36]. The application of *B. melitensis* as a BWA has been tried several times mainly due to low infection doses. The incubation period is relatively long; typically 5–60 days and occasionally even more [37]. The long incubation period was considered as main discriminating parameter for utilizing *B. melitensis* in biological weapon construction. Brucellosis is incapacitating rather than killing. Case fatality is about 2%. Symptoms of brucellosis are nonspecific, sometimes asymptomatic. Some somatic complaints such as weakness, body aches and anorexia could occur. Brucellosis is curable by antibiotic treatment with drugs such as tetracyclines, fluoroquinones, streptomycin and gentamycin [38, 39]. For humans, no vaccine is available but the strains RB-51, RB-19 and REV-1 can be used as a live vaccine for veterinary purposes. A DNA-based vaccine (encoding the outer membrane protein 31) for brucellosis has been recently tested in a mouse model [40]. Although *B. melitensis* was one of the first agents used in biological weapon construction, the CDC enlisted *B. melitensis* into category B, not category A (see above).

Francisella tularensis

F. tularensis is a small, non-motile, Gram-negative bacterium. It is facultative anaerobic. It was firstly isolated in the 1910s near the Californian town Tulare [41]. The human disease was recognized by Edward Francis in 1922 [42]. The name *Francisella tularensis* was chosen as honor to Dr. Francis and the place where it was first isolated. *F. tularensis* belongs to the group of highly infectious pathogens and it is enrolled into CDC category A of BWA. There are several subspecies of *F. tularensis* described in the literature. *F. tularensis* subspecies *tularensis* (type A; also referred to as subspecies *nearctica* by investigators in the former Soviet Union) is the most virulent. It is capable of metabolizing glycerol as well as L-citruline. This subspecies is endemic in North America, and sporadic isolates have been seen in Europe [43, 44]. *F. tularensis* ssp. *holarctica* (type B; formerly referred to as *palaearctica* or *palearctica* in some sources) is less virulent and unable to metabolize glycerol and L-citruline [45, 46]. The other two subspecies, *mediaasiatica* and *novicida* are virulent in only limited scale. The virulence of *F. tularensis mediaasiatica* is very low despite extensive similarity to subspecies *tularensis* [47, 48].

F. tularensis is the cause of the serious zoonotic disease tularemia (sometimes spelled 'tularaemia'). The natural reservoirs of tularemia are rodents and lagomorphs [49–51]. It was found that about 2.1–2.8% of the ticks *Dermacentor reticulatus* are vectors of *F. tularensis holarctica* in the Czech Republic and Austria [52]. Another study proposed that approximately 5% of rodents in China are serologically positive to tularemia [53]. Extreme virulence was documented when 15 people were infected by tularemia disseminated through contaminated fur when a dog shook itself during dinner [54]. Typical manifestations of infection are ulceroglandular, glandular, oculoglandular, oropharyngeal, pneumonic, typhoidal, and septic forms [55]. The long-term mortality in the US for tularemia is estimated to be 1.4% [56]. The immune reaction to tularemia progress is quite fast as the agent has only a short incubation period [57]. Several antibodies are recommended for treatment of tularemia. The antibiotics streptomycin, gentamycin, tetracycline, and chloramphenicol could be applied [58].

Rickettsia prowazekii

R. prowazekii is a small, Gram-negative microorganism. *R. prowazekii* as well as the entire genus *Rickettsia* had been considered for a long time to be a bacterial microorganism, but a lot of oddities were found. *Rickettsia* has a small genome [59] and about a quarter of the genome does not encode for anything. The *Rickettsia* genus has defect metabolizing pathways and is fully dependent on the host cell. For cultivation of *Rickettsia,* procedures typical for virus cultivation are used – infected yolk sacs of embryonated chicken eggs [60, 61]. Investigation of the rRNA genes showed that they are not typical for eubacteria, but extensive similarity to mitochondria of eukaryotic cells was found [62].

R. prowazekii is the causative agent of the most serious variant of typhus – epidemic typhus (also called louse-borne or classic typhus). This disease has been known since ancient times. Outbreaks of epidemic typhus frequently started at prisons, military and refugee camps or in cities with poor hygiene. This disease is transmitted by a body louse (*Pediculus humanus corporis*). In contrast, endemic typhus infections caused by *R. typhi* or *R. felis* are transmitted by fleas. Epidemic typhus is the most serious form of typhus with an extremely high mortality of 10–30%, sometimes even near 70% when the disease remains untreated [63]. The first symptoms start about 10 days after infection. The fever arises quite fast and may reach 40 °C, accompanied by pain, stiffness and headache [64]. After further 5 days a dark red rash appears all over the body. Antibiotics such as tetracycline or chloramphenicol are quite effective against typhus [65]. In this context, it is important to refer to confusing nomenclature. The bacteria *Salmonella typhimurium* and *S. typhi* are the causative agents of typically food-borne diseases which in some form are called typhoid fevers. Typhus and typhoid fever are completely different diseases.

Yersinia pestis

The coccobacillus *Y. pestis* is a non-motile, slowly growing, Gram-negative bacterium from the family *Enterobacteriaceae*. It was also known for a long time as *Pasteurella pestis*. The natural reservoirs of *Y. pestis* are rodents [66]. The transmission of *Y. pestis* is moderated by fleas able to bite humans and other mammals. The fleas known to transmit *Y. pestis* are *Xenopsylla cheopis* and *Ctenocephalides felis* [67–69]. The species *Y. pestis* is divided into three subtypes, or biovars: *antiqua*, *mediaevalis*, and *orientalis*. Each of them is fully pathogenic [70, 71].

Y. pestis is the causative agent of the plague. Plague has strongly influenced human history since ancient times. For instance, the Justinian plague epidemic affected Mediterranean Europe and Egypt in A.D. 541 [72], and the "Black Death" epidemic impact in 1347–1351 resulted in up to 40% casualties across the European populations [73]. Plague has an incubation period of 2–6 days. Typical symptoms are fever, malaise, nausea, vomiting, and diarrhea [74]. Bubonic plague is initiated by the bite an infected flea. One extremely serious form of plague is the pneumonic form; it is transmitted by inhalation of respiratory droplets exhaled by sick individuals [75]. The antibiotics streptomycin and tetracyclines are applicable for treatment; penicillin is partially effective for this form, but completely ineffective for treatment of extended plague [76].

Orthopoxvirus variola

Orthopoxvirus variola (variola virus) is a DNA virus. The virions are relatively large (about 200 nm in diameter) [77]. Even non-enveloped particles are infectious. Virions are released by disruption of the host cell. Virus replication is localized in cytoplasm; the transcription is mediated by a virion-associated DNA-dependent RNA polymerase [78].

The variola virus is the causative agent of the disease smallpox. There are two forms of variola virus: major and minor. The minor form is much milder, with a case fatality rate of about 1%. Variola major is most dangerous, with a case fatality rate of about 30% [79]. Smallpox spread gradually over the whole world. It was introduced to Europe in the early Middle Ages. The year 1796 was a big milestone in known smallpox history. Edward Jenner demonstrated that vaccination with cowpox was able to protect vaccinated individuals against smallpox. A vaccination campaign initiated by the World Health Organization (WHO) in the 1960s has resulted in its eradication. The last case of smallpox was observed in Bangladesh in 1975 [80]. Official eradication was proclaimed on 8 May 1980. Only two laboratories were allowed to keep stocks of variola virus: the Institute of Virus Preparations in the Soviet Union (today Russia) and the CDC in the US.

The disease was typically spread between persons *via* droplets; transmission through direct contact was also possible in some cases. After an incubation period of 7–17 days, high fever commonly with malaise started abruptly. The maculopapular rash appeared after a further 1–2 days. During this phase patients became most infectious. The scabs appeared approximately 25 days after infection. Patients with scabs were no longer a vehicle of infection [81], but remained lifelong immune from further infection. Antiviral substances exerted disputable effect. Applicable drugs were, for example, adenine or cytosine arabinoside [82, 83].

Hemorrhagic fever viruses

Hemorrhagic fever viruses (HFVs) are a group of enveloped RNA viruses and the cause of the so-called viral hemorrhagic fevers (VHFs). They belong to several families [84]: *Arenaviridae* (Venezuelan hemorrhagic fever, Lassa fever, etc.), *Bunyaviridae* (Crimean-Congo hemorrhagic fever – CCHF, Rift Valley fever, etc.), *Filoviridae* (Ebola, Marburg, etc.), *Flaviviridae* (yellow fever, Dengue, Omsk hemorrhagic fever, etc.), *Paramycoviridae* (Hendra virus disease, Nipah virus encephalitis, etc.). VHFs are zoonotic diseases with natural reservoirs in rodents and arthropods such as rats, mice and other rodents, ticks and mosquitoes. VHFs are transmittable to humans *via* contact with contaminated urine, fecal or body excretions or *via* arthropod bites [85]. HFVs are present all over the world including developed countries, but have highest observed incidence in poor countries, especially in Africa [86]. The natural reservoirs as well as the transmission mechanisms are not yet fully known [87].

Symptoms of VHFs are high fever, commonly with exhaustion, and patients with serious progression may bleed under the skin and from body orifices such as mouth, eyes or ears [88, 89]. There is no effective vaccine against VHFs. Treatments with antiviral medication is limited. Partial reduction of mortality caused by Lassa fever and some others *Arenaviruses* has been achieved by applying ribavirin [90]. Continuous effort to prepare effective vaccines is being carried out but as yet with only limited success [91].

Botulinum toxin

Botulinum toxin is a neurotoxic protein produced as secondary metabolite by the obligate anaerobe, spore-forming bacterium *Clostridium botulinum* and some strains of *C. baratii* and *C. butyricum* [92, 93]. Botulinum toxin is one of the most poisonous toxins, with an LD_{50} of 0.001 µg/kg [94]. Its polypeptide structure consists of two chains: the 100 kDa heavy and the 50 kDa light chain. The light chain represents a Zn^{2+}-dependent endopeptidase [95]. Several botulinum toxin types exist: A–G. The toxin blocks acetylcholine release into neurosynapses. Botulinum toxin B, D, F and G interact with synaptobrevin; A, C and E affect SNAP25; and type C affects syntaxin [96]. The toxin is stable in water for several days. On the other side, it can be inactivated by heating at >85 °C for 5 min; moreover, heating could also kill the bacterium *C. botulinum* [97]. The commercial form of botulinum toxin A – Botox, is been used for cosmetic purposes and for medical treatment of blepharospasms and/or hemifacial spasms.

First symptoms of poisoning by botulinum toxin can occur after 2 h, but more typically after 12–72 h [98]. Patients with botulism suffer from neurological impairments of sight, speech and/or swallowing. Muscular paralysis can extend into total weakness, hypotonia and eventually into respiratory distress [99]. Patients are afebrile but secondary infection can occur. Fortunately, botulinum toxin does not penetrate into central nervous parenchyma (brain). Treatment of botulism consists of supportive care and immunization with an anti-toxin [100]. A pentavalent (ABCDE) botulinum toxoid is effective as a vaccine against botulinum toxin [101], and this toxoid is actually distributed by CDC for laboratory staff at risk.

Ricin

Ricin is a toxin from the castor bean plant (*Ricinus communis*). The LD_{50} of ricin is 3–5 µg/kg [102]. The protein (lectin) ricin consists of two parts (A and B), each with molecular mass of about 30 kDa, linked to each other through disulfide bonds. Part A interferes with the ribosome as a glycosidase, thereby blocking translation in the poisoned cell. Part B is necessary for the penetration of part A into the cell [103, 104]. Ricin can be inactivated by heating at 140 °C for 20 min. Its purification from castor beans is simple; aqueous extraction at low pH is followed by sodium sulfate precipitation.

Poisoning by ricin causes inhibition of protein synthesis. Long-term exposure results in organ damage. An immune response to ricin has been described [105]. The effects of ricin are not only disadvantageous. Application of ricin as a treatment for cancer seems possible. Ricin has the capability to induce apoptosis [106]. It acts specifically on malignant cells *in situ* when linked to monoclonal antibodies [107].

Anthrax letters: A recent example of biological weapons menace

Shortly after the World Trade Center tragedy in 2001, the US postal system was abused for the distribution of lethal *B. anthracis* spores [108]. The panic that broke out was surprising. According to the FBI, the perpetrator has not been captured until today. Altogether five letters were sent [109]. The first two letters were sent to NBC television in New York and to the New York Post on 18 September 2001. Nobody died but some people became sick. These letters were not very high-leveled considering purity of the agent; they contained spores with about 10% purity. Here one of the most virulent strains of natural

B. anthracis, the Ames strain was used [110]. Its identity was confirmed subsequently by comparative genome sequencing and single nucleotide polymorphism pattern [111].

The other three letters were sent to Florida's tabloid newspaper 'The Sun' and to the Washington D.C. offices of Senators Leahy and Daschle at 9 October 2001. The most alarming information came from the included particles. Those *B. anthracis* samples contained pure spores (meaning microbial purity, as opposed to vegetative cells) prepared as chemically stabilized homogenous 10-μm particles. The particle size is one of the most critical characteristics for deposition of biological weapons in the lungs with 10 μm being appropriate in this regard. Settling of bacterial cells in lung after envelope opening has been studied in a swine model to explore risk factors [112], and viability of spores in aerosols has also been extensively studied [113]. The preparation by milling was discussed. However, preparation by spray-drying, a more sophisticated method, is more likely. Altogether 5 people died after exposure to manipulated letters and nearly 20 were infected. The letters were tightly closed and the paper served as a filter for aerosol. No connection between the perpetrator and Al Qaida or any totalitarian regime has been proved. One of the suspects, Dr. Steven Hatfill was compensated for accusation in August 2008. The prime suspect Dr. Bruce E. Ivins committed suicide in July 2008. Both suspected scientists were employed in the US Army Medical Research Institute of Infectious Diseases (USA MRIID). Guilt for the anthrax letters has not been unambiguously proven in any case; some conspiratory theories arose [114].

Future trends

The search for methods to protect civilians as well as soldiers against biological weapon fulmination remains current. Some trends are typical in this field. Protective activities can be divided into topics such as biological crisis management, detection and identification, prophylaxis and treatment.

Biological crisis management is a continuous effort to predict crisis events, and to attempt to eliminate technological failures leading to and/or amplifying crisis. The further trends are based on prevention of hysteria accompanying crisis [115]. Sophisticated input data are unnecessary for prediction of biological weapons impact. In particular, infection through aerosolized particles is extensively studied in appropriate models [116, 117] to find effective protection [118]. The safety of civilians in transit and buildings and protection of selected objects is currently being considered by local governments.

Extensive effort is also being made towards early detection and identification of BWA. Improvement of commonly available devices as well as development of new methods are being widely carried out [119, 120]. In particular, methods and parameters of the polymerase chain reaction (PCR) have gradually matured and could provide unique and valuable information [121, 122].

Recent research has also been aimed at construction of biosensors [123]. These devices are considered to be approaches suitable for either detection of BWA [124, 125] or diagnosis of diseases [126–128].

Other approaches broadly considered refer to improvements in treatment, prophylaxis and vaccination. Better vaccines may save lives of the intervening staff. Extensive progress has been made in this field during recent years [129]. Selection of suitable antibiotics and finding of optimal dosage conditions is also being investigated [130].

Gradual improvements in current methods for detection, identification, prophylaxis and treatment are expected in the future. Although no massive armament is perceived at the present time, the challenges of the potential misuse of BWA in the frame of criminal activities as well as naturally occurring epidemics related to these pathogens strongly call for continuation of these research efforts.

Acknowledgments
The project No. FVZ0000604 of the Czech Republic Ministry of Defense is gratefully acknowledged.

References

1 Kortepeter MG, Cieslak TJ, Eitzen EM (2001) Bioterrorism. *J Environ Health* 63: 21–24
2 Agarwal R, Shukla SK, Dharmani S, Gandhi A (2004) Biological warfare – An emerging threat. *J Assoc Physicians India* 52: 733–738
3 Christopher GW, Cieslak TJ, Pavlin JA, Eitzen EM (1997) Biological warfare: A historical perspective. *J Am Med Assoc* 278: 412–417
4 Mayor A (1997) Dirty tricks in ancient warfare. *Mil Hist Quart* 10: 1–37
5 Derbes VJ (1966) De mussis and the Great Plaque of 1348: A forgotten episode in bacteriological war. *J Am Med Assoc* 196: 59–62
6 Poupard JA, Miller LA (1992) History of biological warfare: Catapults to capsomeres. *Ann NY Acad Sci* 666: 9–20
7 Millett PD (2006) The biological and toxin weapons convention. *Rev Sci Tech* 25: 35–52
8 Harris S (1992) Japanese biological warfare research on humans: A case study on microbiology and ethics *Ann NY Acad Sci* 666: 21–52
9 Klietmann WF, Ruoff KL (2001) Bioterrorism: Implications for the clinical microbiologist. *Clin Microbiol Rev* 14: 364–381
10 Torok TJ, Tauxe RV, Wise RP, Livengood JR, Sokolow R, Mauvais S, Birkness KA, Skeels MR, Horan JM, Foster LR (1997) A large community outbreak of salmonellosis caused by international contamination of restaurant salad bars. *J Am Med Assoc* 278: 389–395
11 Olson KB (1999) Aum Shinrikyo: Once and future threat? *Emerg Infect Dis* 5: 513–516
12 Keim P, Kalif A, Schupp J, Hill K, Travis SE, Richmond K, Adair DM, Hugh-Jones, M, Kuske CR, Jackson P (1997) Molecular evolution and diversity in *Bacillus anthracis* as detected by amplified fragment length polymorphism markers. *J Bacteriol* 1979: 818–824
13 Walker DH, Yampolska O, Grinberg LM (1994) Death at Sverdlovsk: What have we learned? *Am J Pathol* 1994: 1135–1141
14 Wilkening DA (2006) Sverdlovsk revisted: Modeling human inhalation anthrax. *Proc Natl Acad Sci USA* 2006: 7589–7594
15 Taylor LH, Latham SM, Woolhouse MEJ (2001) Risk factors for human disease emergence. *Phil Trans R Soc Lond B* 356: 983–989
16 NATO (1996) NATO Handbook on the Medical Aspects of NBC Defensive Operations. Part II – Biological, AMedP-6 (B), Department of the Army, Washington D.C.
17 Kaufmann AF, Meltzer MI, Schmid GP (1997) The economic impact of a bioterrorist attack: Are prevention and postattack intervention programs justifiable? *Emerg Infect Dis* 3: 83–94

18 Bradburne C, Chung MC, Zong Q, Schlauch K, Liu D, Popova T, Popova A, Bailey C, Soppet D, Popov S (2008) Transcriptional and apoptotic responses of THP-1 cells to challenge with toxigenic, and non-toxigenic *Bacillus anthracis*. *BMC Immunol* 13: 9–67

19 Nguyen ML, Crowe SR, Kurella S, Teryzan S, Cao B, Ballard JD, James JA, Farris AD (2009) Sequential B-cell epitopes of *Bacillus anthracis* lethal factor bind lethal toxin-neutralizing antibodies. *Infect Immun* 77: 162–169

20 Griffin KF, Oyston PC, Titball RW (2007) *Francisella tularensis* vaccines. *FEMS Immunol Med Microbiol* 49: 315–323

21 Isherwood KE, Titball RW, Davies DH, Felgner PL, Morrow WJ (2005) Vaccination strategies for *Francisella tularensis*. *Adv Drug Deliv Rev* 57: 1403–1414

22 Turnbull PCB (1999) Definitive identification of *Bacillus anthracis* – A review. *J Appl Microbiol* 87: 237–240

23 Baillie L, Read TD (2001) *Bacillus anthracis*, a bug with attitude! *Curr Opin Microbiol* 4: 78–81

24 Titball RW, Turnbull PCB, Huston RA (1991) The monitoring and detection of *Bacillus anthracis* in the environment. *J Appl Bacteriol Symp* 70: 9–18

25 Riedel S (2005) Anthrax: A continuing concern in the era of bioterrorism. *BUMC Proc* 18: 234–243

26 Mc Sherry J, Kilpatrick R (1992) The plague of Athens. *J R Soc Med* 85: 713–713

27 Theodorides J (1993) The plague of Athens. *J Roy Soc Med* 86: 244–244

28 LaForce FM (1994) Anthrax. *Clin Infect Dis* 19: 1009–1014

29 Patocka J, Splino M (2002) Anthrax toxin characterization. *Acta Med* 45: 3–5

30 Sirard JC, Guidi-Rontani C, Rouet A, Mock M (2000) Characterization of a plasmid region involved in *Bacillus anthracis* toxin production and pathogenesis. *Int J Med Microbiol* 290: 313–316

31 Bhatnagar R, Batra S (2001) Anthrax toxin. *Crit Rev Microbiol* 27: 167–200

32 Guildi-Rontani C, Weber-Levy M, Mock M, Cabiaux V (2000) Translocation of *Bacillus anthracis* lethal and oedema factors across endosome membranes. *Cell Microbiol* 2: 259–264

33 Duesbery NS, Vande Woude GF (1999) Anthrax lethal factor causes proteolytic inactivation of mitogen-activated protein kinase kinase. *J Appl Microbil* 87: 289–293

34 Zhao J, Milne JC, Collier RJ (1995) Effect of anthrax toxin's lethal factor on ion channels formed by the protective antigen. *J Biol Chem* 270: 18626–18630

35 Mujer CV, Wagner MA, Eschenbrenner M, Horn T, Kraycer JA, Redkar R, Hagius S, Elzer P, Delvecchio VG (2002) Global analysis of *Brucella melitensis* proteomes. *Ann NY Acad Sci* 969: 97–101

36 Glynn MK, Lynn TV (2008) Brucellosis. *J Am Vet Med Assoc* 233: 900–908

37 Franco MP, Mulder M, Gilman RH, Smits HL (2007) Human brucellosis. *Lancet Infect Dis* 7: 775–786

38 Al-Tawfiq JA (2008) Therapeutic options for human brucellosis. *Expert Rev Anti Infect Ther* 6: 109–120

39 Pappas G, Papadimitrou P, Christou L, Akritidis N (2006) Future trends in human brucellosis treatment. *Exp Opin Investig Drugs* 15: 1141–1149

40 Gupta VK, Rout PK, Vihan VS (2007) Induction of immune response in mice with a DNA vaccine encoding outer membrane protein (omp31) of *Brucella melitensis* 16 M. *Res Vet Sci* 82: 305–313

41 McCoy GW, Chapin CW (1912) Further observations on a plague like disease of rodents with a plelimiary note on the causative agent, *Bacterium tularense*. *J Infect Dis* 10: 61–72

42 Jellison WL (1972) Tularemia: Dr. Edward Francis and his first 23 isolates of *Francisella tularensis*. *Bull Hist Med* 46: 477–485

43 Nigeovic LE, Wingerter SL (2008) Tularemia. *Infect Dis Clin North Am* 22: 489–504

44 Gurycova D (1998) First isolation of *Francisella tularensis* subsp. *tularensis* in Europe. *Eur J Epidemiol* 14: 797–802

45 Ellis J, Oyston PC, Green M, Titball RW (2002) Tularemia. *Clin Microbiol Rev* 15: 631–646

46 Morner T (1992) The ecology of tularaemia. *Rev Sci Tech* 11: 1123–1130

47 Pavlovich NV, Mishakin BN, Tynkevich NK, Ryzhko IV, Romanova LV, Danilevskaia GI (1991) Comparative characteristics of biological properties of *Francisella tularensis* strains isolated in the USSR. *Antibiot Khimioter* 36: 23–25

48 Broekhuijsen M, Larsson P, Johansson A, Bystrom M, Eriksson U, Larsson E, Prior RG, Sjostedt A, Titball RW (2003) Genome-wide DNA microarray analysis of *Francisella tularensis* strains

demonstrates extensives genetic conservation within the species but identifies regions that are unique to the highly virulent *F. tularensis* subsp. *tularensis*. *J Clin Mircobiol* 41: 2924–2931

49 Pikula J, Treml F, Beklova M, Holesovska Z, Pikulova J (2003) Ecological conditions of natural foci of tularemia in the Czech Republic. *Eur J Epid* 18: 1091–1095

50 Pikula J, Beklova M, Holesovska Z, Treml F (2004) Prediction of possible distribution of tularemia in the Czech Republic. *Vet Med-Czech* 49: 61–64

51 Pikula J, Beklova M, Holesovska Z, Treml F (2004) Ecology of European brown hare and distribution of natural foci of tularaemia in the Czech Republic. *Acta Vet Brno* 73: 267–273

52 Hubalek Z, Sixl W, Halouzka J (1998) *Francisella tularensis* in *Dermacentor reticulatus* ticks from the Czech Republic and Austria. *Wien Klin Wochenschr* 110: 909–910

53 Zhang F, Liu W, Chu MC, He J, Duan Q, Wu X.M, Zhang PH, Zhao QM, Yang H, Xin ZT, Cao WC (2006) *Francisella tularensis* in rodents, China. *Emerg Infect Dis* 12: 994–996

54 Siret V, Barataud D, Prat M, Vaillant V, Ansart S, LeCoustumier A, Vaissaire J, Raffi F, Garre M, Capek I (2006) An outbreak of airborne tularemia in France, August 2004. *Euro Surveill* 11: 58–60

55 Pullen RL, Stuart BM (1945) Tularemia: Analysis of 225 cases. *J Am Med Assoc* 129: 495–500

56 Dennis DT, Iglesby TV, Henderson DA, Bartlett JG, Ascher MS, Eitzen E, Fine AD, Friedlander AM, Hauer J, Layton M, Lillibridge SR, McDade JE, Osterholm MT, O'Toole T, Parker G, Perl TM, Russell PK, Tonat K (2001) Tularemia as a biological wapon – Medical and public health management. *J Am Med Assoc* 285: 2763–2773

57 Pohanka M (2007) Evaluation of immunoglobulin production during tularaemia infection in BALB/c mouse model. *Acta Vet Brno* 76: 579–584

58 Enderlin G, Morales L, Jacobs RF, Cross TJ (1994) Streptomycin and alternative agents for the treatment of tularemia: Review of the literature. *Clin Infect Dis* 19: 42–47

59 Eremeeva EM, Roux V, Raoult D (1993) Determination of genome size and restriction pattern polymorphism of *Rickettsia prowazekii* and *Rickettsia typhi* by pulsed field gel electrophoresis. *FEMS Microbiol Lett* 112: 105–112

60 Weiss E, Coolbaugh JC, Williams JC (1975) Separation of viable *Rickettsia typhi* from yolk sac and L cell host components by Renografin density gradient centrifuation. *Appl Microbiol* 30: 456–463

61 Dasch GA, Samms JR, Weiss E (1978) Biochemical characteristics of typhus group *Rickettsiae* with special attention to the *Rickettsia prowazekii* strains isolated from flying squirrels. *Infect Immun* 19: 676–685

62 Andersson SGE, Zomorodipour A, Winkler HH, Kurland CG (1995) Unusual organization of the rRNA genes in *Rickettsia prowazekii*. *J Bacteriol* 177: 4171–4175

63 Raoult D, Ndihokubwayo JB, Tisson-Dupont H, Roux V, Faugere B, Abegbinni R, Birtles RJ (1998) Outbreak of epidemic typhus associated with trench fever in Burundi. *Lancet* 352: 353–358

64 Bechah Y, Capo C, Mege JL, Raoult D (2008) Epidemic typhus. *Lancet Infect Dis* 8: 417–426

65 Lukin EP, Nesvizhskii IV (2003) Rickettsiosis: State of the art at the turn of the 21st century. *Vestn Ross Akad Med Nauk* 1: 30–35

66 Grygorczuk S, Hermanowska-Szpakowicz T (2002) *Yersinia pestis* as a dangerous biological weapon. *Med Pr* 53: 343–348

67 Shyamal B, Ravi Kumar R, Sohan L, Balakrishnan N, Veena M, Shiv L (2008) Present susceptibility status of rat flea *Xenophsylla cheopis* (Siphonaptera: Pulicidae), vector of plague against organochlorine, organophosphate and synthetic pyrethroids 1. The Nilgiris District, Tamil Nadu India. *J Commun Dis* 40: 41–45

68 Eisen RJ, Wilder AP, Bearden SW, Nontenieri JA, Gage KL (2007) Early-phase transmission of *Yersinia pestis* by unblocked *Xenopsylla cheopis* (Siphonaptera: Pulicidae) is as efficient as transmission by blocked fleas. *J Med Entomol* 44: 678–682

69 Eisen RJ, Borchert JN, Holmes JL, Amatre G, van Wyk K, Enscore RE, Babi N, Atiku LA, Wilder AP, Vetter SM, Bearden SW, Montenieri JA, Gage KL (2008) Early-phase transmission of *Yersinia pestis* by cat fleas (*Ctenocephalides felis*) and their potential role as vectors in a plague-endemic region of Uganda. *Am J Trop Med Hyg* 78: 949–956

70 Achtman M, Zurth K, Morelli C, Torrea G, Guiyoule A, Carniel E (1999) *Yersinia pestis*, the cause of plague, is a recently emerged clone of *Yersinia pseudotuberculosis*. *Proc Natl Acad Sci USA* 96: 14043–14048

71 Guiyoule A, Grimont F, Iteman I, Grimont PAD, Lefevre M, Carniel E (1994) Plague pandemics

investigated by ribotyping of *Yersinia pestis* strains. *J Clin Microbiol* 32: 634–641

72 Russell JC (1968) That earlier plague. *Demography* 5: 174–184

73 Ligon BL (2006) Plague: A review of its history and potential as a biological weapon. *Semin Pediatr Infect Dis* 17: 161–170

74 Reyn CF, Weber NS, Tempest B, Barnes AM, Poland JD, Boyce JM, Zalma V (1977) Epidemiologic and clinical features of an outbreak of bubonic plague in New Mexico. *J Infect Dis* 136: 489–494

75 Craven RB, Maupin GO, Beard ML, Quan TJ, Barnes AM (1993) Reported cases of human plague infections in the United States, 1970–1991. *J Med Entomol* 30: 758–761

76 Crook LD, Tempest B (1992) Plague: A clinical review of 27 cases. *Arch Intern Med* 152: 1253–1256

77 Slifka MK, Hanifin JM (2004) Smallpox: The basics. *Dermatol Clin* 22: 263–274

78 Riedel S (2005) Smallpox and biological warfare: A disease revisited. *BUMC Proc* 18: 13–20

79 Fenner F, Henderson DA, Arita I, Jezek Z, Ladnyi ID (1988) Smallpox and its eradication. *World Health Organization Memorandum* 1460

80 World Health Organization (1975) *Weekly Epidemiol Rec* 38: 325–329

81 Nafziger SD (2005) Smallpox. *Crit Care Clin 21*: 739–746

82 Koplan J, Monsur KA, Foster SO (1975) Treatment of variola major with adenine arabinoside. *J Infect Dis* 131: 34–39

83 Monsur KA, Hossain MS, Huq F, Rahaman MM, Haque MQ (1975) Treatment of variola major with cytosine arabinoside. *J Infect Dis* 131: 40–43

84 Borio L, Inglesby T, Peters CJ, Schmaljohn AL, Hughes JM, Jahrling PB, Ksiazek T, Johnson KM, Meyerhoff A, O'Toole T, Ascher MS, Barlett J, Breman JG, Eitzen EM, Hamburg M, Hauer J, Henderson DA, Johnson RT, Kwik G, Layton M, Lillibridge S, Nabel GJ, Osterholm MT, Perl TM, Russell P, Tonat K (2002) Hemorrhagic fever viruses as biological weapon. *J Am Med Assoc* 18: 2391–2405

85 LeDuc JW (1989) Epidemiology of hemorrhagic fever viruses. *Rev Infect Dis* 11: 730–735

86 Schou S, Hansen AK (2000) Marburg and Ebola virus infection in laboratory nonhuman primates: A literature review. *Comp Med* 50: 108–123

87 Groseth A, Feldmann H, Strong JE (2007) The ecology of Ebola virus. *Trends Microbiol* 15: 408–416

88 Peters CJ, Kuehne RW, Mercado RR, LeBow RH, Spertzel RO, Webb PA (1974) Hemorrhagic fever in Cochabamba, Bolivia, 1971. *Am J Epidemiol* 99: 425–433

89 Slenczka WK (1999) The Marburg virus outbreak of 1967 and subsequent episodes. *Curr Top Microbiol Immunol* 235: 49–75

90 Huggins JW (1989) Prospect for treatment of viral hemorrhagic fevers with ribavirin, a broad-spectrum antiviral drug. *Rev Infect Dis* 11: 750–761

91 Maes P, Clement J, van Ranst M (2009) Recent approaches in hantavirus vaccine development. *Expert Rev Vaccines* 8: 67–76

92 Hall JD, McCroskey LM, Pincomb BJ, Hetheway CL (1985) Isolation of an organism resembling *Clostridium baratii* which produces type F botulinal toxon from an infant with botulism. *J Clin Microbiol* 21: 654–655

93 Aureli P, Fenicia L, Pasolini B, Gianfranceschi M, McCroskey LM, Hatheway CL (1986) Two cases of type E infant botulism caused by neurotoxigenic *Clostridium butyricum* in Italy. *J Infect Dis* 154: 207–211

94 Gill MD (1982) Bacterial toxins: A table of lethal amounts. *Microbiol Rev* 46: 86–94

95 Lacy DB, Tepp W, Cohen AC, DasGupta BR, Stevens RC (1998) Crystal structure of botulinum neurotoxin type A and implications for toxicity. *Nat Struct Biol* 5: 898–902

96 Bach-Rojecky L, Relja M, Filipovic B, Lackovic Z (2007) Botulinum toxin type A and cholinergic system. *Lijec Vjesn* 129: 407–414

97 Fernandez PS, Peck MW (1999) A predictive model that describes the effect of prolonged heating at 70 to 90 degrees C and subsequent incubation at refrigeration temperatures on growth from spores and toxigenesis by nonproteolytic *Clostridium botulinum* in the presence of lysozyme. *Appl Environ Microbiol* 65: 3449–3457

98 Koenig MG, Drutz DJ, Mushlin AI, Schaffner W, Rogers DE (1967) Type B botulism in man. *Am J Med* 42: 208–219

99 Hughes JM, Blumenthal JR, Meson MH, Lombard GL, Dowell VR, Gangarosa EJ (1981) Clinical features of types A and B food-borne botulism. *Ann Intern Med* 95: 442–445

100 Tacket CO, Shandera WX, Mann JM, Hargrett NT, Blake PA (1984) Equine antitoxin use and other factors that predict outcome in type A foodborne botulism. *Am J Med* 76: 794–798

101 Siegel LS (1988) Human immune response to botulinum pentavalent (ABCDE) toxoid determined by a neutralization test and by an enzyme-linked immunosorbent assay. *J Clin Microbiol* 26: 2351–2356

102 Zhan J, Zhou P (2003) A simplified method to evaluate the acute toxicity of ricin and ricinus agglutinin. *Toxicology* 186: 119–123

103 Ippoliti R (2004) Structure and function of the plant toxin ricin, an *N*-glycosidase enzyme. *Ital J Biochem* 53: 92–97

104 Lord MJ, Jolliffe NA, Marsden CJ, Pateman CS, Smith DC, Spooner RA, Watson PD, Roberts LM (2003) Ricin. Mechanisms of cytotoxicity. *Toxicol Rev* 22: 53–64

105 Gonzalez TV, Farrant SA, Mantis NJ (2006) Ricin induces IL-8 secretion from human monocyte/macrophages by activating the p38 MAP kinase pathway. *Mol Immunol* 43: 1920–1923

106 Rao PV, Jayaraj R, Bhaskar AS, Kumar O, Bhattacharya R, Saxena P, Dash PK, Vijayaraghavan R (2005) Mechanism of ricin-induced apoptosis in human cervical cancer cells. *Biochem Pharmacol* 69: 855–865

107 Sun J, Pohl EE, Krylova OO, Krause E, Agapov II, Tonevitsky AG, Pohl P (2004) Membrane destabilization by ricin. *Eur Biophys J* 33: 572–579

108 Canter DA, Gunning D, Rodgers P, O'Connor L, Traunero C, Kempter CJ (2005) Remediation of *Bacillus anthracis* contamination in the U.S. Department of Justice mail facility. *Biosecur Bioterror* 3: 119–127

109 Josefson D (2001) US fear of bioterrorism spreads as anthrax cases increase. *Br Med J* 323: 877–878

110 Higgins JA, Cooper M, Schroeder-Trucker L, Black S, Miller D, Karns JS, Manthey E, Breeze R, Perdue ML (2002) A field investigation of *Bacillus anthracis* contamination of U.S. Department of Agriculture and other Washington, D.C., buildings during the anthrax attack of October 2001. *Appl Environ Microbiol* 69: 593–599

111 Read TD, Salzberg SL, Pop M, Shumway M, Umayam L, Jiang L, Holtzapple E, Busch JD, Smith KL, Schupp JM, Solomon D, Keim P, Fraser CM (2002) Comparative genome sequencing for discovery of novel polymorphisms in *Bacillus anthracis*. *Science* 296: 2028–2033

112 Duncan EJ, Kournikakis B, Ho J, Hill I (2009) Pulmonary deposition of aerosolized *Bacillus atrophaeus* in a Swine model due to exposure from a simulated anthrax letter incident. *Inhal Toxicol* 21: 141–152

113 Duncan S, Ho J (2008) Estimation of viable spores in *Bacillus atrophaeus* (BG) particles of 1 to 9 μm size range. *Clean Soil Air Water* 36: 584–592

114 Gerndt H (2002) Anthrax stories – Theses on legend research in the globalized world. *Österr Z Volkskd* 105: 279–295

115 Benedek DM, Hollway HC, Becker SM (2002) Emergency mental health management in bioterrorism events. *Emerg Med Clin North Am* 20: 393–407

116 Agar SL, Sha J, Foltz SM, Erova TE, Walberg KG, Parham TE, Baze WB, Suarez G, Peterson JW, Chopra AK (2008) Characterization of a mouse model of plague after aerosolization of Yersinia pestis CO92. *Microbiology* 154: 1939–1948

117 Chen PS, Li CS (2007) Real-time monitoring for bioaerosols – Flow cytometry. *Analyst* 132: 14–16

118 Ward M, Siegel JA, Corsi RL (2005) The effectiveness of stand alone air cleaners for shelter-in-place. *Indoor Air* 15: 127–134

119 Eubanks LM, Dickerson TJ, Janda KD (2007) Technological advancements for the detection of and protection against biological and chemical warfare agents. *Chem Soc Rev* 36: 458–470

120 Pohanka M, Hubalek M, Neubauerova V, Macela A, Faldyna M, Bandouchova H, Pikula J (2008) Current and emerging assays for *Francisella tularensis* detection: A review. *Vet Med Czech* 53: 585–594

121 Saikaly PE, Berlaz MA, de Los Reyes FL (2007) Development of quantitative real-time PCR assays for detection and quantification of surrogate biological warfare agents in building debris and lechate. *Appl Environ Microbiol* 73: 6557–6565

122 Edwards KA, Clancy HA, Baeumner AJ (2006) *Bacillus anthracis*: Toxicology, epidemiology and current rapid-detection methods. *Anal Bioanal Chem* 384: 73–84

123 Pohanka M, Skladal P, Kroca M (2007) Biosensors for biological warfare agent detection. *Def Sci J* 57: 185–193

124 Pohanka M, Skladal P (2005) Piezoelectric immunosensor for *Francisella tularensis* detection using immunoglobulin M in a limiting dilution. *Anal Lett* 76: 607–612
125 Pohanka M, Skladal P (2007) Piezoelectric immunosensor for the direct and rapid detection of *Franciella tularensis*. *Folia Microbiol* 52: 325–330
126 Pohanka M, Pavlis O, Skladal P (2007) Diagnosis of tularemia using piezoelectric biosensor technology. *Talanta* 71: 981–985
127 Pohanka M, Treml F, Hubalek M, Bandouchova H, Beklova M, Pikula J (2007) Piezoelectric biosensor biosensor for a simple serological diagnosis of tularemia in infected European brown hares (*Lepus europaeus*). *Sensors* 7: 2825–2834
128 Pohanka M, Skladal P (2007) Serological diagnosis of tularemia in mice using the amperometric immunosensor. *Electroanalysis* 19: 2507–2512
129 Wayne Conlan J, Oyston PC (2007) Vaccines against *Francisella tularensis*. *Ann NY Acad Sci* 1105: 325–350
130 Drusano GL, Okusanva OO, Okusanva A, van Scov B, Brown DL, Kulawy R, Sorgel F, Heine HS, Louie A (2008) Is 60 days of ciprofloxacin administration necessary for postexposure prophylaxis for *Bacillus anthracis*? *Antimicrob Agents Chemother* 52: 3973–3979

Molecular, Clinical and Environmental Toxicology. Volume 2: Clinical Toxicology
Edited by A. Luch
© 2010 Birkhäuser Verlag/Switzerland

Forensic toxicology

Olaf H. Drummer

Victorian Institute of Forensic Medicine, Department of Forensic Medicine, Monash University, Australia

Abstract. Forensic toxicology has developed as a forensic science in recent years and is now widely used to assist in death investigations, in civil and criminal matters involving drug use, in drugs of abuse testing in correctional settings and custodial medicine, in road and workplace safety, in matters involving environmental pollution, as well as in sports doping. Drugs most commonly targeted include amphetamines, benzodiazepines, cannabis, cocaine and the opiates, but can be any other illicit substance or almost any over-the-counter or prescribed drug, as well as poisons available to the community. The discipline requires high level skills in analytical techniques with a solid knowledge of pharmacology and pharmacokinetics. Modern techniques rely heavily on immunoassay screening analyses and mass spectrometry (MS) for confirmatory analyses using either high-performance liquid chromatography or gas chromatography as the separation technique. Tandem MS has become more and more popular compared to single-stage MS. It is essential that analytical systems are fully validated and fit for the purpose and the assay batches are monitored with quality controls. External proficiency programs monitor both the assay and the personnel performing the work. For a laboratory to perform optimally, it is vital that the circumstances and context of the case are known and the laboratory understands the limitations of the analytical systems used, including drug stability. Drugs and poisons can change concentration postmortem due to poor or unequal quality of blood and other specimens, anaerobic metabolism and redistribution. The latter provides the largest handicap in the interpretation of postmortem results.

Introduction

Forensic toxicology represents a number of related disciplines aimed to assist in the detection and interpretation of drugs and poisons for medico-legal purposes. The application of this forensic discipline has evolved substantially over the last two decades and has become a mainstream forensic discipline requiring experienced personnel with high end analytical skills in the use of modern instrumental and isolation techniques and with excellent judgment to tailor an investigation and provide an insight in the possible significance of results. Knowledge of pharmacology and pharmacokinetics are also important to understand the likely effects of any reported results and their time course. This chapter reviews the main elements of forensic toxicology, its applications, the biological specimens and other samples of greatest use, the techniques applied as well as the difficulties and complexities facing the application of the science to case work.

Applications

Criminal matters and death investigations

Traditionally the science was mainly used in postmortem toxicology to detect homicidal poisons. These were often plant-derived poisons such as aconite (aconitine), datura (atropine and scopolamine), hemlock (coniine), deadly nightshade (hyoscyamine and scopolamine), yew (taxines), etc. [1], but also domestic or industrial poisons such as cyanide, thallium and arsenic salts.

In the 21st century few homicides are caused by poisons; however, many people caught up in death investigations consume drugs that have adversely affected their behavior and/or their health. Behavioral changes could include disinhibition, aggression and violence. Adverse effects on health could include seizures, heart disease and even sudden death. These substances may be drugs of abuse (illicit drugs) or legal drugs used in a non-prescribed manner. These are most commonly: amphetamine-type stimulants, cocaine, benzodiazepines and related sedatives, opiates such as heroin, and cannabis products. However, other substances can also be targeted including: other narcotics, barbiturates, ketamine, phencyclidine, muscle relaxants, γ-hydroxybutyrate (GHB), lysergic acid diethylamide (LSD) and many others.

They can also be prescribed drugs, such as the narcotic analgesics (and other analgesics), sedative drugs such as the benzodiazepines, drugs used to treat psychiatric conditions including depression and psychoses, drugs used to treat cardiovascular conditions such as high blood pressure and arrhythmias and drugs used to treat epilepsy. The presence of a prescribed drug in a blood specimen indicates that a medical condition probably exists and that treatment has been sought and obtained. Toxicology will also shed light on whether the drugs have been consumed as recommended or have been abused, or even if an adverse combination of drugs has been prescribed.

Road safety

The application of the science to improve road safety has become a major application both for breath (and blood) alcohol and more recently drugs. For many years some jurisdictions have conducted breath testing for ethanol at a roadside or following an accident. This has been possible due to the close relationship between the concentration of alcohol (ethanol) in alveolar air and blood [2]. Testing in breath involves hand-held devices and any positive result requires subsequent confirmatory testing on another (evidentiary) breath device or by blood testing for alcohol. Excellent reviews on this testing are available including a description of the analytical techniques [3, 4]. This application has been extended to include testing drivers on the spot for drugs using portable devices on small samples of oral fluid taken from the driver [5]. This application is both designed to enforce road safety laws such as driving while impaired by substances and to act as a deterrence to prevent use of impairing drugs while driving and reduce road trauma and mortality [6].

Drugs most likely to impair drivers include the amphetamine-type stimulants, cannabis, cocaine and the benzodiazepines, but can also include a raft of other central nervous system (CNS) active drugs.

In more recent developments involatile metabolites of alcohol can be measured to provide a longer detection period in blood and even more so in hair [7, 8]. The most important of these metabolites is ethyl glucuronide. Concentrations in hair have been correlated with intake of alcohol and can be used to assess degree of alcoholism [8]. This test is also used to provide objective evidence of abstinence to drugs in persons seeking to regain their driving license following an impaired driving conviction.

Workplace and correctional testing

Workplace and correctional drug testing has also grown enormously over the last two decades to stamp out illicit drug use and improve workplace safety. This form of testing has been largely based on urine testing but the development of alternative testing methods now allow use of oral fluid (saliva) rather than urine since drugs are more likely to have been consumed recently and be detectable in oral fluid and are more likely be associated with elevated risks of accidents [5]. Drugs in hair can provide a much longer period of detection than the other specimens and importantly can also provide a weekly or monthly history of drug use [9].

Drug-facilitated crimes

Drug-facilitated crimes have become more popular in recent times, particularly sexual assaults. Forensic toxicology plays a vital role in determining possible exposure to impairing substances hours to weeks after an alleged offence, often using trace analyses [10]. Drugs most commonly used in these crimes are CNS depressant drugs such as the benzodiazepines and related sedatives, GHB, antidepressants, antihistamines, alcohol, etc.

Sports testing

Sports doping has been a well-publicized activity particularly for the Olympic Games and other major international sporting events [11, 12]. Sporting codes are now often monitoring their athletes for use of illicit drugs both in and out of competition. Wider applications in sport include horse and greyhound racing; including testing the animals themselves [13]. This testing is often based on urine but also can involve blood. The type of substances in these applications often focus on anabolic steroids, stimulants, β-blockers, diuretics as well as erythropoietin (blood) and growth hormone (blood) and a long list of other banned substances.

Environmental testing

Increased focus on Governments to regulate and monitor the environment (e.g., air and the waterways) for pollutants leads to corporations and individuals being charged with offences [14]. A number of biomarkers are known and can be used to identify the source of pollution [15]. The evidence against these defendants is often analytical, requiring valid and defendable medico-legal procedures to successfully prosecute cases.

Representative applications encompassing forensic toxicology are listed in Table 1.

Table 1. Key applications of forensic toxicology

Application	Most common specimen[1]
Road safety (alcohol)	Breath, blood, urine
Road safety (drugs of abuse[2])	Blood, oral fluid, urine
Postmortem toxicology	Blood, urine, liver, gastric contents
Clinical forensic toxicology (drug-facilitated crimes, fitness for interview)	Blood, urine
Workplace testing – employment and post incident	Urine, oral fluid
Workplace testing – pre-employment	Hair, urine
Sports testing (humans and veterinary)	Urine, blood
Environmental	Water, air, solids
Custodial programs (prisoners, parolees)	Urine

[1] Listed in approximate rank order
[2] Drugs of abuse include amphetamines, cocaine, cannabis (marijuana), opiates (morphine, heroin) and the benzodiazepines, but can also include other abused drugs such as barbiturates, ketamine, methadone, etc.

Specimens and sampling

One of the features that distinguish forensic toxicology from other toxicology disciplines is the necessity to collect, transport, analyze and store specimens and other samples (exhibits) in such a manner to guarantee chain-of-custody. This means that it is known who handled the exhibit, when and why. This allows the evidence to be tested in a court of law if for any reason there is a concern over the security and propriety of the item examined. This means in practice that all handling of the items must be recorded and the items are transported to the laboratory sealed to ensure no interference has occurred or could be inferred by another party.

There is a large selection of specimens available in forensic toxicology, dependent largely on the type of application [16]. As for clinical toxicology and therapeutic drug monitoring, blood and urine are the most common specimens; however, there are others that can be sampled depending on the application (Tab. 1).

Blood

Blood is the most universally preferred biological specimen if it is available and the collection of the specimen is taken sufficiently close to the event in question. This provides the most direct evidence of a drug in the body and allows toxicologists to infer its likely pharmacological effects. Blood is generally preferred over plasma or serum since most of the forensic literature has results reported in blood; however, some jurisdictions prefer plasma/serum since it can be more easily compared to clinical data. To avoid post collection fermentation and putrefaction at least 1% w/v fluoride should be added to the collection tube. It is preferable to collect two blood specimens. One can be used for alcohol and drug screening and the other for confirmatory tests.

In postmortem situations blood must, wherever possible, be collected from a peripheral site, i.e., in the leg or arm. Collection of blood from the heart or another central site is very likely to be severely contaminated from drugs diffusing from the gastrointestinal tract or neighboring organs (i.e., lungs, heart, stomach). Blood collected from a peripheral site is not immune to drug diffusion (known as redistribution); however, it is likely to be substantially less than at a central site (see section on redistribution).

When deaths have occurred in hospital it will be useful to obtain any specimens taken in hospital for the purpose of biochemical or hematological tests since these will often be closer to the event (causing the forensic interest) than many hours or days later. This will require urgent action to avoid loss of these samples since their retention by hospitals may not be long.

Urine

This specimen is ideal to screen for the presence of drugs since these substances and their metabolites are often present in much higher concentrations than in blood and the volume is not usually limiting. Once drugs are found in urine it is usual practice to analyze blood for the presence of the substances found in urine. Since urine is a waste product stored in the bladder it cannot be used to infer a dose consumed or the likely effects of the drug on the person at the time of sampling.

In cases of drug-facilitated assault, the trace presence of a drug metabolite in urine many hours or days later can be useful evidence of potential exposure [10]. In contrast, workplace drug screening cut-offs are applied to drug screening and confirmation well above the limits of detection of analytical assays [17]. For example, detection limits for benzodiazepines are in the sub-nanogram per milliliter range when attempting to detect clandestine exposure to these substances in victims [18]. However, in workplace, drug testing urine cut-offs for benzodiazepines are around 300 ng/mL [19]. Urine is the most common specimen used in workplace testing.

Water loading is often employed to dilute urine-based drug tests. For this reason urinary creatinine is measured to determine the likelihood of this occurring [20].

Hair

Hair provides an ideal specimen to provide a history of exposure to substances. Drugs and poisons are deposited in hair as hair grows out of the follicle and remains in that location until the hair is cut off. Consequently, analyses for content along the shaft of the hair can provide a history of exposure [9, 21].

Drugs bind primarily to the melanin pigment in hair; hence persons with black hair will generally have higher concentrations than individuals with non-pigmented hair particularly for basic drugs (e.g., amphetamines, antidepressants, opiates). As a rule acidic drugs tend to have much lower concentrations than basic drugs (e.g., benzodiazepines); however, modern instrumental techniques based on tandem mass spectrometry (MS/MS) have sufficient sensitivity for even a small number of strands of hair.

It is important to remember that drugs are also present in sweat and sebaceous secretions. Consequently, small amounts of drugs can diffuse into the external shaft of the hair. Hence the interpretation may not be straightforward unless there are clear "spikes" in the concentrations along the shaft and/or concentrations are moderate to high.

Hair grows at about 1 cm per month, but can vary from about 0.7 to 1.4 cm per month and can exist in either the anagen (active growing stage), catagen (transition stage), or telogen (resting stage) phases [22, 23]. Hair taken from the nape of the head has the most constant growth and tends to be present in most persons (Fig. 1).

Oral fluid

There are a number of glands that secrete fluids in the mouth. They all contain drugs depending on the characteristics of the drug, pH and degree of protein binding in blood and the oral fluid [24, 25]. For the most part there is a relationship between drug concentration in oral fluid to that in blood; however,

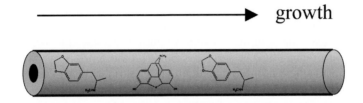

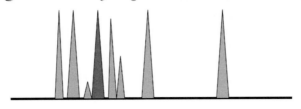

Figure 1. Diagrammatic hair shaft showing how segmental analysis can provide a time line of exposure.

drugs may be locally deposited into the mucosa of the mouth if drugs are smoked (e.g., cannabis, cocaine, methamphetamine) or tablets are retained in the mouth for a period of time [25]. One of the advantages of this specimen is that it can be collected with little infringement of privacy in the view of the collector thus avoiding potential issues of adulteration and substitution sometimes seen with urine tests.

This specimen is used to detect recent use of illicit drugs in drivers through on-site tests [26, 27] as well as in workplaces to detect past use of illicit drugs [28, 29].

Postmortem specimens

While blood, urine and hair can also be collected in deceased persons and indeed should be part of a routine collection in all cases subjected to a medicolegal death investigation, there are a number of specimens unique to postmortem toxicology. The most common are gastric contents, liver and vitreous humor [16, 30].

Gastric contents can provide useful information in relation to the degree of oral administration if an overdose is suspected, and if positive for large amounts of drugs can supplement data obtained on blood. It is essential that the contents are quantified since a distinction needs to be made from trace amounts from a previous non-toxic ingestion and from a significant ingestion. Unless the whole contents are submitted for analysis the results will have limited relevance.

A section of liver is useful when the significance of the concentration of drug in blood is marginal and additional information is required to determine a possible role of the drug in the death. In putrefied bodies blood may not be available, hence there will be greater reliance on data from solid tissues. The section of liver should be taken from the right side of the body to minimize diffusion of drugs from the intestines near the left lobe.

Vitreous humor is a most useful fluid and should be collected in all cases, particularly if significant postmortem changes or trauma are likely to have occurred. For example, alcohol concentrations in vitreous humor are little higher than in blood and helps to substantiate the reliability of blood alcohol concentrations. The measurement of glucose is useful in cases of significant hyperglycemia, and urea and chloride are useful to determine possible kidney dysfunction and/or dehydration.

Other specimens may at times be useful depending on the circumstance but these tend to be exceptional compared to those already mentioned. These include lungs (or lung fluid in cases of exposure to volatile substances), brain, kidneys, bone and bone marrow.

Techniques

This chapter cannot hope to review all techniques applicable to forensic toxicology; rather this section provides a snapshot of the most common methods and some of the more recent developments in analytical methodology [31]. The first step in any analysis is the isolation of drugs from the matrix. There are a number of isolation techniques used depending on the sample, substances being screened and the detection method used.

Isolation procedures

A small aliquot of specimen (<0.1 mL) is usually applied directly to immunoassay-based procedures, i.e., urine or blood, but when chromatographic procedures are used some form of clean-up is inevitably required. Typically these are either liquid-liquid or solid-phase procedures.

Liquid-liquid extraction (LLE) is the oldest technique and is still the most commonly used. This technique involves the extraction of the analyte(s) from the biological material or solubilized solid material with an organic solvent. The aqueous phase is buffered or pH adjusted to ensure the analyte(s) are not in an ionized form, i.e., acidic pH is used for acids and basic pH for basic substances. Common solvents include butyl chloride, hexane, ethyl or butyl acetate or solvent combinations such chloroform/2-propanol (3:1), hexane: isoamyl alcohol (98:2), dichloromethane:isopropanol:ethyl acetate (1:1:3) [32]. Solvents of high polarity may have higher extraction efficiencies but give much dirtier extracts and should be avoided, e.g., ethyl acetate. Diethyl ether is an effective solvent but is too volatile and is potentially explosive. It should be avoided. The retained solvent is then removed from the mixture and is evaporated to dryness, or further treated to remove extraneous substances. The residue is then re-constituted into a solvent suitable for analysis, usually chromatographic separation on a liquid chromatography (LC) or gas chromatography (GC) system.

Solid-phase extraction (SPE) methods are also widely used and are based on the absorption of the analyte(s) onto a solid support that allows selective absorption. The excess fluid containing the analyte(s) is washed through the mini-column and the retained substances are then eluted off with a suitable solvent. Most common supports are alkyl-bonded silica mini-columns, such as C18 or mixed-phase columns [33].

This and other solid-phase or solvent-less methods such as solid-phase microextraction, single-drop microextraction, hollow-fiber liquid-phase microextraction, and sub-critical water extraction are also used [34, 35]. The choice of the preferred isolation method is not simple and is usually obtained empirically. For urine analyses, LLE has been shown to be superior using acetylation and hydrolysis compared to other LLE isolation and extraction methods and SPE [36]. This will not necessarily be the case for other specimens or detection methods. Each application needs to be assessed for efficiency and accuracy.

There are a large number of detection techniques that can be used in forensic toxicology; however, by far the most common can be grouped into immunoassay and chromatography-based methods.

Immunoassays

Immunoassay screening techniques rely on the competition of the analyte and the labeled antigen with an antibody showing selectivity for a class of related drugs. This can be performed on urine using one of a number of different kits relying on different chemical principles, such as enzyme multiplied immunoassay (EMIT), fluorescence polarization (FPIA), cloned enzyme donor immunoassay (CEDIA) and kinetic interaction of microparticles in solution (KIMS). Drugs that are predominately present in urine as conjugates (sulfates and glucuronides) require prior hydrolysis before being subjected to immunoassay, e.g., benzodiazepines and opiates. This technique can be automated allowing large batches of tests to be conducted very quickly.

Drugs of abuse can be tested with microplate enzyme-linked immunosorbent assay (ELISA) tests. These also represent a quick and convenient method for the analysis of drugs in blood, hair extracts and tissue homogenates. Sensitivities to drugs will vary from kit to kit due to manufacturer, chemical principle used for identification and batch of antibodies used. Drug classes targeted most commonly include the amphetamines, barbiturates, benzodiazepines, cannabinoids, cocaine metabolites and opiates. Kits for other drugs are also available and include 6-acetylmorphine (6-AM), lysergic acid diethyl-amide (LSD), fentanyl, methadone and phencyclidine. The range of drugs and drug classes tested will depend on their local availability and use.

The performance of immunoassays can be adversely affected by sample quality. For example, in postmortem cases significant putrefaction can lead to false results. This can be reduced by the use of a purification technique such as methanol treatment. False positives are common for the amphetamines due to amine putrefactive products [37].

Substances added to urine to avoid drug detection are well known and cause strong interferences. Each kit is likely to be affected differently depending on the chemical principle used. Adulterants include glutaraldehyde, detergent, bleach, lemon juice, vinegar, sodium hydroxide, bicarbonate, and salts such as sodium chloride [38].

Chromatography-based methods

High-performance LC and GC have become the mainstay of chromatographic methods. The use of phase-bonded capillary columns with GC enables the chromatography of a large range of drugs underivatized. These include the amphetamines, barbiturates, cocaine, some benzodiazepines and other hyp-notics, some opioids (e.g., codeine, heroin, methadone and oxycodone), most antidepressants and antipsychotics; many others are often included. Highly polar compounds can be made amenable to GC by suitable derivatization. These include morphine, benzoylecgonine and some benzodiazepines [32]. The most common detector used in forensic toxicology is the nitrogen phos-phorous detector (NPD) due to its selectivity for nitrogenous compounds (as well as the uncommon phosphorous containing compounds). The flame ion-ization detector (FID) is mainly used for ethanol determination.

When using GC, less volatile substances or substances with poor thermal stability can be derivatized to stabilize the substance and facilitate improved chromatography. The most common derivatizing agents for amines include perfluorinated anhydrides (e.g., trifluoroacetic anhydride or pentafluoropropi-onic anhydride) or silyl derivatives. Carboxyl groups can be derivatized with activated silyl agents, diazomethane, iodobutane or a perfluorinated alcohol in the presence of a perfluorinated anhydride. The latter compounds can also be used to derivatize amino, hydroxyl and carboxyl groups.

Forensic laboratories now use mass spectrometry (MS) as the detector of choice. This produces spectroscopic data of peaks that allow an identification to be made, which is not possible with other detectors where only retention time can be used to presume the presence of a drug [39] (Fig. 2).

LC was a very popular technique in the 1970s and 1980s until capillary col-umn GC and later GC-MS became the chromatographic technique of choice. In this period ultraviolet detectors and multi-wavelength or photodiode array de-tectors were common and relatively inexpensive; some specific analytes could

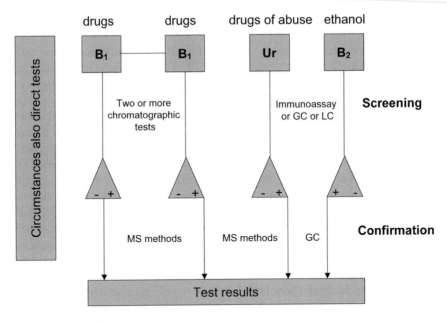

Figure 2. Scheme illustrating drug tests conducted in a typical forensic toxicology case. B, blood; Ur, urine; GC, gas chromatography; LC, liquid chromatography.

be detected using electrochemical (e.g., morphine and some other opiates) or fluorescence detectors (e.g., quinine, propranolol, morphine). Over the last 10 years LC-MS instruments became more readily available to forensic laboratories and are now arguably more popular than GC-based instruments. The ability to separate both polar and slightly polar compounds in one chromatographic system underivatized is an advantage both in terms of time and cost.

The availability of tandem MS (MS/MS or MS^n) has further revolutionized analytical toxicology. In general, tandem MS has a higher specificity than MS alone, since spectra are obtained from a characteristic ion formed in the first stage MS. Ion-trap instruments operate somewhat differently in that all ions are produced in one chamber; however, the net effect is derivative MS. This instrument can produce ions to the third or forth generation if required. Usually, small bore LC columns allow relatively quick chromatography enabling a high throughput of samples on LC-MS/MS using automated sample injectors. Reverse-phase systems are frequently used with an aqueous-alcohol based system buffered to a particular pH. Columns are hydrocarbon-linked chains (e.g., C18, C8, phenyl-alkyl) to fine silica beads packed into 2- or 4-mm i.d. stainless steel tubes that can accommodate high pressures.

Time of flight (TOF) MS provides high accuracy masses that can be used to identify unknown substances in biological extracts, particularly urine [40, 41]. Two-dimensional chromatography has also been employed and offers improved separation characteristics compared to one-dimensional techniques [42,

43]. Capillary electrophoresis (CE) in its various forms [32, 44] has been used successfully to detect a range of drugs. However, sensitivity is limiting so that it has found more use in illicit drug analyses of powders and reaction mixtures from clandestine laboratory investigations [45–47]. Thin-layer chromatography (TLC) is still used in a few laboratories since it is inexpensive and can cover a range of common drugs and poisons. Its sensitivity is limited and is usually restricted to urine extracts due to the relatively high concentration of drugs and metabolites and the large volume of specimen available. However, the use of over-pressurized TLC can be used for liver extracts [48]. More recently matrix-assisted laser desorption/ionization TOF MS (MALDI-TOF) has been used on TLC "spots" as an experimental technique [49].

Screening and confirmation

It is also vital that a distinction is made from screening tests and confirmatory tests. Screening, or initial tests, provide an indication of the absence or presence of a drug or drug class, but does not provide unequivocal proof of the presence of a drug or drug class. For example, drug screening using immunoassays, no matter how good the antibody, cannot provide a medico-legal proof of presence of any targeted substance. Unless mass spectrometry (MS) has been used and the obtained spectra are sufficiently unique for unequivocal identification, drugs (and other chemical substances) are not confirmed as present in a sample (Tab. 2).

The usual practice is to conduct two independent tests before a result is reported in a medico-legal environment. In situations where testing is restricted to common drugs of abuse, immunoassays are often used as the initial test to see if any drugs from those classes are present and then mass spectrometry is used to identify the drug. Initial tests could include other techniques such as TLC, LC using ultraviolet or multi-wavelength detectors, or GC using NPD, for example. Initial tests also help to eliminate quickly (and relatively cheaply) the negative samples from the smaller number of positive samples.

Table 2. Methods in forensic toxicology

Screening methods	Confirmatory methods
Immunoassays	
GC-NPD	GC-MS
GC-MS	GC-MS/MS or GC-MS^n
LC-UV (DAD)	LC-MS/MS or LC-MS^n
TLC	
TOF-MS	

GC, gas chromatography; LC, liquid chromatography; MS, mass spectrometry; NPD, nitrogen phosphorous detector; UV, ultraviolet detector; DAD, photodiode array detector; TLC, thin layer chromatography; TOF, time-of-flight.

The performance of two tests conducted at different times, and possibly also by a different person can provide a further surety that no sample mix-up has occurred in the laboratory while preparing the tubes for analysis. While initial tests are not always confirmed, it is good practice to investigate cases where confirmatory results are not consistent with the initial test.

The use of more sophisticated analytical equipment available to some laboratories makes it feasible to both screen and confirm samples for drugs in one step. This applies particularly to tandem MS either connected to a GC (GC-MS/MS) or an LC (LC-MS/MS). This approach is best suited to targeted analyses in which characteristic product ions from a specific number of analytes are scanned at relevant retention times, and post-analysis macros allow relatively rapid interrogation of the acquired data. While MS/MS is usually more specific than MS alone, it is essential that at least two product ions are chosen in the last MS stage to ensure sufficient identification power [50]. One-point or a limited number of calibration standards is used to semi-quantify any drug present.

Performance of assays

An often neglected area of forensic toxicology is to ensure assays are not only fully validated but also each assay is monitored for performance. Validation refers to a process to establish that the assay works sufficiently well to meet the intended purpose and that any interference or inaccuracies are evaluated and preferably minimized. This means establishing adequate detection limits, defining the concentration response curve (i.e., linearity or otherwise), determining precision at different concentrations within an assay and between assays and ensuring it is robust and can perform equally well with different analysts. Importantly, the specificity needs to be established to ensure no interferences occur [51].

Once the assay is validated and documentation can be provided to support this work, day-to-day performance of routine assay batches must be monitored by way of quality controls. These controls use the same matrix as the unknown samples (i.e., blood for blood specimens) and contain drug(s) at a predetermined concentration. The acceptance range of each batch of controls is then determined and used to establish the acceptability of a particular batch assay. Typically acceptance ranges are ± 2 SD but can be ±15% or 20% depending on the analyte and method used. For alcohol determination in blood the relative SD (RSD) (SD/mean) is often around 2%, requiring much tighter acceptance limits. The use of multiple controls at the same concentration or different concentrations enables a better statistical treatment of results that fall outside the acceptance limit, such as the Westgard rules [52].

Since recoveries of analytes will vary from specimen to specimen, it is essential that matrix matching is employed. This means that calibration samples are performed in the same matrix as the unknown sample. This can create problems if a particular drug needs to be quantified in various tissues in a case, i.e., blood, liver, vitreous humor, etc. Although use of deuterated internal standards can compensate for variable recoveries, it is prudent to validate this approach against true matrix matching.

Quality control materials are available from organizations including the College of American Pathologists (CAP), the United Kingdom National External Quality Assessment Scheme (UKNEQAS) for therapeutic drug assays and the Dutch Association for Quality Assessment in therapeutic drug monitoring and clinical toxicology (KKGT). Various in-house national programs also exist in many jurisdictions. Proficiency programs are also used to independently monitor laboratory performance for both identification of foreign substances and for quantitative accuracy [53, 54]. Proficiency programs have also been made for hair [55] and oral fluid analyses [56]. These data also provide a guide over the spread of results for particular drugs over many laboratories often using different techniques.

Toxicology testing policies

All laboratories, whether they are publicly funded organizations especially designed for forensic work in the jurisdiction or private laboratories, that engaged in contract work need to have developed a policy (and procedure) for drug testing that is both clear to their clients and most relevant for the case submitted. Case is defined here as a test or series of tests on a specimen or collection of specimens pertaining to a matter.

The concept of performing a drug screen (on a sample) infers that the tests conducted cover a wide range of drugs (and possibly poisons); however, no laboratory is able to cover all substances. The laboratory (and client) needs to be realistic in the scope of drug testing, but not to cover too small a range of substances as to render the testing wholly inadequate. For example, if the drug screening is meant to cover "drugs of abuse", then those substances targeted should be clearly defined. Similarly, if other drugs are included in the screen, then some indication of the extent of these tests needs to be made so that it is both clear to the client and satisfies the purpose of the testing in the first place. While this can be done during contract negotiations, it is also vital that the test certificate or report provides sufficient information to the reader on what tests have been conducted, even if the result is negative for substances.

The preferred approach in forensic toxicology cases is to perform a drug screen that covers as large a range of substances as feasible for the jurisdiction and laboratory. This approach is sometimes termed "general unknown screen" (GUS) or "systematic toxicological analysis" (STA). This might include the range of substances listed in the Table 3.

Those drug or drug classes on the left side of Table 3 are commonly abused and can cause significant behavioral changes, even if an overdose is not expected. Those on the right are less commonly examined in forensic cases

Table 3. Target substances in systematic toxicological analyses

Common target drugs	Other target drugs
Alcohol (ethanol)	Anticonvulsants (e.g., carbamazepine, lamotrigine, phenytoin, valproate, etc.)
Amphetamine and related stimulants including ecstasy	Cardiovascular drugs (e.g., β-blockers, digoxin, other antiarrhythmics, etc.)
Cocaine (including at least benzoylecgonine)	Antidiabetics (orally active)
Benzodiazepines and related hypnotics (i.e., zolpidem, zopiclone)	High potency opioids (e.g., fentanyl, hydromorphone, buprenorphine, etc.)
Cannabis (Δ^9-tetrahydrocannabinol in blood)	γ-Hydroxybutyrate (GHB)
Opiates/opioids [e.g., morphine, 6-acetyl-morphine (6-AM), oxycodone, methadone, etc.]	Muscle relaxants, i.e., carisoprodol, quinine
Antidepressants	Barbiturates and related anxiolytics
Antipsychotic drugs	Volatile substances (e.g., hydrocarbons)

but can be important to rule out exposures to these substances. Both sides of Table 3 include drugs used in therapeutic settings, e.g., anticonvulsants, antidepressants, benzodiazepines, most opioids, etc. The detection of these substances assists in understanding what ailments the person might have had and whether the concentration of drug detected indicates compliance to prescribed medication.

Skills and qualifications

There is no universally accepted minimum qualification or skill level for forensic toxicologists. It is preferable for practitioners to have had experience in analytical chemistry before becoming forensic toxicologists. This allows a greater breadth of experience and applications than those traditionally practiced in a toxicology laboratory. It is also preferable that practitioners have knowledge of pharmacology and pharmacokinetics since this allows them to better tailor their analytical tests and most importantly enables them to provide an interpretation of the results for clients and courts.

Traditionally practitioners have entered the discipline from an analytical chemistry or biochemistry background or from a background of pharmacy or pharmacology in which analytical chemistry is a major. Increasingly persons with higher degrees, particularly doctoral degrees, are sought since these graduates have a higher skills base and are able to work better independently on case investigations or method development than those without a research background. In some jurisdictions local organizations assist in the training and development of toxicologists and provide a level of certification. For example, the American Board of Forensic Toxicology (ABFT) and the German Society of Toxicological and Forensic Chemistry (GTFCh) certifies toxicologists through an examination process.

Interpretation of toxicology data

The process of obtaining a valid result in a case can be long and complex, particularly if a number of tests were conducted to exclude a large range of substances and any detected substances are confirmed by another method. This is not the end of the line for the laboratory: the result(s) must be given some interpretation to guide the investigator (e.g., police officer, medical examiner and coroner), and, potentially, other stakeholders.

It is far too easy to refer to a published database of toxicological information to guide such interpretations. However, these databases rarely, if at all, provide the context of the case from which the data derive, or whether the data refer to single exposure to a substance or multiple exposures, or even if other factors influence the resultant response.

Heroin or other potent opioids can easily cause death in certain circumstance, particularly if a person is unaccustomed to the dose being administered or there are other drugs consumed that also depress the CNS and cause cardio-respiratory arrest. On the other hand, persons regularly exposed to opioids will develop substantial tolerance and can easily tolerate doses (and consequently blood and tissue concentrations) that would kill an opioid-naïve person. Without knowledge of the circumstances of drug use, a blood concentration cannot be usefully interpreted, no matter how high a concentration is. A user of opioids who suffered a fatal gun shot wound is likely to have died from the injury, not the drug, presuming of course the person was alive at the time of the shooting. This situation applies effectively to all drugs. It is therefore vital that the context of the case, i.e., the circumstances, are known and are considered in any interpretation of results. If the context of the case is not known then no interpretation is possible.

More often than not in forensic toxicology more than one substance is detected. The interpretation must consider the role of these other drugs. Furthermore, deaths do not always occur during the apparent peak concentration of drugs; indeed many deaths due to drugs can be delayed. Coma can occur for many hours before death ensures. In this situation the blood concentration may be quite low due to continuing drug clearance before death ultimately occurs. This applies particularly to opioids.

Artifacts

Analysts need to be aware that artifacts can occur that affect the blood concentration. These can occur before sample collection and after due to instability of the analyte or other processes that can affect the concentration. Table 4 summarizes the most common reasons.

Table 4. Artifacts affecting concentration of analytes

Before sample collection	After sample collection
Instability of analyte	Instability of analyte
Quality of specimen (particularly postmortem due to putrefaction or inhomogeneity of blood)	Blood:plasma concentration ratios
Diffusion of analyte from neighboring tissues in deceased persons (redistribution)	Recovery of drug from specimen not corrected in calculations (e.g., absence of internal standard)
Contamination of analyte from gastric or intestinal contents in deceased persons	
Postmortem metabolism (anaerobic) of susceptible drugs	

Instability and anaerobic metabolism

Some analytes are instable for physiochemical reasons, leading to progressive loss of these drugs with time. Examples include cocaine, cyanide, fenoterol, heroin, salicylate, olanzapine and some benzodiazepines. These losses are variable and can be reduced by the use of ultra-low temperature freezers (–60 °C or lower) [37, 57–60]. Some drugs can be metabolized in the body after death or in collection tubes due to anaerobic bacteria. These include dothiepin, thioridazine, flunitrazepam, clonazepam, nitrazepam and morphine conjugates [61–63]. The use of fluoride in collection tubes prevents bacterial-mediated metabolism post collection [64]. Unfortunately, fluoride can accelerate losses for organophosphates, leading to rapid degradation of dichlorvos and possibly related poisons [65].

Blood:plasma ratios

Blood concentrations are rarely the same as those in plasma/serum. This fact is often not considered when comparing results with published data performed in other blood products. For example, Δ^9-tetrahydrocannabinol (THC) concentrations in blood are almost half that of plasma since almost all of the THC is found in plasma [66]. Moreover, these ratios are variable. Studies have shown a mean blood:plasma ratio of 0.39 with a range of 0.28–0.48 [66]. Similarly, variable ratios have been observed for the antipsychotic clozapine and its metabolite norclozapine [67].

Hydroxychloroquine used in the treatment of rheumatoid arthritis has blood concentrations several times that of plasma [68]. However, most drugs do have ratios within a factor of two; however, even this difference can impact on an interpretation. Most pharmacokinetics studies have measurements performed in plasma or serum. These studies can be useful to determine the relevance of a blood concentration in a forensic or clinical toxicology case providing the blood:plasma ratio is known.

Quality of specimen

In postmortem cases blood settles in the body causing an uneven distribution of red blood cells and serum and indeed other bodily fluids. Blood may therefore not be of a composition typical of the body as a whole thereby producing variable results depending on where the blood was sampled. The variation in alcohol concentration in different sites is illustrative of this problem [69, 70]. Blood:plasma ratios that are not close to unity will further compound these regional variations in deceased cases.

Delays in sampling are inevitable in deceased cases since bodies are not always discovered and transferred to the mortuary within hours of the death. Putrefactive changes will occur quite quickly depending on the ambient temperature and storage conditions. Consequently, the quality of the specimens obtained will be affected. In some circumstances bacteria can produce poisonous substances, e.g., ethanol and cyanide [37]. γ-Hydroxybutyrate (GHB) sometimes known as fantasy is a more recent drug of abuse. In living persons small amounts are produced naturally and appear in blood and urine, usually in concentrations under 10 mg/L. It can also be produced postmortem in the body and even in the collection tube if fluoride preservative is not present. Concentrations produced can easily exceed those considered potentially toxic, particularly if blood collected is not peripheral (>100 mg/L) [71].

Redistribution

The diffusion of drug from a higher concentration in tissue surrounding blood vessels into pooled blood in vessels leads to an elevation in the concentration of drug in that vessel (Fig. 3). This process of redistribution is widespread and unless proven otherwise should be considered to have occurred for all drugs postmortem. This phenomenon is greatest for drugs with high lipid solubility or high tissue concentrations relative to blood. Drugs showing increases of over 200% are numerous with reports of increases of 10-fold in some situations (Tab. 5). The worst offenders are digoxin, (dextro)propoxyphene, methadone, tricyclic antidepressants and many antipsychotic drugs and possibly THC [72–80].

Water-soluble morphine shows little change in blood concentration after death in humans [81, 82]. The same is true for most benzodiazepines and cocaine metabolites since these have relatively low lipid solubility [83]. However, the concentrations of more lipid soluble opioids can show significant increases after death. The rate and extent of these changes are quite variable

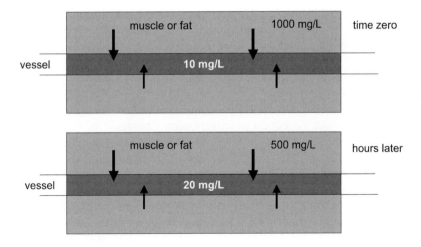

Figure 3. Scheme illustrating process of redistribution. Diffusion of drug occurs from high concentration in muscle or fat to a lower concentration in blood vessel.

Table 5. Extent of postmortem redistribution for selected drugs

Drugs	Extent of redistribution
Antipsychotic drugs (e.g., fluoxetine, quetiapine, etc.) Tricyclic antidepressants (e.g., amitriptyline) Chloroquine Digoxin Hydroxychloroquine Ketamine Fat soluble opioids (methadone, propoxyphene, etc.) Serotonin reuptake inhibitors (fluoxetine, paroxetine, sertraline, venlafaxine) MDMA (3,4-methylene dioxy methamphetamine, "ecstasy") and other fat soluble amphetamines including methamphetamine	Moderate to high > 200%
Amphetamine Barbiturates (most) Benzodiazepines (most) Cocaine and metabolites Pethidine (meperidine) Morphine and 6-acetylmorphine (6-AM) Cocaine Zolpidem and zopiclone	Low ≤ 200%

and cannot be estimated for a particular situation when only blood measurements are conducted postmortem.

While peripheral blood shows fewer changes than blood taken from the central sites, changes still occur in the postmortem period. These processes also take place in liver and lung tissue since these tissues have reserves of drugs and are well served by blood vessels. Nevertheless, if sampling is appropriate, liver can complement the interpretation of a blood result. Therefore, it is recommended that concentrations of drugs are also quantified in liver (and other tissues depending on the circumstance) when blood results are marginally high and may, or may not, be subject to redistributive changes.

Selected case reports

To illustrate the complexity of forensic toxicology in a death investigation consider the following:

Case 1

A 45-year woman was found deceased in her bed in the morning. She had been on narcotic analgesics in the form of oxycodone (sustained release) 20 mg twice daily for chronic back pain. An autopsy found no significant natural disease or injuries that could explain her death; however, she was found to have heavy lungs (edema). Peripheral blood, a section of her right liver lobe and her gastric contents were taken during her postmortem examination. Systematic toxicological analyses on her blood found oxycodone at 0.15 mg/L using a combination of immunoassay (drugs of abuse), GC screen and LC-MS/MS analysis and confirmation for over 100 common drugs and poisons. Her liver results were consistent with the blood concentration. The concentration of this drug was consistent with therapeutic use and would not be expected to cause death given the use of this analgesic for many months. Examination of her medication found in her bedroom indicated that she had taken 20 oxycodone tablets in the 10 days since her last visit to her medical practitioner who had prescribed her next months' doses. This reconciliation of medication indicated compliance to her prescribed medication.

The toxicological analysis also detected 0.4 mg/L methadone in her blood as well as 0.2 mg/L codeine and 40 mg/L paracetamol (acetaminophen). Gastric contents found only traces of methadone, codeine and paracetamol. These results were unexpected, particularly the methadone which is a potent long-acting narcotic analgesic that not only requires a prescription but also requires the treating physician to apply for a patient permit. Examination of her medical records showed that she had visited a specialist pain doctor who had prescribed the methadone. While she was meant to have ceased her oxycodone she had continued to take this drug while starting on methadone. Deaths are well known in persons starting methadone therapy who do not have sufficient tolerance to the drug [84–86]. She should have been tolerant to oxycodone given her weeks of therapy and it is likely that the additional metha-done was too much causing her death from respiratory depression. Slowing of respiration during sleep causes fluid build-up in the lungs, leading to slowly developing coma and eventual death, invariably during sleep. The use of over-the-counter codeine preparation (also containing paracetamol) would have contributed to her death. It was not apparent why the methadone tablets were not discovered in her home but they may have been stored in another room.

The performance of a systematic drug screen, being to able to reconcile her medications and being able to obtain information on her medical history pro-vided relevant evidence that led to a coroners finding of accidental death from drug toxicity.

Case 2

A 45-year old man was found deceased in his home. He had been shot in the chest some hours earlier by a woman who claimed she had been assaulted by her "crazy" boy friend who had accused her of seeing someone else. The post-mortem examination confirmed the gunshot wound as the cause of death and found no significant natural disease. Peripheral blood was taken from the upper thigh for toxicology as well as vitreous humor and urine. The forensic toxicol-ogy laboratory conducted wide-ranging drug screens using immunoassays for drugs of abuse in urine and GC-MS on a basic/neutral blood extract. These found methamphetamine in blood at 1.2 mg/L, amphetamine at 0.2 mg/L, alprazolam at 0.5 mg/L. Urinalysis confirmed the presence of methamphet-amine and alprazolam. Alcohol was not detected in blood and urine.

The deceased had a known history of violence and drug use and had become increasingly paranoid and aggressive in recent months. Methamphetamine-associated violence in long-term users is well known and can be associated with paranoid psychoses. The presence of methamphetamine proved a recent moderate dose; low dose use usually has blood concentrations below 0.2 mg/L. The toxicology does not prove the behavior occurred but does support the cir-cumstances alleged by the accused. Alprazolam is commonly seen in "drug users" and, while it is often used to soften the rough edges caused by amphet-amine use, it actually can increase disinhibitive and violent behavior.

Conclusion

Forensic toxicology is an important science that supports a range of medico-legal applications. Foremost for the practitioner is to have a strong background in analytical chemistry including isolation, separation and detection tech-niques particularly those involving MS. The selection of the appropriate range of samples will depend on the application but will always require proper doc-umentation, transport and storage to guarantee the integrity of the items for analysis. Knowledge of drug effects and pharmacokinetics, together with an appreciation of possible limitations in the interpretation of results, ensures credible evidence that has not been overstated.

References

1 Beyer J, Drummer OH, Maurer HH (2009) Analysis of toxic alkaloids in body samples. *Forensic Sci Int* 185: 1–9
2 Hlastala MP (1998) The alcohol breath test – A review. *J Appl Physiol* 84: 401–408
3 Mason MF, Dubowski KM (1976) Breath-alcohol analysis: Uses, methods, and some forensic problems – Review and opinion. *J Forensic Sci* 21: 9–41
4 Kugelberg FC, Jones AW (2007) Interpreting results of ethanol analysis in postmortem specimens: A review of the literature. *Forensic Sci Int* 165: 10–29
5 Drummer OH (2006) Drug testing in oral fluid. *Clin Biochem Rev* 27: 147–159
6 Boorman M, Owens K (2009) The Victorian legislative framework for the random testing drivers at the roadside for the presence of illicit drugs: An evaluation of the characteristics of drivers detected from 2004 to 2006. *Traffic Inj Prev* 10: 16–22
7 Palmer RB (2009) A review of the use of ethyl glucuronide as a marker for ethanol consumption in forensic and clinical medicine. *Semin Diagn Pathol* 26: 18–27
8 Yegles M, Labarthe A, Auwarter V, Hartwig S, Vater H, Wennig R, Pragst F (2004) Comparison of ethyl glucuronide and fatty acid ethyl ester concentrations in hair of alcoholics, social drinkers and teetotallers. *Forensic Sci Int* 145: 167–173
9 Musshoff F, Madea B (2007) New trends in hair analysis and scientific demands on validation and technical notes. *Forensic Sci Int* 165: 204–215
10 LeBeau MA (2008) Guidance for improved detection of drugs used to facilitate crimes. *Ther Drug Monit* 30: 229–233
11 Trout GJ, Kazlauskas R (2004) Sports drug testing – An analyst's perspective. *Chem Soc Rev* 33: 1–13
12 Thevis M, Schanzer W (2007) Mass spectrometry in sports drug testing: Structure characterization and analytical assays. *Mass Spectrom Rev* 26: 79–107
13 Yu NH, Ho EN, Tang FP, Wan TS, Wong AS (2008) Comprehensive screening of acidic and neutral drugs in equine plasma by liquid chromatography–tandem mass spectrometry. *J Chromatogr A* 1189: 426–434
14 Murphy B, Morrison R (2007) *Introduction to Environmental Forensics,* 2nd edn., Academic Press, New York, 776
15 Simoneit BR (1999) A review of biomarker compounds as source indicators and tracers for air pollution. *Environ Sci Pollut Res Int* 6: 159–169
16 Flanagan RJ, Connally G, Evans JM (2005) Analytical toxicology: Guidelines for sample collection postmortem. *Toxicol Rev* 24: 63–71
17 Verstraete AG, Pierce A (2001) Workplace drug testing in Europe. *Forensic Sci Int* 121: 2–6.
18 ElSohly MA, Gul W, Murphy TP, Avula B, Khan IA (2007) LC-(TOF) MS analysis of benzodiazepines in urine from alleged victims of drug-facilitated sexual assault. *J Anal Toxicol* 31: 505–514
19 Lu NT, Taylor BG (2006) Drug screening and confirmation by GC-MS: Comparison of EMIT II and Online KIMS against 10 drugs between US and England laboratories. *Forensic Sci Int* 157: 106–116
20 Arndt T (2009) Urine-creatinine concentration as a marker of urine dilution: Reflections using a cohort of 45,000 samples. *Forensic Sci Int* 186: 48–51
21 Kintz P (2007) Bioanalytical procedures for detection of chemical agents in hair in the case of drug-facilitated crimes. *Anal Bioanal Chem* 388: 1467–1474
22 Balikova M (2005) Hair analysis for drugs of abuse. Plausibility of interpretation. *Biomed Pap Med Fac Univ Palacky Olomouc Czech Repub* 149: 199–207
23 Kintz P, Villain M, Cirimele V (2006) Hair analysis for drug detection. *Ther Drug Monit* 28: 442–446
24 Aps JK, Martens LC (2005) The physiology of saliva and transfer of drugs into saliva. *Forensic*

Sci Int 150: 119–131

25 Drummer OH (2005) Pharmacokinetics of illicit drugs in oral fluid. *Forensic Sci Int* 150: 133–142

26 Verstraete AG (2005) Oral fluid testing for driving under the influence of drugs: History, recent progress and remaining challenges. *Forensic Sci Int* 150: 143–150

27 Drummer OH, Gerostamoulos D, Chu M, Swann P, Boorman M, Cairns I (2007) Drugs in oral fluid in randomly selected drivers. *Forensic Sci Int* 170: 105–110

28 Bush DM (2008) The U.S. Mandatory Guidelines for Federal Workplace Drug Testing Programs: Current status and future considerations. *Forensic Sci Int* 174: 111–119

29 Drummer OH (2008) Introduction and review of collection techniques and applications of drug testing of oral fluid. *Ther Drug Monit* 30: 203–206

30 Drummer OH (2004) Postmortem toxicology of drugs of abuse. *Forensic Sci Int* 142: 101–113

31 Drummer OH (2007) Requirements for bioanalytical procedures in postmortem toxicology. *Anal Bioanal Chem* 388: 1495–1503

32 Drummer OH (1999) Chromatographic screening techniques in systematic toxicological analysis. *J Chromatogr B Biomed Sci Appl* 733: 27–45

33 Degel F (1996) Comparison of new solid-phase extraction methods for chromatographic identification of drugs in clinical toxicological analysis. *Clin Biochem* 29: 529–540

34 Nerin C, Salafranca J, Aznar M, Batlle R (2009) Critical review on recent developments in solventless techniques for extraction of analytes. *Anal Bioanal Chem* 393: 809–833

35 Pragst F (2007) Application of solid-phase microextraction in analytical toxicology. *Anal Bioanal Chem* 388: 1393–1414

36 Peters FT, Drvarov O, Lottner S, Spellmeier A, Rieger K, Haefeli WE, Maurer HH (2009) A systematic comparison of four different workup procedures for systematic toxicological analysis of urine samples using gas chromatography–mass spectrometry. *Anal Bioanal Chem* 393: 735–745

37 Skopp G (2004) Preanalytic aspects in postmortem toxicology. *Forensic Sci Int* 142: 75–100

38 Wu AH, Forte E, Casella G, Sun K, Hemphill G, Foery R, Schanzenbach H (1995) CEDIA for screening drugs of abuse in urine and the effect of adulterants. *J Forensic Sci* 40: 614–618

39 Maurer HH (1992) Systematic toxicological analysis of drugs and their metabolites by gas chromatography–mass spectrometry. *J Chromatogr* 580: 3–41

40 Gergov M, Boucher B, Ojanpera I, Vuori E (2001) Toxicological screening of urine for drugs by liquid chromatography/time-of-flight mass spectrometry with automated target library search based on elemental formulas. *Rapid Commun Mass Spectrom* 15: 521–526

41 Ojanpera S, Pelander A, Pelzing M, Krebs I, Vuori E, Ojanpera I (2006) Isotopic pattern and accurate mass determination in urine drug screening by liquid chromatography/time-of-flight mass spectrometry. *Rapid Commun Mass Spectrom* 20: 1161–1167

42 Song SM, Marriott P, Kotsos A, Drummer OH, Wynne P (2004) Comprehensive two-dimensional gas chromatography with time-of-flight mass spectrometry (GC × GC-TOFMS) for drug screening and confirmation. *Forensic Sci Int* 143: 87–101

43 Lowe RH, Karschner EL, Schwilke EW, Barnes AJ, Huestis MA (2007) Simultaneous quantification of Δ^9-tetrahydrocannabinol, 11-hydroxy-Δ^9-tetrahydrocannabinol, and 11-nor- Δ^9-tetrahydrocannabinol-9-carboxylic acid in human plasma using two-dimensional gas chromatography, cryofocusing, and electron impact-mass spectrometry. *J Chromatogr A* 1163: 318–327

44 Maurer HH (1999) Systematic toxicological analysis procedures for acidic drugs and/or metabolites relevant to clinical and forensic toxicology and/or doping control. *J Chromatogr B Biomed Sci Appl* 733: 3–25

45 Tagliaro F, Bortolotti F, Pascali JP (2007) Current role of capillary electrophoretic/electrokinetic techniques in forensic toxicology. *Anal Bioanal Chem* 388: 1359–1364

46 Lurie IS (1997) Application of micellar electrokinetic capillary chromatography to the analysis of illicit drug seizures. *J Chromatogr A* 780: 265–284

47 Tagliaro F, Turrina S, Pisi P, Smith FP, Marigo M (1998) Determination of illicit and/or abused drugs and compounds of forensic interest in biosamples by capillary electrophoretic/electrokinetic methods. *J Chromatogr B Biomed Sci Appl* 713: 27–49

48 Pelander A, Backstrom D, Ojanpera I (2007) Qualitative screening for basic drugs in autopsy liver samples by dual-plate overpressured layer chromatography. *J Chromatogr B Analyt Technol Biomed Life Sci* 857: 337–340

49 Santos LS, Haddad R, Hoehr NF, Pilli RA, Eberlin MN (2004) Fast screening of low molecular weight compounds by thin-layer chromatography and "on-spot" MALDI-TOF mass spectrometry. *Anal Chem* 76: 2144–2147

50 Sauvage FL, Gaulier JM, Lachatre G, Marquet P (2008) Pitfalls and prevention strategies for liquid chromatography–tandem mass spectrometry in the selected reaction-monitoring mode for drug analysis. *Clin Chem* 54: 1519–1527

51 Peters FT, Drummer OH, Musshoff F (2007) Validation of new methods. *Forensic Sci Int* 165: 216–224

52 http://www.westgard.com/mltrule.htm. [accessed 18 April 2009]

53 Clarke J, Wilson JF (2005) Proficiency testing (external quality assessment) of drug detection in oral fluid. *Forensic Sci Int* 150: 161–164

54 Flanagan RJ, Whelpton R (2009) *Quality Management. Encyclopedia of Forensic Science*, Wiley, London, *in press*

55 Lee S, Park Y, Han E, Choe S, Lim M, Chung H (2008) Preparation and application of a fortified hair reference material for the determination of methamphetamine and amphetamine. *Forensic Sci Int* 178: 207–212

56 Ventura M, Ventura R, Pichini S, Leal S, Zuccaro P, Pacifici R, Langohr K, de la Torre R (2008) ORALVEQ: External quality assessment scheme of drugs of abuse in oral fluid: Results obtained in the first round performed in 2007. *Forensic Sci Int* 182: 35–40

57 Al-Hadidi KA, Oliver JS (1995) Stability of temazepam in blood. *Sci Justice* 35: 105–108

58 Levine B, Blanke RV, Valentour JC (1983) Postmortem stability of benzodiazepines in blood and tissues. *J Forensic Sci* 28: 102–115

59 Drummer OH, Gerostamoulos J (2002) Postmortem drug analysis: Analytical and toxicological aspects. *Ther Drug Monit* 24: 199–209

60 Couper FJ, Drummer OH (1999) Postmortem stability and interpretation of β2-agonist concentrations. *J Forensic Sci* 44: 523–526

61 Robertson MD, Drummer OH (1998) Stability of nitrobenzodiazepines in postmortem blood. *J Forensic Sci* 43: 5–8

62 Batziris HP, McIntyre IM, Drummer OH (1999) The effect of sulfur-metabolising bacteria on sulfur-containing psychotropic drugs. *Int Biodeter Biodegrad* 44: 111–116

63 Moriya F, Hashimoto Y (1997) Distribution of free and conjugated morphine in body fluids and tissues in a fatal heroin overdose: Is conjugated morphine stable in postmortem specimens? *J Forensic Sci* 42: 736–740

64 Robertson MD, Drummer OH (1995) Postmortem drug metabolism by bacteria. *J Forensic Sci* 40: 382–386.

65 Moriya F, Hashimoto Y, Kuo TL (1999) Pitfalls when determining tissue distributions of organophosphorus chemicals: Sodium fluoride accelerates chemical degradation. *J Anal Toxicol* 23: 210–215

66 Schwilke EW, Karschner EL, Lowe RH, Gordon AM, Cadet JL, Herning RI, Huestis MA (2009) Intra- and intersubject whole blood/plasma cannabinoid ratios determined by 2-dimensional, electron impact GC-MS with cryofocusing. *Clin Chem* 55: 1188–1195

67 Flanagan RJ, Yusufi B, Barnes TR (2003) Comparability of whole-blood and plasma clozapine and norclozapine concentrations. *Br J Clin Pharmacol* 56: 135–138

68 Brocks DR, Skeith KJ, Johnston C, Emamibafrani J, Davis P, Russell AS, Jamali F (1994) Hematologic disposition of hydroxychloroquine enantiomers. *J Clin Pharmacol* 34: 1088–1097

69 Briglia EJ, Bidanset JH, Dal Cortivo LA (1992) The distribution of ethanol in postmortem blood specimens. *J Forensic Sci* 37: 991–998

70 Sylvester PA, Wong NA, Warren BF, Ranson DL (1998) Unacceptably high site variability in postmortem blood alcohol analysis. *J Clin Pathol* 51: 250–252

71 Berankova K, Mutnanska K, Balikova M (2006) Gamma-hydroxybutyric acid stability and formation in blood and urine. *Forensic Sci Int* 161: 158–162

72 Barnhart FE, Fogacci JR, Reed DW (1999) Methamphetamine – A study of postmortem redistribution. *J Anal Toxicol* 23: 69–70

73 Hilberg T, Rogde S, Morland J (1999) Postmortem drug redistribution – Human cases related to results in experimental animals. *J Forensic Sci* 44: 3–9

74 Jaffe P (1997) *The Distribution and Redistribution of Four Serotonin Reuptake Inhibitors in Postmortem Specimens*, Monash University, Melbourne

75 Moriya F, Hashimoto Y (2000) Redistribution of methamphetamine in the early postmortem period. *J Anal Toxicol* 24: 153–155

76 Pounder DJ, Jones GR (1990) Postmortem drug redistribution – A toxicological nightmare. *Forensic Sci Int* 45: 253–263

77 Moriya F, Hashimoto Y (1999) Redistribution of basic drugs into cardiac blood from surrounding tissues during early-stages postmortem. *J Forensic Sci* 44: 10–16

78 Drummer OH (2008) Postmortem toxicological redistribution In: GN Rutty (ed.): *Essentials of Autopsy Practice*, Volume 4, Springer-Verlag, Berlin pp. 1–21

79 Rodda KE, Drummer OH (2006) The redistribution of selected psychiatric drugs in post-mortem cases. *Forensic Sci Int* 164: 235–239

80 Caplehorn JR, Drummer OH (2002) Methadone dose and post-mortem blood concentration. *Drug Alcohol Rev* 21: 329–333

81 Logan BK, Smirnow D (1996) Postmortem distribution and redistribution of morphine in man. *J Forensic Sci* 41: 37–46

82 Gerostamoulos J, Drummer OH (2000) Postmortem redistribution of morphine and its metabolites. *J Forensic Sci, in press*

83 Robertson MD, Drummer OH (1998) Postmortem distribution and redistribution of nitrobenzodiazepines in man. *J Forensic Sci* 43: 9–13

84 Caplehorn JR, Drummer OH (1999) Mortality associated with New South Wales methadone programs in 1994: Lives lost and saved. *Med J Aust* 170: 104–109

85 Drummer OH, Syrjanen M, Opeskin K, Cordner S (1990) Deaths of heroin addicts starting on a methadone maintenance programme. *Lancet* 335: 108

86 Milroy CM, Forrest ARW (2000) Methadone deaths: A toxicological analysis. *J Clin Pathol* 53: 277–281

Glossary

AAPCC	American Association of Poison Control Centers
AC	activated charcoal
AChE	acetylcholinesterase
ACTX	atracotoxin
ADH	alcohol dehydrogenase
AFB_1	aflatoxin B_1
ALI	acute lung injury
6-AM	6-acetylmorphine (= 6-MAM)
APAP	N-acetyl-p-aminophenol (acetaminophen, paracetamol)
APCI	atmospheric pressure chemical ionization
ARDS	acute respiratory distress syndrome
ASP	amnesic shellfish poisoning
AST	aspartate aminotransferase
ATA	alimentary toxic aleukia
AUC	area under the curve
AZA	azaspiracid
BAL	British anti-lewisite (2,3-dimercaptopropanol, dimercaprol)
BIA	benzylisoquinoline alkaloid
BLL	blood lead level
BoNT	botulinum neurotoxin
BTX	PbTX, brevetoxin
BUN	blood urea nitrogen
BWA	biological warfare agents
CBC	complete blood count
Cdt	cytolethal distending toxin
CE	capillary electrophoresis
CFTR	cystic fibrosis transmembrane conductance regulator
CIRL	calcium-independent receptor for latrotoxin
CK	creatine kinase
CNS	central nervous system
COMT	catechol O-methyltransferase
COPD	chronic obstructive pulmonary disease
CPK	creatinine phosphokinase
CPR	cardio-pulmonary resuscitation
CT	computed tomography
CTX	ciguatoxin
CWA	chemical warfare agents
DAD	diode-array detection

DIC	disseminated intravascular coagulation
DMSA	2,3-dimercaptosuccinic acid
DMSO	dimethyl sulfoxide
DON	deoxynivalenol
DSP	diarrheic shellfish poisoning
DTX	dinophysistoxin
ECG	electrocardiogram
ED	emergency department
EDTA	ethylenediamintetraacetic acid
EEG	electroencephalogram
EI	electron ionization
ELISA	enzyme-linked immunosorbent assay
EMIT	enzyme multiplied immunoassay technique
EPA	U.S. Environmental Protection Agency
ERK	extracellular signal-regulated kinase
ESI	electrospray ionization
FDA	U.S. Food and Drug Administration
FID	flame ionization detector
FUM	fumonisin
GABA	γ-aminobutyric acid
Gb	gambierol
GC	gas chromatography
GCS	Glascow coma score
GHB	γ-hydroxybutyrate
GI	gastrointestinal
GOT	glutamic oxaloacetic transaminase
GPCR	G protein-coupled receptor
GPT	glutamic pyruvic transaminase
GSH	glutathione
HAB	harmful algal bloom
Hb	hemoglobin
HBV	hepatitis B virus
HCC	human hepatocellular carcinoma
Hck	hematopoietic cell kinase
HCN	hydrogen cyanide
HFV	hemorrhagic fever virus
HIET	high-dose insulin euglycemia therapy
HMWPT	high-molecular weight protein toxins
HPLC	high-performance liquid chromatography
5-HT_3	5-hydroxytryptamine (serotonin)
i.c.	intracutaneous
i.m.	intramuscular
i.p.	intraperitoneal
i.v.	intravenous
IARC	International Agency for Research on Cancer

IC_{50}	inhibitory concentration 50%
IFN	interferon
Ig	immunoglobulin
IL	interleukin
INH	isoniazid
IP_3	inositol triphosphate
IPCS	International Programme on Chemical Safety
IR	infrared spectroscopy
JNK	c-Jun N-terminal protein kinase
LAAO	L-amino acid oxidase
LC	liquid chromatography
LD_{50}	lethal dose 50%
LDH	lactate dehydrogenase
LLE	liquid-liquid extraction
LOD	limit of detection
LSD	D-lysergic acid diethylamide
LTX	latrotoxin
mAb	monoclonal antibody
MAHA	microangiopathic haemolytic anaemia
MALDI-TOF	matrix-assisted laser desorption/ionization time-of-flight
6-MAM	6-monoacetylmorphine (= 6-AM)
MAM	methylazoxy-methanol
MAPK	mitogen-activated protein kinase
MDAC	multiple-dose AC
MDMA	3,4-methylenedioxymethamphetamine
MHC	major histocompatibility complex
MRM	multiple-reaction monitoring
MS	mass spectrometry
MTX	maitotoxin *or* methotrexate
NAC	*N*-acetylcysteine
NAPQI	*N*-acetyl-*p*-benzoquinone imine
NICI	negative ion chemical ionization
NIDA	U.S. National Institute of Drug Abuse
NIV	nivalenol
NMDA	*N*-methyl-D-aspartate
NMR	nuclear magnetic resonance
NRU	neutral red uptake
NSAID	non-steroidal anti-inflammatory drug
NSCC	non-selective cation channels
NSP	neurotoxic shellfish poisoning
OA	okadaic acid
OEL	occupational exposure limits
OTA	ochratoxin A
OTC	ornithine transcarbamylase
PA	pyrrolizidine alkaloid

PBM	peripheral blood mononuclear (cells)
PBTK	physiologically based toxicokinetic (model)
PbTX	brevetoxin, BTX
PCP	phencyclidine
PDB	Protein Databank
PEEP	positive end-expiratory pressure
PEG	polyethylene glycol
PEPCK	phosphoenolpyruvate carboxy kinase
PFT	pore-forming toxin
PKA	protein kinase A
PKC	protein kinase C
PKS	polyketide synthases
PLA$_2$	phospholipase A$_2$
PLC	phospholipase C
PlTX	palytoxin
PM	particulate matter
PPase	phosphoprotein phosphatase
PSP	paralytic shellfish poisoning
PTX	pectenotoxin
QSAR	quantitative structure-activity relationship
RBC	red blood cell
REACH	Registration, Evaluation, Authorization and Restriction of Chemicals
RIA	radioimmunoassays
ROS	reactive oxygen species
s.c.	subcutaneous
SAg	superantigen
SAR	structure activity relationship
SD	standard deviation
SEB	staphylococcal enterotoxin B
SIM	selected-ion monitoring
SNARE	soluble N-ethylmaleimide-sensitive factor attachment receptor
SPE	solid-phase extraction
SPME	solid-phase microextraction
STX	saxitoxin
SVDK	snake venom detection kit
TCA	tricyclic antidepressant
TCM	Traditional Chinese Medicine
TCR	T cell receptor
TDM	therapeutic drug monitoring
TEM	transmission electron microscopy
TeNT	tetanus neurotoxin
THC	Δ^9-tetrahydrocannabinol
TLC	thin-layer chromatography
TNF	tumor necrosis factor

| TSS | toxic shock syndrome |
| WBI | whole bowel irrigation |

TSS	toxic shock syndrome
TTX	tetrodotoxin
UDS	urine drug screening
UV	ultraviolet
VGNC	voltage-gated sodium channel
VOC	volatile organic compound
VPA	valproic acid
WBCT	whole blood clotting time
WBI	whole bowel irrigation
WHO	World Health Organization
YTX	yessotoxin

Index

The EXS-Series
Experientia Supplementum

Experientia Supplementum (EXS) is a multidisciplinary book series originally created as supplement to the journal *Experientia* which appears now under the cover of *Cellular and Molecular Life Sciences*. The multi-authored volumes focus on selected topics of biological or biomedical research, discussing current methodologies, technological innovations, novel tools and applications, new developments and recent findings.
The series is a valuable source of information not only for scientists and graduate students in medical, pharmacological and biological research, but also for physicians as well as practitioners in industry.

Forthcoming titles:

Molecular, Clinical and Environmental Toxicology, Volume 3, EXS 101, A. Luch (Editor), 2010
Galanin, EXS 102, T. Hökfelt (Editor), 2010

Published volumes:

Proteomics in Functional Genomics, EXS 88, P. Jollès, H. Jörnvall (Editors), 2000
New Approaches to Drug Development, EXS 89, P. Jollès (Editor), 2000
The Carbonic Anhydrases, EXS 90, Y.H. Edwards, W.R. Chegwidden, N.D. Carter (Editors), 2000
Genes and Mechanisms in Vertebrate Sex Determination, EXS 91, G. Scherer, M. Schmid (Editors), 2001
Molecular Systematics and Evolution: Theory and Practice, EXS 92, R. DeSalle, G. Giribet, W. Wheeler (Editors), 2002
Modern Methods of Drug Discovery, EXS 93, A. Hillisch, R. Hilgenfeld (Editors), 2003
Mechanisms of Angiogenesis, EXS 94, M. Clauss, G. Breier (Editors), 2004
NPY Family of Peptides in Neurobiology, Cardiovascular and Metabolic Disorders: from Genes to Therapeutics, EXS 95, Z. Zukowska, G.Z. Feuerstein (Editors), 2006
Cancer: Cell Structures, Carcinogens and Genomic Instability, EXS 96, L.P. Bignold (Editor), 2006
Plant Systems Biology, EXS 97, S. Baginsky, A.R. Fernie (Editors), 2006
Neurotransmitter Interactions and Cognitive Function, EXS 98, E.D. Levin (Editor), 2006
Molecular, Clinical and Environmental Toxicology, Volume 1, EXS 99, A. Luch (Editor), 2009

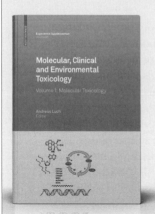

EXPERIENTIA SUPPLEMENTUM

Molecular, Clinical and Environmental Toxicology

Vol.1: Molecular Toxicology

Luch, A., Federal Institute for Risk Assessment, Berlin, Germany (Ed.)

2009. XIV, 470 p. 90 illus.
Hardcover
ISBN 978-3-7643-8335-0
EXS – Experientia
Supplementum,
Volume 99

Molecular Toxicology is the first volume of a three-volume set on molecular, clinical and environmental toxicology that offers a comprehensive and in-depth response to the increasing importance and abundance of chemicals in daily life. By providing intriguing insights far down to the molecular level, this work covers the entire range of modern toxicology with special emphasis on recent developments and achievements. It is written for students and professionals in medicine, science, public health and engineering who are demanding reliable information on toxic or potentially harmful agents and their adverse effects on the human body.

Contents:
- Historical milestones and discoveries that shaped the toxicology sciences.
- Physiologically based toxicokinetic models and their application in human exposure and internal dose assessment.
- The role of biotransformation and bioactivation in toxicity.
- Genotoxicity: damage to DNA and its consequences.
- Role of DNA repair in the protection against genotoxic stress.
- On the impact of the molecule structure in chemical carcinogenesis.
- Chemical induced alterations in p53 signaling.
- Molecular pathways involved in cell death after chemically induced DNA damage.
- The aryl hydrocarbon receptor at the crossroads of multiple signaling pathways.
- Mapping the epigenome – impact for toxicology.
- Receptors mediating toxicity and their involvement in endocrine disruption.
- Toxicogenomics: transcription profiling for toxicology assessment.
- The role of toxicoproteomics in assessing organ specific toxicity.
- High-throughput screening for analysis of *in vitro* toxicity.

www.birkhauser.ch